Social Cognition in Schizophrenia

Social Cognition in Schizophrenia

From Evidence to Treatment

EDITED BY DAVID L. ROBERTS

DAVID L. PENN

OXFORD
UNIVERSITY PRESS

OXFORD
UNIVERSITY PRESS

Oxford University Press is a department of the University of Oxford.
It furthers the University's objective of excellence in research, scholarship,
and education by publishing worldwide.

Oxford   New York
Auckland   Cape Town   Dar es Salaam   Hong Kong   Karachi
Kuala Lumpur   Madrid   Melbourne   Mexico City   Nairobi
New Delhi   Shanghai   Taipei   Toronto

With offices in
Argentina   Austria   Brazil   Chile   Czech   Republic   France   Greece
Guatemala   Hungary   Italy   Japan   Poland   Portugal   Singapore
South Korea   Switzerland   Thailand   Turkey   Ukraine   Vietnam

Oxford is a registered trademark of Oxford University Press in the UK and in certain other countries

Published in the United States of America by
Oxford University Press
198 Madison Avenue, New York, New York 10016, United States of America

Library of Congress Cataloging-in-Publication Data
Social cognition in schizophrenia : from evidence to treatment / edited by David L. Roberts,
David L. Penn.
      p. cm.
Includes bibliographical references and index.
ISBN 978-0-19-977758-7
1. Schizophrenia.   2. Social perception.   3. Schizophrenia – Treatment.   I. Roberts, David L.,
1973-   II. Penn, David L.
RC514.S592 2013
616.89'8—dc23
2012024752

9 8 7 6 5 4 3 2 1
Printed in the United States of America on acid-free paper

CONTENTS

Contributors   ix

Introduction   1
Shannon M. Couture and David L. Penn

PART ONE: FOUNDATIONS OF HUMAN SOCIAL COGNITION

1. The Development of Social Cognition in Theory and Action   19
Kristen E. Lyons and Melissa A. Koenig

2. Social Cognition: Social Psychological Insights from Normal Adults   41
Kristjen Lundberg

3. Cross-Cultural Variation in Social Cognition and the Social Brain   69
Shihui Han

4. The Social Cognitive Brain: A Review of Key Individual Difference
Parameters with Relevance to Schizophrenia   93
*Amy M. Jimenez, Dylan G. Gee, Tyrone D. Cannon,
and Matthew D. Lieberman*

5. Social Cognitive Neuroscience: Clinical Foundations   120
Oana Tudusciuc and Ralph Adolphs

PART TWO: DESCRIPTIVE AND EXPERIMENTAL RESEARCH

6. Social Cognition and Functional Outcome in Schizophrenia   151
William P. Horan, Junghee Lee, and Michael F. Green

7. Emotion Processing in Schizophrenia   173
Christian G. Kohler, Elizabeth Hanson, and Mary E. March

8. Characteristics of Theory of Mind Impairments in Schizophrenia   196
Ahmad Abu-Akel and Simone G. Shamay-Tsoory

 9. Social Cognition and the Dynamics of Paranoid Ideation   215
     Richard P. Bentall and Alisa Udachina

10. Social Cognition Early in the Course of the Illness   245
     Jean Addington and Danijela Piskulic

11. The Social Cognitive Neuroscience of Schizophrenia   263
     Amy E. Pinkham

PART THREE: TREATMENT APPROACHES

12. Introduction to Social Cognitive Treatment Approaches for
     Schizophrenia   285
     Joanna M. Fiszdon

13. Integrated Neurocognitive Therapy   311
     Daniel R. Mueller, Stefanie J. Schmidt, and Volker Roder

14. Cognitive Enhancement Therapy   335
     Shaun M. Eack

15. Metacognitive Training in Schizophrenia: Theoretical Rationale and
     Administration   358
     *Steffen Moritz, Ruth Veckenstedt, Francesca Bohn, Ulf Köther,
     and Todd S. Woodward*

16. Social Cognition and Interaction Training   384
     Dennis R. Combs, Johanna Torres, and Michael R. Basso

Conclusion: The Future of Social Cognition in Schizophrenia: Implications
     from the Normative Literature   401
     David L. Roberts and Amy E. Pinkham

Index   415

CONTRIBUTORS

Ahmad Abu-Akel
Independent
Los Angeles, California

Jean Addington, Ph.D.
Hotchkiss Brain Institute
Department of Psychiatry
University of Calgary
Calgary, Canada

Ralph Adolphs, Ph.D.
Division of Humanities and
    Social Sciences
California Institute of Technology
Pasadena, California

Michael R. Basso, Ph.D.
Department of Psychology
University of Tulsa
Tulsa, Oklahoma

Richard P. Bentall, Ph.D.
Institute of Psychology, Health &
    Society
University of Liverpool
Liverpool, United Kingdom

Francesca Bohn
University Medical Center
    Hamburg-Eppendorf
Department of Psychiatry and
    Psychotherapy
Hamburg, Germany

Tyrone D. Cannon, Ph.D.
Departments of Psychology and
    Psychiatry & Biobehavioral Sciences
University of California
Los Angeles, California

Dennis R. Combs, Ph.D.
Department of Psychology
University of Texas
Tyler, Texas

Shannon M. Couture, Ph.D.
Department of Psychology
University of Southern California
Los Angeles, California

Shaun M. Eack, Ph.D.
School of Social Work
University of Pittsburgh
Pittsburgh, Pennsylvania

Joanna M. Fiszdon, Ph.D.
VA Connecticut Healthcare System
Yale University School of Medicine
West Haven, Connecticut

Dylan G. Gee, M.A.
Department of Psychology
University of California
Los Angeles, California

Michael F. Green, Ph.D.
VA Desert Pacific Mental Illness
   Research, Education and Clinical
   Center
UCLA Semel Institute for
   Neuroscience and Human
   Behavior
Los Angeles, California

Shihui Han, Ph.D.
Department of Psychology
Peking University
Beijing, China

Elizabeth Hanson
Department of Psychiatry
University of Pennsylvania
Philadelphia, Pennsylvania

William P. Horan, Ph.D.
VA Desert Pacific Mental Illness
   Research, Education and Clinical
   Center
UCLA Semel Institute for
   Neuroscience and Human
   Behavior
Los Angeles, California

Amy M. Jimenez, M. A.
Department of Psychology
University of California
Los Angeles, California

Melissa A. Koenig, Ph.D.
Institute of Child Development
University of Minnesota
Minneapolis, Minnesota

Christian G. Kohler, M.D.
Department of Psychiatry
University of Pennsylvania
Philadelphia, Pennsylvania

Ulf Köther
University Medical Center Hamburg-
   Eppendorf
Department of Psychiatry and
   Psychotherapy
Hamburg, Germany

Junghee Lee, Ph.D.
VA Desert Pacific Mental Illness
   Research, Education and Clinical
   Center
UCLA Semel Institute for
   Neuroscience and Human Behavior
Los Angeles, California

Matthew D. Lieberman, Ph.D.
Departments of Psychology and
   Psychiatry & Biobehavioral Sciences
University of California
Los Angeles, California

Kristjen Lundberg
Department of Psychology
University of North Carolina
Chapel Hill, North Carolina

Kristen E. Lyons, Ph.D.
Institute of Child Development
University of Minnesota
Minneapolis, Minnesota

Mary E. March, M.S.
Department of Psychiatry
University of Pennsylvania
Philadelphia, Pennsylvania

Steffen Moritz, Ph.D.
University Medical Center Hamburg-
   Eppendorf
Department of Psychiatry and
   Psychotherapy
Hamburg, Germany

Daniel R. Mueller, Ph.D.
University Hospital of Psychiatry
University of Bern
Bern, Switzerland

David L. Penn, Ph.D.
Department of Psychology
University of North Carolina
Chapel Hill, North Carolina

Amy E. Pinkham, Ph.D.
Department of Psychology
Southern Methodist University
Dallas, Texas

Danijela Piskulic, Ph.D.
Hotchkiss Brain Institute
Department of Psychiatry
University of Calgary
Calgary, Canada

David L. Roberts, Ph.D.
Department of Psychiatry
University of Texas Health Science
   Center
San Antonio, Texas

Volker Roder, Ph.D
University Hospital of Psychiatry
University of Bern
Bern, Switzerland

Stefanie J. Schmidt, M.Sc.
University Hospital of Psychiatry
University of Bern
Bern, Switzerland

Simone G. Shamay-Tsoory, Ph.D.
Department of Psychology
Haifa University
Haifa, Israel

Johanna Torres, B.A.
Department of Psychology
University of Texas
Tyler, Texas

Oana Tudusciuc, M.D., Ph.D.
Division of Humanities and Social
   Sciences
California Institute of Technology
Pasadena, California

Alisa Udachina, Ph.D.
School of Psychology
University of Sheffield
Sheffield, United Kingdom

Ruth Veckenstedt, Ph.D.
University Medical Center Hamburg-
   Eppendorf
Department of Psychiatry and
   Psychotherapy
Hamburg, Germany

Todd S. Woodward, Ph.D.
Department of Psychiatry
University of British Columbia
BC Mental Health and Addictions
   Research Institute
Vancouver, Canada

INTRODUCTION

SHANNON M. COUTURE AND DAVID L. PENN ■

There is clear consensus that individuals with schizophrenia and related disorders experience marked functioning deficits in the community. Problems with independent living, social skills, obtaining and maintaining employment, and establishing rewarding relationships with others are well documented (e.g., Hooley, 2010) and a central focus of recovery-oriented models of treatment (Bellack, 2006). Widespread recognition of the importance of enhancing functional outcomes in schizophrenia has led researchers to focus on which factors underlie and contribute to poor functioning. Over the years, various models of functioning in schizophrenia have been proposed, and social cognition has emerged as a promising predictor of functional status (Couture et al., 2006; Fett et al., 2011; discussed in depth in Chapter 6). The clinical vignettes below illustrate how social cognitive deficits can impact the social relationships and occupational functioning of individuals with schizophrenia.

Vignette 1

Susan is a 53-year-old woman with chronic schizophrenia. Since the onset of her illness, she has struggled with interpreting others' social cues. This has persisted even though her symptoms have stabilized and she has been able to maintain part-time work baking homemade pies. For example, she recently delivered pies to the home of a customer. The customer, upon taking the pies, remarked, "Thanks so much Susan, your pies have surprised me again!" Susan mistook the customer's comment (and smile) for disappointment (rather than her true feeling of always being surprised that Susan outdid herself again) and said "I'm sorry that I disappointed you, perhaps you should order pies from someone else" and walked off. This isn't the first time that Susan has reacted this way to a customer.

Vignette 2

Tom is a 35-year-old man who works for a local company. He was diagnosed with schizophrenia when he was 24 and has worked intermittently since then. He tends to struggle in relating to others when stressed, which also leads to poor sleep (and which, in turn, augments his stress levels). Tom almost got fired when he blamed others in the office for taking his pens and office supplies; a paranoid type of attributional style. This followed a period in which he would read too much into e-mail messages at work. For example, when a colleague didn't respond to his e-mail right away, he assumed that the colleague was angry with him. Another time, a colleague suggested that he help Tom with an assignment, which Tom felt was due to the colleague thinking that he was incompetent. These sort of issues have led Tom to be estranged from colleagues at work.

WHAT IS SOCIAL COGNITION?

Several definitions of social cognition have been proposed in the diverse literatures of social psychology, evolutionary psychology, biological psychiatry, and clinical psychology. Fiske and Taylor (1991) defined social cognition as the "way in which people make sense of other people" (p.1), and Ostrom's (1984) definition stated that social cognition is the "domain of cognition that involves the perception, interpretation, and processing of social information" (p. 176). However, the most comprehensive definitions are those that link social cognitive abilities to real-world functioning. Brothers' (1990) definition described social cognition as the "mental operations underlying social interactions, which include the human ability and capacity to perceive the intentions and dispositions of others" (p. 28). Similarly, Adolphs (2001) identified social cognition as "the ability to construct representations of the relation between oneself and others and to use those representations flexibly to guide social behavior" (p. 231).

Thus, most definitions of social cognition share the idea that social cognition is a set of related neurocognitive processes applied to the recognition, understanding, accurate processing, and effective use of social cues and information in real-world situations (Penn et al., 1997). Can neurocognitive deficits account for the social cognitive deficits observed in schizophrenia? This question has been raised in numerous studies of social cognition in schizophrenia, typically presented as an argument for a generalized performance deficit in schizophrenia versus a specific deficit in social cognition (e.g., Bryson et al., 1997; Hooker & Park, 2002; Johnston et al., 2001; Kucharska-Pietura et al., 2005; Penn et al., 2000; Vauth et al., 2004; van Hooren et al., 2008).

IS SOCIAL COGNITION DISTINCT FROM NEUROCOGNITION?

We believe that substantial accumulating evidence demonstrates social cognition and neurocognition are related, but separable, constructs. Four lines of research support this notion: (1) neurocognitive and social cognitive tasks are dissociable, (2) neurocognition and social cognition are reliably distinguished statistically, (3) social cognition contributes to functioning above the influence of neurocognition and likely serves as a mediator between neurocognition and functioning, and (4) neurocognition and social cognition appear to have different neurobiological substrates.

Neurocognitive and Social Cognitive Tasks Are Dissociable

First, neurocognitive and social cognitive tasks can be dissociated from each other using a variety of techniques. For example, Brunet and colleagues (2003) demonstrated that individuals with schizophrenia were able to complete sequences of physical causality, but not causality due to intentionality (i.e., theory of mind [ToM]), thus highlighting the specificity of ToM deficits, rather than a general difficulty with linking causal events (Brunet et al., 2003). Similarly, Cutting and Murphy (1990) asked participants questions about social information (i.e., social knowledge) and general knowledge, and discovered that those with schizophrenia demonstrated the greatest impairment on the social knowledge task.

Interestingly, Pomarol-Clotet and colleagues (2010) recruited individuals with schizophrenia with average IQs (thereby "controlling" for general cognitive impairment). The average-IQ schizophrenia patients were still impaired, relative to controls, in identifying emotional intensity despite performing similarly on the simpler task of emotion labeling. Kucharska-Pietura et al. (2005) replicated prior findings suggesting individuals with schizophrenia are impaired on both nonemotional facial perception and facial emotion perception tasks (e.g., Hooker & Park, 2002), suggestive of a generalized performance deficit. However, they found that even after controlling for impairment in nonemotional facial perception, individuals with schizophrenia still demonstrated marked deficits on emotion perception tasks. These results indicate that although individuals with schizophrenia are indeed impaired on a variety of tasks, they do demonstrate a specific impairment in emotion perception (Kucharska-Pietura et al., 2005).

Neurocognition and Social Cognition Are Statistically Separable

Modestly sized statistical relationships between neurocognition and social cognition demonstrate that the two constructs do not completely overlap in shared variance. For instance, affect recognition has been found to have a moderate relationship with various memory processes, as bivariate correlations range from .23 (Silver & Shlomo, 2001) to .50 (Schneider et al., 1995), with several other studies supporting correlation estimates within this range (Bryson et al., 1997; Kohler et al., 2000; Sachs et al., 2004). Similarly, attention has shown a significant association with affect perception in some studies (r = .20 to .60; Bryson et al., 1997; Combs & Gouvier, 2004; Kee et al., 1998; Kohler et al., 2000; Penn et al., 1993), but not others (Penn et al., 1996). Furthermore, executive functioning or cognitive flexibility also had a modest relationship with affect perception in some studies (r = .29 to .50; Kohler et al., 2000; Sachs et al., 2004; Schneider et al., 1995), but again, not in others (Penn et al., 1996).

Within ToM, the relationship between memory and ToM is generally small, with one study finding no relationship (Mazza et al., 2001) and another suggesting that memory accounts for 8% of the variance in ToM abilities (Greig et al., 2004). Interestingly, recent reviews of ToM in schizophrenia have suggested that ToM impairment cannot be explained by general cognitive impairment or executive function impairment (Brune, 2005; Harrington et al., 2005; Pickup, 2008; Sprong et al., 2007).

More recently, studies have begun using advanced statistical techniques to determine the amount of overlap between neurocognition and social cognition. Using structural equation modeling, Vauth et al. (2004) demonstrated that although neurocognition accounted for substantial variance in social cognition (83% in their study), in order to model the covariances properly, it was essential to keep neurocognition and social cognition as separate constructs. That is, using a one-dimensional model did not fit the data well, thus indicating the neurocognition and social cognition were best conceptualized as distinct. (Of note, other studies have found less robust overlap; 22.5% in Bell et al. [2009] and 17.3% in Couture et al. [2011]). Sergi et al. (2007) also found that a two-factor model (i.e., neurocognition and social cognition as separate, but correlated, factors) fit the data significantly better than did a one-factor model. Likewise, van Hooren and colleagues (2008) argued that the results from exploratory factor analyses indicated social cognition and neurocognition were distinct constructs, and Williams et al. (2008) also found a separable factor for social cognition using principal components analysis.

Thus, the statistical differentiation of neurocognition and social cognition, combined with differential task designs, indicates nonoverlapping, but related, constructs.

Social Cognition as an Independent, Likely Mediational, Contributor to Functioning

Several studies have suggested that social cognition contributes to functioning beyond the influence of neurocognition and may mediate the pathway between neurocognition and functioning. Social cognition demonstrated a stronger relationship with functional outcome than with neurocognition in a number of studies (Brune et al., 2007; Penn et al., 1996; Pollice et al., 2002; Vauth et al., 2004), including in a recent meta-analysis of 52 studies (Fett et al., 2011). Other research has shown that the relationship between social cognition and functional outcome cannot be explained by neurocognitive factors (Corrigan & Toomey, 1995; Meyer & Kurtz, 2009; Poole et al., 2000) and that both domains appear to make an independent or equal contribution to functional outcomes (Addington et al., 2005; Brune, 2005; Combs et al., 2011; Mancuso et al., 2010; Pinkham & Penn, 2006; Roncone et al., 2002). For example, Mancuso et al. (2010) found that a social cognitive factor comprised of "lower-order" processes (emotion and social perception, detection of lies) predicted significant variance in role-play performance and a measure of functional capacity above and beyond the influence of the Measurement and Treatment Research to Improve Cognition in Schizophrenia (MATRICS) neurocognitive battery and negative symptoms. Brune et al. (2007) found that despite the relatively robust relationship between executive functioning and social behavior ($r = -.436$), when entered into a regression model, ToM accounted for 50% of the variance in social behavior, whereas executive functioning did not enter the stepwise regression model.

Moreover, several studies have suggested social cognition may serve as a mediator between neurocognition and functioning in schizophrenia (Addington et al., 2006; Bell et al., 2009; Couture et al., 2011; Meyer & Kurtz, 2009; Sergi et al., 2006; Vauth et al., 2004), although one study suggested social cognition was best conceptualized as a moderator rather than a mediator (Nienow et al., 2006). Thus, this line of research suggests that social cognition may be one mechanism by which neurocognitive impairment affects functioning in the community, consistent with prior conjectures (Green et al., 2000) that social cognition is more directly tied to functioning, given that it is theoretically more proximal to social interactions than is neurocognition. Although these findings have not yet been demonstrated in longitudinal work required for a stringent test of mediation, they clearly provide support both for the importance of social cognition, as well as for its ability to be distinguished from neurocognition.

Different Neural Substrates for Neurocognition Versus Social Cognition

Investigations into the neural substrates underlying neurocognition and social cognition have suggested that two brain systems are involved in the processing of emotions: a ventral system, including the amygdala, ventral anterior cingulate gyrus, and ventral prefrontal cortex, which plays a role in identifying emotion; and a dorsal system, including the hippocampus, dorsal regions of the anterior cingulate gyrus, and the dorsal prefrontal cortex, which is involved in the allocation of attention, planning, and effortful behavior (Bozikas et al., 2004; Phillips et al., 2003). Furthermore, some researchers have concluded that there is evidence to support the presence of a "social cognitive neural circuit," incorporating the amygdala, fusiform gyrus, superior temporal sulcus, and prefrontal cortices (Adolphs, 2001; Blakemore & Frith, 2004; Lee et al., 2004; Phillips et al., 2003; Pinkham et al., 2003; Pinkham et al., 2008a, 2008b; Winston et al., 2004). The amygdala, in particular, has been found to play an important role in responses to emotional stimuli, particularly in the identification of the emotional significance of stimuli in general (Adolphs et al., 1999, 2002; Aleman & Kahn, 2005; Phillips, 2003), and negatively-valenced emotions in particular (Adolphs & Tranel, 2003). It appears the amygdala may be most accurately characterized as involved in automatic processing, which may then bias social cognitive processing, rather than being recruited specifically for the cognitive processes involved in social cognition (Adolphs, 2009). Thus, it appears that certain neural structures show greater activation during social cognitive than neurocognitive processing, which again lends support for the relative distinction between these constructs (Phillips et al., 2003).

These results are further supported by findings from research on individuals with brain damage and other neuropsychiatric disorders. For example, individuals with frontal lobe damage (Anderson et al., 1999; Blair & Cipolotti, 2000; Fine et al., 2001) or prosopagnosia (Kanwisher, 2000) show significantly impaired performance in varying areas of social cognition, such as ToM and facial processing, but have intact discrimination of other types of nonsocial stimuli. In contrast, individuals with Williams syndrome tend to show a relative strength in social cognitive abilities, such as the detection of basic emotions from faces and normal performance on first-order ToM tasks (Jones et al., 2000), but have marked deficits in other aspects of neurocognition (Tager-Flusberg et al., 1998; reviewed in Pinkham et al., 2003). Thus, there appears to be consensus among social cognitive neuroscientists that social information is processed differently in the brain than is nonsocial information; that is, that there is something unique about the way the brain responds to social cognitive stimuli (Adolphs, 2009; Insel, 2010).

The foregoing indicates that neurocognition and social cognition can be differentiated across a range of study methodologies. However, it is also clear that neurocognitive ability plays a role in social cognition. The next section highlights the domains of social cognition that will serve as a focus of this book.

DOMAINS OF SOCIAL COGNITION

In schizophrenia, the most commonly studied domains of social cognition include emotion perception, social perception, attributional style, and ToM (Green et al., 2005, 2008; Green & Horan, 2010; Pinkham et al., 2003). Each of these domains will be discussed in more depth in later chapters. Briefly, emotion perception (also called emotion recognition, affect recognition, or affect perception) is the ability to ascertain emotional information (i.e., what the other person is feeling) from facial expressions, vocal inflections (i.e., prosody), body movement, or some combination of these. Social perception is typically defined as the ability to use social cues and context to ascertain social roles or interpersonal aspects of the social situation (e.g., intimacy or status). Attributional style refers to stylistic modes of explaining social events, such as whether the event occurred as a consequence of the individual's actions, other's actions, or due to features of the situation. Theory of mind involves both the ability to understand that others have mental states different from one's own and the capability to make inferences about the content of those mental states (e.g., others' intentions).

Although these constructs have yielded useful measures and relatively consistent findings that individuals with schizophrenia are deficient in these abilities (e.g., Bora et al., 2009; Kohler et al., 2010; Sprong et al., 2007), there has been no unifying model of social cognition within schizophrenia. Thus, the domains previously studied were not selected via empirical means to determine whether they capture the full extent of social cognitive ability. Notably, some researchers consider emotion perception, including the National Institute of Mental Health (NIMH) MATRICS group, to be part of a larger construct called emotion processing (Green et al., 2008). Emotion processing involves emotion perception plus additional components, such as understanding how to effectively manage emotions, differentiating between the usefulness of emotions, or expressing emotions (Green et al., 2008; Phillips & Seidman, 2008). The emphasis on understanding emotions in a broader sense than being able to perceive emotions correctly in others is reflected in the incorporation of the Mayer-Salovey-Caruso Emotional Intelligence Test (MSCEIT) managing emotions subtest as part of the MATRICS battery as the measure to assess social cognition. This choice is in contrast to prior approaches that did not conceptualize social cognition as encompassing emotional regulation components (for a full discussion of emotion processing, see Chapter 7). This point relates to the fact that there has been little empirical exploration of the structure of social cognition or the relations among the domains purported to comprise it, or consideration of additional domains neglected in prior research.

As such, this volume takes a broader perspective and includes chapters written by experts from social psychology, social cognitive neuroscience, developmental psychopathology, and cross-cultural psychology in addition to experts from the field of social cognition in schizophrenia. For example, the field of social psychology has a more expansive definition of social cognition involving self-relevant cognitive processing, motivated/emotional effects on cognition, and heuristics and biases, as well as a distinction between automatic and controlled processing similar to social neuroscience perspectives (Lieberman, 2007) (see Chapter 2 for a description of social psychology's perspectives on social cognition). In addition, recent research by Stefan Moritz and Todd S. Woodward has also expanded social cognition in schizophrenia to include *metacognition*, or thinking about one's thinking. Their basic and treatment research has demonstrated that individuals with schizophrenia have problems with understanding methods for problem solving and decision making resulting from problems with jumping to conclusions, attributional biases, and ToM (see Chapter 15).

ISSUES IN THE MEASUREMENT OF SOCIAL COGNITION IN SCHIZOPHRENIA

Although issues relevant to the measurement of social cognition and the description of specific tasks will be covered in more detail elsewhere in this volume, we will briefly discuss some of the critical methodological and measurement issues that impact much of social cognitive research in schizophrenia.

Structure of Social Cognition

First and foremost, it is important to note that the structure of social cognition is generally unknown (Green et al., 2008; Mancuso et al., 2010; Sergi et al., 2007). That is, there are little data on the relationships among proposed facets of social cognition (i.e., emotion perception, ToM, attributional style), and almost no data on whether these facets appear to be a part of the underlying latent construct of social cognition. One recent study found social cognition to be comprised of three subfactors: one for attributional style, one for "lower-order" processing (emotion perception and detecting lies), and one for "higher-order" processing (managing emotions and detecting sarcasm) (Mancuso et al., 2010). The factor for attributional style was relatively uncorrelated with the other two factors, which were modestly associated with one another ($r = .26$). An interesting point to note here is that many social cognitive tasks, particularly those for emotion perception and ToM, are typically based on an index of performance accuracy, whereas attributional style measures are scored based on a characteristic way of responding or bias. It is reasonable that methodological differences between tasks such as this one may impact the strength of the relationship among social cognitive tasks.

Other research also supports the proposal that social cognition is comprised of distinct, but related, subconstructs. Specifically, Njomboro and colleagues (2008) found that in brain lesioned patients, the perception of emotions from facial displays was intact, but ToM reasoning was impaired. These findings suggest that these two components of social cognition may be distinct constructs under the umbrella of social cognition. However, some of the tasks developed to assess social cognitive ability are less clearly differentiated. For instance, the Eyes Test (Baron-Cohen et al., 2001) is a prime example of conceptual overlap within tasks. During the Eyes Test, participants are shown 36 pairs of eyes and asked to select, from four responses, the choice that most accurately reflects what the person is thinking or feeling. Although it is generally considered a test of ToM (Bora et al., 2009), it clearly includes elements of emotion perception as well.

An additional problem in considering the structure of social cognition is the development of new tasks that do not readily fit into previously established categories. Judgments about trustworthiness from viewing static facial displays (e.g., as used in Baas et al., 2008; Couture et al., 2010) do not fit with other domains of social cognition, but do seem to relate to the construct of social cognition more broadly. Within the domain of ToM, new approaches have been developed based on neuroscience research suggesting that ToM may be separable into two components: social-perceptual (detection of mental states from readily available cues like facial expression and body movement) and social-cognitive (reasoning about the content of another's mental state) ToM (Bora et al., 2008; Sabbagh, 2004).

Little is known about how some of these new developments relate to more established social cognitive tasks and domains.

These problems all relate to one general point: No clear agreement has been reached about the domains of social cognition to consider in schizophrenia, nor on the tasks that should be used in research. Tasks for particular studies are often based on researcher impressions and opinion rather than on clear empirical grounding, and often research groups develop their own task to suit their study's purpose. Theory of mind tasks, in particular, are widely variable. Two recent meta-analyses subdivided ToM tasks into multiple categories, ranging from four (Sprong et al., 2007) to seven (Bora et al., 2009). Despite having multiple categories, both meta-analyses had to exclude studies that used tasks that did not fit into any of these categories. Task variability has implications for comparing results across studies (Harrington et al., 2005; Yager & Ehmann, 2006).

Psychometric Properties

Few studies report psychometric data for social cognitive tasks (Green et al., 2008; Yager & Ehmann, 2006). Commonly used tasks, such as the Facial Emotion Identification and Discrimination Tasks (FEIT, FEDT; Kerr & Neale, 1993), have demonstrated poor internal consistency when evaluated (e.g., Kee et al., 2004; Penn et al., 2000). It is noteworthy that establishing internal consistency for these types of tasks may be somewhat complicated by uncertainty regarding universal impairment on all emotions (Marwick & Hall, 2008). In other words, if individuals with schizophrenia are more impaired on some emotions compared to others, how might this impact internal consistency? Should we expect high internal consistency across emotions, within emotions, or both? Although this conceptual wrinkle deserves consideration, it is clear that most published studies do not present these data and, thus, much is unknown about the internal consistency of social cognitive measures.

Even less data are available on other psychometric variables, such as test–retest reliability, floor and ceiling effects, normality of distributions, construct validity, predictive validity, or norms. The little data available do suggest that ceiling effects or limited range of scores may be problematic for at least some social cognitive measures (Bora et al., 2009; Corcoran & Frith, 2003; Green et al., 2008; Kohler et al., 2003; Versmissen et al., 2008). Given the recent focus on developing treatments to address social cognitive deficits (as discussed in Part III of this book), the lack of data on the utility of measures for repeated assessment and their susceptibility to practice effects is especially concerning.

Ecological Validity

Given the important role social cognition plays in functioning, the ability of tasks to approximate real-life social situations is critical. Many tasks consist of static displays, often of faces alone, and information is typically presented only in one sensory modality. Little consideration is given to how individuals with schizophrenia incorporate multiple cues and consider context in their understanding of social situations. In addition, tasks often use posed facial expressions (as opposed to genuine expressions) and hypothetical scenarios that may have limited relevance in the lives of individuals with schizophrenia (Aarke et al., 2009; Beese & Stratton, 2004; Johnston et al., 2008). Many of these issues can be attributed to the difficulty inherent in balancing the conflicting demands of internal validity and ecological validity; however, it is important that subsequent research begin to develop a more sophisticated approach to assessing social cognitive ability in schizophrenia in an effort to further refine our interventions.

CONCLUSION AND INTRODUCTION TO TRANSLATIONAL THEME OF THIS BOOK

The field of social cognition in schizophrenia has expanded rapidly in recent decades (Green & Leitman, 2008), reflecting evidence suggesting that social cognition plays an important role in functioning (Couture et al., 2006; Fett et al., 2011) and its potential as a point of intervention in schizophrenia (Penn et al., 2007). It is important to acknowledge that although this rapid expansion has contributed to our understanding of schizophrenia, many of the constructs of interest were borrowed from other fields and operationalized in a variety of ways before consensus on which constructs should be included in social cognitive schizophrenia research. This book synthesizes and integrates findings not only from the field of schizophrenia, but also from experts in related fields. Integration of findings from basic science and experimental psychopathology approaches in Parts I and II will provide a clear picture of current knowledge and provide directions for future research. Part III translates findings from Parts I and II to provide treatment approaches for clinicians.

The ensuing chapters in this book expand upon many of the topics mentioned in the preceding sections. Part I focuses on broad topics in the basic science of social cognition across disorders and normal development. Chapter 1 provides an overview of the acquisition of social cognitive skills in childhood and the role that failure to acquire appropriate skills plays in the development of psychopathology. Chapter 2 explores social cognitive skills in adults from the perspective of social psychology. The cross-cultural applicability of social cognition is described in Chapter 3. Chapters 4 and 5 provide important insights from the field of social cognitive neuroscience.

In Part II, we turn our focus to social cognition within schizophrenia. Chapter 6 addresses the important topic of the link between social cognition and social functioning in schizophrenia, and addresses some of the concerns raised in this chapter about the unique contribution of social cognition above and beyond neurocognition to functioning. Chapters 7, 8, and 9 focus on major components of social cognition within schizophrenia (emotion processing, ToM, and attributional style) and summarize the state-of-the-science in these domains. Given the importance of early intervention in schizophrenia, Chapter 10 focuses on social cognition early in the course of schizophrenia. Chapter 11 follows from Chapters 4 and 5 in Part I by describing social cognitive neuroscience findings in schizophrenia.

Part III provides the practical implications of research findings from Parts I and II. Chapter 12 provides an overview of social cognitive approaches to treatment in schizophrenia. It is followed by descriptions of current treatments available for social cognitive deficits in schizophrenia: Integrated Neurocognitive Therapy (Chapter 13), Cognitive Enhancement Therapy (Chapter 14), Metacognitive Training (Chapter 15), and Social Cognition and Interaction Training (Chapter 16). In the Conclusion, an integrative summary of the book's contents and implications for future research are discussed.

REFERENCES

Aakre, J.M., Seghers, J.P., St-Hilaire, A., & Docherty, N. (2009). Attributional style in delusional patients: A comparison of remitted paranoid, remitted nonparanoid, and current paranoid patients with nonpsychiatric controls. *Schizophrenia Bulletin, 35*(5), 994–1002.

Addington, J., Saeedi, H., & Addington, D. (2005). The course of cognitive functioning in first episode psychosis: Changes over time and impact on outcome. *Schizophrenia Research, 78*, 35–43.

Adolphs, R. (2001). The neurobiology of social cognition. *Current Opinion in Neurobiology, 11*(2), 231–239.

Adolphs, R. (2009). The social brain: Neural basis of social knowledge. *Annual Review of Psychology, 6*, 693–716.

Adolphs, R., Baron-Cohen, S., & Tranel, D. (2002). Impaired recognition of social emotions following amygdala damage. *Journal of Cognitive Neuroscience, 14*(8), 1264–1274.

Adolphs, R., & Tranel, D. (2003). Amygdala damage impairs emotion recognition from scenes only when they contain facial expressions. *Neuropsychologia, 41*, 1281–1289.

Adolphs, R., Tranel, D., Hamann, S., Young, A. W., Calder, A. J., Phelps, E. A., et al. (1999). Recognition of facial emotion in nine individuals with bilateral amygdala damage. *Neuropsychologia, 37*, 1111–1117.

Aleman, A., & Kahn, R. S. (2005). Strange feelings: Do amygdala abnormalities dysregulate the emotional brain in schizophrenia? *Progress in Neurobiology, 77*, 283–298.

Anderson, S. W., Bechara, A., Damasio, H., Tranel, D., & Damasio, A. R. (1999). Impairment of social and moral behavior related to early damage in the human prefrontal cortex. *Nature Neuroscience, 2*(11), 1032–1037.

Baas, D., van't Wout, M., Aleman, A., & Kahn, R.S. (2008). Social judgement in clinically stable patients with schizophrenia and healthy relatives: Behavioural evidence of social brain dysfunction. *Psychological Medicine, 38*, 747–754.

Baron-Cohen, S., Wheelwright, S., Hill, J., Raste, Y., & Plumb, I. (2001). The "reading the mind in the eyes" test revised version: A study with normal adults, and adults with Asperger syndrome or high-functioning autism. *Journal of Child Psychology and Psychiatry, 42*(2), 241–251.

Beese, A.G., & Stratton, P. (2004). Causal attributions in delusional thinking: An investigation using qualitative methods. *British Journal of Clinical Psychology, 43*, 267–283.

Bell, M., Tsang, H.W.H., Greig, T.C., & Bryson, G.J. (2009). Neurocognition, social cognition, perceived social discomfort, and vocational outcomes in schizophrenia. *Schizophrenia Bulletin*, *35*(4), 738–747.

Bellack, A. S. (2006). Scientific and consumer models of recovery in schizophrenia: Concordance, contrasts, and implications. *Schizophrenia Bulletin*, *32*, 432–442.

Blair, R. J. R., & Cipolotti, L. (2000). Impaired social response reversal: A case of "acquired sociopathy." *Brain*, *123*, 1122–1141.

Blakemore, S. J., & Frith, C. D. (2004). How does the brain deal with the social world? *Neuroreport*, *15*(1), 119–128.

Bora, E., Gokcen, S., Kayahan, B., & Veznedaroglu, B. (2008). Deficits of social-cognitive and social-perceptual aspects of theory of mind in remitted patients with schizophrenia: Effect of residual symptoms. *Journal of Nervous and Mental Disease*, *196*, 95–99.

Bora, E., Yucel, M., & Pantelis, C. (2009). Theory of mind impairment in schizophrenia: Meta-analysis. *Schizophrenia Research*, *109*, 1–9.

Bozikas, V.P., Kosmidis, M.H., Anezoulaki, D., Giannakou, M., & Karavatos, A. (2004). Relationship of affect recognition with psychopathology and cognitive performance in schizophrenia. *Journal of the International Neuropsychological Society*, *10*, 549–558.

Brothers, L. (1990). The social brain: A project for integrating primate behavior and neurophysiology in a new domain. *Concepts in Neuroscience*, *1*, 27–61.

Brune, M. (2005). "Theory of mind" in schizophrenia: A review of the literature. *Schizophrenia Bulletin*, *31*, 21–42.

Brune, M., Abdel-Hamid, M., Lehmkamper, C., & Sonntag, C. (2007). Mental state attribution, neurocognitive functioning, and psychopathology: What predicts poor social competence in schizophrenia best? *Schizophrenia Research*, *92*, 151–159.

Brunet, E., Sarfati, Y., & Hardy-Boyle, M. (2003). Reasoning about physical causality and other's intentions in schizophrenia. *Cognitive Neuropsychiatry*, *8*(2), 129–139.

Bryson, G., Bell, M. D., & Lysaker, P. H. (1997). Affect recognition in schizophrenia: A function of global impairment or a specific cognitive deficit. *Psychiatry Research*, *71*, 105–113.

Combs, D. R., & Gouvier, W. D. (2004). The role of attention in affect perception: An examination of Mirsky's four factor model of attention in chronic schizophrenia. *Schizophrenia Bulletin*, *3*, 727–738.

Combs, D. R., Waguspack, J., Chapman, D., Basso, M. R., & Penn, D. L. (2011). An examination of social cognition, neurocognition, and symptoms as predictors of social functioning in schizophrenia. *Schizophrenia Research*, *128*, 177–178.

Corcoran, R., & Frith, C. D. (2003). Autobiographical memory and theory of mind: Evidence of a relationship in schizophrenia. *Psychological Medicine*, *33*(5), 897–905.

Corrigan, P. W., & Toomey, R. (1995). Interpersonal problem solving and information processing in schizophrenia. *Schizophrenia Bulletin*, *21*(3), 395–403.

Couture, S. M., Penn, D. L., & Roberts, D. L. (2006). The functional significance of social cognition in schizophrenia: A review. *Schizophrenia Bulletin*, *32*(S1), S44–S63.

Couture, S. M., Granholm, E. L., & Fish, S. C. (2011). A path model investigation of neurocognition, theory of mind, social competence, negative symptoms and real-world functioning in schizophrenia. *Schizophrenia Research*, *125*, 152–160.

Couture, S. M., Penn, D. L., Losh, M., Adolphs, R., Hurley, R., & Piven, J. (2010). Comparison of social cognitive functioning in schizophrenia and high-functioning autism: More convergence than divergence. *Psychological Medicine*, *40*, 569–579.

Cutting, J., & Murphy, D. (1990). Impaired ability of schizophrenics, relative to manics or depressives, to appreciate social knowledge about their culture. *British Journal of Psychiatry*, *157*, 355–358.

Fett, A. J., Viechtbauer, W., Dominguez, M., Penn, D. L., van Os, J., & Krabbendam, L. (2011). The relationship between neurocognition and social cognition with functional outcomes in schizophrenia: A meta-analysis. *Neuroscience and Biobehavioral Reviews, 35,* 573–588.

Fine, C., Lumsden, J., & Blair, R. J. R. (2001). Dissociation between "theory of mind" and executive functions in a patient with early left amygdala damage. *Brain, 124,* 287–298.

Fiske, S. T., & Taylor, S. (1991). *Social cognition* (2nd ed.). New York: McGraw-Hill.

Green, M. F., & Horan, W. P. (2010). Social cognition in schizophrenia. *Current Directions in Psychological Science, 19,* 243–248.

Green, M. F., Kern, R. S., Braff, D. L., & Mintz, J. (2000). Neurocognitive deficits and functional outcome in schizophrenia: Are we measuring the "right stuff"? *Schizophrenia Bulletin, 26*(1), 119–136.

Green, M. F., Olivier, B., Crawley, J. N., Penn, D. L., & Silverstein, S. (2005). Social cognition in schizophrenia: Recommendations from the MATRICS New Approaches Conference. *Schizophrenia Bulletin, 31,* 882–887.

Green, M. F., Penn, D. L., Bentall, R., Carpenter, W. T., Gaebel, W., Gur, R. C., et al. (2008). Social cognition in schizophrenia: An NIMH workshop on definitions, assessment, and research opportunities. *Schizophrenia Bulletin, 34*(6), 1211–1220.

Greig, T. C., Bryson, G., & Bell, M. D. (2004). Theory of mind performance in schizophrenia: Diagnostic, symptom, and neuropsychological correlates. *The Journal of Nervous and Mental Disease, 192,* 12–18.

Harrington, L., Siegert, R. J., & McClure, J. (2005). Theory of mind in schizophrenia: A critical review. *Cognitive Neuropsychiatry, 10,* 249–286.

Hooker, C., & Park, S. (2002). Emotion processing and its relationship to social functioning in schizophrenia patients. *Psychiatry Research, 112,* 41–50.

Hooley, J. M. (2010). Social factors in schizophrenia. *Current Directions in Psychological Science, 19*(4), 238–242.

Insel, T. R. (2010). The challenge of translation in social neuroscience: A review of oxytocin, vasopressin, and affiliative behavior. *Neuron, 65*(6), 768–779.

Johnston, P. J., Katsikitis, M., & Carr, V. (2001). A generalised deficit can account for problems in facial emotion recognition in schizophrenia. *Biological Psychiatry, 58,* 203–227.

Johnston, L., Miles, L., & McKinlay, A. (2008). A critical review of the Eyes Test as a measure of social-cognitive impairment. *Australian Journal of Psychology, 60*(3), 135–141.

Jones, W., Bellugi, U., Lai, Z., Chiles, M., Reilly, J., Lincoln, A., et al. (2000). II. Hypersociability in Williams Syndrome. *Journal of Cognitive Neuroscience, 12,* 30–46.

Kanwisher, N. (2000). Domain specificity in face perception. *Nature Neuroscience, 3*(8), 759–763.

Kee, K. S., Horan, W. P., Mintz, J., & Green, M. F. (2004). Do the siblings of schizophrenia patients evidence affect perception deficits? *Schizophrenia Research, 67,* 87–94.

Kee, K. S., Kern, R. S., & Green, M. F. (1998). Perception of emotion and neurocognitive functioning in schizophrenia: What's the link? *Psychiatry Research, 81,* 57–65.

Kerr, S. L., & Neale, J. M. (1993). Emotion perception in schizophrenia: Specific deficit or further evidence of generalized poor performance? *Journal of Abnormal Psychology, 102,* 312–318.

Kohler, C., Bilker, W. B., Hagendoorn, M., Gur, R. E., & Gur, R. C. (2000). Emotion recognition deficit in schizophrenia: Association with symptomatology and cognition. *Biological Psychiatry, 48,* 127–136.

Kohler, C. G., Turner, T. H., Bilker, W. B., Brensinger, C. M., Siegel, S. J., Kanes, S. J., et al. (2003). Facial emotion recognition in schizophrenia: Intensity effects and error pattern. *American Journal of Psychiatry, 160,* 1768–1774.

Kohler, C. G., Walker, J. B., Martin, E. A., Healey, K. M., & Moberg, P. J. (2010). Facial emotion perception in schizophrenia: A meta-analytic review. *Schizophrenia Bulletin, 36*(5), 1009–1019.

Kucharska-Pietura, K., David, A. S., Masiak, M., & Phillips, M. L. (2005). Perception of facial and vocal affect by people with schizophrenia in early and late stages of illness. *British Journal of Psychiatry, 187*, 523–528.

Lee, K. H., Farrow, T. F. D., Spence, S. A., & Woodruff, P. W. R. (2004). Social cognition, brain networks, and schizophrenia. *Psychological Medicine, 34*, 391–400.

Lieberman, M. D. (2007). Social cognitive neuroscience: A review of core processes. *Annual Review of Psychology, 58*, 259–289.

Mancuso, F., Horan, W. P., Kern, R. S., & Green, M. F. (2010). Social cognition in psychosis: Multidimensional structure, clinical correlates, and relationship with functional outcome. *Schizophrenia Research.* doi: 10.1016/j.schres.2010.11.007

Marwick, K., & Hall, J. (2008). Social cognition in schizophrenia: A review of face processing. *British Medical Bulletin, 88*, 43–58.

Mazza, M., DeRisio, A., Surian, L., Roncone, R., & Casacchia, M. (2001). Selective impairments of theory of mind in people with schizophrenia. *Schizophrenia Research, 47*, 299–308.

Meyer, M. B., & Kurtz, M. M. (2009). Elementary neurocognitive function, facial affect recognition, and social skills in schizophrenia. *Schizophrenia Research, 110*, 173–179.

Nienow, T. M., Docherty, N. M., Cohen, A. S., & Dinzeo, T. J. (2006). Attentional dysfunction, social perception, and social competence: What is the nature of their relationship? *Journal of Abnormal Psychology, 115*(3), 408–417.

Njomboro, P., Deb, S., & Humpreheys, G. W. (2008). Dissociation between decoding and reasoning about mental states in patients with theory of mind reasoning impairments. *Journal of Cognitive Neuroscience, 20*(9), 1557–1564.

Ostrom, T. M. (1984). The sovereignty of social cognition. In R.S. Wyer & T.K. Srull (Eds.), *Handbook of social cognition* (Vol. 1, pp. 1–37). Hillsdale, NJ: Erlbaum.

Penn, D. L., Combs, D. R., Ritchie, M., Francis, J., Cassisi, J., Morris, S., & Townsend, M. (2000). Emotion recognition in schizophrenia: Further investigation of generalized versus specific deficit models. *Journal of Abnormal Psychology, 109*(3), 512–516.

Penn, D. L., Corrigan, P. W., Bentall, R. P., Racenstein, J. M., & Newman, L. (1997). Social cognition in schizophrenia. *Psychological Bulletin, 121*(1), 114–132.

Penn, D. L., Roberts, D. L., Combs, D., & Sterne, A. (2007). Best practices: The development of the social cognition and interaction training program for schizophrenia spectrum disorders. *Psychiatric Services, 58*, 449–451.

Penn, D. L., Spaulding, W., Reed, D., & Sullivan, M. (1996). The relationship of social cognition to ward behavior in chronic schizophrenia. *Schizophrenia Research, 20*(3), 327–335.

Penn, D. L., van der Does, A., Spaulding, W. D., Garbin, C., Linszen, D., & Dingemans, P. (1993). Information processing and social cognitive problem solving in schizophrenia: Assessment of interrelationships and changes over time. *Journal of Nervous and Mental Disease, 181*(1), 13–20.

Phillips, L. K., & Seidman, L. J. (2008). Emotion processing in persons at risk for schizophrenia. *Schizophrenia Bulletin, 34*(5), 888–903.

Phillips, M. L. (2003). Understanding the neurobiology of emotion perception: Implications for psychiatry. *British Journal of Psychiatry, 182*, 190–192.

Phillips, M. L., Drevets, W. C., Rauch, S. L., & Lane, R. D. (2003). Neurobiology of emotion perception I: The neural basis of normal emotion perception. *Biological Psychiatry, 54*, 504–514.

Pickup, G. J. (2008). Relationship between theory of mind and executive function in schizophrenia: A systematic review. *Psychopathology, 41,* 206–213.

Pinkham, A. E., Hopfinger, J. B., Pelphrey, K. A., Piven, J., & Penn, D. L. (2008a). Neural bases for impaired social cognition in schizophrenia and autism spectrum disorders. *Schizophrenia Research, 99,* 164–175.

Pinkham, A. E., Hopfinger, J. B., Ruparel, K., & Penn, D. L. (2008b). An investigation of the relationship between activation of a social cognitive neural network and social functioning. *Schizophrenia Bulletin, 34*(4), 688–697.

Pinkham, A. E., & Penn, D. L. (2006). Neurocognitive and social cognitive predictors of interpersonal skill in schizophrenia. *Psychiatry Research, 143,* 167–178.

Pinkham, A. E., Penn, D. L., Perkins, D. O., & Lieberman, J. (2003). Implications for the neural basis of social cognition for the study of schizophrenia. *American Journal of Psychiatry, 160,* 815–824.

Pollice, R., Roncone, R., Falloon, I. R. H., Mazza, M., DeRisio, A., Necozione, S., et al. (2002). Is theory of mind in schizophrenia more strongly associated with clinical and social functioning than with neurocognitive deficits? *Psychopathology, 35,* 280–288.

Pomarol-Clotet, E., Hynes, F., Ashwin, C., Bullmore, E. T., McKenna, P. J., & Laws, K. R. (2010). Facial emotion processing in schizophrenia: A non-specific neuropsychological deficit? *Psychological Medicine, 40*(6), 911–919.

Poole, J. H., Tobias, F. C., & Vinogradov, S. (2000). The functional relevance of affect recognition errors in schizophrenia. *Journal of the International Neuropsychological Society, 6,* 649–658.

Roncone, R., Falloon, I. R. H., Mazza, M., DeRisio, A., Pollice, R., Necozione, S., Morosini, P., & Casacchia, M. (2002). Is theory of mind in schizophrenia more strongly associated with clinical and social functioning than with neurocognitive deficits? *Psychopathology, 35*(5), 280–288.

Sabbagh, M. A. (2004). Understanding orbitofrontal contributions to theory-of-mind reasoning: Implications for autism. *Brain and Cognition, 55,* 209–219.

Sachs, G., Steger-Wuchse, D., Krypsin-Exner, I., Gur, R. C., & Katschnig, H. (2004). Facial recognition deficits and cognition in schizophrenia. *Schizophrenia Research, 68*(1), 27–35.

Schneider, F., Gur, R. C., Gur, R. E., & Shtasel, D. L. (1995). Emotional processing in schizophrenia: Neurobehavioral probes in relation to psychopathology. *Schizophrenia Research, 17,* 67–75.

Sergi, M. J., Rassovsky, Y., Nuechterlein, K. H., & Green, M. F. (2006). Social perception as a mediator of the influence of early visual processing on functional status in schizophrenia. *American Journal of Psychiatry, 163,* 448–454.

Sergi, M. J., Rassovsky, Y., Widmark, C., Reist, C., Erhart, S., Braff, D. L., et al. (2007). Social cognition in schizophrenia: Relationships with neurocognition and negative symptoms. *Schizophrenia Research, 90,* 316–324.

Silver, H., & Shlomo, N. (2001). Perception of facial emotions in chronic schizophrenia does not correlate with negative symptoms but correlates with cognitive and motor dysfunction. *Schizophrenia Research, 52*(3), 265–273.

Sprong, M., Schothorst, P., Vos, E., Hox, J., & van Engeland, H. (2007). Theory of mind in schizophrenia: Meta-analysis. *British Journal of Psychiatry, 191,* 5–12.

Tager-Flusberg, H., Boshart, J., & Baron-Cohen, S. (1998). Reading the windows into the soul: Evidence for domain-specific sparing in Williams syndrome. *Journal of Cognitive Neuroscience, 10*(5), 631–639.

van Hooren, S., Versmissen, D., Janssen, I., Myin-Germeys, I., Campo, J., Mengelers, R., et al. (2008). Social cognition and neurocognition as independent domains in psychosis. *Schizophrenia Research, 103*, 257–265.

Vauth, R., Rusch, N., Wirtz, M., & Corrigan, P. W. (2004). Does social cognition influence the relation between neurocognitive deficits and vocational functioning in schizophrenia? *Psychiatry Research, 128*, 155–165.

Versmissen, D., Janssen, I., Myin-Germeys, I., Mengelers, R., Campo, J., van Os, J., & Krabbendam, L. (2008). Evidence for a relationship between mentalising deficits and paranoia over the psychosis continuum. *Schizophrenia Research, 99*, 103–110.

Williams, L. M., Whitford, T. J., Flynn, G., Wong, W., Liddell, B. J., Silverstein, S., et al. (2008). General and social cognition in first episode schizophrenia: Identification of separable factors and prediction of functional outcome using the IntegNeuro test battery. *Schizophrenia Research, 99*, 182–191.

Winston, J. S., Henson, R. N., Fine-Goulden, M. R., & Dolan, R. J. (2004). fMRI adaptation reveals dissociable neural representations of identity and expression in face perception. *Journal of Neurophysiology, 92*(3), 1830–1839.

Yager, J. A., & Ehmann, T. S. (2006). Untangling social function and social cognition: A review of concepts and measurement. *Psychiatry, 69*(1), 47–68.

Foundations of Human Social Cognition

PART ONE

Foundations of Human
Social Cognition

The Development of Social Cognition in Theory and Action

KRISTEN E. LYONS AND MELISSA A. KOENIG ∎

Humans are highly social beings. From our earliest moments, our lives are deeply and intricately intertwined with those of our caregivers. As children develop, their social world expands to include siblings, relatives, peers, and the vast number of individuals that they encounter throughout their daily lives, from neighbors and friends to co-workers and clients. To make sense of this social world and to navigate daily interactions effectively, individuals must have an appreciation of the unobservable psychological forces that underlie others' behavior. Understanding that another's actions are driven by that person's thoughts, desires, and beliefs, and that these internal mental states are shaped by that person's previous experience, enables us to predict how others are likely to act and how others will likely view or respond to our actions. The goal of this chapter is to provide an overview of how typically developing individuals come to understand the nuances of the psychological world.

The term *theory of mind* (ToM) refers to the framework that informs children's and adults' understanding of behavior (Flavell, 2004b; Wellman & Liu, 2004). Core elements of this understanding include the notions that (a) other people have intentions, desires, and beliefs; (b) these internal mental states motivate other people's behavior; (c) mental states and processes are based on an individual's previous experience; and (d) mental representations may differ between individuals and from reality. Over the last 25 years, much has been learned about the typical trajectory of children's developing ToM. However, rigorous debate continues over the mechanisms of change, and developmental scientists have only recently begun to investigate how children, increasingly with age, use their ToM understanding in their learning and social interactions.

THE DEVELOPMENTAL COURSE OF THEORY OF MIND

In typically developing children, ToM emerges gradually, with rapid improvement being observed in the first 5 years of life (Wellman & Liu, 2004), although subtle and important improvements are observed throughout childhood (Baron-Cohen, O'Riordan, Stone, Jones, & Plaisted, 1999; Dumontheil, Apperly, & Blakemore, 2010; Perner & Wimmer, 1985), and individual differences in ToM are even detected in adults (Baron-Cohen, Wheelwright, Hill, Raste, & Plumb, 2001). There is general consensus that three key milestones in the development of social cognition are achieved in a staggered timeline, with understanding of intentions preceding understanding of desires, followed by an understanding of belief (Sodian & Kristen, 2010; Wellman & Liu, 2004).

Before a child can analyze the different ways in which a person's mind relates to facts of the world, they begin with a basic appreciation that others have a mental life (Meltzoff, 1988). When asking whether infants construe others as having a psychological life, we are asking if infants treat the behavior of inanimate objects or machines as distinct from the behavior of people. Research demonstrates that infants indeed expect people, but not inanimate entities, to engage in certain types of behavior. For example, young infants anticipate that human hands cause other objects to move, but blocks or trains do not (Leslie, 1984; Saxe, Tzelnic, & Carey, 2007). Infants also expect that humans, but not robots, balls, or inanimate objects, will begin to move without causal contact with another entity (Kosugi, Ishida, & Fujita, 2003; Legerstee, 1992; Spelke, 2003).

Young infants even appear to appreciate, at some level, that human action is motivated by intentions. That is to say, rather than viewing human behavior as random movements through space, infants perceive and encode human actions as goal-directed (e.g., a person reaching for a toy) (Flavell, 2004b). For example, using a habituation paradigm, Woodward (1998) showed 6-month-old infants scenes taking place on a small stage that had two toys (e.g., a teddy bear on the left side of the stage and a ball on the right side of the stage). During the habituation phase, a hand repeatedly moved across the stage and grasped one of two toys (e.g., the teddy bear). During the test phase, the locations of the two toys were switched (e.g., so that the teddy bear was on the right and the ball was on the left). Infants were then shown two new scenes: the hand following the same path to grasp the other toy ("new goal events"), and the hand following a different path to grasp the same toy ("new path events"). Infants looked longer when the hand grasped a new object, suggesting that they viewed this scene (in which the hand displayed a different intention) as more novel and interesting than the alternative scene (in which the hand displayed the same intention but displayed dissimilar spatiotemporal properties). Notably, this pattern was not observed when an inanimate grasping rod was used, nor when the hand was covered by a sparkly glove, nor when the back of the hand flopped near the object, thus suggesting that infants attribute goals (and perhaps intentions) to the well-defined actions of human actors.

In efforts to explain the source of this intentional attribution, some have suggested that the ability to view human action as intentional is dependent upon one's own first-hand experience in engaging in similar acts (Sommerville, Woodward, & Needham, 2005). Infants younger than 5–6 months of age (who are not yet physically capable of self-directed reaching and grasping) do not discriminate between new goal and new path events at test. However, providing young infants with only a few minutes of reaching experience by putting sticky Velcro mittens on their hands (that allow them to "pick up" toys simply by touching them) causes infants as young as 3 months to preferentially look at the new goal scene compared to the scene with the new path (Sommerville, et al., 2005). Taken together, the results suggest that a nascent framework for understanding human action may be available very early in human development and that the development of such a framework may depend, in part, upon one's own first-hand experience with the actions one is perceiving.

Imitation studies provide further evidence that very young children look beyond the surface features of a scene to extract the underlying mental motivation. Infants as young as 14 months of age readily imitate the actions of adults (e.g., Meltzoff, 1988). However, they are discriminate in their choice of the action to imitate, selectively imitating only intended actions. In one study, for example, 14- to 18-month-old infants imitated a majority of actions that were marked by an adult as intentional (i.e., actions that were followed by the adult saying "There!"), but imitated less than half of the actions that were marked as accidental (i.e., actions that were followed by adults saying "Oops!") (Carpenter, Akhtar, & Tomasello, 1998). In another study, 18-month-old children viewed adults attempting but failing to perform an action (e.g., attempting to pull apart a dumb-bell). When they were given an opportunity to play with each of the objects themselves, infants tended to execute the intended action (which they had never seen), rather than the observed failed actions (Meltzoff, 1995). Taken together, these results suggest that during the second half of the first year through the second year of life, children robustly extract others' intent from the surface features of their actions.

The second major milestone in ToM development is typically achieved midway through the second year. At this age, children begin to exhibit an appreciation that others' behavior is motivated by their desires, and that others may have desires that differ from one's own. To test whether young children could reason in this way about desires, Repacholi and Gopnik (1997) conducted an experiment with 14- and 18-month-old children. The experimenter tasted two types of foods (e.g., crackers and broccoli), expressing delight about one of the foods and expressing disgust at the other. Then, she placed her hand out and asked the participants to give her one more. Although older participants offered the experimenter the food for which she expressed a preference, the younger participants offered whichever food they preferred. These results show that during the toddler years, children come to understand that another person may desire something (e.g., broccoli) that differs from one's own preference (e.g., crackers). This represents a major achievement—the ability to reason about the unobservable psychology of another person (Repacholi & Gopnik, 1997; Wellman & Liu, 2004)—and has typically been viewed as the first step in developing a ToM. Understanding of desires continues to mature throughout the preschool years. By 3 years of age (Wellman & Woolley, 1990), children predict that another person will act in accordance with that person's desires (e.g., that someone who prefers to go swimming will choose to go to the pool rather than going to the park to play soccer), even if they conflict with one's own. However, the ability to predict that actions follow from desires appears to be hampered when the others' desire is more distant from one's own (e.g., when children are told that the other person prefers a clearly unattractive sticker over a clearly attractive one) (Moore, Jarrold, Russell, Lumb, Sapp, & MacCallum, 1995). Four-year-olds show a similar difficulty in predicting the emotions of story protagonists who receive their desired or undesired selections when those selections conflict with the child's own. It is not until age 5 that children consistently judge that others' will be happy to receive their desired selection of a snack or a toy, even if it conflicts with the child's own preference (Rieffe, Terwogt, Koops, Stegge, & Oomen, 2001). Thus, although children begin to understand the mental world of desires before their second birthday, more robust understanding of the role of desires in motivating behavior is not observed until much later in the preschool years.

The third major milestone in the development of ToM concerns children's developing understanding of knowledge and belief (Sodian & Kristen, 2010; Wellman & Liu, 2004). Between the ages of 4 and 5 years, most children come to appreciate that (a) in order to know something, a person must have had some kind of perceptual access to that information; (b) others may hold beliefs that differ from one's own; and (c) beliefs are mere approximations of reality and thus may be false (Wellman & Liu, 2004).

A rudimentary appreciation of the connection between perceiving and knowing likely begins to emerge during infancy (Flavell, 2004b; Onishi & Baillargeon, 2005), and, by 3 years, children demonstrate a basic understanding that, in order to know something (e.g., what object is hidden inside a box), a person must have had access to that information (Pillow, 1989; Pratt & Bryant, 1990). However, in spite of such early beginnings, preschoolers persist in exhibiting striking limitations in their ability to reason about knowledge and belief. During the preschool years, dramatic developmental improvement is observed in children's understanding about *how* people come to acquire different kinds of knowledge (e.g., information about the color vs. the weight of an object). Three-year-olds perform much more poorly than older children when they are asked to judge which puppet would know the appearance (or the texture) of a hidden object: the puppet who looked inside a tunnel or the puppet who felt inside the tunnel (O'Neill, Astington, & Flavell, 1992). Similar limitations are observed when young children are asked how they themselves came to acquire knowledge (e.g., via touching, seeing, or hearing an adult describe an object hidden in a box), even just a few moments after learning the information (O'Neill & Gopnik, 1991). This failure to encode the mode through which information was learned suggests that young preschoolers lack awareness of their ongoing mental operations, as well as an understanding of the function of different perceptual operations.

In the later preschool years, children begin to appreciate that past experiences may influence individuals' perceptions or beliefs about ambiguous stimuli or events. For example, many 4- and 5-year-old children report that a puppet who has only seen a small portion of a drawing will know what is in the drawing. In contrast, the majority of 6-year-olds correctly report that the puppet would not know what is in the drawing, and would be likely to misinterpret it based on his or her previous experiences (Pillow & Henrichon, 1996).

Developmental changes are also observed between the ages of 3 and 5 in children's appreciation of their own previously incorrect beliefs. For example, Gopnik and Astington (1988) presented children with objects that appeared to be one thing (e.g., a rock) but in reality were another (e.g., a sponge). After showing children the true nature of the objects, children were asked what they previously thought the object was, and what the object was really. The majority of 3-year-olds failed to report their previous belief (based on the appearance of the object—i.e., a rock), instead reporting on their current mental representation (of what the object was in reality—i.e., a sponge). In contrast, by age 5, the vast majority of children were able to report on their previous false mental representation of the objects. The passing of such a test marks a critical change in children's understanding of the mental world: the conceptual understanding that mental representations are subjective approximations of reality, and that mental representations of the same object may differ (between individuals or even between one's own past and current mental states).

This understanding is at the core of the last major milestone in ToM development: the understanding of false belief. The false-belief task originated from the comparative psychology literature (Premack & Woodruff, 1978) as a thought experiment about what kind of a task would be sufficient to show that an individual understood the mental state of another. The basic premise of the false-belief task is as follows: An individual sees an object hidden in location A. When that individual is absent, the object is moved to location B. The participant is then prompted to predict where the individual will search for the object—in location A (where it was previously seen) or location B (where the object is really). If children answer this question simply based on reasoning about the other's desire to obtain the object, then they will say location B (i.e., where the character would have to look to find the object). If children answer this question based on their own perspective of the situation, they will say location B (i.e., where the child knows the object to be located). Children will only give the correct search location if they understand that the subject of the story has a different mental state than their own, one that is based on subjective, limited, and, in this case, incorrect information. Wimmer and Perner (1983) were the first to develop a human version of this task and examined developmental changes in performance between 4 and 9 years. In their version of the task, a boy puts his chocolate in one cupboard, but his mother moves it to another location while the boy is absent. When asked where the boy would search for his chocolate, half of the 4-year-old children failed this test, stating that the boy would look in the new location. In contrast, the vast majority of older children answered the question correctly, saying the boy would look for his chocolate where he last left it. A meta-analysis of 178 studies using various versions of false-belief tasks showed that this pattern of developmental change is observed in across-task manipulations (e.g., whether the participant is involved in deceiving the story character or someone else is involved in moving the object) and in children with different countries of origin (Wellman, Cross,

& Watson, 2001). Taken together, these findings suggest that the passing of the false-belief task marks an important conceptual change in children's understanding of the mental world and that this change typically occurs in the later preschool years. Experimental evidence indicates that children typically demonstrate competence in reasoning about beliefs only after they demonstrate a competent ability to reason about desires (Wellman & Liu, 2004), and in naturalistic observations of children's language development, words referring to desires (e.g., want) typically appear in speech before language referring to beliefs (e.g., think) (Bartsch & Wellman, 1995).

It is important to note, however, that recent infant research, using looking time as the dependent measure, has found evidence that infants as young as 15 months of age may have an implicit understanding of false belief (Onishi & Baillergeon, 2005; Scott & Baillargeon, 2009; Song, Onishi, Baillargeon, & Fisher, 2008; Surian, Caldi, & Sperber, 2007). In the original study by Onishi and Baillargeon (2005), infants viewed adults acting out scenarios analogous to the false-belief task (i.e., watching an adult hide an object in location A, and, when the adult was absent, viewing the object being moved to location B). Infants looked longer when the adult searched in location B than when they searched in location A, suggesting that the adults' searching behavior violated their expectations (that the adult would search in location A, where the object was initially hidden). Like all infant data, diverse research groups have interpreted these findings differently. The authors argued that these findings suggest that even very young children understand that others' beliefs are based on their experiences and that beliefs may be false. More conservative interpretations have contended that perhaps lower-level associative processes can explain the results. For example, Ruffman and Perner (2005) countered that children may use a form of statistical learning to predict where others will search for objects (e.g., people typically look for an object in the location where it was last seen) rather than a higher-order mental attribution (e.g., the woman should search in location A because she does not know the object was moved to location B and instead thinks the object is in location A) (for a response, see Baillargeon, Scott, & He, 2010). Issues of interpretation aside, it is important to note that, like many other types of ToM reasoning, it appears that understanding beliefs may have its roots in infancy and gradually develop over the course of the preschool years.

However, ToM development is *not* complete at age 5. Subtle but important changes in children's awareness and understanding of mental states continue throughout childhood and into adolescence. Around age 7, children develop *second-order ToM understanding*, understanding that others (e.g., John) mentally represent what third parties (e.g., Mary) are thinking (Perner & Wimmer, 1985). Children's understanding of faux pas and nonliteral meaning improves between ages 7 and 9 (Baron-Cohen et al., 1999; Creusere, 2000), although it is still not at ceiling levels of performance even at this age, thus suggesting that understanding the ways in which language relates to the mind of the speaker continues to improve throughout middle childhood. Using more complex visual perspective-taking tasks, developmental improvements in ToM reasoning have been observed into adolescence (Dumontheil et al., 2010), and individual differences in the ability to reason about ToM are even observed in adults (Baron-Cohen et al., 2001; Birch & Bloom, 2007; Keysar, Lin, & Barr, 2003; Meins et al., 2003; Nickerson, 1999).

Hence, although false-belief understanding is often taken as the hallmark of having a ToM, social cognition requires understanding a much wider variety of mental states and processes, as well as how they are causally related to each other (Flavell, 2004b). Although the seeds of social understanding appear to sprout during infancy, and substantial improvement in ToM is observed during the preschool years, full competence in understanding others' mental states and processes is not observed until adolescence.

THEORIES OF THEORY OF MIND DEVELOPMENT

It is often noted that an understanding of mental states may be one of the more difficult domains for young children to master because mental states cannot be directly observed (Wellman, 2002). Accordingly, much attention has been focused on elucidating the mechanisms that permit children to learn about the psychological world and drive developmental changes in social cognition.

Theories of ToM development can be categorized under two main classes: *domain-general accounts* and *domain-specific accounts*. Domain-general accounts posit that developmental improvements in children's ability to reason about and attribute mental states to others are driven by broader improvements in children's cognitive abilities. These generalized improvements in cognition are thought to promote improvements in ToM understanding by equipping children with the basic skills needed to accurately reason about mental states. One prevalent domain-general account is that improvements in ToM are driven by improvements in executive function, or children's ability to consciously control their thoughts and actions (including improvements in inhibitory control, working memory, and attentional flexibility). Correlational research indicates that individual differences in executive function are robustly correlated with children's false-belief understanding (Carlson & Moses, 2001). This relation may be at least partially due to the fact that successful performance on false-belief tasks requires that children *inhibit* their own knowledge, *flexibly shift their attention* to another character's perspective, while *maintaining in working memory* the conditions that the other character has experienced. Data from a recent study investigating the neural correlates of ToM reasoning are consistent with this notion. Liu and colleagues (Liu, Sabbagh, Gehring, & Wellman, 2009) recorded event-related potentials (ERPs) while 4- to 6-year-old children and adults completed a false-belief task. During the task, participants were asked to reason about characters' mistaken beliefs (false-belief trials) and to reason about the true location of a hidden object (control trials). Children who passed the false-belief tasks and adults (who also passed the tasks) showed a late slow wave over left prefrontal cortex (which was greater for false-belief compared to control trials) in a region previously documented to be critically important for working memory. Children who failed the false-belief task did not exhibit ERP waveforms that differentiated the two trial types. Thus, there is some evidence to suggest that executive function skills (i.e., working memory) are necessary for children to be able to reason about the psychological states of others.

However, executive function skills are correlated with ToM performance even when the executive function demands of the false-belief task are reduced, thus suggesting that the correlation between executive function and ToM cannot fully be explained by task demands (Perner, Lang, & Kloo, 2002). It has alternatively been proposed that executive function skills may not simply help children to pass false-belief tasks; they may also help children to take advantage of interactions in their daily lives to learn about the psychological world. That is to say, children who have better executive function skills may be able to flexibly shift their attention and inhibit their own thoughts to take on the perspectives of others in their interactions with parents and peers. Practicing these skills may lead to better performance on ToM as tested at later time points. Consistent with this proposal are the results of longitudinal research showing that executive function skills at age 2 predict ToM at age 3 and age 4 (Hughes & Ensor, 2007), above and beyond earlier ToM skills and language ability.

A second domain-general account is that ToM development critically hinges on the development of representational understanding (Perner, 1991; Perner & Leekam, 2008). This account posits that, in order to reason about mental states (i.e., *mental* representations of the state of the world), children must have a general conceptual understanding of representation. Namely, children must understand that representations are meant to approximate reality, but they do not necessarily correspond to reality. To test this hypothesis, a false-sign task was developed as a non-mental analogue to the false-belief task. In this task, children are shown a drawing of a town, including a sign indicating that the ice cream truck has driven to a location behind the church. Participants are told that, later, the ice cream truck drives away from the church and over to the school, but the driver forgets to change the sign. Children are then asked, "Where does the sign say the ice-cream truck is?" As in the false-belief task, to answer the question correctly, children must set aside their knowledge of reality to reason about how the sign (a *physical* representation) represents the location of the object. Performance on this task correlates with performance on the standard false-belief task, suggesting a common source of difficulty (Perner & Leekam, 2008). Specifically, these findings have been interpreted as showing that younger children's inability to reason about mental representations is due to a general inability to appreciate that (physical or mental) representations of objects in the world may not correspond with reality. Only when children come to learn that a representation may be false (i.e., the ice cream truck is really in location B, but the sign says it is in location A) can they come to appreciate the subjective nature of mental representations.

A third domain-general account of ToM holds that language development plays a critical role in promoting ToM (Harris, 2006). As mental states cannot be directly observed, conversations with others (especially older siblings or parents) may be a crucial inroad to learning about mental states. Consistent with this notion are findings from research with children who lack the ability to communicate with their parents in their early years (e.g., deaf children born to hearing parents). Such children show significant delays in ToM compared to children who are able to communicate with their parents from an early age (e.g., hearing children or deaf children born to deaf parents; Meristo, Falkman, Hjelmuist, Tedoldi, Surian, & Siegal, 2007). These delays are observed even when nonverbal ToM tasks are employed (Figueras-Costa & Harris, 2001), suggesting that it is not language per se that limits children's ability to reason successfully on ToM tasks, but rather the opportunity to converse with others through language that facilitates the development of ToM. Further evidence consistent with this notion is research showing that maternal talk about the mind is correlated with children's ToM ability concurrently (Moeller & Schick, 2006) and longitudinally (Ruffman, Slade, & Crowe, 2002).

Language may also play a critical role in the development of ToM by changing the way that children think about the world. In line with a Whorfian hypothesis, this domain-general account of ToM development posits that mastering more complex forms of syntax allows children to think in terms of conditional structures that are necessary to understand mental representations. For example, once children can use two clauses in conjunction with one another, they can then understand that Max thinks the chocolate is in cupboard X, but the chocolate is really in cupboard Y (Astington & Jenkins, 1999; Watson, Painter, Bornstein, 2001). Evidence from a training study is consistent with this hypothesis. Lohmann and Tomasello (2003) randomly assigned 3-year-olds to one of several training conditions. In one condition, children were simply exposed to deceptive objects, such as those used in appearance reality tests, and their deceptive nature was revealed using minimal verbal input from the experimenter. In a second condition, the experimenter discussed the objects using stories in which sentential complementary syntax was emphasized, but the deceptive nature of the objects was never revealed. In a third condition, both of these elements were combined. The sentential complement training condition, but not the simple exposure to the deceptive objects training, improved children's performance on change of location false-belief tasks. Moreover, individual differences in the improvement in comprehension of complex syntax predicted improvements in false-belief understanding, suggesting that developmental improvements with specific linguistic constructions may be critically important to children's developing an ability to reason about the mental world.

A second class of accounts contends that developmental changes in ToM are due to changes specific to this domain. One of these views holds that reasoning about the psychological world is supported by a specialized system of knowing that comes online very early in life (Carey, 2009; Leslie, 2005). In essence, this perspective posits that infants are born with basic core knowledge about the social world (e.g., that humans and other animate beings are sentient and agentic, whereas objects are not). This core knowledge equips infants to (through their experiences and interactions with others) learn about the mental world. With this experience, core knowledge solidifies and becomes more refined (Carey, 2009; Carey &

Spelke, 1994). Support for this proposal comes from studies of social understanding in very young children, including the findings that 6-month-old infants view hands as acting with intention (Leslie, 1984), and Onishi and Baillargeon's (2005) looking-time study of false-belief expectations in 15-month-old infants. Recent neuroimaging studies showing that there may be a specialized neural network involved in social reasoning (see Saxe, Carey, & Kanwisher [2004] for a review, and also Chapter 4 in this book) are also consistent with the proposal that ToM development may be driven by the maturation of a specialized ToM mechanism (Leslie, 2005).

An alternative domain-specific account posits that ToM development operates like the development of a scientific theory (Gopnik & Wellman, 1992; Wellman & Gelman, 1998). The "theory theory" of ToM development contends that children come to understand others' minds by first forming a folk hypothesis about why other people act the way that they do and then gathering additional information by observing others and adjusting their hypotheses based on this evidence. With development, these hypotheses are tested against the available evidence, tailored in ways that are responsive to the evidence, and bolstered into theories about the psychological motivations behind others' behavior. Thus, the psychological world comes to be understood through a set of predictions and explanations about what might be operating in others' minds based on an objectively derived understanding of how internal states motivate behavior. Support for this proposal comes from a recent computational modeling study of the development of false-belief (Goodman et al., 2006), showing that children's false-belief reasoning can be explained in terms of rational inferences.

In contrast, the simulation theory of ToM development holds that children come to learn about others' mental activities by first gaining an appreciation of their own mental states and reactions in different situations. They then use this insight to project mental states to others (Harris, 1992). From this perspective, children use their self-knowledge to predict how or why others act the way that they do (e.g., when I am in situation X and I do Y, it is because I feel Z. Since my brother is acting the same way in the same context, he probably also feels Z.) Support for this theory comes from research on pretend play and ToM development. Specifically, individual differences in children's engagement in role-playing with others is correlated with their ToM performance, but other kinds of play (e.g., solitary play) are not (Harris, 2000; Schwebel, Rosen, & Singer, 1999). Among other benefits, these experiences may provide children with the opportunity to practice taking on other roles and the opportunity to observe how others' behavior differs when they have taken on a given perspective (Lillard, 2001), thus leading to an enhanced ability to simulate the minds of others in the real world.

The questions of which account best specifies the initial state, which account best explains sequential changes, and which account best characterizes the learning mechanisms involved is a topic of active debate. For example, it is likely that numerous sociocultural factors contribute to the development of ToM, as well as to maturationally specified developments of the brain. Thus, elements of many of the theories discussed likely contribute to the development of social cognition.

Elucidating the unique contribution of each factor and how each operates in conjunction with one another is a critical task for ongoing and future research.

THEORY OF MIND IN ACTION

Much of what developmental scientists have learned about ToM development comes from studies of children (or adolescents) predicting the beliefs, emotions, or actions of characters in stories. Although the experimental control afforded by this approach allows us to elucidate the mental states that children of different ages can or cannot appreciate, it provides little information about how children develop the ability to use their understanding of the psychological world in their social interactions. Thus, there is a growing interest in understanding the processes through which children's developing understanding of the psychological world gives rise to changes in their behavior.

Some have argued that even infants use social understanding to guide their responding in the context of communication. During the first year of life, infants begin to follow others' gazes, looking to the location where parents or other adults are looking (Brooks & Meltzoff, 2005; Hood, Willen, & Driver, 1998; Farroni, Csibra, Simion, & Johnson, 2002; Flavell, 2004b). By 10 months of age, they begin to do so more discriminately, only shifting their gaze when the experimenter's eyes are open, but not when the experimenter's eyes are closed (Brooks & Meltzoff, 2005). By 12 months of age, infants will physically change their position in order to see an object that they currently cannot see when an experimenter expresses interest in it, suggesting that, at this young age, even infants appreciate that the experimenter is viewing something of interest (Moll & Tomasello, 2004; Tomasello & Haberl, 2003). Around 12 months of age, infants also engage in social referencing—looking to their caregivers when they are faced with novel or potentially threatening situations. For example, when infants are placed on a visual cliff (a glass-topped table that appears to have a deep drop), infants look to their mothers (on the other side of the table) and respond in accordance with the mother's emotional expression (e.g., crossing the table when positive emotions are expressed and avoiding crossing the table when negative emotions are expressed) (Klinnert, Emde, Butterfield, & Campos, 1986; Vaish & Striano, 2004).

Some have interpreted these behaviors richly, arguing that they show that very young children appreciate the ongoing mental intentions and beliefs of others, whereas others have argued for a much leaner interpretation of these behaviors, suggesting that these early behaviors are driven by more bottom-up factors (e.g., learning that others' eyes are often directed at interesting or important stimuli, or that when infants feel afraid, they seek contact with their caregivers). Although further research is needed to clarify the capacities that motivate and explain early social communication, these interactions no doubt provide an important foundation for children's learning about the psychological world and the mental states of others (Flavell, 2004b).

Early understanding of the mental world also appears to be critically important to learning. Specifically, appreciating that gaze indicates attention may be crucial to the ability to map words onto objects. Experimental evidence shows that when infants hear a novel label from an adult, they attach that label to the object at which the adult was looking, rather than to the object that captured the infant's attention (Baldwin, 1991; Baldwin & Moses, 2001; Woodward & Markman, 1998). Indeed, infants who exhibit more advanced social competence in these early markers of social understanding (e.g., gaze following) showcase advantages in early vocabulary acquisition, being better able to identify which object an adult is labeling (Brooks & Meltzoff, 2005; Morales, Mundy, & Rojas, 1998). Thus, the ability to attend to and engage in social interactions with others appears to facilitate early learning.

The evaluation of speakers' mental states likely continues to influence word learning in later periods as well. In particular, as young children begin to understand the conditions that lead to knowledge, they become more discriminating in when, and from whom, they accept word labels. For example, in one study, when a speaker expressed doubt about what a novel object was called, 3- and 4-year-olds were much less likely to learn a novel object's label compared to when that speaker expressed knowledge and certainty about what a novel object was called (Sabbagh & Baldwin, 2001). Four-year-olds were also more likely to learn the labels for novel objects when the speaker had created the object, compared to when someone else created it, suggesting a rather sophisticated appreciation of the speaker's knowledge about the object. In contrast, 3-year-olds failed to differentiate between these instances.

Developing an understanding of the psychological world does not simply allow children to learn about the transient mental states of others, such as perceptually based beliefs and intentions. It should also afford them ability to reason about more stable differences in other people's knowledge or expertise (Heyman, 2008; Koenig & Harris, 2005a; Lutz & Keil, 2002). Tracking stable differences in others' competence and using this knowledge to decide whether one should trust them, and in what contexts, is therefore critically important (Koenig & Harris, 2005b). For example, biology teachers typically know more about science than do math teachers, parents know more about family history than do friends, and Dutch speakers know Dutch words whereas English speakers do not. Children and adults rely on the testimony of others for much of what they know about the world and, given this dependence, should evaluate the expertise of others in order to know when these others are likely to be offering a competent, informed judgment as opposed to a biased or misinformed one (e.g., Keil, 2006, 2008).

Recent evidence suggests that children show considerable sophistication in their efforts to evaluate people as potential sources of information. Not only do children prefer to learn from reliable more than from less-reliable individuals (Birch, Vauthier, & Bloom, 2008; Jaswal & Neely, 2006; Koenig & Harris, 2005a,b; Sabbagh & Baldwin, 2001), they form enduring profiles of an informant's prior accuracy and continue to use this information when evaluating new testimony after a week has passed (Corriveau & Harris, 2009). The ability to use an individual's epistemic reliability to guide learning and imitation appears to be an early emerging competence (Birch, Akmal, & Frampton, 2010; Chow, Poulin-Dubois, & Lewis, 2008; Koenig & Woodward, 2010; Poulin-Dubois & Chow, 2009). By age 4, children monitor the relative magnitude of a person's errors and assess incorrect information for "how wrong" it is (Einav & Robinson, 2010). Furthermore, children are capable of revising their judgments in light of new evidence bearing on an individual's reliability (Scofield & Behrend, 2008) and, by 4 years of age, monitor the relative frequency of errors made by two informants (Pasquini, Corriveau, Koenig, & Harris, 2007). This line of research thus documents a general competence that infants and young children display when learning from others and indicates an early sensitivity to an impressive range of cues used to make these selective judgments.

Children's ability to attend to the competence of a source and avoid those that seem misinformed or ignorant has obvious epistemic advantages in that it helps children manage the risks of misinformation. However, the potential problems of communicated information may not simply arise from the incompetence of others, but also from their interests and their (dis)honesty. One recent study (Vanderbilt, Liu, & Heyman, 2011) found that 3-year-olds readily trusted the advice of a puppet (about where to search for a sticker) that had previously been helpful and also readily trusted a puppet that had previously been tricky (providing children with wrong information). Four-year-olds were less trusting overall but still failed to differentiate between the previously helpful versus tricky informant. Only 5-year-olds were significantly more likely to trust the information provided by the helpful puppet. The difference in selective trusting was associated with children's ToM understanding (as measured via the 2004 battery developed by Wellman and Liu), thus suggesting that children's developing understanding of the psychological world facilitates their ability to reason about the more stable mental intentions and likely actions of others.

The ability to track and detect differences in informants appears to emerge even earlier in the context of more conventional tasks, in which young children have more a priori knowledge to use when evaluating the reliability of others. For example, on novel word learning tasks, children as young as 24 months are more likely to accept novel labels from speakers who have previously labeled common objects correctly (e.g., labeling a shoe as "shoe") than from speakers who have previously labeled common objects incorrectly (e.g., labeling a shoe as "boat") (Koenig & Woodward, 2010; see also Poulin-Dubois & Chow, 2009). The tendency to selectively trust informants based on their accuracy appears to be related to children's ability to explicitly track differences in the quality of an informant. For example, Koenig, Clément, and Harris (2004) found that children who were able to report which of two speakers said the right things and which of two speakers said the wrong things systematically accepted novel labels from the more reliable speaker to a greater degree. Children who could not report on this difference performed at chance levels. Thus, it appears that when children are able to track a speaker's past reliability, they use this insight to determine whether that individual should be trusted.

However, to truly show that selective trust is based on understanding of differences in knowledge, expertise, or intentions, it is necessary to rule out the possibility that children are using a lower level cue, such as avoiding any speaker who says something incorrect. Although some evidence of a halo effect has been observed in children (5-year-olds judge previously accurate speakers as being more knowledgeable about words, general facts, and being nicer in future scenarios than previously inaccurate speakers), this effect does not generalize to all domains (such as talents, preferences, or situation-specific knowledge), suggesting that a discriminate extension of trust is observed in children (Brosseau-Liard & Birch, 2010). More recently, Koenig and Jaswal (2011) found evidence that preschoolers were not more likely to trust an expert outside of his or her domain of expertise (e.g., a dog expert labeling novel objects) compared to a neutral informant, consistent with the notion that preschoolers are not overly general in their positive attributions of knowledge to a previously accurate informant. However, a second experiment found that when children were told about a speaker who was incompetent at naming dogs, their distrust of this speaker generalized to other domains. Thus, although children did not overattribute knowledge to a dog expert, there appeared to be a "pitchfork effect," such that children discounted information across domains from an incompetent source. These findings suggest that when judging what someone else is likely to know (or not know), the scope of children's inferences differ depending on whether the individual showed herself to be knowledgeable or incompetent.

Of course, mature reasoning about psychological traits must also take the context into consideration, including situational factors that may limit a person's ability to exhibit his or her knowledge or expertise. Preschoolers appear to take into account the situational factors that may constrain an individual's ability to provide accurate information (Nurmsoo & Robinson, 2009; Robinson & Whitcombe, 2003). Three- to five-year-olds preferentially trust a knowledgeable informant, but only when that informant has the ability to select his or her response willingly. For example, Kushnir, Gelman, and Wellman (2008) presented preschoolers with informants who were either knowledgeable about how a toy worked (i.e., who had played with the toy before and who knew which blocks made the toy light up) or an ignorant informant (who had not previously played with the toy). Preschoolers trusted the knowledgeable informant's selection of a block more frequently than the ignorant informant's selection; however, no preference was observed when the knowledgeable informant was blindfolded and therefore could not purposefully select that block. In other research, preschoolers have been found to consider whether informants' errors could be explained by the presence of physical constraints (e.g., the person had to label an object when they were blindfolded; Nurmsoo & Robinson, 2009), suggesting that preschoolers consider a number of causally-related cues when determining how to extend their trust (Koenig, 2010).

Children's developing understanding of the psychological world likely becomes increasingly important as their social networks expand and they begin to form relationships with peers. Correlational research indicates that young children (preschoolers and kindergartners) who are more advanced in their ToM understanding are rated by their teachers as having better social skills and higher popularity (Cassidy, Werner, Rourke, Zubernis, & Balaraman, 2003; Watson, Nixon, Wilson, & Capage, 1999), and preadolescents who have better scores on tests of social understanding are rated by their teachers and peers as being more socially competent (Bosacki & Astington, 1999).

Although increased social understanding has generally been linked with reduced aggression (Dodge & Crick, 1990), greater insight into how one's actions will affect others may also facilitate actions aimed at harming or deceiving others (Arsenio & Lemerise, 2001). Theory-of-mind skills are associated with *increased* proactive aggression in early elementary school-aged children who have been victimized by their peers (Renouf, Brendgen, Séguin, Vitar, Boivin, & Dionne, 2010), and in older children, some subtypes of bullying have been linked to increased social cognition skills (Sutton, Smith, & Swettenham, 1999). Thus, there appears to be a complex interaction between social cognition and children's peer relations: Children who have difficulty understanding others may be more prone to misunderstand the intentions of others, perhaps leading to a tendency to respond with inappropriate levels of aggression. Children who are more adept at understanding others may generally have more positive interactions with their peers, leading to reductions in the tendency to respond aggressively. However, when socially competent children do decide to respond aggressively, they may be able to inflict greater harm because they have a better understanding of their peers' underlying thoughts, emotions, and motivations, and hence may be better able to "push their buttons."

Competence with deception is often viewed as a developmental achievement since, to tell lies effectively, children need to take into account the mental states of listeners while appreciating that the goal of lying is to intentionally create a false belief in the mind of another (Sodian, 1991). Both producing and comprehending acts of deception undergo change in the preschool years (Carlson, Moses, & Hix, 1998; Couillard & Woodward, 1999; Jaswal, Carrington Croft, Setia, & Cole, 2011; Russell, Mauthner, Sharpe, & Tidswell, 1991). Lying about a transgression increases between ages 3 and 5, and the lies that children tell become increasingly sophisticated and consistent with the evidence of their transgressions during this period. These improvements are associated with improved ToM and executive function skills (Evans, Xu, & Lee, 2011). In research with older children, individual differences in the ability to effectively lie (i.e., to tell a story and answer questions consistent with one's previous lie) are associated with individual differences in second-order ToM ability (Talwar, Gordon, & Lee, 2007). Thus, as children become increasingly expert in the psychological world, they become increasingly able to use this knowledge to their advantage (for benevolent or more nefarious purposes).

CONCLUSION

Understanding of the social world begins to emerge during the first year of life, improves rapidly during the first 5 years, and continues to develop through childhood and into adolescence. Age-related improvements in knowledge about the psychological world and in the ability to reason online about other people's intentions, desires, perspectives, and beliefs may be driven by a host of factors, including improvements in executive function, language, and conceptual understanding of representation.

Future research is needed to elucidate the specific contributions of each of these factors and how they may interact with more domain-specific mechanisms of social cognition, the formation of reasoned theories about psychological mechanisms, and the simulation of mental states. Doing so will provide key insight into the forces that shape typically developing individuals' understanding of the psychological world and the influences that may cause typical development to go awry.

Much has been learned about the development of children's ability to predict how characters in stories will think, feel, or act. Less is known about children's ability to use this insight online in their interactions with others. Recent research suggests that the development of social cognition may be critically important to learning and the quality of peer relations. Continuing this line of work in future research that investigates how children's developing knowledge of the psychological world influences their behavior in their social interactions with others may provide critical new insight into the consequences of atypical social cognition and how to intervene to improve social functioning in a wide range of individuals.

REFERENCES

Arsenio, W. F., & Lemerise, E. A. (2001). Varieties of childhood bullying: Values, emotion processes, and social competence. *Social Development, 10,* 59–73.

Astington, J. W., & Jenkins, J. M. (1999). A longitudinal study of the relation between language and theory-of-mind development. *Developmental Psychology, 35,* 1311–1320.

Baillargeon, R., Scott, R. M., & He, Z. (2010). False belief understanding in infants, *Trends in Cognitive Science, 14,* 110–118.

Baldwin, D. A. (1991). Infants' contribution to the achievement of joint reference. *Child Development, 62,* 875–890.

Baldwin, D. A., & Moses, L. J. (2001). Links between social understanding and early word learning: Challenges to current accounts. *Social Development, 10,* 309–329.

Baron-Cohen, S., O'Riordan, M., Stone, V., Jones, R., & Plaisted, K. (1999). Recognition of faux pas by normally developing children with Asperger syndrome or high-functioning autism. *Journal of Autism and Developmental Disorders, 29,* 407–418.

Baron-Cohen, S., Wheelwright, S., Hill, J., Raste, Y., & Plumb, I. (2001). The "reading the mind in the eyes" test revised version: A study with normal adults, and adults with Asperger syndrome or high-functioning autism. *Journal of Child Psychology and Psychiatry, 42,* 241–251.

Bartsch, K., & Wellman, H. M. (1995). *Children talk about the mind.* New York: Oxford University Press.

Birch, S. A. J., Akmal, N., & Frampton, K. L. (2010). Two-year-olds are vigilant of others non-verbal cues to credibility. *Developmental Science, 13,* 363–369.

Birch, S. A. J., & Bloom, P. (2007). The curse of knowledge in reasoning about false beliefs. *Psychological Science, 18*, 382–386.

Birch, S. A. J., Vauthier, S. A., & Bloom, P. (2008). Three- and four-year-olds spontaneously use others' past performance to guide their learning. *Cognition, 107*, 1018–1034.

Bosacki, S., & Astington, J. W. (1999). Theory of mind in preadolescence: Relations between social understanding and social competence. *Social Development, 8*, 237–255.

Brooks, R., & Meltzoff, A. N. (2005). The development of gaze following and its relation to language. *Developmental Science, 8*, 535–543.

Brosseau-Liard, P. E., & Birch, S. A. J. (2010). "I bet you know more and are nicer too!": What children infer from others' accuracy. *Developmental Science, 13*, 772–778.

Carey, S. (2009). *The origin of concepts.* New York: Oxford University Press.

Carey, S., & Spelke, E. (1994). Domain-specific knowledge and conceptual change. In L. A. Hirschfeld, & S. A. Gelman (Eds.), *Mapping the mind: Domain specificity in cognition and culture.* (pp. 169–200). New York: Cambridge University Press.

Carlson, S. M., & Moses, L. J. (2001). Individual differences in inhibitory control and children's theory of mind. *Child Development, 72*, 1032–1053.

Carlson, S. M., Moses, L. J., & Hix, H. R. (1998). The role of inhibitory processes in young children's difficulties with deception and false belief. *Child Development, 69*(3), 672–691.

Carpenter, M., Akhtar, N., & Tomasello, M. (1998). Fourteen- through 18–month-old infants differentially imitate intentional and accidental actions. *Infant Behavior & Development, 21*, 315–330.

Cassidy, K. W., Werner, R. S., Rourke, M., Zubernis, L. S., & Balaraman, G. (2003). The relationship between psychological understanding and positive social behaviors. *Social Development, 12*, 198–221.

Chow, V., Poulin-Dubois, D., & Lewis, J. (2008). To see or not to see: Infants prefer to follow the gaze of a reliable looker. *Developmental Science, 11*, 761–770.

Corriveau, K., & Harris, P. L. (2009). Preschoolers continue to trust a more accurate informant 1 week after exposure to accuracy information. *Developmental Science, 12*, 188–193.

Couillard, N. L., & Woodward, A. L. (1999). Children's comprehension of deceptive points. *British Journal of Developmental Psychology, 17*, 515–521.

Creusere, M. A. (2000). A developmental test of theoretical perspectives on the understanding of verbal irony: Children's recognition of allusion and pragmatic insincerity. *Metaphor and Symbol, 15*, 29–45.

Dodge, K. A., & Crick, N. R. (1990). Social information-processing bases of aggressive behavior in children. *Personality and Social Psychology Bulletin. Special Issue: Illustrating the Value of Basic Research, 16*, 8–22.

Dumontheil, I., Apperly, I. A., & Blakemore, S. (2010). Online usage of theory of mind continues to develop in late adolescence. *Developmental Science, 13*, 331–338.

Einav, S., & Robinson, E. J. (2010). Children's sensitivity to error magnitude when evaluating informants. *Cognitive Development, 25*, 218–232.

Evans, A. D., Xu, F., & Lee, K. (2011). When all signs point to you: Lies told in the face of evidence. *Developmental Psychology, 47*, 39–49.

Farroni, T., Csibra, G., Simion, F., & Johnson, M. H. (2002). Eye contact detection in humans from birth. *Proceedings of the National Academy of Sciences, 99*, 9602–9605.

Figueras-Costa, B., & Harris, P. (2001). Theory of mind development in deaf children: A nonverbal test of false-belief understanding. *Journal of Deaf Studies and Deaf Education, 6*, 92–102.

Flavell, J. H. (2004a). Development of knowledge about vision. In D. T. Levin (Ed.), *Thinking and seeing: Visual metacognition in adults and children.* (pp. 13–36). Cambridge, MA: MIT Press.

Flavell, J. H. (2004b). Theory-of-mind development: Retrospect and prospect. *Merrill-Palmer Quarterly: Journal of Developmental Psychology. Special Issue: The Maturing of the Human Developmental Sciences: Appraising Past, Present, and Prospective Agendas, 50,* 274–290.

Goodman, N.D., Baker, C.L, Bonawitz, E.B., Mansinghka, V.K., Gopnik, A., Wellman, H., et al. (2006). Intuitive Theories of Mind: A Rational Approach to False Belief. *Proceedings of the Twenty-Eighth Annual Conference of the Cognitive Science Society.* Vancouver, Canada.

Gopnik, A., & Astington, J. W. (1988). Children's understanding of representational change and its relation to the understanding of false belief and the appearance-reality distinction. *Child Development,59,* 26–37.

Gopnik, A., & Wellman, H. M. (1992). Why the child's theory of mind really is a theory. *Mind & Language, 7*(1–2), 145–171.

Harris, P. L. (1992). From simulation to folk psychology: The case for development. *Mind & Language,7,* 120–144.

Harris, P. L. (2000). *The work of the imagination.* Malden: Blackwell Publishing.

Harris, P. L. (2006). *Social cognition.* Hoboken, NJ: John Wiley & Sons Inc.

Hughes, C., & Ensor, R. (2007). Executive function and theory of mind: Predictive relations from ages 2 to 4. *Developmental Psychology, 43,* 1447–1459.

Heyman, G. D. (2008). Children's critical thinking when learning from others. *Current Directions in Psychological Science, 17,* 344–347.

Hood, B. M., Willen, J. D., & Driver, J. (1998). Adult's eyes trigger shifts of visual attention in human infants, *Psychological Science, 9,* 53–56.

Jaswal, V. K., Carrington Croft, A., Setia, A. R., & Cole, C. A. (2010). Young children have a specific, highly robust bias to trust testimony. *Psychological Science, 21,* 1541–1547.

Jaswal, V. K., & Neely, L. A. (2006). Adults don't always know best: Preschoolers use past reliability over age when learning new words. *Psychological Science, 17,* 757–758.

Keil (2006). Doubt, deference and deliberation. In J. Hawthorne and T. Gendler (Eds.), *Oxford Studies in Epistemology.* Oxford: Oxford University Press.

Keil (2008). Getting to the truth: Grounding incomplete knowledge. *Brooklyn Law Review, 73,* 1035–1052.

Keysar, B., Lin, S., & Barr, D. J. (2003). Limits on theory of mind use in adults. *Cognition, 89,* 25–41.

Klinnert, M. D., Emde, R. N., Butterfield, P., & Campos, J. J. (1986). Social referencing: The infant's use of emotional signals from a friendly adult with mother present. *Developmental Psychology, 22,* 427–432.

Koenig, M. A. (2010). Selective trust in testimony: Children's evaluation of the message, the speaker and the speech act. In T. Gendler & J. Hawthorne (Eds.), *Oxford studies in epistemology* (Vol. 3). Oxford: Oxford University Press.

Koenig, M. A., Clément, F., & Harris, P. L. (2004). Trust in testimony: Children's use of true and false statements. *Psychological Science, 15,* 694–698.

Koenig, M. A., & Harris, P. L. (2005a). Preschoolers mistrust ignorant and inaccurate speakers. *Child Development, 76,* 1261–1277.

Koenig, M. A., & Harris, P. L. (2005b). The role of social cognition in early trust. *Trends in Cognitive Sciences, 9,* 457–459.

Koenig, M. A., & Jaswal, V. K. (2011). Characterizing children's expectations about expertise and incompetence: Halo or pitchfork effects? *Child Development, 82,* 1634–1637.

Koenig, M. A., & Woodward, A. L. (2010). Sensitivity of 24–month-olds to the prior inaccuracy of the source: Possible mechanisms. *Developmental Psychology, 46,* 815–826.

Kosugi, D., Ishida, H., & Fujita, K. (2003). 10–month-old infants' inference of invisible agent: Distinction in causality between object motion and human action. *Japanese Psychological Research, 45,* 15–24.

Kushnir, T., Wellman, H. M., & Gelman, S. A. (2008). The role of preschoolers' social understanding in evaluating the informativeness of causal interventions. *Cognition, 107,* 1084–1092.

Legerstee, M. (1992). A review of the animate–inanimate distinction in infancy: Implications for models of social and cognitive knowing. *Early Development & Parenting, 1,* 59–67.

Leslie, A. M. (1984). Infant perception of a manual pick-up event. *British Journal of Developmental Psychology, 2,* 19–32.

Leslie, A. M. (2005). Developmental parallels in understanding minds and bodies. *Trends in Cognitive Sciences, 9,* 459–462.

Liu, D., Sabbagh, M. A., Gehring, W. J., & Wellman, H. M. (2009). Neural correlates of children's theory of mind development. *Child Development, 80,* 318–326.

Lillard, A. (2001). Pretend play as twin earth: A social-cognitive analysis. *Developmental Review, 21,* 495–531.

Lohmann, H., & Tomasello, M. (2003). The role of language in the development of false belief understanding: A training study. *Child Development, 74,* 1130–1144.

Lutz, D. J., & Keil, F. C. (2002). Early understanding of the division of cognitive labor. *Child Development, 73,* 1073–1084.

Meins, E., Fernyhough, C., Wainwright, R., Clark-Carter, D., Gupta, M. D., Fradley, E., & Tuckey, M. (2003). Pathways to understanding mind: Construct validity and predictive validity of maternal mind-mindedness. *Child Development, 74,* 1194–1211.

Meltzoff, A. N. (1988). Infant imitation and memory: Nine-month-olds in immediate and deferred tests. *Child Development, 59,* 217–225.

Meltzoff, A. N. (1995). Understanding the intentions of others: Re-enactment of intended acts by 18-month-old children. *Developmental Psychology, 31,* 838–850.

Meristo, M., Falkman, K. W., Hjelmquist, E., Tedoldi, M., Surian, L., & Siegal, M. (2007). Language access and theory of mind reasoning: Evidence from deaf children in bilingual and oralist environments. *Developmental Psychology, 43,* 1156–1169.

Moeller, M. P., & Schick, B. (2006). Relations between maternal input and theory of mind understanding in deaf children. *Child Development, 77,* 751–766.

Moll, H., & Tomasello, M. (2004). 12- and 18-month-old infants follow gaze to spaces behind barriers. *Developmental Science, 7,* 1–9.

Moore, C., Jarrold, C., Russell, J., Lumb, A., Sapp, F., & MacCallum, F. (1995). Conflicting desire and the child's theory of mind. *Cognitive Development, 10,* 467–482.

Morales, M., Mundy, P., & Rojas, J. (1998). Following the direction of gaze and language development in 6-month-olds. *Infant Behavior & Development, 21,* 373–377.

Nickerson, R. S. (1999). How we know—and sometimes misjudge—what others know: Imputing one's own knowledge to others. *Psychological Bulletin, 125,* 737–759.

Nurmsoo, E., & Robinson, E. J. (2009). Identifying unreliable informants: Do children excuse past inaccuracy? *Developmental Science, 12,* 41–47.

O'Neill, D. K., Astington, J. W., & Flavell, J. H. (1992). Young children's understanding of the role that sensory experiences play in knowledge acquisition. *Child Development, 63,* 474–490.

O'Neill, D. K., & Gopnik, A. (1991). Young children's ability to identify the sources of their beliefs. *Developmental Psychology, 27,* 390–397.

Onishi, K. H., & Baillargeon, R. (2005). Do 15-month-old infants understand false beliefs? *Science, 308,* 255–258.

Pasquini, E. S., Corriveau, K. H., Koenig, M., & Harris, P. L. (2007). Preschoolers monitor the relative accuracy of informants. *Developmental Psychology, 43,* 1216–1226.

Perner, J. (1991). *Understanding the representational mind.* Cambridge, MA: MIT Press.

Perner, J., Lang, B., & Kloo, D. (2002). Theory of mind and self-control: More than a common problem of inhibition. *Child Development, 73,* 752–767.

Perner, J., & Leekam, S. (2008). The curious incident of the photo that was accused of being false: Issues of domain specificity in development, autism, and brain imaging. *The Quarterly Journal of Experimental Psychology, 61,* 76–89.

Perner, J., & Wimmer, H. (1985). "John thinks that Mary thinks that …": Attribution of second-order beliefs by 5- to 10-year-old children. *Journal of Experimental Child Psychology, 39,* 437–471.

Pillow, B. H. (1989). Early understanding of perception as a source of knowledge. *Journal of Experimental Child Psychology, 47,* 116–129.

Pillow, B. H., & Henrichon, A. J. (1996). There's more to the picture than meets the eye: Young children's difficulty understanding biased interpretation. *Child Development, 67,* 803–819.

Poulin-Dubois, D., & Chow, V. (2009). The effect of a looker's past reliability on infants' reasoning about beliefs. *Developmental Psychology, 45,* 1576–1582.

Pratt, C., & Bryant, P. (1990). Young children understand that looking leads to knowing (so long as they are looking into a single barrel). *Child Development, 61,* 973–982.

Premack, D., & Woodruff, G. (1978). Does the chimpanzee have a theory of mind? *Behavioral and Brain Sciences, 1,* 515–526.

Renouf, A., Brendgen, M., Séguin, J. R., Vitaro, F., Boivin, M., & Dionne, G. (2010). Interactive links between theory of mind, peer victimization, and reactive and proactive aggression. *Journal of Abnormal Child Psychology, 38,* 1109–1123.

Repacholi, B. M., & Gopnik, A. (1997). Early reasoning about desires: Evidence from 14- and 18-month-olds. *Developmental Psychology, 33,* 12–21.

Rieffe, C., Terwogt, M. M., Koops, W., Stegge, H., & Oomen, A. (2001). Preschoolers' appreciation of uncommon desires and subsequent emotions. *British Journal of Developmental Psychology, 19,* 259–274.

Robinson, E. J., & Whitcombe, E. L. (2003). Children's suggestibility in relation to their understanding about sources of knowledge. *Child Development, 74,* 48–62.

Ruffman, T., & Perner, J. (2005). Do infants really understand false belief? *Trends in Cognitive Sciences, 9,* 462–463.

Ruffman, T., Slade, L., & Crowe, E. (2002). The relation between children's and mothers' mental state language and theory-of-mind understanding. *Child Development, 73,* 734–751.

Russell, J., Mauthner, N., Sharpe, S., & Tidswell, T. (1991). The "windows task" as a measure of strategic deception in preschoolers and autistic subjects. *British Journal of Developmental Psychology. Special Issue: Perspectives on the Child's Theory of Mind: II, 9,* 331–349.

Saxe, R., Carey, S., & Kanwisher, N. (2004). Understanding other minds: Linking developmental psychology and functional neuroimaging. *Annual Review of Psychology, 55,* 87–124.

Saxe, R., Tzelnic, T., & Carey, S. (2007). Knowing who dunnit: Infants identify the causal agent in an unseen causal interaction. *Developmental Psychology, 43,* 149–158.

Sabbagh, M. A., & Baldwin, D. A. (2001). Learning words from knowledgeable versus ignorant speakers: Links between preschoolers' theory of mind and semantic development. *Child Development,72,* 1054–1070.

Schwebel, D. C., Rosen, C. S., & Singer, J. L. (1999). Preschoolers' pretend play and theory of mind: The role of jointly constructed pretence. *British Journal of Developmental Psychology, 17,* 333–348.

Scofield, J., & Behrend, D. A. (2008). Learning words from reliable and unreliable speakers. *Cognitive Development, 23,* 278–290.

Scott, R. M., & Baillargeon, R. (2009). Which penguin is this? Attributing false beliefs about object identity at 18 months. *Child Development, 80,* 1172–1196.

Sodian, B. (1991). The development of deception in young children. *British Journal of Developmental Psychology. Special Issue: Perspectives on the Child's Theory of Mind: I, 9,* 173–188.

Sodian, B., & Kristen, S. (2010). Theory of mind. In B. M. Glatzeder, V. Goel, & A. von Muller (Eds.), *Towards a theory of thinking* (pp. 189–201). Berlin: Springer-Verlag.

Sommerville, J. A., Woodward, A. L., & Needham, A. (2005). Action experience alters 3-month-old infants' perception of others' actions. *Cognition, 96,* 1–11.

Song, J., Onishi, K. H., Baillargeon, R., & Fisher, C. (2008). Can an agent's false belief be corrected by an appropriate communication? Psychological reasoning in 18-month-old infants. *Cognition, 109,* 295–315.

Spelke, E. S. (2003). Core knowledge. In N. Kanwisher & J. Duncan (Eds.). *Attention and performance: Functional neuroimaging of visual cognition* (vol. 20). Oxford: Oxford University Press.

Surian, L. Caldi, S., & Sperber, D. (2007). Attribution of beliefs by 13-month-old infants. *Psychological Science, 18,* 580–586.

Sutton, J., Smith, P. K., & Swettenham, J. (1999). Social cognition and bullying: Social inadequacy or skilled manipulation? *British Journal of Developmental Psychology, 17,* 435–450.

Talwar, V., Gordon, H. M., & Lee, K. (2007). Lying in the elementary school years: Verbal deception and its relation to second-order belief understanding. *Developmental Psychology, 43,* 804–810.

Tomasello, M., & Haberl, K. (2003). Understanding attention: 12- and 18-month-olds know what is new for other persons. *Developmental Psychology, 39,* 906–912.

Vaish, A., & Striano, T. (2004). Is visual reference necessary? contributions of facial versus vocal cues in 12-month-olds' social referencing behavior. *Developmental Science, 7,* 261–269.

Vanderbilt, K. E., Liu, D, & Heyman, G. D. (2011). The development of distrust. *Child Development, 82,* 1372–1380.

Watson, A. C., Nixon, C. L., Wilson, A., & Capage, L. (1999). Social interaction skills and theory of mind in young children. *Developmental Psychology, 35,* 386–391.

Watson, A. C., Painter, K. M., & Bornstein, M. H. (2001). Longitudinal relations between 2-year-olds' language and 4-year-olds' theory of mind. *Journal of Cognition and Development, 2,* 449–457.

Wellman, H. M. (2002) Understanding the psychological world: Developing a theory of mind. In U. Goswami (Ed.), *Handbook of childhood cognitive development* (pp. 167–187). Oxford: Blackwell.

Wellman, H. M., Cross, D., & Watson, J. (2001). Meta-analysis of theory-of-mind development: The truth about false belief. *Child Development, 72,* 655–684.

Wellman, H. M., & Gelman, S. A. (1998). Knowledge acquisition in foundational domains. In W. Damon (Ed.), *Handbook of child psychology: Volume 2: Cognition, perception, and language.* (pp. 523–573). Hoboken, NJ: John Wiley & Sons Inc.

Wellman, H. M., & Liu, D. (2004). Scaling of theory-of-mind tasks. *Child Development, 75,* 523–541.

Wellman, H. M., & Woolley, J. D. (1990). From simple desires to ordinary beliefs: The early development of everyday psychology. *Cognition, 35,* 245–275.

Wimmer, H., & Perner, J. (1983). Beliefs about beliefs: Representation and constraining function of wrong beliefs in young children's understanding of deception. *Cognition, 13,* 103–128.

Woodward, A. L. (1998). Infants selectively encode the goal object of an actor's reach. *Cognition, 69,* 1–34.

Woodward, A. L., & Markman, E. M. (1998). Early word learning. In W. Damon (Ed.), *Handbook of child psychology: Volume 2: Cognition, perception, and language.* (pp. 371–420). Hoboken, NJ: John Wiley & Sons Inc.

2

Social Cognition

Social Psychological Insights from Normal Adults

KRISTJEN LUNDBERG ■

Normal adults often have difficulty navigating a complex social world. Perhaps we have looked foolish at the office because we misinterpreted a co-worker's careless error as an action involving malicious intent, or perhaps we have mistakenly inferred that a stranger's haste in ending a conversation with us in a supermarket checkout line was evidence for extreme dislike. The cognitive, emotional, and behavioral processes by which people come to understand themselves and others in the social world is known as *social cognition*. The study of social cognition originated within social psychology during the general "cognitive revolution" (Sperry, 1993) of the 1960s and early 1970s. Social cognition as a construct within social psychology is used to describe a generalized, broad theoretical paradigm focusing on how people process information within social contexts. It includes many specific topics, such as person perception, making causal attributions about self and others, arriving at social judgments, and the dynamics of decision making, among numerous other topics (Augoustinos, Walker, & Donaghue, 2006; Fiske & Taylor, 2008; Kunda, 1999; Moskowitz, 2005; Smith & Semin, 2004). These social cognitive operations may occur at automatic or controlled levels of processing and may be further influenced by various motivational biases (Chaiken & Trope, 1999).

Potential difficulties in understanding the social world are compounded in patients with schizophrenia, who experience several social cognitive deficits. Thus, it is perhaps unsurprising that both social psychologists and schizophrenia researchers, each with interests in people's functioning relative to other people in the social world, have arrived at the common conclusion that social cognition is of critical importance. The purpose of this chapter is to briefly describe some areas of social cognition research conducted by social psychologists, primarily using normal adults, with an eye toward providing insights that may be valuable to schizophrenia researchers. In the first section, I suggest that social psychologists and schizophrenia researchers may be defining social cognition slightly differently, and I outline four characteristics of social cognition as viewed by social psychologists. Recognizing these differences may help lessen potential confusion.

In the second section, I describe social psychological social cognition research on topics that have been of interest to schizophrenia researchers, namely, attribution biases, emotion processing, social perception, and theory of mind (ToM). My second suggestion is that, even within these topics, other phenomena studied by social psychologists in greater depth also may be usefully examined by schizophrenia researchers. Discussion of these phenomena may further enlighten what is known about the disorder. In the last section, I draw some conclusions and offer additional speculations for future research. My final suggestion is that a wider breadth of social cognition topics studied by social psychologists may be relevant to schizophrenia researchers but have thus far received relatively less attention.

DIFFERING DEFINITIONS OF SOCIAL COGNITION

It is useful to note at the outset that social psychologists and schizophrenia researchers appear to define the construct of social cognition in slightly different ways. For schizophrenia researchers, social cognition is used more commonly to define particular types of social processing, such as the ability to draw causal inferences, process emotions, understand others' actions, and take another's perspective (Green & Horan, 2010). For social psychologists, in contrast, social cognition is seen as more of a general paradigm or perspective from which to conduct psychological research (Carlston, 2010; also see Sherman, Judd, & Park, 1989). Although commonalities exist between the two perspectives (e.g., interests in person perception and causal inferences), for social psychologists, social cognition is not a specific topic area of investigation per se, but rather an approach to doing research that can be used to investigate a wide variety of topic areas (Augoustinos et al., 2006; Smith & Semin, 2004). What characterizes social cognition for social psychologists? According to Fiske and Taylor (2008), there are four common features to social cognition research: unabashed mentalism, process orientation, interdisciplinary cross-fertilization, and real-world applications.

Unabashed Mentalism

The first feature is what Fiske and Taylor (2008) term "unabashed mentalism," a focus on people's mental representations, such as *schemas*. Schemas are organized sets of ideas, such as a person's conceptualization of him- or herself, attitudes and beliefs concerning racial groups, or notions about the physical properties of the external world. Once schemas are activated and accessible, they have far-reaching consequences, such as when inferring whether someone is a threat or when deciding whether to continue a romantic relationship. This mentalism contrasts, for example, with the behaviorist tradition of dismissing internal mental states as a topic of study (Watson, 1930; Skinner, 1963; Thorndike, 1940). In this sense, social cognition stems from social psychology's historically "cognitive" focus, exemplified in the classic works of Asch (1946) on trait-based impressions, Hovland and colleagues on attitude change (Hovland, Janis, & Kelley, 1953), and Festinger (1957) on cognitive dissonance. This broader rejection within social psychology of behaviorism's antimentalist approach was met with a groundswell of interest in the study of cognitive processes, as well as with a new set of methods and metaphors (e.g., the brain as a computer) borrowed from cognitive psychology. This confluence of factors endowed social cognitive researchers with opportunities to open the "black box" and explore not only the contents of the mind, but also thinking and reasoning processes themselves (e.g., attention, encoding, and memory), as well as their impact on behavior.

Process Orientation

A second feature is that social cognition is *process oriented*. From a social cognitive perspective, examining cognitive processes is of pivotal importance. It is not enough to know a person's response to a stimulus, but rather one must also know the underlying mechanism by which the person arrived at that response. Sometimes these evaluations and responses occur quite automatically, with little conscious deliberation or intention, whereas, at other times, evaluations and responses occur in a more deliberative, controlled fashion. This distinction between automatic and controlled processing has become one of the main theoretical perspectives in social cognition research. *Automatic processes* are generally defined as unintentional, uncontrollable, efficient, and occurring largely outside of conscious awareness, whereas *controlled processes* are generally defined as intentional, controllable, effortful, and conscious (for reviews see Chaiken & Trope, 1999; Fiske & Taylor, 2008).

Social cognition research has become heavily informed by advances in understanding automatic and often *implicit* processes, with an emphasis on rapid, unconscious reactions to environmental stimuli of which people may not be aware (Bargh, 1994). Researchers have utilized and adapted increasingly sophisticated methods ranging from reaction timing to brain imaging to assess the impact of automatic cognitive processes on evaluative and behavioral responses (Cacioppo et al., 2002). In particular, social cognition researchers have developed a variety of "implicit" measures to examine automatic associations between attitudes and behaviors (Fazio & Olson, 2003; see also Gawronski & Payne, 2010). Because such measures do not require conscious introspection and are designed to capture automatic responses, they may provide information that explicit measures cannot. For example, although explicit expressions of prejudice against blacks may not always be observed publicly (Bobo, 2001), the persistence of racial disparities would lead many to doubt that prejudice itself has disappeared. Instead, individuals simply may be unable or unwilling to report their automatic evaluative responses. Measures of implicit attitudes (e.g., the affect misattribution procedure [AMP; Payne, Cheng, Govorun, & Stewart, 2005], the Implicit Association Test [IAT; Greenwald, McGhee, & Schwartz, 1998]) have been used to address these limitations, and have been shown to be predictive of a diverse range of outcome measures, such as less friendly nonverbal behavior in intergroup interactions (e.g., Dovidio, Kawakami, & Gaertner, 2002) and biased judgments in social perception and judgment (e.g., Gawronski, Geschke, & Banse, 2003; Lambert, Payne, Ramsey, & Schaffer, 2005).

The fact that people with schizophrenia typically have deficits in important domains of controlled processing, such as executive functioning, may lead them to overly rely on automatic information processing (e.g., "environmental dependency"; Lhermitte, 1986; Velligan et al., 2008, 2009). Thus, distinctions between automatic and controlled processes in producing evaluative and behavioral outcomes may be of particular interest to schizophrenia researchers. Indeed, as evidence for this interest, some schizophrenia researchers already have begun adopting implicit measures to assess constructs such as implicit self-esteem and attentional biases in schizophrenia samples (for a review, see Teachman, Cody, & Clerkin, 2010).

Interdisciplinary Cross-Fertilization

Third, social cognition is characterized by interdisciplinary approaches and *cross-fertilization* of ideas. Not only is there an obvious melding of social with traditional cognitive psychology but also a melding with other fields, such as developmental psychology, clinical psychology, and neuroscience. For example, neuroscientific approaches have found that specific brain regions are activated in response to social decision making (see Jimenez et al. [2013], Chapter 4, this volume). The striatum, which is active for basic rewards, also is involved in encoding more abstract social rewards, such as positive feelings produced by mutual cooperation (Sanfey, 2007). Interdisciplinary cross-fertilization is particularly evident between social and clinical psychology. The last three decades have witnessed a burgeoning interest in applying social psychological concepts to better understand, diagnose, and treat emotional and behavioral problems; in using the study of clinical phenomena to inform our understanding of intra- and interpersonal processes in healthy populations; and in uncovering the underlying mechanisms of constructs that are of common interdisciplinary interest (e.g., subjective well-being, self-esteem; see Kowalski & Leary, 2003). This current book is itself testament to the interdisciplinary cross-fertilization between social and clinical psychology, with schizophrenia researchers adopting the construct of social cognition in order to better understand the nature of the disorder, and to inform treatments to improve functional outcomes for people with schizophrenia.

Real-World Applications

Finally, social cognition researchers are concerned with *real-world applications*. One particularly interesting example of such application is that social cognition research has been used to inform legal decisions of the U.S. Supreme Court (Fiske,

Bersoff, Borgida, Deaux, & Heilman, 1991). Researchers have been called upon as expert witnesses to testify to the antecedent conditions, indicators, consequences, and remedies of stereotyping, with testimony influencing the outcomes in prejudice and discrimination cases. Although it may be commonplace for schizophrenia researchers to be concerned with real-world applications, particularly those who are involved in clinical practice, real-world applications are not always of concern for many psychological researchers, particularly those with cognitive leanings, who instead may be more interested in theory-building. Such a lack of concern for real-world applications is *not* generally the case for social cognition researchers. Interest in real-world applications from both social cognition and schizophrenia researchers can thus augment and inform both areas. Schizophrenia researchers can employ the theories, ideas, and methods of social cognition to better understand the disorder, and social psychologists might better understand limitations to their theorizing in learning what goes wrong when severe social cognitive deficits lead judgments astray.

Summary

Although commonalties exist between perspectives, social psychologists and schizophrenia researchers may be using the construct of social cognition in slightly different ways. For social psychologists, social cognition is not a specific topic (or set of topics) of investigation per se, but instead encompasses a broader way of thinking about and doing research, characterized by unabashed mentalism, process orientation, interdisciplinary cross-fertilization, and concern for real-world applications. Schizophrenia researchers, in contrast, more often use the construct of social cognition to study specific abilities and processes that are problematic for people with this disorder. Recognizing this distinction at the outset may help to diminish potential confusion that may result among social psychologists, schizophrenia researchers, and others when discussing what is meant by the term *social cognition* (see also Green et al., 2008).

INCREASING DEPTH OF TOPICS IN SCHIZOPHRENIA RESEARCH

Researchers interested in utilizing a social cognition approach to better understand and treat schizophrenia have consistently identified four topics of primary interest: attribution biases, emotion processing, social perception, and theory of mind (ToM) (e.g., Green et al., 2008). Social psychologists also have long-standing interests in these topics, but with a somewhat increased depth of perspective. By discussing social cognition research related to these four topics from a social psychological perspective, I suggest that even within topics already of interest to schizophrenia researchers there are other phenomena that may be worthy of examination. I note that the categories of research described in this section are not necessarily mutually exclusive. For example, making causal attributions (attribution biases) can involve inferring others' emotions (emotion processing), and this inference may affect how others are perceived (social perception).

Attribution Biases

As described in the opening examples of this chapter, we have all made mistakes when inferring the causes of our own as well as other people's behaviors. Inferring causes is known as making *causal attributions*. For example, imagine you are driving down the highway in bumper-to-bumper rush-hour traffic and you are forced suddenly to slam on the brakes because a shiny silver sports car cuts directly in front of you. Why did this driver do this? Was she unaware that that you were behind her? Was she trying to avoid an encroaching car in another lane? Or, was she simply a reckless jerk? Countless times a day, we are confronted with events such as these that beg for explanations, events that prompt us to ask (and to answer) the question: *Why?* The importance of making causal attributions lies in the fact that subjectively different answers to "why" questions, despite objectively similar actions (e.g., getting cut-off in traffic), can evoke very different responses. That is, if we had inferred that the driver of the sports car just did not see us or was avoiding another automobile, then we might more readily excuse the behavior, although it does not change it. However, if we had instead inferred that the driver was simply a reckless jerk rushing home from work, endangering our life without concern, then the response evoked may be one of anger, rage, or even retaliation.

But we are not even-handed when making causal attributions. Decades of social psychological research have shown that people are consistently biased in making attributions. Generally, we are more likely to infer causality as being due to another's internal dispositions (e.g., personality, attitudes, or traits). This tendency is known as the *correspondence bias* or, because it is so pervasive, the *fundamental attribution error* (Ross, 1977; see also Ross, Amabile, & Steinmetz, 1977; Snyder & Frankel, 1976). Although present in normal adults, this bias in attributing causal fault to people's internal qualities may be taken to extremes in some people with schizophrenia. For example, some people with schizophrenia may have a paranoid or hostile attributional bias, whereby they see mainly negative qualities in other people. Alternatively, people with schizophrenia who are experiencing self-stigma or comorbid depression may be biased toward attributing negative social events to their own failings.

To fully understand attribution biases, one must understand the processes by which people make attributions in the first place. Within social psychology, the genesis of attribution theory is considered to lie in Fritz Heider's (1958) classic book, *The Psychology of Interpersonal Relations*. Among Heider's numerous contributions was the distinction between attributions made to the actor's personality or disposition (i.e., *internal* attributions) versus those made to the situation (i.e., *external* attributions). As early as 1944, Heider foreshadowed the correspondence bias, noting that, although "changes in the environment are almost always caused by acts of persons in combination with other factors, the tendency exists to ascribe the changes *entirely to persons*" (1944, p. 361, emphasis added). The bias toward internal, dispositional attributions was echoed and formalized in the subsequent theorizing of Kelley's (1967, 1972, 1973) covariation model and Jones and Davis's (1965) correspondent inference theory.

According to Kelley, an observer will use three types of information to determine the cause of another person's (i.e., the actor's) behavior. The first, *consensus*, refers to the extent to which other actors respond in the same way to the same stimulus (i.e., person or situation). The second, *distinctiveness*, refers to the extent to which the actor has responded in a unique way to this particular stimulus. And the final piece of information, *consistency*, refers to the extent to which the same actor responds in the same way to the same stimulus over time. For example, imagine a situation in which you and your friend Robert attend a party together, but then Robert spends the entire night talking to everyone except you. Why did Robert ignore you? How might you explain his behavior? According to Kelley's model, you will look for three specific pieces of evidence and draw your conclusion on the basis of the particular pattern you find. For instance, if this situation has low consensus (no one else ignores you at parties), low distinctiveness (Robert has been known to do such things to other people besides you), and high consistency (Robert always ignores you at parties), then you might conclude that the action is due to Robert's disposition (e.g., perhaps he is not very considerate) (see also McArthur, 1972).

Jones and Davis (1965), in their correspondent inference theory, likewise focused on the extent to which observers' attributions are made to internal or external factors. The default assumption was that observers normally infer that an actor's behavior corresponds to her or his stable personality traits—hence the name correspondent inference—unless other information overrides this assumption. Jones and Davis identified several factors that may lead an observer to be more or less likely to make an internal attribution, including: (a) how desirable the consequences of the behavior are (i.e., if an outcome is desirable to the actor, it is more likely that an internal attribution will be made), (b) what is unique or non-normative about the action compared to alternatives that the actor did not pursue (i.e., if it is unique or non-normative, it is more likely that an internal attribution will be made), and (c) the hedonic relevance of the action to the actor (i.e., if it is seen as promoting the goals of the actor, it is more likely that an internal attribution will be made). As an example, imagine that a candidate were to send you an e-mail of thanks following a job interview. To the extent that this behavior is standard for job candidates (i.e., normative), you would likely attribute the act of doing so to social norms and not infer anything particular about the disposition of the actor. However, if the job candidate were to deliver a handwritten note of thanks, whether you view the action as very thoughtful or a bit obsequious, you are likely to infer that the candidate's disposition is the cause, rather than attributing the behavior to social norms.

Formal social psychological models of attribution, such as Kelley's covariation model and Jones and Davis's correspondent inference theory, could be of value to schizophrenia researchers who study attribution biases. For example, perhaps patients with schizophrenia are unable to use consensus, distinctiveness, and consistency information in the way that healthy adults do, and as Kelley's attribution model would predict. Similarly, it may be that patients with schizophrenia severely fail to adjust for situational factors when determining the causes of people's actions, particularly when actions have perceived negative consequences, and are more likely to arrive at dispositional inferences—an extreme version of Jones and Davis's predictions. Compounding these possibilities is that one main reason why normal adults often fall prey to a bias toward internal attributions is simply because it is easier to make such inferences, whereas it requires more cognitive effort to take situational factors into account (Gilbert, 1989; Gilbert, Pelham, & Krull, 1988). Because patients with schizophrenia have cognitive processing deficits, these patients may be particularly prone to making internal attributions relative to normal adults. This possibility could help to explain some of the attribution biases exhibited by patients with schizophrenia and suggests that treatments to improve attributional bias may need to address the issue of cognitive deficits.

Emotion Processing

Schizophrenia researchers use the term "emotion processing" to refer "broadly to perceiving and using emotions adaptively" (Green & Horan, 2010, p. 244). How people with schizophrenia perceive the emotions of others, and how they may be inaccurate in these emotion perceptions, has received considerable attention from schizophrenia researchers (Horan, Kern, Green, & Penn, 2008). For example, inaccurately inferring that a stranger is angry at you because she abruptly ended a conversation, without considering other possibilities like her being in a hurry or having a bad day at work, could result in your experiencing unwarranted hostility, disdain, or even paranoia. It is thus perhaps quite natural that schizophrenia researchers have a strong interest in how people might accurately perceive the emotions of others. Social psychological researchers also are interested in understanding how normal adults perceive others' emotions, but they have an additional long-standing interest in how a person's own emotional experiences shape—and often cloud—social cognition. Below, we discuss both of these issues.

The early years of social cognition research were dominated by a focus on cognition—after all, the perspective was called social *cognition*—and left little room for emotions (Fiske & Taylor, 2008). However, there have always been proponents who have asserted the importance, even the primacy, of emotions (e.g., Zajonc, 1980), and emotions are now considered to be one of the primary drivers of people's processing of social information. For example, one view of the role of emotion in social cognition focuses on the idea of *congruence* and suggests that specific emotions influence attention, perception, memory, and evaluation in emotion-specific ways. From this perspective, one's current emotion may serve as a prime, alerting one to attend to emotion-consistent objects in the environment, prompting associated items to be recalled from memory, and so on. To illustrate the idea of congruence, participants induced to feel specific emotions were faster at identifying emotion-congruent words than they were at identifying emotion-incongruent, neutral, and even valence-congruent/emotion-incongruent words (Niedenthal & Setterlund, 1994). In other words, a happy person would likely be faster to identify the word *delight* (positive, happy related) than she would be to identify *weep* (negative, sad related), *crime* (negative, sad unrelated), *colony* (neutral), and even *luck* (positive, happy unrelated). The idea that emotions influence cognitive processing in a congruent manner may be relevant to patients with schizophrenia, some of whom may be experiencing relatively consistent negative emotions, confirming and reinforcing their views that the world is a negative place.

Other accounts of the relationships between emotions and social cognition concentrate on the role of emotion in determining *what* we think. For example, one prominent account of how emotions influence social judgments is the *feelings-as-information* approach (for reviews, see Schwarz & Clore, 1996, 2007). From this perspective, emotions are seen as a source of information when making evaluations (see also Keltner, Ellsworth, & Edwards, 1993). In one classic experiment (Schwarz & Clore, 1983), researchers telephoned participants to ask about their perceived level of life satisfaction and found that their responses were correlated with the weather: On overcast days, participants reported lower average levels of satisfaction. That is, bad moods, presumably induced by the bad weather, were used as information when judging overall life satisfaction ("my life is unsatisfying"). Tellingly, in other conditions in which participants were first explicitly asked about the weather before answering questions about life satisfaction, moods did not influence judgments. In other words, participants who did not have the weather brought to their attention used emotions by default when evaluating their lives, whereas those who first had the weather brought to their attention discounted it as a relevant piece of evidence ("I'm feeling bad because of the weather not because I'm generally unsatisfied").

These *misattributions*, or mistakes in identifying the true source of our feelings, are known to impact a broad array of judgments and decisions. Hikers are more likely to be attracted to a confederate if they meet while crossing a precarious bridge (misattributing the arousal of fear for the arousal of attraction) versus after a period of rest (Dutton & Aron, 1974). Those who have been induced to experience anger make more optimistic estimates of risk, whereas those experiencing fear are more cautious in their judgments (Lerner & Keltner, 2001). Furthermore, extraneous feelings of disgust lead to more severe moral judgments (Schnall, Haidt, Clore, & Jordan, 2008; Wheatley & Haidt, 2005). For example, Schnall et al. (2008) found that participants exposed to a disgusting smell expressed more severe condemnations in response to moral vignettes (e.g., marriage between first cousins). Although incidental emotions may cloud everyone's judgments, it may be that patients with schizophrenia have a particularly hard time identifying sources of their feelings, with their judgments being pervasively overinfluenced by the emotions they are experiencing at any given time.

Schizophrenia researchers and social psychologists are also interested in how people perceive the emotions of others. Classically, in his 1872 publication

The Expression of Emotions in Man and Animals, Darwin (1872/1998) argued for a biological basis to emotional expressiveness. From this perspective, facial and bodily movements associated with particular emotions are considered remnants of adaptive behaviors. For example, expressions of disgust—the wrinkled nose, raised upper lip, and narrowed eyes—might prepare the body to expel noxious substances, and may also signal that one should avoid such substances in the first place (Rozin & Fallon, 1987; Rozin, Haidt, & McCauley, 2000). This adaptive value of emotional expressiveness suggests that particular expressions of emotion may be universal. Indeed, Paul Ekman and his colleagues found evidence supporting the idea of cross-cultural universality in emotional expressions (Ekman, 1971; Ekman & Friesen, 1971; see also Izard, 1971). Their work, as well as that of their successors, has demonstrated that people throughout the world both express and recognize the same distinct patterns of emotional facial expressions. Although Ekman's research originally identified six basic emotional expressions (happiness, sadness, fear, anger, surprise, disgust), subsequent work has continued to expand the list of emotional expressions having unique, universal displays to include contempt (Ekman & Friesen, 1986), as well as shame, embarrassment, and guilt (Keltner, 1997).

These findings may have particularly relevant implications for researchers who are interested in schizophrenia since patients with schizophrenia often have significant difficulty in reading and decoding others' emotions (Hooley, 2010; see Kohler, Hanson, & March (2013), Chapter 7, this volume). According to the *social-functional perspective* (Frijida & Mesquita, 1994; Keltner & Haidt, 1999), one of the primary functions of emotions is to direct and facilitate one's social interactions and relationships. Although identifying and responding to one's own emotions is an integral aspect of those interactions and relationships (e.g., recognizing one's own sense of guilt may prompt one to make amends), accurately identifying and responding to the emotions of others (e.g., detecting the anger of someone who is a real threat or the expression of contempt that indicates our violation of an important social norm) is also vital to a wide range of individual and social goals. For example, recognizing others' fear may provide you with information about threatening objects in the environment (Mineka & Cook, 1993). Another person's distress may evoke sympathetic responses and further your intentions to engage in helpful behaviors (Eisenberg et al., 1989). Facial expressions of emotion also have been shown to moderate verbal communication in predicting socially cooperative behaviors (Stouten & De Cremer, 2010). Other underlying mechanisms by which we infer the mental states of others (including emotions) are discussed later in the section on ToM.

Social Perception

Social perception (also known as person perception) is a term used broadly by social psychological researchers to refer to processes by which people come to view themselves and other people. In this sense, as described previously, the categories within social cognition that we have outlined are not necessarily mutually exclusive. That is, attribution biases and emotion processing, as well as ToM (described later), are all related in a more general way to how we come to perceive ourselves and others in a social context. Schizophrenia researchers use the term "social perception" to refer to abilities to identify social roles, societal rules, and social contexts (Green & Horan, 2010), all of which individuals with schizophrenia show deficits in doing. However, both social psychologists and schizophrenia researchers have common interests in specific aspects of social perception, such as interpreting nonverbal communications and ambiguous features in social situations as we form impressions of other people.

A great deal of information is exchanged via nonverbal behavior, regularly proceeding without conscious intention or even awareness on the part of both sender and receiver. These nonverbal communiqués are often working in the service of our social goals. For example, nonverbal displays of status and power may elicit compliance or submissive behavior from others (Ellsworth, Carlsmith, & Henson, 1972), whereas nonconscious mimicry of others may result in increased liking for the mimicker by those being mimicked (Chartrand & Bargh, 1999). In normal adults, the ability to infer information from nonverbal behavior often results in astonishingly accurate judgments, even though the exact cues that were used to arrive at such conclusions may remain outside of conscious awareness. For example, Chawla and Krauss (1994) presented participants with conversations that had been taped either spontaneously or after having been rehearsed by actors. Those viewing both the video and the audio of the conversations were able to identify which were spontaneous and which had been rehearsed with about 80% accuracy. Further, participants' responses were correlated with the use of certain hand gestures and pauses in speech that are indicative of trouble with lexical access (e.g., searching for the right word), a sign of extemporaneous speech. In other words, although further probes indicated that participants were unable to articulate their awareness of using such information, they nevertheless were nonconsciously attending to it and using it to make judgments.[1]

The impressive abilities of normal adults to make accurate social judgments is perhaps most apparent in research on *thin slicing*. In a typical thin slicing study, observers are briefly exposed (for as little as 50 ms) to a nonverbal behavior stimulus, such as a static photograph, silent video clip, or audio recording (filtered so as to make specific words unidentifiable), and are subsequently asked to make judgments regarding a range of social variables. Despite such limited exposure to stimuli, participants have shown remarkable accuracy in judgments of characteristics as varied as extraversion (e.g., Borkenau & Liebler, 1992), sexual orientation (e.g., Rule, Ambady, & Hallett, 2009; Johnson, Gill, Reichman, & Tassinary, 2007), political party affiliation (e.g., Rule & Ambady, 2010), and job performance (e.g., Ambady, Krabbenhoft, & Hogan, 2006; Rule & Ambady, 2008). Further, there is evidence to suggest that the impressions we form in those first moments go on to guide subsequent judgments and decisions with substantial real-world implications. For example, Ambady and Rosenthal (1993) demonstrated that ratings of teachers' nonverbal behaviors (e.g., confidence, enthusiasm; based on exposure to 30 s or less of a silent video clip) were predictive of end-of-semester student evaluations and principals' ratings.

Although using thin slicing to draw inferences about others can be remarkably accurate, it can also sometimes lead us astray. For example, Correll, Park, Wittenbrink, and Judd (2002) had participants view pictures of black and white individuals holding either guns or neutral objects (e.g., a wallet) and instructed them to determine as quickly as possible whether or not to "shoot." Participants chose to "shoot" as a response in this experiment more quickly if the target was a black individual holding a gun than if he was white and to "not shoot" more quickly when the target was an unarmed white individual than if he was black (see also Payne, 2001, 2006). Thus, accuracy in using thin slicing was moderated by the race of the person in question, reinforcing people's stereotypic judgments.

Another long-standing tradition in social perception has shown that *priming*, the simple activation of constructs or schemas through prior exposure, can influence how one perceives and evaluates another person (e.g., Higgins, Rholes, & Jones, 1977; Srull & Wyer, 1979). For example, Higgins et al. (1977) asked participants to read a description of a man named Donald who behaved ambiguously, in ways that could be construed as positive or negative (e.g., "He felt he didn't really need to rely on anyone"). Participants who had been primed with positive trait terms (e.g., *independent, self-confident*) were more likely to evaluate Donald positively, whereas those primed with negative trait terms (e.g., *aloof, conceited*) were more likely to evaluate him negatively. Other priming research leads to similar conclusions. For example, an ambiguously behaving target is more likely to be perceived as hostile by people who have been primed with words related to an African American stereotype (e.g., *musical*; Devine, 1989). A group of people at an office water cooler is more likely to be perceived as gossiping if they are women or as talking about sports if they are men (Dunning & Sherman, 1997; see also Kunda & Sherman-Williams, 1993). Also, the evidence from a mock trial is more likely to be deemed supportive of a conviction if a defendant has a Hispanic name than an Anglo name, although only if the stereotype is activated before any evidence is considered (Bodenhausen, 1988).

Some schemas can be *chronically* accessible and therefore affect not only the judgments made but also what information is attended to in the first place (Bargh & Pratto, 1986). Because the use of schemas in social perception is an efficient process, requiring fewer cognitive resources (Fiske & Neuberg, 1990; Macrae, Milne, & Bodenhausen, 1994), they are used more often when cognitive resources are scarce (e.g., Bodenhausen, 1990). To the extent that certain constructs (e.g., threats, hostility) may be more chronically accessible to some people with schizophrenia, who are already laboring under diminished cognitive control, the accessibility of those constructs may facilitate a tendency to disproportionally see threatening, hostile figures and behavior everywhere.

Theory of Mind

Social psychologists have a strong history of investigating people's inferences about the mental states of others, although the specific construct of ToM has probably received more direct attention within developmental than social psychology (e.g., determining how and when children begin to understand the internal states of others; see Lyons & Koenig [2013], Chapter 1, this volume). Within social psychology, inferring the mental states of others has been regarded typically as a building block of both causal attribution and social perception, although it is telling that the fifth and latest volume of the *Handbook of Social Psychology* devotes a separate chapter to the topic of *mind perception* (Epley & Waytz, 2010), which the authors refer to as a "preattributional process" (p. 499) and as distinct from person perception (Macrae & Quadflieg, 2010). This process of inferring the mental states of others—beliefs, goals, and intentions—is also sometimes referred to as *mentalizing* (Frith & Frith, 2003).

Inferring others' states of mind is of critical importance to virtually every social interaction. For example, if we are to ensure our own safety and well-being, we must attempt to judge the intentions of others to determine if they are friend or foe. If we are to influence others, we must first understand their current perspective, their personal goals, and what persuasive messages they might find most compelling. If we are to love and care for another in a close relationship, we must be responsive to their emotional states, their needs, and the many other intricacies of human intimacy. Importantly, we must do all of these things and more without having direct access to the inner workings of the minds of others. Instead, we must infer these inner workings by relying on various cues in behavior and speech, our own knowledge and experiences, and naïve theories about people and the social world.

One means of better understanding what ToM entails is by reviewing a classic test of it called the *false-belief paradigm* (Wimmer & Perner, 1983; see also Baron-Cohen, Leslie, & Frith, 1985). In this procedure, participants are told a story about a boy named Maxi who places some chocolate in a blue cupboard before going out to play. While he is gone, Maxi's mother moves the chocolate from the blue cupboard to the green cupboard. Participants are then asked where Maxi will look for the chocolate when he returns. Correctly identifying the blue cupboard indicates the participant's ability to both (a) represent Maxi's mind and beliefs about the world as distinct from one's own, and (b) understand that beliefs (e.g., the chocolate is in the blue cupboard) may diverge from reality (e.g., the chocolate is now in the green cupboard). Although infants and young children may demonstrate an understanding of other important mental representations, such as goals and intentions (Phillips, Wellman, & Spelke, 2002; Warneken & Tomasello, 2006), it is not until the approximate age of 4 years that the more complex inference skills that are associated with ToM begin to appear and children are consistently able to choose the correct cupboard where Maxi will look (for a review of false-belief paradigms, see Wellman, Cross, & Watson, 2001).

Theory of Mind phenomena are found in complex real-world scenarios as well. Imagine that a close work colleague has just received bad news. How is she feeling? Angry or shocked or sad? How should you respond? With a comforting touch, an offer for after-work drinks, or by giving her some space to be left alone? Research on ToM suggests that you will use several pieces of information when determining your colleague's state of mind, which will in turn dictate how you will respond to her. In addition to the verbal and nonverbal information offered through your colleague's behavior and speech, you are likely to rely on two primary sources of information: your own mental states or experiences (*simulation theory*) and your naïve theories about other minds (*theory theory*). Examples of the latter strategy are described elsewhere in this chapter, as theory theory could be said to encompass much of the research in causal attributions and person perception, in which it is assumed that people can reason about other minds independently of our own mental states.

Simulation theory suggests that individuals use their own thoughts, emotions, and mental states as the most immediate means of insight regarding the thoughts, emotions, and mental states of others. (Some research I previously described on emotion processing, such as that on congruence and feelings-as-information, similarly suggests that one's own current states—in those cases emotions—can influence reasoning and judgment.) For example, research on the *false consensus effect* finds that people use their own performance as diagnostic of how their peers would perform on the same test (Alicke & Largo, 1995); overestimate the extent to which others share their political and social views (Goethals, Allison, & Frost, 1979; Mullen & Goethals, 1990); and believe their own level of endorsement of personality inventory statements (e.g., "I like to let people know where I stand on things") to be normative in the population (Krueger & Clement, 1994). This "egocentric" bias even extends to attempts to determine how others view oneself. Chambers, Epley, Savitsky, and Windschitl (2008) asked participants to speculate about how observers would evaluate their performance and found people were unable to discount the impact of their privately held knowledge about their own past performance on the same task (see also Gilovich, Kruger, & Medvec, 2002). Work from social neuroscience has demonstrated that the same neural region—the medial prefrontal cortex (mPFC)—is implicated in both mentalizing about others and self-reflection (Mitchell, Banaji, & Macrae, 2005; see Jimenez et al. [2013], Chapter 4, this volume). Further, developments in the study of *mirror neurons* (for a review, see Rizzolatti & Craighero, 2004) also suggest that we may even be simulating the experiences of others at a neurophysiological level (Gallese & Goldman, 1998).

But what if you perceive another person to be quite different from you? In that case, one's own mind is likely not as useful a piece of information. Normal adults do, in fact, take the perceived similarity between self and others into account, relying less on self-reflection when encountering a dissimilar other (Ames, 2004; Mitchell, Macrae, & Banaji, 2006; Todd, Hanko, Galinsky, & Mussweiler, 2011). Further, humans undoubtedly possess the ability to distinguish between our own minds and the minds of others to some extent, as doing so is clearly an essential component of the false-belief procedure (i.e., "Just because I know the chocolate is in the green cupboard doesn't mean that Maxi will know"). Thus, a related issue is *perspective taking*, or actively considering the viewpoints of others. Interestingly, perspective taking may function, at times, not by considering others as distinct from oneself, but by considering others *as* the self. For example, Galinsky and Moskowitz (2000) found that when participants were asked to write an essay about an outgroup member (e.g., an elderly person) and were also asked to engage in perspective taking, they were less likely to use stereotypes. These positive consequences are in line with research indicating that other positive behaviors are associated with perspective taking, such as acting prosocially (e.g., Richardson, Hammock, Smith, Gardner, & Signo, 1994; Toi & Batson, 1982; but see Epley, Caruso, & Bazerman, 2006). Yet, one explanation that Galinsky and Moskowitz found for this positive change in behavior is that the essay writers were describing the elderly person using more self-relevant characteristics (see also Davis, Conklin, Smith, & Luce, 1996; Galinsky & Ku, 2004). In other words, the prosocial behavior that perspective taking often fosters may actually be considered a form of pro-*self* behavior! Failure to overcome this egocentric bias has been identified as one of the key barriers to accuracy in perspective taking (for a review, see Epley & Caruso, 2008). For example, Kruger and colleagues found that although message recipients were better able to distinguish between sincere and sarcastic tones when messages were delivered by telephone rather than e-mail, the *senders* of those messages failed to predict a difference in recipients' accuracy based on mode of communication (Kruger, Epley, Parker, & Ng, 2005). That is, the senders were unable to accurately adjust for the privately held knowledge of their intentions.

These findings may have important implications for schizophrenia researchers (see Abu-Akel & Shamay-Tsoory [2013], Chapter 8, this volume). First, as interventions that are designed to address perspective taking deficits in schizophrenic patients are investigated (see Part III of this volume), it may be useful to note that the egocentric biases in perspective taking that are present in normal adult populations may be exacerbated in people with schizophrenia, especially given the cognitively effortful nature of perspective taking (see Epley & Caruso, 2008), paired with the overreliance on automatic processing exhibited by schizophrenic patients. This combination presents an additional obstacle that must be overcome for effective treatment. Second, another side to speculating about the minds of others is being able to speculate about what others think about us, which can result in a tendency to overexaggerate the extent to which others are attending to and evaluating us (e.g., Gilovich, Medvec, & Savitsky, 2000). This hyperattentiveness to the evaluations of others, when taken to extremes, could possibly account for some of the more severe persecutory delusions that are characteristic of schizophrenia (Martin & Penn, 2001), an idea that supports the speculation that people with schizophrenia actually possess an overactive ToM (Abu-Akel, 1999; Badcock, 2004; see Abu-Akel & Shamay-Tsoory [2013], Chapter 8, this volume). Such possibilities are a fruitful direction for future research on social cognition and schizophrenia.

Summary

Schizophrenia researchers have emphasized four social cognition topics of primary interest: attribution biases, emotion processing, social perception, and ToM. Yet, even within these topics already of interest to schizophrenia researchers, there are other phenomena that may be usefully examined. For example, several social psychological theories suggest how people draw causal inferences, and schizophrenia researchers may benefit by more fully examining how various pieces of information are used by people with schizophrenia. Additionally, schizophrenia researchers may examine not only perceiving the emotions of others, but also focus more on how current emotional states can influence judgments. It may also be beneficial to examine how people with schizophrenia use thin slices of information when drawing conclusions about others and how they may struggle to simulate other minds due to intensified egocentric biases, as well as how these deficits and biases may be exacerbated because patients often have limited cognitive resources.

INCREASING BREADTH OF TOPICS IN SCHIZOPHRENIA RESEARCH

Just as insights may be gained from more thoroughly exploring social cognition topics that are already of interest to schizophrenia researchers, insights also may be gained from exploring additional social cognition topics studied by social psychologists. In this concluding section, I suggest that other topics studied by social psychological researchers may also be relevant to schizophrenia researchers but have thus far received relatively less attention. As examples, I discuss three topic areas: dual processing models, metacognitive experiences, and experiences of conscious will. Of course, this is not meant to be an exhaustive list of topics that may be potentially relevant to schizophrenia researchers. Rather, I hope to give a flavor for a greater breadth of other potentially relevant issues that schizophrenia researchers may draw on when exploring social cognition in schizophrenia.

Dual-Processing Models

Throughout this chapter, I have made reference to several forms of judgmental conclusions that may be arrived at automatically (i.e., via a process that is unintentional, uncontrollable, efficient, and occurring largely outside of conscious awareness) versus those that require more controlled (i.e., intentional, controllable, effortful, and conscious) processing. For example, research indicates that dispositional (internal) causal attributions may be arrived at more automatically, whereas adjusting for situational (external) causes may require more controlled cognitive effort. The use of current emotions in judgments may occur more automatically by default, whereas correcting for or discounting the effect of current emotions in judgments requires more effortful thought. Priming affects people's social perceptions relatively automatically, without much need for conscious awareness of prime exposure. And, people use their own minds as a guide to the mental states of others in an automatic way, without any deliberation.

Various dual-process models began emerging within social psychology throughout the 1980s and early 1990s to account for domain-specific phenomena, including those in the areas of causal attribution (Gilbert, 1991; Trope, 1986), person perception (Brewer, 1988; Fiske & Neuberg, 1990), and persuasion (Chaiken, 1980; Petty & Cacioppo, 1986), among many others (for a review, see Chaiken & Trope, 1999). However, as automatic and controlled processing may be relevant to numerous topic-specific domains, several attempts have been made to articulate general dual-processing models (for reviews, see Kahneman, 2003; Smith & DeCoster, 2000; Strack & Deutsch, 2004). Considering ideas about dual-processing modes may be particularly relevant to researchers attempting to better understand schizophrenia and improve functional outcomes for schizophrenic individuals. As we have noted, the deficits in important domains of controlled processing, such as executive functioning, exhibited by those with schizophrenia may result in an overdependence on automatic processing. This tendency may result in more extreme versions of attribution biases, inaccurate emotion processing and social perception, and a greater inability to understand what others are thinking than that exhibited in normal adult populations. An inability to exert control certainly presents problems if the default response is unhealthy or self-defeating. But, of course, automatic processes are not always *wrong* (i.e., do not always necessitate a correction). Therefore, one means of circumventing the potential problems associated with schizophrenic patients' general reliance on automatic processing may be to harness its power positively by encouraging the automatization of healthy habits and responses (e.g., Roberts, Kleinlein, & Stevens, 2012; Velligan et al., 2008, 2009).

Metacognitive Experiences

Metacognitive experiences are subjective experiences that accompany all cognitive operations and include experiential information, such as the ease or difficulty of recall or association and the feeling of thought-confidence (for a review, see Schwarz, Sanna, Skurnik, & Yoon, 2007). Social cognition researchers have found that, although people certainly do form judgments based on the content of their thoughts (what they are thinking about), metacognitive experiences can also strongly influence judgments. For example, if one attempts to retrieve examples supporting another's trustworthiness but finds this task subjectively difficult to accomplish (the experience of thinking of trustworthy actions is hard), one may ironically infer that the other is in fact *un*trustworthy. Reliance on metacognitive experiences for making judgments is heightened under conditions of limited cognitive resources (e.g., distraction, load, or impairment; Schwarz et al., 1991), which are common in schizophrenia. Thus, processes such as these may have paradoxical implications, as in the common technique of "generating alternatives" used in cognitive therapy for psychosis. For example, a patient may report that she saw a long, dark limousine in front of her house and is certain that the CIA is after her. This assertion may lead the therapist to suggest that the person think of other possible reasons why the car was parked there. However, cognitive deficits may make this process such an effortful one for the person that, even if she can generate other possibilities, she may ironically conclude that the belief must be very true (because the other reasons do not readily come to mind), further entrenching a delusion of persecution. It is as if she is saying, "It was so difficult for me to imagine other explanations that my original judgment must be true."

Schizophrenia researchers have recently begun developing promising interventions aimed at increasing awareness and countering the influence of cognitive biases (see Combs et al. [2013], Chapter 16, this volume, and Moritz [2013], Chapter 15, this volume). Additional investigation of the influence of subjective experiences, particularly those of various types of fluency (see Schwarz & Clore, 2007), in people with schizophrenia and how they may be harnessed to promote adaptive thinking and behavior may prove to be a fruitful area for future research.

Experiences of Conscious Will

Schizophrenia is characterized by a range of symptoms involving aberrant experiences of intentionality or conscious will, including delusions of control, thought broadcasting and withdrawal, and auditory verbal hallucinations (Roberts, Stutes, & Hoffman, in press). The processes by which people infer that the self is—or is not—the cause of an action, utterance, or event have also been studied by social psychological researchers in normal adults. Research using normal adult populations has found that people routinely, and rather consistently, make the same mistakes of over- and underattributing agency to conscious will that many patients with schizophrenia do, albeit to a much lesser degree.

One prime example is a line of research by Daniel Wegner and his colleagues on the essential components and processes of *apparent mental causation*, which has contributed much to our understanding of the circumstances under which the self is viewed as a causal agent, as well as the implications of these findings for the idea of conscious will (Wegner, 2002; Wegner & Wheatley, 1999). For example, it has been shown that normal adults may come to believe that they have affected the outcome of an athletic competition (involving a confederate trained to make successful shots in a mock basketball set-up) after having simply been induced to generate prior thoughts that are consistent with the outcome (e.g., "the shooter releases the ball and it swooshes through the net"; Pronin, Wegner, McCarthy, & Rodriguez, 2006). In other words, normal adults in these experiments display an exaggerated sense of will in that they believe their thoughts cause events, despite the fact that our normal ideas about the logic of causality would suggest otherwise. People also have been shown to misattribute their own actions to another.

To illustrate this, Wegner and colleagues conducted a series of experiments modeled on the practice of facilitated communication, a technique in which communication-impaired clients are assisted at a computer keyboard by facilitators who attempt to sense the clients' responses and inclinations by bracing their hands as they type (Wegner, Fuller, & Sparrow, 2003). Participants ("facilitators") placed their hands over those of a confederate ("communicators") and were instructed to sense their partner's answers to a series of questions. Despite the fact that the confederates were not privy to the questions asked, the participants tended to provide correct answers to the questions and to report that their partner's inclinations had influenced the answers they provided. That is, normal adults in these experiments exhibited systematic mistakes in believing that their own actions had been caused by another. Thus, it may be interesting for future researchers to directly compare normal adult and schizophrenia samples in how they experience conscious will and apparent mental causation. Again, it may be that schizophrenic patients exhibit more extreme versions of those biases found in normal adult populations, perhaps contributing to aberrant intentionality symptoms in schizophrenia. In short, investigating elements that indicate agency or authorship, such as visual action feedback and the presence of action-relevant thoughts (Wegner & Sparrow, 2004), in both people with schizophrenia and healthy adult populations may help inform both areas and explain pathologies that may develop when the normal inference processes of healthy adults go awry.

CONCLUSION

Social psychologists and schizophrenia researchers share common interests in illuminating the social cognitive processes by which people come to understand themselves and others. We have offered three primary observations and made suggestions that may be valuable to schizophrenia researchers interested in social cognition. First, social psychologists and schizophrenia researchers may conceive of social cognition differently, and recognizing this difference may help alleviate confusion and facilitate more cross-disciplinary collaboration. Second, within the topic areas already of interest to schizophrenia researchers, social psychology has produced in-depth theorizing that may enrich the schizophrenia literature. Third, there are domains of social cognition research in social psychology that have promising implications for schizophrenia research but have received little attention. That said, social psychologists may also have much to learn from schizophrenia researchers. For example, learning more about what cognitive and emotional skills may be most critical to healthy social interactions, understanding where current social cognitive process models may be incomplete, and clarifying how judgments made by people with extreme impairments differ from the "impairments" (biases, errors, mistakes) made routinely in normal adult populations. By examining social cognition in schizophrenia, social psychologists and schizophrenia researchers would be continuing the tradition of interdisciplinary collaboration from which social cognition research first arose.

ACKNOWLEDGMENTS

I thank the editors of this book for their helpful comments on this chapter.

NOTE

1. It is worthwhile to note that, in some cases, consciously attempting to utilize these otherwise nonconscious nonverbal behaviors may be quite difficult and even antithetical to one's goals. For example, studies have shown that mimicry attempts can backfire when explicitly detected, resulting in more negative evaluations of the mimicker (Bailenson, Yee, Patel, & Beall, 2008; Bourheis, Giles, & Lambert, 1975)—a finding that has cautionary implications for attempting to teach those with social deficits to intentionally engage in mimicry to improve social interactions. Yet, many of the experimental findings on nonconscious mimicry relied on confederates who were instructed to mimic another (e.g., Chartrand & Bargh, 1999), which suggests a more nuanced view of the benefits and consequences of spontaneous versus intentional mimicry. Regardless, it is interesting to speculate that applying and investigating mimicry as part of social skills training for schizophrenia patients may help to inform an understanding of the relative importance of automatic versus controlled processes in acquiring and using nonverbal behavioral skills.

REFERENCES

Abu-Akel, A. (1999). Impaired theory of mind in schizophrenia. *Pragmatics and Cognition*, *7*, 247–282.

Abu-Akel, A., & Shamay-Tsoory, S. G. (2013). Characteristics of theory of mind impairments in schizophrenia. In D. L. Roberts & D. L. Penn (Eds.), *Social cognition in schizophrenia: From evidence to treatment* (Chapter 8). New York: Oxford University Press.

Alicke, M. D., & Largo, E. L. (1995). The role of the self in the false consensus effect. *Journal of Experimental Social Psychology*, *31*, 28–47.

Ambady, N., Krabbenhoft, M. A., & Hogan, D. (2006). The 30-sec. sale: Using thin slices to evaluate sales effectiveness. *Journal of Consumer Psychology*, *16*, 4–13.

Ambady, N., & Rosenthal, R. (1993). Half a minute: Predicting teacher evaluations from thin slices of nonverbal behavior and physical attractiveness. *Journal of Personality and Social Psychology*, *64*, 431–441.

Ames, D. R. (2004). Strategies for social inference: A similarity contingency model of projection and stereotyping in attribute prevalence estimates. *Journal of Personality and Social Psychology*, *87*, 573–585.

Asch, S. E. (1946). Forming impressions of personality. *Journal of Abnormal and Social Psychology*, *41*, 1230–1240.

Augoustinos, M., Walker, I., & Donaghue, N. (2006). *Social cognition: An integrated introduction* (2nd ed.). London: Sage.

Badcock, C. R. (2004). Mentalism and mechanism: The twin modes of human cognition. In C. Crawford & C. Salmon (Eds.), *Human nature and social values: Implications of evolutionary psychology for public policy* (pp. 99–116). Mahwah, NJ: Erlbaum.

Bailenson, J. N., Yee, N., Patel, K., & Beall, A. C. (2008). Detecting digital chameleons. *Computers in Human Behavior, 24,* 66–87.

Bargh, J. A. (1994). The four horsemen of automaticity: Awareness, efficiency, intention, and control in social cognition. In R. S. Wyer, Jr., & T. K. Srull (Eds.), *Handbook of social cognition* (2nd ed., pp. 1–40). Hillsdale, NJ: Erlbaum.

Bargh, J. A., & Pratto, F. (1986). Individual construct accessibility and perceptual selection. *Journal of Experimental Social Psychology, 22,* 293–311.

Baron-Cohen, S., Leslie, A. M., & Frith, U. (1985). Does the autistic child have a "theory of mind"? *Cognition, 21,* 37–46.

Bobo, L. (2001). Racial attitudes and relations at the close of the twentieth century. In N. Smelser, W. J. Wilson, & F. Mitchell, F. (Eds.), *America becoming: Racial trends and their consequences* (pp. 262–299). Washington, DC: National Academy Press.

Bodenhausen, G. (1988). Stereotypic biases in social decision making and memory: Testing process models of stereotype use. *Journal of Personality and Social Psychology, 55,* 726–737.

Bodenhausen, G. V. (1990). Stereotypes as judgmental heuristics: Evidence of circadian variations in discrimination. *Psychological Science, 1,* 319–322.

Borkenau, P., & Liebler, A. (1992). Trait inferences: Sources of validity at zero acquaintance. *Journal of Personality and Social Psychology, 62,* 645–657.

Bourhis, R. Y., Giles, H., & Lambert, W. E. (1975). Social consequences of accommodating one's style of speech: A cross-national investigation. *International Journal of the Sociology of Language, 6*(5), 5–71.

Brewer, M. B. (1988). A dual process model of impression formation. In T. K. Srull & R. S. Wyer Jr. (Eds.), *Advances in social cognition* (Vol. 1, pp. 1–36). Hillsdale, NJ: Erlbaum.

Cacioppo, J. T., Berntson, G. G., Adolphs, R., Carter, C. S., Davidson, R. J., McClintock, M. K., et al. (Eds.). (2002). *Foundations in social neuroscience.* Cambridge, MA: MIT Press.

Carlston, D. (2010). Social cognition. In R. F. Baumeister & E. J. Finkel (Eds.), *Advanced social psychology: The state of the science* (pp. 63–99). New York: Oxford University Press.

Chaiken, S. (1980). Heuristic versus systematic information processing and the use of source versus message cues in persuasion. *Journal of Personality and Social Psychology, 39,* 752–66.

Chaiken, S., & Trope, Y. (Eds.). (1999). *Dual-process theories in social psychology.* New York: Guilford Press.

Chambers, J. R., Epley, N., Savitsky, K., & Windschitl, P. D. (2008). Knowing too much: Using private knowledge to predict how one is viewed by others. *Psychological Science, 19,* 542–548.

Chartrand, T. L., & Bargh, J. A. (1999). The chameleon effect: The perception-behavior link and social interaction. *Journal of Personality and Social Psychology, 76,* 893–910.

Chawla, P., & Krauss, R. M. (1994). Gesture and speech in spontaneous and rehearsed narratives. *Journal of Experimental Social Psychology, 30,* 580–601.

Combs, D. R., Torres, J., & Basso, M. R. (2013). Social cognition and interaction training. In D. L. Roberts & D. L. Penn (Eds.), *Social cognition in schizophrenia: From evidence to treatment* (Chapter 16). New York: Oxford University Press.

Correll, J., Park, B., Judd, C. M., & Wittenbrink, B. (2002). The police officer's dilemma: Using ethnicity to disambiguate potentially threatening individuals. *Journal of Personality and Social Psychology, 83,* 1314–1329.

Darwin, C. (1872/1998). *The expression of the emotions in man and animals.* Oxford: Oxford University Press. (Original work published 1872)

Davis, M. H., Conklin, L., Smith, A., & Luce, C. (1996). Effect of perspective taking on the cognitive representation of persons: A merging of self and other. *Journal of Personality and Social Psychology, 70*, 713–726.

Devine, P. G. (1989). Stereotypes and prejudice: Their automatic and controlled components. *Journal of Personality and Social Psychology, 56*, 5–18.

Dovidio, J., Kawakami, K., & Gaertner, S. (2002). Implicit and explicit prejudice and interracial interaction. *Journal of Personality and Social Psychology, 82*, 62–68.

Dunning, D., & Sherman, D. A. (1997). Stereotypes and tacit inference. *Journal of Personality and Social Psychology, 73*, 459–471.

Dutton, D. G., & Aron, A. P. (1974). Some evidence for heightened sexual attraction under conditions of high anxiety. *Journal of Personality and Social Psychology, 30*, 510–517.

Eisenberg, N., Fabes, R. A., Miller, P. A., Fultz, J., Shell, R., Mathy, R. M., & Reno, R. R. (1989). Relation of sympathy and distress to prosocial behavior: A multimethod study. *Journal of Personality and Social Psychology, 57*, 55–66.

Ekman, P. (1971). Universals and cultural differences in facial expressions of emotion. In J. K. Cole (Ed.), *Nebraska symposium on motivation* (Vol. 18, pp. 207–283). Lincoln: University of Nebraska Press.

Ekman, P., & Friesen, W. V. (1971). Constants across cultures in the face and emotion. *Journal of Personality and Social Psychology, 17*, 124–129.

Ekman, P., & Friesen, W. V. (1986). A new pan-cultural facial expression of emotion. *Motivation and Emotion, 10*, 159–168.

Ellsworth, P. C., Carlsmith, J. M., & Henson, A. (1972). The stare as a stimulus to flight in human subjects: A series of field experiments. *Journal of Personality and Social Psychology, 21*, 302–311.

Epley, N., & Caruso, E. M. (2008). Perspective taking: Misstepping into others' shoes. In K. D. Markman, W. M. P. Klein, & J. A. Suhr (Eds.), *The handbook of imagination and mental simulation* (pp. 295–309). New York: Psychology Press.

Epley, N., Caruso, E. M., & Bazerman, M. H. (2006). When perspective taking increases taking: Reactive egoism in social interaction. *Journal of Personality and Social Psychology, 91*, 872–889.

Epley, N., & Waytz, A. (2010). Mind perception. In S. T. Fiske, D. T. Gilbert, & G. Lindzey (Eds.), *Handbook of social psychology* (Vol. 5, pp. 498–541). Hoboken, NJ: John Wiley & Sons.

Fazio, R. H., & Olson, M. A. (2003). Implicit measures in social cognition research: Their meaning and use. *Annual Review of Psychology, 54*, 297–327.

Festinger, L. (1957). *A theory of cognitive dissonance*. Stanford, CA: Stanford University Press.

Fiske, S. T., Bersoff, D. N., Borgida, E., Deaux, K., & Heilman, M. E. (1991). Social science research on trial: The use of sex stereotyping research in Price Waterhouse v. Hopkins. *American Psychologist, 46*, 1049–1060.

Fiske, S. T., & Neuberg, S. L. (1990). A continuum of impression formation, from category-based to individuating processes: Influences of information and motivation on attention and interpretation. In M. P. Zanna (Eds.), *Advances in experimental social psychology* (Vol. 23, pp. 1–74). New York: Academic Press.

Fiske, S. T., & Taylor, S. E. (2008). *Social cognition: From brains to culture*. Boston, MA: McGraw-Hill.

Frijda, N. H., & Mesquita, B. (1994). The social roles and functions of emotions. In K. Shinobu & H. R. Markus (Eds.), *Emotion and culture: Empirical studies of mutual influence* (pp. 51–87). Washington, DC: American Psychological Association.

Frith, U., & Frith, C. (2003). Development and neurophysiology of mentalizing. *Philosophical Transactions of the Royal Society of London B, 358*, 459–473.

Galinsky, A. D., & Ku, G. (2004). The effects of perspective-taking on prejudice: The moderating role of self-evaluation. *Personality and Social Psychology Bulletin, 30*, 594–604.

Galinsky, A. D., & Moskowitz, G. B. (2000). Perspective taking: Decreasing stereotype expression, stereotype accessibility and in-group favoritism. *Journal of Personality and Social Psychology, 78*, 708–724.

Gallese, V., & Goldman, A. (1998). Mirror neurons and the simulation theory of mind-reading. *Trends in Cognitive Sciences, 12*, 493–501.

Gawronski, B., Geschke, D., & Banse, R. (2003). Implicit bias in impression formation: Associations influence the construal of individuating information. *European Journal of Social Psychology, 33*, 573–589.

Gawronski, B., & Payne, B. K. (Eds.). (2010). *Handbook of implicit social cognition: Measurement, theory, and applications.* New York: Guilford Press.

Gilbert, D. T. (1989). Thinking lightly about others: Automatic components of the social inference process. In J. S. Uleman & J. A. Bargh (Eds.), *Unintended thought* (pp. 189–211). New York: Guilford Press.

Gilbert, D. T. (1991). How mental systems believe. *American Psychologist, 46*, 107–119.

Gilbert, D. T., Pelham, B. W., & Krull, D. S. (1988). On cognitive busyness: When person perceivers meet persons perceived. *Journal of Personality and Social Psychology, 54*, 733–739.

Gilovich, T., Kruger, J., & Medvec, V. H. (2002). The spotlight effect revisited: Overestimating the manifest variability in our actions and appearance. *Journal of Experimental Social Psychology, 78*, 211–222.

Gilovich, T., Medvec, V. H., & Savitsky, K. (2000). The spotlight effect in social judgment: An egocentric bias in estimates of the salience of one's own actions and appearance. *Journal of Personality and Social Psychology, 78*, 211–222.

Goethals, G. F., Allison, S. J., & Frost, M. (1979). Perception of the magnitude and diversity of social support. *Journal of Experimental Social Psychology, 15*, 570–581.

Green, M. F., & Horan, W. P. (2010). Social cognition in schizophrenia. *Current Directions in Psychological Science, 19*, 243–248.

Green, M. F., Penn, D. L., Bentall, R., Carpenter, W. T., Gaebel, W., Gur, R. C., et al. (2008). Social cognition in schizophrenia: An NIMH workshop on definitions, assessment, and research opportunities. *Schizophrenia Bulletin, 34*, 1211–1220.

Greenwald, A. G., McGhee, D. E., & Schwartz, J. L. K. (1998). Measuring individual differences in implicit cognition: The Implicit Association Test. *Journal of Personality and Social Psychology, 74*, 1464–1480.

Heider, F. (1944). Social perception and phenomenal causality. *Psychological Review, 51*, 358–374.

Heider, F. (1958). *The psychology of interpersonal relations.* New York: Wiley.

Higgins, E. T., Rholes, W. S., & Jones, C. R. (1977). Category accessibility and impression formation. *Journal of Experimental Social Psychology, 13*, 141–154.

Hooley, J. M. (2010). Social factors in schizophrenia. *Current Directions in Psychological Science, 19*, 238–242.

Horan, W. P., Kern, R. S., Green, M. F., & Penn, D. L. (2008). Social cognition training for individuals with schizophrenia: Emerging evidence. *American Journal of Psychiatric Rehabilitation, 11*, 205–252.

Hovland, C. I., Janis, I. L., & Kelley, H. H. (1953). *Communication and persuasion.* New Haven, CT: Yale University Press.

Izard, C. E. (1971). *The face of emotion.* New York: Appleton-Century-Crofts.

Jimenez, A. M., Gee, D. G., Cannon, T. D., & Lieberman, M. D. (2013). The social cognitive brain: A review of key individual differences parameters with relevance to schizophrenia. In D. L. Roberts & D. L. Penn (Eds.), *Social cognition in schizophrenia: From evidence to treatment* (Chapter 4). New York: Oxford University Press.

Johnson, K. L., Gill, S., Reichman, V., & Tassinary, L. G. (2007). Swagger, sway, and sexuality: Judging sexual orientation from body motion and morphology. *Journal of Personality and Social Psychology, 98,* 321–334.

Jones, E. E., & Davis, K. E. (1965). From acts to dispositions: The attribution process in person perception. In L. Berkowitz (Ed.), *Advances in experimental social psychology* (Vol. 2, pp. 219–266). New York: Academic Press.

Kahneman, D. (2003). A perspective on judgment and choice. *American Psychologist, 58,* 697–720.

Kelley, H. H. (1967). Attribution theory in social psychology. In D. Levine (Ed.), *Nebraska symposium on motivation* (Vol. 15, pp. 192–238). Lincoln: University of Nebraska Press.

Kelley, H. H. (1972). Attribution in social interaction. In E. E. Jones, D. E. Kanouse, H. H. Kelley, R. E. Nisbett, S. Valins, & B. Weiner (Eds.), *Attribution: Perceiving the causes of behavior* (pp. 1–26). Morristown, NJ: General Learning Press.

Kelley, H. H. (1973). The process of causal attribution. *American Psychologist, 28,* 107–128.

Keltner, D. (1997). Signs of appeasement: Evidence for the distinct displays of embarrassment, amusement, and shame. In P. Ekman & E. L. Rosenberg (Eds.), *What the face reveals: Basic and applied studies of spontaneous expression using the Facial Action Coding System (FACS)* (pp. 133–160). London: Oxford University Press.

Keltner, D., Ellsworth, P. C., & Edwards, K. (1993). Beyond simple pessimism: Effects of sadness and anger on social perception. *Journal of Personality and Social Psychology, 4,* 740–752.

Keltner, D., & Haidt, J. (1999). Social functions of emotions at four levels of analysis. *Cognition & Emotion, 13,* 505–521.

Kohler, C. G., Hanson, E., & March, M. E. (2013). Emotion processing in schizophrenia. In D. L. Roberts & D. L. Penn (Eds.), *Social cognition in schizophrenia: From evidence to treatment* (Chapter 7). New York: Oxford University Press.

Kowalski, R. M., & Leary, M. R. (Eds.) (2003). *Key readings in social-clinical psychology.* New York: Psychology Press.

Krueger, J., & Clement, R. W. (1994). The truly false consensus effect: An eradicable and egocentric bias in social perception. *Journal of Personality and Social Psychology, 67,* 596–610.

Kruger, J., Epley, N., Parker, J., & Ng, Z. (2005). Egocentrism over email: Can we communicate as well as we think? *Journal of Personality and Social Psychology, 89,* 925–936.

Kunda, Z. (1999). *Social cognition: Making sense of people.* Cambridge, MA: MIT Press.

Kunda, Z., & Sherman-Williams, B. (1993). Stereotypes and the construal of individuating information. *Personality and Social Psychology Review, 103,* 284–308.

Lambert, A. J., Payne, B. K., Ramsey, S., & Shaffer, L. M. (2005). On the predictive validity of implicit attitude measures: The moderating effect of perceived group variability. *Journal of Experimental Social Psychology, 41,* 114–128.

Lerner, J. S., & Keltner, D. (2001). Fear, anger, and risk. *Journal of Personality and Social Psychology, 81,* 146–159.

Lhermitte, F. (1986). Human autonomy and the frontal lobes. Part II: Patient behavior in complex and social situations: The "environmental dependency syndrome." *Annals of Neurology, 19,* 335–343.

Lyons, K. E., & Koenig, M. A. (2013). The development of social cognition in theory and action. In D. L. Roberts & D. L. Penn (Eds.), *Social cognition in schizophrenia: From evidence to treatment* (Chapter 1). New York: Oxford University Press.

Macrae, C. N., Milne, A. B., & Bodenhausen, G. V. (1994). Stereotypes as energy-saving devices: A peek inside the cognitive toolbox. *Journal of Personality and Social Psychology, 66,* 37–47.

Macrae, C. N., & Quadflieg, S. (2010). Perceiving people. In S. T. Fiske, D. T. Gilbert, & G. Lindzey (Eds.), *Handbook of social psychology* (Vol. 5, pp. 428–463). Hoboken, NJ: John Wiley & Sons.

Martin, J. A., & Penn, D. L. (2001). Social cognition and sub-clinical paranoid ideation. *British Journal of Clinical Psychology, 40,* 261–265.

McArthur, L. A. (1972). The how and what of why: Some determinants and consequences of causal attribution. *Journal of Personality and Social Psychology, 22,* 171–193.

Mineka, S., & Cook, M. (1993). Mechanisms involved in the observational conditioning of fear. *Journal of Experimental Psychology: General, 122,* 22–28.

Mitchell, J. P., Banaji, M. R., & Macrae, C. N. (2005). The link between social cognition and self-referential thought in the medial prefrontal cortex. *Journal of Cognitive Neuroscience, 17,* 1306–1315.

Mitchell, J. P., Macrae, C. N., & Banaji, M. R. (2006). Dissociable medial prefrontal contributions to judgments of similar and dissimilar others. *Neuron, 50,* 655–663.

Moritz, S. Veckenstedt, R., Vitzthum, F., Köther, U., & Woodward, T. S. (2013). Metacognitive training in schizophrenia: Theoretical rationale and administration. In D. L. Roberts & D. L. Penn (Eds.), *Social cognition in schizophrenia: From evidence to treatment* (Chapter 15). New York: Oxford University Press.

Moskowitz, G. B. (2005). *Social cognition: Understanding self and others.* New York: Guilford.

Mullen, B., & Goethals, G. R. (1990). Social projection, actual consensus, and valence. *British Journal of Social Psychology, 29,* 279–282.

Niedenthal, P. M., & Setterlund, M. B. (1994). Emotion congruence in perception. *Personality and Social Psychology Bulletin, 20,* 401–411.

Payne, B. K. (2001). Prejudice and perception: The role of automatic and controlled processes in misperceiving a weapon. *Journal of Personality and Social Psychology, 81,* 181–192.

Payne, B. K. (2006). Weapon bias: Split second decisions and unintended stereotyping. *Current Directions in Psychological Science, 15,* 287–291.

Payne, B.K., Cheng, C. M., Govorun, O., & Stewart, B. (2005). An inkblot for attitudes: Affect misattribution as implicit measurement. *Journal of Personality and Social Psychology, 89,* 277–293.

Petty, R. E., & Cacioppo, J. T. (1986). The elaboration likelihood model of persuasion. In L. Berkowitz (Ed.), *Advances in experimental social psychology* (Vol. 19, pp. 123–205). New York: Academic Press.

Phillips, A. T., Wellman, H. M., & Spelke, E. S. (2002). Infants' ability to connect gaze and emotional expression to intentional action. *Cognition, 85,* 53–78.

Pronin, E., Wegner, D. M., McCarthy, K., & Rodriguez, S. (2006). Everyday magical powers: The role of apparent mental causation in the overestimation of personal influence. *Journal of Personality and Social Psychology, 91*, 218–231.

Richardson, D. R., Hammock, G. S., Smith, S.M., Gardner, W., & Signon, S. (1994). Empathy as a cognitive inhibitor of interpersonal aggression. *Aggressive Behavior, 20*, 275–289.

Rizzolatti, G., & Craighero, L. (2004). The mirror-neuron system. *Annual Review of Neuroscience, 27*, 169–192.

Roberts, D. L., Kleinlein, P., & Stevens, B. J. (2012). An alternative to generating alternative interpretations in cognitive therapy for psychosis. *Behavioural and Cognitive Psychotherapy, 40*, 491–495.

Roberts, D. L., Stutes, D., & Hoffman, R. (in press). Alien intentionality in schizophrenia. In A. Mishara, M. Schwartz, P. Corlett, & P. Fletcher (Eds.), *Phenomenological neuropsychiatry: Bridging the clinic with clinical neuroscience.*

Ross, L. (1977). The intuitive psychologist and his shortcomings: Distortions in the attribution process. In L. Berkowitz (Ed.), *Advances in experimental social psychology* (Vol. 10, pp. 173–220). New York: Academic Press.

Ross, L., Amabile, T. M., & Steinmetz, J. L. (1977). Social roles, social control, and biases in social-perception processes. *Journal of Personality and Social Psychology, 35*, 484–494.

Rozin, P., & Fallon, A. E. (1987). A perspective on disgust. *Psychological Review, 94*, 23–41.

Rozin, P., Haidt, J., & McCauley, C. R. (2000). Disgust. In D. Levinson, J. Ponzetti, & P. Jorgenson (Eds.), *Encyclopedia of human emotions* (Vol. 1, 2nd ed., pp. 188–193). New York: Macmillan.

Rule, N. O., & Ambady, N. (2008). The face of success: Inferences from chief executive officers' appearance predict company profits. *Psychological Science, 19*, 109–111.

Rule, N. O., & Ambady, N. (2010). Democrats and republicans can be differentiated from their faces. *PLoS ONE, 5*(1), e8733. doi: 10.1371/journal.pone.0008733.

Rule, N. O., Ambady, N., & Hallett, K. C. (2009). Female sexual orientation is perceived accurately, rapidly, and automatically from the face and its features. *Journal of Experimental Social Psychology, 45*, 1245–1251.

Sanfey, A. G. (2007). Decision neuroscience: New directions in studies of judgment and decision-making. *Current Directions in Psychological Science, 16*, 151–155.

Schnall, S., Haidt, J., Clore, G. L., & Jordan, A. H. (2008). Disgust as embodied moral judgment. *Personality Social Psychology Bulletin, 34*, 1096–1109.

Schwarz, N., Bless, H., Strack, F., Klumpp, G., Rittenauer-Schatka, H., & Simons, A. (1991). Ease of retrieval as information: Another look at the availability heuristic. *Journal of Personality and Social Psychology, 61*, 195–202.

Schwarz, N., & Clore, G. L. (1983). Mood, misattribution, and judgments of well-being: Informative and directive functions of affective states. *Journal of Personality and Social Psychology, 45*, 513–523.

Schwarz, N., & Clore, G. L. (1996). Feelings and phenomenal experiences. In E. T. Higgins & A. Kruglanski (Eds.), *Social psychology: Handbook of basic principles* (pp. 433–465). New York: Guilford.

Schwarz, N., & Clore, G. L. (2007). Feelings and phenomenal experiences. In A. W. Kruglanski & E. T. Higgins (Eds.), *Social psychology: Handbook of basic principles* (2nd ed., pp. 385–407). New York: Guilford Press.

Schwarz, N., Sanna, L. J., Skurnik, I., & Yoon, C. (2007). Metacognitive experiences and the intricacies of setting people straight: Implications for debiasing and public information campaigns. *Advances in Experimental Social Psychology, 39*, 127–161.

Sherman, S. J., Judd, C. M., & Park, B. (1989). Social cognition. *Annual Review of Psychology, 40*, 281–326.

Skinner, B. F. (1963). Operant behavior. *American Psychologist, 18*, 503–515.

Smith, E. R., & DeCoster, J. (2000). Dual-process models in social and cognitive psychology: Conceptual integration and links to underlying memory systems. *Personality and Social Psychology Review, 4*, 108–131.

Smith, E. R., & Semin, G. R. (2004). Socially situated cognition: Cognition in its social context. In M. P. Zanna (Ed.), *Advances in experimental social psychology* (Vol. 36, pp. 53–116). San Diego, CA: Elsevier Academic Press.

Snyder, M. L., & Frankel, A. (1976). Observer bias: A stringent test of behavior engulfing the field. *Journal of Personality and Social Psychology, 36*, 1202–1212.

Sperry, R. W. (1993). The impact and promise of the cognitive revolution. *American Psychologist, 48*, 878–885.

Srull, T. K., & Wyer, R. S., Jr. (1979). The role of category accessibility in the interpretation of information about persons: Some determinants and implications. *Journal of Personality and Social Psychology, 37*, 1660–1672.

Stouten, J., & De Cremer, D. (2010). 'Seeing is believing': The effects of facial expressions of emotion and verbal communication in social dilemmas. *Journal of Behavioral Decision Making, 23*, 271–287.

Strack, F., & Deutsch, R. (2004). Reflective and impulsive determinants of social behavior. *Personality and Social Psychology Review, 8*, 220–247.

Teachman, B. A., Cody, M. W., & Clerkin, E. M. (2010). Clinical applications of implicit social cognition theories and methods. In B. Gawronski & B. K. Payne (Eds.), *Handbook of implicit social cognition: Measurement, theory, and applications* (pp. 489–521). New York: Guilford Press.

Thorndike, E. L. (1940). *Human nature and the social order.* New York: Macmillan.

Todd, A. R., Hanko, K., Galinsky, A. D., & Mussweiler, T. (2011). When focusing on differences leads to similar perspectives. *Psychological Science, 22*, 134–141.

Toi, M., & Batson, C. D. (1982). More evidence that empathy is a source of altruistic motivation. *Journal of Personality and Social Psychology, 43*, 281–292.

Trope, Y. (1986). Identification and inferential processes in dispositional attribution. *Psychological Review, 93*, 239–257.

Velligan, D. I., Diamond, P. M., Maples, N. J., Mintz, J., Li, X., Glahn, D. C., & Miller, A. L. (2008). Comparing the efficacy of interventions that use environmental supports to improve outcomes in patients with schizophrenia. *Schizophrenia Research, 102*, 312–319.

Velligan, D. I., Diamond, P. M., Mueller, J. Li, X., Maples, N. J., Wang, M., & Miller, A. L. (2009). The short-term impact of generic versus individualized environmental supports on functional outcomes and target behaviors in schizophrenia. *Psychiatry Research, 168*, 94–101.

Warneken, F., & Tomasello, M. (2006). Altruistic helping in human infants and young chimpanzees. *Science, 31*, 1301–1303.

Watson, J. (1930). *Behaviorism.* New York: Norton.

Wegner, D. M. (2002). *The illusion of conscious will.* Cambridge, MA: MIT Press.

Wegner, D. M., Fuller, V. A., & Sparrow, B. (2003). Clever hands: Uncontrolled intelligence in facilitated communication. *Journal of Personality and Social Psychology, 85*, 5–19.

Wegner, D. M., & Sparrow, B. (2004). Authorship processing. In M. Gazzaniga (Ed.), *The cognitive neurosciences* (3rd ed., pp. 1201–1209). Cambridge, MA: MIT Press.

Wegner, D. M., & Wheatley, T. P. (1999). Apparent mental causation: Sources of the experience of will. *American Psychologist, 54*, 480–492.

Wellman, H. M., Cross, D., & Watson, J. (2001). Meta-analysis of theory-of-mind development: The truth about false belief. *Child Development, 72*, 655–684.

Wimmer, H., & Perner, J. (1983). Beliefs about beliefs: Representations and constraining function of wrong beliefs in young children's understanding of deception. *Cognition, 13,* 103–128.

Wheatley, T., & Haidt, J. (2005). Hypnotically induced disgust makes moral judgments more severe. *Psychological Science, 16*, 780–784.

Zajonc, R. B. (1980). Feeling and thinking: Preferences need no inferences. *American Psychology, 35*(2), 151–175.

3

Cross-Cultural Variation in Social Cognition and the Social Brain

SHIHUI HAN ■

SOCIAL COGNITION AND THE SOCIAL BRAIN IN SOCIOCULTURAL CONTEXTS

Humans are essentially social animals. An individual begins to react to others immediately after birth and develops through interacting with others. One of the most significant parts of a person's life is to join others in a variety of social activities and to seek specific social goals. Consequences of social interactions may be either positive or negative, and one can suffer severely by merely being isolated from social environments. Current state-of-art techniques for communication have increased the number of individuals that one may interact with in society. This has resulted in large-scale, rapid social interactions among people from diverse geographical and cultural regions and backgrounds.

To navigate in social environments efficiently, people have to think about themselves and others frequently and to understand themselves and others correctly. The processing of social information about oneself and others, referred to as *social cognition*, provides a basis for appropriate social behaviors and an avenue to achieve social goals. Some social information, such as facial expression, can be perceived directly, whereas other social information, such as intentions and beliefs, have to be inferred based on the analysis of perceived information. An important feature of social cognition is context dependence—that is, what and how social information is processed relies heavily on whom an individual interacts with and in which social context such interactions occur. For example, people may think of and treat others in dominance and in subordination differently, and the way individuals interact with those who sit high or low in the social hierarchy may vary greatly from one society to another (Triandis & Gelfand, 1998). Based on cross-cultural comparisons, psychological findings have formulated several variations of standard social cognitive processes in different cultural contexts, such as causal attribution (Choi, Nisbett, & Norenzayan, 1999), self-construals (Markus & Kitayama, 1991, 2010), and affect valuation (Tsai, Knutson, & Fung, 2006).

Cross-cultural variation in social cognition may reflect, to a certain degree, the difference in cognitive styles between different cultures. It has been proposed that the human mind can be characterized by either "a context-independent processing style—aggregating and integrating across situations, ignoring situational variance in one's thoughts, feelings, and responses" or "a context-dependent processing style—paying attention to specific social contexts" (Kühnen & Oyserman, 2002, p. 492). Specifically, people in many Western cultural contexts are inclined to focus exclusively on the *focal object* during cognitive processes, such as visual perception and causal attributions of social and physical events. In contrast, people in many East Asian cultural contexts are more likely to pay attention to *contexts* during perception, causal attribution, and other cognitive tasks (Ji, Peng, & Nisbett, 2000; Masuda & Nisbett, 2001; Nisbett, Peng, Choi, & Norenzayan, 2001; Nisbett & Masuda, 2003). These findings of cultural differences in cognitive styles change the classic psychological and philosophical views that the basic processes of human cognition are universal.

A key function of the human brain is to deal with the social world. From an evolutionary perspective, the brain evolves to cope with a complexity of social interactions, such that the relative neocortex volume increases as a function of the mean social group size (Dunbar & Shultz, 2007), suggesting that more complex and larger scale social interactions require more neural resources in the primate brain. Humans have evolved specific patterns of brain activity to deal with complicated information relating to the self and others. Recent brain imaging studies have accumulated ample data that help to uncover the function of different brain regions in social cognition (Lieberman, 2010; also see Jimenez, Gee, Cannon, & Lieberman [2013], Chapter 4, this volume). Plasticity is part of the intrinsic nature of the brain (Pascual-Leone, Amedi, Fregni, & Merabet, 2005), and this allows, during adolescence, for the development of neural mechanisms that are adapted to the context-dependent nature of social cognition (Blakemore, 2008).

Culture provides a framework for social interactions by building social values and norms and by assigning meaning to social events. Given the diversity of sociocultural contexts across the world, the human brain may develop neural mechanisms to mediate social interactions in specific sociocultural contexts. In this sense, culture may also function to shape neural correlates of social cognition in the human brain. Indeed, recent research has shown increasing evidence that neural activity involved in specific social cognitive processes may differ between individuals who grow up in different cultural contexts (Chiao & Ambady, 2007; Han & Northoff, 2008; Kitayama & Uskul, 2011). The increasing transcultural brain imaging findings have given birth to a new discipline—*cultural neuroscience*, which investigates mutual interactions between cultural values, practices, and beliefs and human brain function, and provides[1] a new perspective on the functional organization of the human brain associated with social cognition. The new discipline is manifested in several published special issues of journals (e.g.,

Social Affective and Cognitive Neuroscience, 2011; *Progress in Brain Research*, 2009) and edited books (e.g., Han & Pöppel, 2011).

This chapter reviews previous psychological findings of cross-cultural varia-tions in social cognition and recent brain imaging findings of cross-cultural varia-tions in the neural substrates underlying social cognition. This literature review outlines what aspects of social cognition vary across cultures and to what degree the underlying neural mechanisms are shaped by sociocultural contexts. This chapter will also discuss the implications of transcultural imaging findings for mental health and raise future questions regarding the cultural diversity of social cognitive processes and their underlying neural mechanisms.

CROSS-CULTURAL VARIATION IN THE PROCESSING OF OTHERS

In most cases, social interactions aim to realize specific social goals through cooperation between members of a social group. To make social cooperation possible and effective, one has to coordinate his or her behaviors with others, based on predictions of what others are going to do. Understanding others' minds, such as their thoughts and feelings, is necessary for cooperative and competitive social activities. Thinking about others' minds constitutes a key component of social cognition, and the underlying neurocognitive processes have been of great interest among psychologists and neuroscientists. Increasing psychological and brain imaging evidence suggests that social cognition can be, by and large, decomposed into *cognitive capacity*, which primarily supports the understanding of others' intentions, beliefs, desires, and the like, and *affective capacity*, which principally mediates the understanding and sharing of others' feelings and emotional states. Studies of cross-cultural psychology and tran-scultural brain imaging have shown evidence that distinct neurocognitive pro-cesses are involved in cognitive and affective capacities and that these exhibit cross-cultural variations.

Perspective Taking

Multiple processes aimed at understanding others are engaged during social inter-actions and communication with others (Frith & Frith, 2010). One has to realize that others have the power or authority to act with specific social goals and to ascribe mental states to others in order to explain and predict their actions. One cognitive capacity of social cognition is to know that what others see may be dif-ferent from what is perceived by oneself. Perceiving a visual scene from another person's viewpoint or taking others' perspectives is critical for understanding oth-ers' minds during social communication and for coordinating behaviors between oneself and others. How is the ability of perspective taking influenced by cul-tural contexts? In accordance with the assertion that people in a Western cultural context have an independent view of the self and focus attention on the self, whereas people in an East Asian cultural context have an interdependent view of the self and focus attention on contexts and connections with others (Markus & Kitayama, 1991, 2010; Kühnen & Oyserman, 2002, Nisbett et al., 2001; Nisbett & Masuda, 2003), it seems likely that East Asians may be better perspective takers compared to Westerners.

This idea was tested in a study that compared eye-track measures and behavioral performance between Chinese and American participants in a game that required distinction between one's own knowledge and that of another person (Wu & Keysar, 2007). In this game, a "director" sits opposite a participant at a table with objects placed in a grid and instructs the subject to move certain objects. The director's and participant's perspectives differ as some objects are occluded from the director's perspective and the participant knows that he or she will not be asked to move the occluded objects (competitors). The critical test is how eye fixation and reaction times to move the target object, which can be seen by both the director and the participant, are influenced by the occluded competitor, which is identical to the target object but can be seen only by the participant. If Chinese participants pay closer attention to others' perspectives than Americans do, their eye fixation and reaction times would be influenced by the occluded object to a much lesser degree compared to those of Americans. Indeed, it was found that Americans fixated on the competitor more than twice as often as they fixated on a neutral baseline object, whereas Chinese participants fixated on the competitor only slightly more than they fixated on the baseline object. In addition, it took Americans much longer to identify the correct target when the competitor was present compared to a baseline condition, whereas the competitor caused virtually no delay for the Chinese participants. These results suggest that, relative to Americans, Chinese individuals may be more attuned to the perspective of others during social interactions.

The neural substrates of perspective taking have also been investigated in a few studies that combined functional magnetic resonance imaging (fMRI) and different paradigms. For example, taking an avatar's perspective activated the mesial superior parietal and right premotor cortex (Vogeley et al., 2004). Watching video clips depicting simple hand or foot actions filmed from the third-person perspective increased activity in the lingual gyrus (Jackson, Meltzoff, & Decety, 2006). The medial part of the superior frontal gyrus, left superior temporal sulcus, left temporal pole, and right inferior parietal lobe showed increased activity when medical students responded to a list of health-related questions from the perspective of a lay person (Ruby & Decety, 2003). It appears that distinct brain regions are engaged during taking others' perspectives, depending on whether tasks require visuospatial or conceptual transformations between the self and others. However, because most previous brain imaging studies of perspective taking recruited participants in the Western cultural contexts, neural mechanisms underlying perspective taking that are sensitive to cultural influences remain unknown (see also Jimenez et al. [2013], Chapter 4, this volume).

Mental State Reasoning

In addition to knowing that others have different perspectives, humans also consider others' mental states (e.g., intentions, desires and beliefs) in order to interpret and predict their behavior. This ability, referred to as *theory of mind* (ToM) or *mentalizing*, has been studied extensively in developmental psychology (see Lyons & Koenig [2013], Chapter 1, this volume). Children are able to understand that others can have false beliefs and to distinguish between their knowledge and that of others after age 4 (e.g., Perner, 1991; Wellman, Cross, & Watson, 2001). Moreover, children from different cultures seem to show similar developmental trajectories of ToM ability. Chinese and American children start to understand others' false beliefs at the same age (Sabbagh, Xu, Carlson, Moses, & Lee, 2006). However, brain imaging studies suggest that the neural bases of mentalizing may vary across different cultural contexts. Kobayashi et al. (2006) found that, relative to judgments of event outcomes based on an understanding of physical-causal reasoning, judgments about others' false beliefs activated the right dorsal medial prefrontal cortex (DMPFC), right anterior cingulate cortex (ACC), right middle frontal gyrus, and dorsal lateral prefrontal cortex in both American English-speaking monolingual adults and Japanese-English late bilingual adults. However, judgments of mental states in monolingual Americans produced greater activation in the right insula, bilateral temporoparietal junction (TPJ), and right DMPFC relative to bilingual Japanese participants, who showed greater brain activity in the right orbital frontal gyrus. The same group also found increased activity in the DMPFC and precuneus in American English-speaking monolingual children and Japanese bilingual children aged 8 to 11 years when they performed cartoon-based or word-based ToM tasks (Kobayashi, Glover, & Temple, 2007). However, the word-based ToM task generated greater activity in the left superior temporal sulcus in American than in Japanese children, whereas enhanced activity was identified in the left inferior temporal gyrus in Japanese compared to American children. In addition, stronger activation in the right TPJ in the cartoon-based ToM task was observed in American compared to Japanese children. In the cartoon-based ToM task, Japanese children showed stronger activation in the left anterior superior temporal sulcus and temporal pole than did American children. These results suggest that cultural differences in ToM-related neural activity are not the same in adults and children, suggesting that, although children may acquire ToM ability by the age of 4, acculturation still shapes the underlying neural substrates during later development.

Recent studies using the Reading the Mind in the Eyes (RME) test (Baron-Cohen, Wheelwright, Hill, Raste, & Plumb, 2001) also showed evidence for cultural influences on the neural substrates of ToM. The RME test consists of photographs depicting only the eye region of a face. Four mental state terms accompanying each stimulus are presented at each corner of the photograph, and participants have to identify the term that matches the mental state of the eyes. Adams et al. (2010) found that, relative to a gender discrimination task, the RME task induced increased activity in the bilateral superior temporal sulci (STS) and bilateral inferior frontal gyrus in both European Americans and Japanese individuals. Culture-specific neural responses to mental state reasoning was observed in the bilateral posterior STS, where the neural activity showed an intracultural advantage; that is, greater response to eyes from the same culture compared to eyes from the other culture, in both the European Americans and Japanese. The intracultural advantage was also evident in responses to mental state judgments, with participants being more accurate in judging eyes from the same, compared to other, cultures. Taken together, these findings suggest that recruitment of neural circuits associated with ToM varies across different ToM tasks and is modulated by cultural group membership; this effect is similar for different cultural groups. Cultural influences on neurocognitive processes involved in mentalizing may occur early during development.

Gesture Understanding

Because humans use gestures to communicate expressively, and gestures are highly culture-specific, neural mechanisms underlying gesture understanding may also be culturally specific. To test how motor resonance (i.e., increased corticospinal excitability [CSE] during observation of gestures) is affected by cultural familiarity, Molnar-Szakacs et al. (2007) used transcranial magnetic stimulation (TMS) to measure CSE during observation of emblems (i.e., gestures that convey conventionalized meaning without accompanying speech) with culture-specific meanings. They found that European Americans showed higher CSE during observations of an American compared to a Nicaraguan actor. However, Nicaraguan and American emblems elicited similar CSE when performed by the American actor, whereas Nicaraguan emblems performed by the Nicaraguan actor yielded higher CSE than did American emblems. The results suggest an interaction effect between perceptual and cultural factors on the motor resonance of observed gestures.

A recent fMRI study showed further evidence that the mentalizing and mirror neuron regions, which are associated with the understanding of others' mental states and with perception of others' physical actions, respectively, may be differentially involved in gesture understanding, depending on the cultural familiarity of the gestures (Liew, Ma, Han, & Aziz-Zadeh, 2011). Specifically, Chinese participants showed greater activity in the brain areas associated with mentalizing (e.g., the posterior cingulate cortex, DMPFC, and the bilateral TPJ) to culturally familiar than unfamiliar gestures, whereas unfamiliar gestures more strongly activated the posterior mirror neuron regions (e.g., the left inferior parietal lobe, left postcentral gyrus, dorsal region of the postcentral gyrus, and ventral portion of the supramarginal gyrus). Thus, distinct brain regions in the mentalizing and mirror neuron systems may be engaged in social communication for understanding culturally familiar and unfamiliar gestures.

Bodily Expression

Perception of others' bodily expressions helps people to understand both mental states and social status, which helps to guide appropriate behaviors in social hierarchies and to determine behavioral consequences. Bodily expressions give signals of dominance (marking higher status) and signals of subordination (marking lower status) (Hall, Coats, & LeBeau, 2005). However, bodily expressions can be assigned different cultural values. For example, the American culture generally encourages dominance (Triandis & Gelfand, 1998), whereas the Japanese culture generally encourages subordination (Yamaguchi, Kuhlman, & Sugimori, 1995). Would distinct values assigned to bodily expressions be associated with culturally specific neural underpinnings? Freeman et al. (2009) assessed this by conducting brain scans of American and Japanese individuals during the perception of figural outlines of body displays that implicate dominance or subordination. Self-report showed a tendency in Americans of performing more behaviors to dominate others. On the contrary, Japanese participants reported preference of more subordinate behaviors so as to be dominated by others. Moreover, dominant stimuli activated the caudate nucleus, bilaterally, and the medial prefrontal cortex in Americans, whereas these were activated by subordinate stimuli in Japanese individuals. The results suggest that the cultural tuning of tendencies in social behaviors can be accomplished by way of the mesolimbic reward system. Moreover, the cultural values placed on social status lead to specific neural representations of culturally preferred bodily expression.

Causal Attribution

In most cases, causes of human behaviors are not obvious and are beyond perception. Cultural psychology has accumulated evidence for cultural differences in causal attribution of both social behaviors and physical events. It has been shown that East Asians are more sensitive to contextual constraints, whereas European Americans are more prone to individuals' internal dispositions when making causality judgments on social behaviors (Choi et al., 1999; Morris & Peng, 1994). Cultural differences are also observed in causal attribution of physical events. Peng and Knowles (2003) found that American and Chinese students with no formal physics education emphasized different causes when explaining physical events. Americans were more likely to attribute the causes of physical events to dispositional factors (e.g., weight), whereas Chinese participants were more likely to attribute causes of the same events to contextual factors (e.g., a medium). The cultural difference in causal attribution of physical events has been associated with culture-specific patterns of neural activity. Han et al. (2011) first scanned Chinese participants during causality or motion direction judgments when viewing animations of object collisions. They identified a neural circuit related to causal attribution consisting of the medial/lateral prefrontal cortex and left parietal/temporal cortex by contrasting causality versus motion direction judgments. They showed further that the medial prefrontal activity was sensitive to the demand to infer causes of physical events whereas the left parietal activity was modulated by the contextual complexity of physical events. More interestingly, Han et al. (2011) found that the medial prefrontal activity involved in causality judgments was comparable in American and Chinese participants, whereas the left parietal activity associated with causality judgments was stronger in Chinese than in Americans, regardless of whether participants attended to the contextual information. These findings indicate that activity in the medial prefrontal cortex may be universally implicated in causal reasoning, whereas the contextual processing in the left parietal cortex is sensitive to cultural differences in causality perception.

EMOTION

There has been evidence for both universality and cultural variation of emotional processes. For example, emotional categories in terms of valence and arousal are universal (Russell, 1994), whereas the process of learning to control emotional expression may be dependent on cultural factors (Matsumoto, 1989). Both behavioral and brain imaging studies suggest that cultural experiences may influence emotion recognition. Markham and Wang (1996) found that both Chinese and Australian children showed higher recognition accuracy of emotional faces from their own cultural group than of those from another cultural group. Recent fMRI research investigated whether culture affects the neural mechanisms that underlie emotion processing. Chiao et al. (2008) scanned native Japanese participants in Japan and Caucasians in the United States while they perceived photos of Japanese and Caucasian faces expressing fearful or nonfearful (e.g., angry, happy, neutral) emotions. They found that fearful faces from the participants' own cultural group induced greater activation in the left and right amygdala compared with fearful faces from another culture. Moreover, this "cultural tuning" of automatic neural responses was evident only for fearful faces. The findings suggest heightened arousal to or vigilance for fear expressed by members of one's own cultural group.

EMPATHY

Empathy refers to the capacity to understand and share the emotional states of others, which may provide a proximate mechanism for prosocial behaviors such as cooperation and altruism (de Waal, 2008). Both behavioral and brain studies show evidence that empathic concerns for others are strongly influenced by social relations between observers and targets. Johnson et al. (2002) found that white university students reported greater feelings of empathy for white compared to black defendants, suggesting a bias in empathy for racial in-group members. Recent brain imaging studies demonstrate that the racial bias in empathy occurs not only with black individuals but also with other racial groups. Xu et al. (2009) found that, when perceiving painful stimulation applied to Caucasian or Chinese faces, Caucasians and Chinese participants reported similar subjective feelings of pain suffered by racial in-group and out-group members.

However, empathic neural responses in the ACC decreased significantly to racial out-group compared to in-group faces, and this was evident in both Caucasians and Chinese participants. Similarly, Avenanti et al. (2010) found that observing painful stimulation applied to the hands of racial in-group models elicited sensorimotor empathic responses in black and white individuals, whereas no such vicarious mapping of the pain occurred when perceiving racial out-group models. Moreover, the medial prefrontal activity in response to pain expressed by in-group relative to out-group members predicted greater empathy and altruistic motivation for racial in-group members (Mathur, Haradi, Lipke, & Chiao, 2010).

It appears that multiple aspects of empathy for pain are modulated by racial intergroup relations. However, it should be noted that the bias in empathic neural responses does not take place just for specific racial groups, indicating that the bias in empathy does not simply arise from the skin color of a target person. The factor that essentially determines the bias in empathy is the group relation between an observer and a target; the concept of "social groups" is a product of social experiences and practices and appears to be common in different sociocultural contexts. The current findings suggest that culturally universal concepts of racial intergroup relations may play an important role in shaping the neural activity underlying empathy.

CROSS-CULTURAL VARIATIONS IN THE PROCESSING OF ONESELF

Self-concept has been studied widely in philosophy, psychology, and neuroscience, and has been assigned with discrepant meanings in different cultures. From the cognitive perspective, the self refers to an entity that provides a basis for perception of the outside world. However, self-concept varies greatly across sociocultural contexts, and the cultural variations in self-concept may generate consequences for other social cognitive processes. To date, most researchers have investigated cultural variations in self-concept in a framework proposed by social psychologists that differentiates between self-construals in Western and East Asian cultural contexts (Markus & Kitayama, 1991; Triandis, 1989). A basic assumption is that many Western cultures encourage the individualism that views people as entities who are independent of one another whereas many non-Western (e.g., East Asian) cultures emphasize the fundamental connectedness of human beings to each other. Consequently, Western cultures foster independent self-construals that view the self as an autonomous entity with a unique configuration of internal attributes, one inclined to privilege self-focused attention and to organize behaviors primarily with reference to internal attributes. By contrast, East Asian cultures emphasize interdependent self-construals that are sensitive to information related to significant others and are inclined to privilege attention toward intimate others as much as to the self and to organize behaviors primarily with reference to others.

Self-Face Recognition

The processing of self-related information is a key component of human social cognition. In the perceptual domain, self-related processing is manifested in self-face recognition, and recent research illustrates distinct cross-cultural differences in the processing of one's own face. Initial behavioral studies examined unique processes of self-face recognition by measuring reaction times (RTs) to self-face in different tasks. Tong and Nakayama (1999) observed shorter RTs when searching for self-face compared to a stranger's face among distractor faces. Keenan et al. (1999) found faster responses to self-face than to faces of familiar or unfamiliar others in a face identification task. The early observation of self-advantage in behavioral responses during face recognition was obtained in participants in a Western (American) cultural context and was explained by perceptual mechanisms, such as robust representations for overlearned familiar faces (Tong & Nakayama, 1999). Subsequent research similarly found self-face advantages in participants in an East Asian (Chinese) cultural context. However, when comparing RTs to self-face and a friend's face in a face orientation judgment task between British and Chinese participants, it was found that the self-face advantage was much more salient in British than in Chinese (Sui, Liu, & Han, 2009), consistent with the proposition that enhanced self-focused attention in individuals in Western cultural contexts facilitates self-face recognition, relative to those in Eastern cultural contexts.

Recent research proposed a social cognitive mechanism to connect the self-concept with behavioral responses to self-face. To test whether priming that constitutes a threat to one's positive view of the self influences self-face recognition, Ma and Han (2010) first asked participants to judge if a number of negative personal traits were appropriate to describe themselves in order to reduce the implicit positive association with the self. This self-concept threat priming may reduce the self-face advantage if the latter is facilitated by positive views of the self. They found that, although RTs were shorter to the identification of self-face compared to familiar faces in a control priming condition, the self-concept threat priming reduced the self-face advantage greatly, even leading to faster responses to familiar faces than to self-face. This finding supports the idea that self-face recognition may activate positive attributes in self-concept, which facilitates behavioral responses to self-face. In addition, Ma and Han (2010) found that the effect of self-concept threat priming on RTs to self-face was greater in Chinese than in American participants. This supports the idea that self-concept in individuals who grow up in Western cultural contexts resist external influences more strongly, relative to individuals who grow up in East Asian cultural contexts.

Cultural differences in self-face recognition were also evident when considering how social contexts modulate behavioral performance during self-face recognition. Ma and Han (2009) first tested if the self-face advantage can be reduced in Chinese participants in a social context with someone who is dominant in the social hierarchy. They asked Chinese graduate students to identify orientations of self-face intermixed with either their faculty advisor's face or with the face of another faculty member. Interestingly, it was found that, although participants responded faster to self-face than to the faculty member's face, they responded slower to self-face compared to the advisor's face. To further assess if the self-face disadvantage (or the "boss effect") was associated with negative evaluations from advisors that may constitute threats to self-esteem, Ma and Han quantified the relation between social threats and RTs to self-face. They found that differential RTs to self-face and advisor's face correlated with individuals' subjective ratings of fear of negative evaluations from the advisor. Although the findings provide evidence that social threat in real social situations may influence self-face recognition in Chinese participants, one may predict that such an effect may be reduced in a Western cultural context in which self-concept depends on others' opinions to a much lesser degree. This was tested in a follow-up study that replicated Ma and Han's (2009) experiment in American participants. Liew et al. (2011) found that, unlike Chinese participants, European Americans did not show a "boss effect"; that is, they responded faster to self-face compared to their advisors' faces. Moreover, differential RTs to self-face versus advisor's face correlated with subjective ratings of the advisor's perceived social status. The comparison between the "boss effects" in Chinese and Americans indicates a strong cultural modulation of self-face processing in social contexts. In addition, the findings suggest that perception of self-face in social contexts is strongly influenced by threats to self-concept in Chinese cultural context but is modulated by general social dominance in the American cultural context, suggesting that the very concept of a "boss" may be significantly different in relation to the self in Western and East Asian cultures.

Are neural correlates of self-face recognition influenced by sociocultural contexts? Early fMRI studies of self-face recognition explored the neural mechanisms that differentiated between the processing of self-face and the faces of familiar/unfamiliar others, but did not consider cross-cultural variation of the underlying neural substrates. Accumulating evidence now suggests that a widely distributed network is engaged during self-face recognition (Platek, Wathne, Tierney, & Thomson, 2008). For example, studies of American college students found increased activation in the right frontal cortex during self-face processing compared to familiar famous face processing (Platek, Keenan, Gallup, & Mohamed, 2004), and in the right inferior parietal lobule, inferior frontal gyrus, and inferior occipital gyrus when contrasting morphed face images containing more self than those containing more familiar others (Uddin, Kaplan, Molnar-Szakacs, Zaidel, & Iacoboni, 2005). Belgian college students also showed increased activity in the right frontal cortex and right anterior insula during perception of self-face versus a familiar face (Devue et al. 2007). Similarly, studies of Japanese college students found that perception of self-face versus unfamiliar faces increased activity in the right occipito-temporo-parietal junction, right frontal operculum, and the left fusiform gyrus (Sugiura et al., 2005). A recent fMRI study of Chinese college students dissociated the functional significance of the left and right fusiform gyrus by showing evidence that the left fusiform gyrus is sensitive to self-face physical properties and the right fusiform gyrus is sensitive to self-face identity (Ma & Han, 2012).

Because these brain imaging studies respectively scanned participants in different cultural contexts, little can be known about the cross-cultural variations of neural correlates of self-face recognition without directly comparing different cultural groups using the same procedure and task in the same study. Given that independent self-construals promote self-focused attention and interdependent self-construals stress one's connection with others, there may be distinct neural mechanisms of self-face recognition in cultural contexts that facilitate different self-construals. To test this, Sui et al. (2009) recorded event-related brain potentials (ERPs) to self-face and a friend's face from participants in Western (British) and East Asian (Chinese) cultural contexts. They found that, in British participants, judgments of head orientations of their own face elicited a negative activity at 280–340 ms over the frontal-central area (N2) with larger amplitudes to self-face relative to a friend's face. In contrast, Chinese participants showed larger N2 amplitudes to a friend's face compared to self-face. In addition, there was a significant correlation between the self-advantage in behavioral responses and the differential N2 amplitudes to self-face versus a friend's face: The larger the differential N2 amplitudes to self-face versus a friend's face, the greater the self-face advantage in RTs. As the anterior N2 is associated with deeper processing of faces to benefit individuation of faces (Kubota & Ito, 2007), the culture-specific N2 modulation suggests that, relative to Chinese participants, British individuals with independent self-construals may pay more attention to information about the self than about others. In contrast, Chinese participants with interdependent self-construals may assign high social salience to a friend's face compared to self-face.

To directly test if culture-specific self-construals influence the neural substrates involved in self-face recognition, Sui and Han (2007) combined self-construal priming and self-face recognition tasks in an fMRI study. Self-construal priming refers to a procedure developed by Gardner et al. (1999) that asks participants to read essays including independent or interdependent pronouns (e.g., "I" or "We"). Behavioral performances suggest that one's self-construal formed chronically by an individual culture can be temporarily shifted by priming tasks of searching independent or interdependent pronouns in essays (Gardner et al., 1999). If independent self-construals facilitate self-face recognition, one may predict greater neural activity to self-face after independent compared to interdependent self-construal priming. Indeed, Sui and Han (2007) found that, although the neural activity in the right middle frontal cortex was increased to self-face compared to familiar faces, the right frontal activity differentiating between the self and familiar faces was enlarged by the independent relative to interdependent self-construal priming. The increased right frontal activity was also associated with faster responses to self-face than to familiar faces, suggesting that the neural correlates of self-face recognition can be modulated by temporary shifts of self-construals from one style to another. Together, studies that employed cross-cultural comparisons and self-construal priming indicate that self-perception is strongly affected by cultural patterns of independence or interdependence.

Self-Related Memory

In addition to the findings of cultural differences in self-face recognition, there has been increasing evidence for cross-cultural variation of self-related processing in the memory domain. A well-known paradigm to study self-specific memory processes is a self-reference task developed by Rogers et al. (1977). This task first asks participants to make judgments on whether a list of trait adjectives can describe the self or others. After this encoding phase, participants have to recognize as many of the words as they can. A typical finding of this paradigm is that participants better remember self-descriptive traits than other-descriptive traits (the self-reference effect) (Klein, Loftus, & Burton, 1989). Interestingly, whereas Westerners showed the self-reference effect over close others, such as one's mother and best friends (Heatherton et al., 2006; Klein et al., 1989), Chinese remembered equally well the trait adjectives associated with the self and close others (e.g., mother, Qi & Zhu, 2002; Zhu & Zhang, 2002). Wang and Conway (2004) also found that European Americans frequently focused on memories of personal experiences and placed a great emphasis on their feelings and personal roles in the memory events. In contrast, Chinese participants were more likely to describe memories of social and historical events and focused more on social interactions and the roles of other people. The findings of these behavioral studies support the dissociation in memory processes between the self and close others in Western cultures but not in East Asian cultures.

Following the early behavioral studies, the self-reference task was used in fMRI research to explore the neural correlates of the self-reference effect and potential cross-cultural variation. Kelley et al. (2002) scanned American participants while they performed trait judgments on the self and a public person. It was found that, relative to judgments of a public person, self-judgments were associated with activation in the ventral medial prefrontal cortex (VMPFC); VMPFC activity associated with self-judgments was decreased relative to the resting state but was greater compared to that associated with public-person judgments. The finding of increased VMPFC activity during judgments of one's own traits has been repeatedly demonstrated in subsequent studies in the Western cultural context (Northoff et al., 2006). VMPFC activity linked to self-trait judgments was even stronger than that associated with trait judgments of a close other (e.g., best friend) in American participants (Heatherton et al., 2006). The VMPFC may play an important role in coding self-relevance of stimuli, since trait words rated high versus low in self-relevance increased VMPFC activity (Moran, Macrae, Heatherton, Wyland, & Kelley, 2006) and VMPFC activity correlated with memory performances on recall of self-related trait words (Ma & Han, 2011 Macrae, Moran, Heatherton, Banfield, & Kelley, 2004).These brain imaging findings suggest a good paradigm for assessing the neural representation of the self in relation to others, one that may be useful for investigating cross-cultural variation of self-representation in the human brain. If, according to Markus and Kitayama (1991, 2010), the self is dissociated from close others in self-construals in many Western cultures, one would predict that the neural representation of the self in the VMPFC may be separated from that of a close other. In contrast, neural representations of the self and close others may partially overlap in the VMPFC to mediate interdependent self-construals in East Asian cultural contexts. Thus, VMPFC activity related to trait judgments of the self and close others can be used to test the psychological model of cross-cultural variation of self-construals.

An early study tested this hypothesis by scanning Chinese individuals and English-speaking Wester individuals during trait judgments of the self, one's mother, and a public person (Zhu, Zhang, Fan, & Han, 2007). The critical issue addressed in this study was whether the self and mother share neural representations in the VMPFC in individuals in the Chinese cultural context but are dissociated from each other in the VMPFC in individuals in the Western cultural context. A memory test after the scanning showed that Chinese participants remembered equally well the trait adjectives related to the self and mother, whereas Westerners remembered better the trait adjectives related to the self than those related to mother, replicating the findings of the earlier studies (e.g., Qi & Zhu, 2002; Zhu & Zhang, 2002). In addition, although both Chinese and Westerners showed greater VMPFC activity to self- than public-person-judgments, Chinese participants also demonstrated stronger VMPFC activity to mother judgments compared to public-person judgments. Directly comparing self- and mother judgments did not show any significant activation differences in the VMPFC, suggesting comparable neural representations of the self and mother in the VMPFC. In contrast, in Westerners, mother judgments failed to activate the VMPFC relative to public-person judgments, and self-judgments gave rise to increased VMPFC activation compared with mother judgments, indicating the hypothesized dissociation between the self and mother in the VMPFC in Westerners. The results provide the first evidence for cross-cultural variations in neural substrates underlying self representations in relation to close others and a neuroscience account of the psychological model of Western versus East Asian cultural differences in self-construals.

As the neural substrates of self-face recognition showed dynamic variations as a consequence of cultural value priming (Sui & Han, 2007), one may expect similar influences of cultural priming on the neural representation of one's own personality traits—the mental aspects of self-concept. Specifically, for those with two cultural systems in their minds (bicultural individuals), it is likely that self and close other representations may overlap in the VMPFC after East Asian cultural values are activated, whereas self and close others may be dissociated in the VMPFC after Western cultural values are activated. Indeed, Ng et al. (2010) showed that, after being primed with pictures of Chinese cultural icons, Westernized Chinese participants living in Hong Kong showed increased VMPFC to both the self and mother during the trait judgment task. However, after being primed with pictures of Western cultural icons, VMPFC activity to mother judgments was decreased, whereas VMPFC activity to self-judgments was enhanced. These findings provide evidence for dynamic cognitive and neural representations of the self in relation to close others in bicultural individuals. In addition, the finding of temporal dynamic variations of neural representations of the self is consistent with the observed differences in self-representations in Chinese and Westerners that reflects the accumulated influences of cultural values and practice over time.

Cultural influences on neural representations of self-concept are also manifested during the processing of general and contextual self-judgments. Chiao and colleagues (2009) scanned Japanese and Caucasian Americans during a general self-referential task that required responses to questions such as "In general, does this sentence describe you?" and a contextual self-referential task that required responses to questions such as "Does this sentence describe you when you are talking to your mother?" Although this study did not report differences in the neural correlates of self-judgments between Japanese and Caucasian American participants, the authors classified participants, in terms of self-report on the Singelis (1994) self-construal scale, into individualist and collectivist groups. It was found that individualists showed significantly greater VMPFC activation for general self-descriptions relative to contextual self-descriptions, whereas collectivists demonstrated significantly greater activation for contextual self-descriptions compared to general self-descriptions. Moreover, the degree of VMPFC response to self-judgments (contextual minus general) correlated positively with the degree of differential collectivism versus individualism. A follow-up study from the same group (Chiao et al., 2010) scanned bicultural participants (e.g., Asian Americans) while they performed the general/contextual self tasks. Half of the participants were primed with cultural values of individualism and half with cultural values of collectivism prior to self-judgments. The priming procedure consisted of a Sumerian warrior story task and a similarities and differences with family and friends (SDFF) task (Trafimow, Triandis, & Goto, 1991) that have been shown to influence self-construals. The bicultural participants primed with individualistic values showed increased activation in the VMPFC and posterior cingulate cortex (PCC) during general relative to contextual self-judgments. In contrast, bicultural participants primed with collectivistic values showed increased responses within the MPFC and PCC during contextual relative to general self-judgments. Thus, neural representations of a general self and a contextual self in the MPFC appear to be shaped by cultural values of individualism and collectivism.

Cross-cultural variations in other aspects of self-concept have been documented in social psychological research. For example, using the Rosenberg Self-Esteem Scale (Rosenberg, 1965), Schmitt and Allik (2005) reported higher levels of self-competence (i.e., feeling you are confident, capable, and efficacious) in individualistic cultures than in collectivistic cultures, but higher levels of self-liking (i.e., feeling you are good, socially relevant, and maintain group harmony) in collectivistic cultures than in individualistic cultures. However, to date, little is known about the neural correlates of self-esteem and potential cross-cultural variations, which should be investigated in the future. Taken together, both psychological and brain imaging studies have shown evidence for cross-variations in the cognitive and neural processing of self-related information. The cultural influences on self-related processing take place in perceptual, memory, and social domains and show a coherent pattern.

In summary, individualistic cultural contexts and cultural priming facilitates self-construals that emphasize the self as an independent entity, one that behaves in accordance with one's own internal traits and thoughts and independently of others' thoughts and feelings. In contrast, collectivistic cultural contexts and cultural priming promote self-construals that view the self primarily in relation to others and particularly to close others. The observed cultural differences reflect the consequences of social practices and interactions on how the human brain thinks of the self in relation to others.

HOW DO CROSS-CULTURAL VARIATIONS IN SOCIAL COGNITION AND THE SOCIAL BRAIN OCCUR?

Plasticity is an intrinsic property of the human brain, and it enables the nervous system to adapt to environmental pressures and experiences (Pascual-Leone et al., 2005). There is robust evidence that brain function is modulated by sensory experiences. For example, the occipital cortex, which is commonly involved in visual processing in sighted humans, can be engaged in auditory processing— such as being activated by heard sounds or words (Burton, Snyder, Diamond, & Raichle, 2002; Gougoux et al., 2009)—in blind individuals. VMPFC activity engaged in self-referential processing is also sensitive to sensory experiences, as sighted individuals showed VMPFC activation during self-judgments on visually but not aurally presented trait words, whereas congenitally blind individuals showed VMPFC activity during self-judgments on aurally presented trait words (Ma & Han, 2011). Auditory deprivation results in the recruitment of the primary auditory cortex in the processing of vibrotactile stimuli (Levanen, Jousmaki, & Hari, 1998) and sign language (Nishimura et al., 1999) in deaf humans. Thus, sensory experiences substantially shape the function of the primary sensory cortex to adapt to the processing of information from different modalities.

Similarly, the brain regions involved in social cognition can be shaped profoundly by social experiences due to the human rearing environment, human preference for social interactions, and developmental properties of the brain. First, humans create the most complex and varied social environments on earth, including massive social components and influences from extended families, communities (e.g., schools and institutes), and nation states (Wexler, 2011). People in different social environments behave differently during social interactions, and unique styles of social interactions also create distinct features of social contexts. Second, human infants show strong intentions to communicate and interact with others from early on. Within hours of birth, infants show interest in looking at the human face (Goren, Sarty, & Wu, 1975). Within 2 days of birth, they imitate others' actions using their tongues and heads (Meltzoff & Moore, 1977). Third, most of these social cognitive processes engage the anterior frontal and temporal lobes of the brain, and these brain regions take the longest time to mature, giving them ample time to be influenced by cultural and personal experiences. A longitudinal MRI study showed that gray matter density starts to decrease in the primary sensorimotor areas; such change then spreads over the frontal, parietal, and temporal cortices, and this process lasts until the age of 21 years (Gogtay et al., 2004). This provides a long time for the brain to adapt to varying sociocultural contexts. Fourth, brain regions engaged in social cognition undergo substantial functional and structural development during adolescence. Prefrontal activity increases between childhood and adolescence and then decreases between early adolescence and adulthood, possibly related to structural development in this area (Blakemore, 2008). Finally, variation of brain structure and function may correlate directly with social behaviors. For example, orbital prefrontal cortex volume correlates with social cognitive competence (Powell, Lewis, Dunbar, García-Fiñana, & Roberts, 2010), and amygdala volume correlates with the size and complexity of social networks in adults (Bickart, Wright, Dautoff, Dickerson, & Barrett, 2011).

Together, the plasticity of the brain, importance of social interactions, and variety of social environments provide a framework for the human brain to develop specific neurocognitive strategies to afford social interactions in different sociocultural contexts. Human cognition and the brain may also undergo modulation by sociocultural contexts even during adulthood in order to adapt to new environments. This is possible because cultural priming studies have shown that temporary activation of specific cultural values and knowledge is able to modulate cognitive strategies (Hong, Morris, Chiu, & Benet-Martinez, 2000) and the underlying brain mechanisms that support them (Chiao et al., 2010; Ng et al., 2010; Sui & Han, 2007). Therefore, it is highly possible that functional reorganization of the brain may occur in immigrants after moving to a new country with a different cultural context and living there for an extended period of time. Shaping the neural activity associated with social cognition in different cultural contexts is helpful for acculturation and in learning appropriate social behaviors in new sociocultural contexts.

IMPLICATIONS FOR MENTAL HEALTH

The findings of cross-cultural variations in social cognition and the social brain have many implications for mental health. Each individual has his or her own cultural identity that defines oneself in relation to a cultural group. Cultural identity also influences how an individual thinks of and interacts with others in social environments. The influences of cross-cultural variations in social cognition on mental health may come from both general cultural values/norms and relationships between individuals. In most cases, people behave in accordance with their cultural values/norms and expect positive feedback from others during social interactions. This is important for one's mental health and well-being. Given the cross-cultural variation in how people think of the self and others, one has to adjust his or her own behaviors when moving to a new cultural context to get positive feedback from others. In addition, people must be aware of cultural differences in the way people think of the self and others when trying to build relationship between themselves and others.

Cross-cultural variations in social cognition may be associated with specific mental disorders that lead to the impairment of normal social interactions. Heinrichs et al. (2006) found that people who hold collectivistic values are more accepting toward socially reticent and withdrawn behaviors than are those who hold individualistic values. These cultural value differences may be associated with culture-specific social anxiety disorders that are characterized by persistent fear of social or performance situations in which a person is exposed to unfamiliar people or to possible scrutiny by others. Dinnel et al. (2002) found that a fear of displeasing or embarrassing others varies across people with different self-construals, being more likely to be expressed by individuals who construe themselves low on independence but high on interdependence. To date, it is unknown how cultural difference in neural substrates underlying self-construals is associated with cross-cultural variations of social anxiety disorder. Future research may combine cultural neuroscience and psychopathology approaches to investigate the cognitive and neural bases of mental problems such as social anxiety disorder. Findings of the neurocognitive bases of culture-specific mental disorders may help to develop culture-specific treatments.

FUTURE QUESTIONS

Many important fundamental questions regarding cross-cultural variations in social cognition and the social brain remain to be answered. From the neuroscience perspective, the findings of cross-cultural variation in social cognition and the social brain raise the question of the flexibility of the cognitive system and its underlying neural substrates. The current cultural neuroscience studies mainly depend upon functional brain imaging techniques that are limited by spatial resolution. The cultural neuroscience findings suggest cross-cultural variations of large-scale neural networks (i.e., brain regions) but tell little about neural mechanisms at an individual neuron level, which is a challenge for future cultural neuroscience researchers to tackle. Another important fundamental question is whether and how culture and genes interact and lead to the co-determination of cognitive and neural processes involved in social cognition. This can be tested by comparing two subject groups with different genotypes in different cultural contexts.

Findings of cross-cultural variations in social cognition and the social brain also raise clinical issues regarding deficits in social cognition and related treatments. How are cultural differences in neurocognitive processing of social information related to other mental problems? Do we expect that the same neurocognitive mechanisms mediate psychiatric disorders, such as schizophrenia and depression, across cultures? Finding answers to these questions is critical for the understanding of appropriate treatments for mental disorders in different cultural contexts.

ACKNOWLEDGMENTS

This work was supported by National Natural Science Foundation of China (Project 30910103901, 91024032), National Basic Research Program of China (973 Program 2010CB833903). I am grateful to Sook-Lei Liew and Yina Ma for comments on an early draft of this chapter.

REFERENCES

Adams, R. B. Jr., Rule, N. O., Franklin, R. G., Jr., Wang, E., Stevenson, M. T., Yoshikawa, S., et al. (2010). Cross-cultural reading the mind in the eyes: An fMRI investigation. *Journal of Cognitive Neuroscience, 22*, 97–108.

Avenanti, A., Sirigu, A., & Aglioti, S. M. (2010). Racial bias reduces empathic sensorimotor resonance with other-race pain. *Current Biology, 20*, 1018–1022.

Baron-Cohen, S., Wheelwright, S., Hill, J., Raste, Y., & Plumb, I. (2001). The "reading the mind in the eyes" test revised version: A study with normal adults, and adults with Asperger syndrome or high-functioning autism. *Journal of Child Psychology and Psychiatry, 42*, 241–251.

Bickart, K. C., Wright, C. I., Dautoff, R. J., Dickerson, B. C., & Barrett, L. F. (2011). Amygdala volume and social network size in humans. *Nature Neuroscience, 14*, 163–164.

Blakemore, S. J. (2008). The social brain in adolescence. *Nature Review Neuroscience, 9*, 267–277.

Burton, H., Snyder, A. Z., Diamond, J. B., & Raichle, M. E. (2002). Adaptive changes in early and late blind: A FMRI study of verb generation to heard nouns. *Journal of Neurophysiology, 88*, 3359–3371.

Chiao, J. Y., & Ambady, N. (2007). Cultural neuroscience: Parsing universality and diversity across levels of analysis. In S. Kitayama & D. Cohen (Eds.), *Handbook of cultural psychology* (pp. 237–254). New York: Guilford Press.

Chiao, J. Y., Iidaka, T., Gordon, H. L., Nogawa, J., Bar, M., Aminoff, E., et al. (2008). Cultural specificity in amygdala response to fear faces. *Journal of Cognitive Neuroscience, 20*, 2167–2174.

Chiao, J. Y., Harada, T., Komeda, H., Li, Z., Mano, Y., Saito, D., et al. (2010). Dynamic cultural influences on neural representations of the self. *Journal of Cognitive Neuroscience, 22*, 1–11.

Chiao, J. Y., Harada, T., Komeda, H., Li, Z., Mano, Y., Saito, D., et al. (2009). Neural basis of individualistic and collectivistic views of self. *Human Brain Mapping, 30*, 2813–2820.

Choi, I., Nisbett, R. E., & Norenzayan, A. (1999). Causal attribution across cultures: Variation and universality. *Psychological Bulletin, 125*, 47–63.

Devue, C., Collette, F., Balteau, E., Degueldre, C., Luxen, A., Maquet, P., et al. (2007). Here I am: The cortical correlates of visual self-recognition. *Brain Research, 1143*, 169–182.

de Waal, F. B. M. (2008). Putting the altruism back into altruism: The evolution of empathy. *Annual Review of Psychology, 59*, 279–300.

Dinnel, D. L., Kleinknecht, R. A., & Tanaka-Matsumi, J. (2002). A cross-cultural comparison of social phobia symptoms. *Journal of Psychopathology and Behavioral Assessment, 24*, 75–84.

Dunbar, R. I., & Shultz, S. (2007). Evolution in the social brain. *Science, 17*, 1344–1347.

Freeman, J. B., Rule, N. O., Adams, R. B. Jr., & Ambady, N. (2009). Culture shapes a mesolimbic response to signals of dominance and subordination that associates with behavior. *Neuroimage, 47,* 353–359.

Frith, U., & Frith, C. (2010). The social brain: Allowing humans to boldly go where no other species has been. *Philosophical Transactions of the Royal Society Biological Sciences, 365,* 165–176.

Gardner, W. L., Gabriel, S., & Lee, A. Y. (1999). "I" value freedom, but "we" value relationships: Self-construal priming mirrors cultural differences in judgment. *Psychological Science, 10,* 321–326.

Gogtay, N., Giedd, J. N., Lusk, L., Hayashi, K. M., Greenstein, D., Vaituzis, A. C., et al. (2004). Dynamic mapping of human cortical development during childhood through early adulthood. *Proceedings of the National Academy of Sciences, USA, 101,* 8174–8179.

Goren, C. C., Sarty, M., & Wu, P. Y. K. (1975). Visual following and pattern discrimination of face-like stimuli by newborn infants. *Pediatrics, 56,* 544–549.

Gougoux, F., Belinb, P., Vossa, P., Leporea, F., Lassondea, M., & Zatorre, R. J. (2009). Voice perception in blind persons: A functional magnetic resonance imaging study. *Neuropsychologia, 47,* 2967–2974.

Hall, J. A., Coats, E. J., & LeBeau, L. S. (2005). Nonverbal behavior and the vertical dimension of social relations: A meta-analysis. *Psychological Bulletin, 131,* 898–924.

Han, S., & Northoff, G. (2008). Culture-sensitive neural substrates of human cognition: A transcultural neuroimaging approach. *Nature Review Neuroscience, 9,* 646–654.

Han, S., Mao, L., Qin, J., Friederici, A. D., & Ge, J. (2011). Functional roles and cultural modulations of the medial prefrontal and parietal activity associated with causal attribution. *Neuropsychologia, 49,* 83–91

Han, S., & Pöppel, E. (Eds.). (2011). *Culture and neural frames of cognition and communication (on thinking).* Berlin: Springer.

Heatherton, T. F., Wyland, C. L., Macrae, C. N., Demos, K. E., Denny, B. T., & Kelley, W. M. (2006). Medial prefrontal activity differentiates self from close others. *Social Cognitive and Affective Neuroscience, 1,* 18–25.

Heinrichs, N., Rapee, R. M., Alden, L.A., Bögels, S., Hofmann, S. G., Ja Oh, K., et al. (2006). Cultural differences in perceived social norms and social anxiety. *Behaviour Research and Therapy, 44,* 1187–1197.

Hong, Y., Morris, M., Chiu, C., & Benet-Martinez, V. (2000). Multicultural minds: A dynamic constructivist approach to culture and cognition. *American Psychologist, 55,* 709–720.

Jackson, P. L., Meltzoff, A. N., & Decety, J. (2006). Neural circuits involved in imitation and perspective-taking. *NeuroImage, 31,* 429–439.

Ji, L., Peng, K., & Nisbett, R. E. (2000). Culture, control, and perception of relationships in the environment. *Journal of Personality and Social Psychology, 78,* 943–955.

Jimenez, A. M., Gee, D. G., Cannon, T. D., & Lieberman, M. D. (2013). The social cognitive brain: A review of key individual differences parameters with relevance to schizophrenia. In D. L. Roberts & D. L. Penn (Eds.), *Social cognition in schizophrenia: From evidence to treatment* (Chapter 4). New York: Oxford University Press.

Johnson, J. D., Simmons, C. H., Jordan, A., MacLean, L., Taddei, J., & Thomas, D. (2002). Rodney King and O. J. revisited: The impact of race and defendant empathy induction on judicial decisions. *Journal of Applied Social Psychology, 32,* 1208–1223.

Keenan, J. P., McCutcheon, B., Freund, S., Gallup, G. G., Sanders, G., & Pascal-Leone, A. (1999). Left hand advantage in a self-face recognition task. *Neuropsychologia, 37,* 1421–1425.

Kelley, W. M., Macrae, C. N., Wyland, C. L., Caglar, S., Inati, S., & Heatherton, T. F. (2002). Finding the self? An event-related fMRI study. *Journal of Cognitive Neuroscience, 14,* 785–794.

Kitayama, S., & Uskul, A.K. (2011). Culture, mind, and the brain: Current evidence and future directions. *Annual Review of Psychology, 62,* 419–449.

Klein, S. B., Loftus, J., & Burton, H. A. (1989).Two self-reference effects: The importance of distinguishing between self-descriptiveness judgments and autobiographical retrieval in self-referent encoding. *Journal of Personality and Social Psychology, 56,* 853–865.

Kobayashi, C., Glover, G. H., & Temple, E. (2006). Cultural and linguistic influence on neural bases of "theory of mind": An fMRI study with Japanese bilinguals. *Brain and Language, 98,* 210–220.

Kobayashi, C., Glover, G. H., & Temple, E. (2007). Cultural and linguistic effects on neural bases of "theory of mind" in American and Japanese children. *Brain Research, 1164,* 95–107.

Kubota, J. T., & Ito, T. A. (2007). Multiple cues in social perception: The time course of processing race and facial expression. *Journal of Experimental Social Psychology, 43,* 738–752.

Kühnen, U., & Oyserman, D. (2002). Thinking about the self influences thinking in general: Cognitive consequences of salient self-concept. *Journal of Experimental Social Psychology, 38,* 492–499.

Levanen, S., Jousmaki, V., & Hari, R. (1998). Vibration-induced auditory-cortex activation in a congenitally deaf adult. *Current Biology, 8,* 869–872.

Lieberman, M. D. (2010). Social cognitive neuroscience. In S. T. Fiske, D. T. Gilbert, & G. Lindzey (Eds.), *Handbook of social psychology* (5th ed., pp. 143–193). New York: McGraw-Hill.

Liew, S. L., Ma, Y., Han, S., & Aziz-Zadeh, L. (2011). Who's afraid of the boss: Cultural differences in social hierarchies modulate self-face recognition in Chinese and Americans. *PLoS ONE, 6,* e16901.

Liew, S., Han, S., & Aziz-Zadeh, L. (2011). Familiarity modulates mirror neuron and mentalizing regions during intention understanding. *Human Brain Mapping, 32,* 1986–1997.

Lyons, K. E., & Koenig, M. A. (2013). The development of social cognition in theory and action. In D. L. Roberts & D. L. Penn (Eds.), *Social cognition in schizophrenia: From evidence to treatment* (Chapter 1). New York: Oxford University Press.

Ma, Y., & Han, S. (2009). Self-face advantage is modulated by social threat—Boss effect on self-face recognition. *Journal of Experimental Social Psychology, 45,* 1048–1051.

Ma, Y., & Han, S. (2010). Why respond faster to the self than others? An implicit positive association theory of self advantage during implicit face recognition. *Journal of Experimental Psychology: Human Perception and Performance, 36,* 619–633.

Ma, Y., & Han, S. (2011). Neural representation of self-concept in sighted and congenitally blind adults. *Brain 134,* 235–246.

Ma, Y., & Han, S. (2012. Functional dissociation of the left and right fusiform gyrus in self-face recognition. *Human Brain Mapping,* in press.

Macrae, C. N., Moran, J. M., Heatherton, T. F., Banfield, J. F., & Kelley, W. M. (2004). Medial prefrontal activity predicts memory for self. *Cerebral Cortex 14,* 647–654.

Markham, R., & Wang, L. (1996). Recognition of emotion by Chinese and Australian children. *Journal of Cross-Cultural Psychology, 27,* 616–643.

Markus, H. R., & Kitayama, S. (1991). Culture and the self: Implication for cognition, emotion and motivation. *Psychological Review, 98,* 224–253.

Markus, H. R., & Kitayama, S. (2010). Cultures and selves: A cycle of mutual constitution. *Perspective on Psychological Science, 5*, 420–430.

Masuda, T., & Nisbett, R. E. (2001). Attending holistically versus analytically: Comparing the context sensitivity of Japanese and Americans. *Journal of Personality and Social Psychology, 81*, 922–934.

Mathur, V. A., Harada, T., Lipke, T., & Chiao, J. Y. (2010). Neural basis of extraordinary empathy and altruistic motivation. *Neuroimage, 51*, 1468–1475.

Matsumoto, D. (1989). Cultural influences on the perception of emotion. *Journal of Cross-Cultural Psychology, 20*, 92–105.

Meltzoff, A. N., & Moore, M. K. (1977). Imitation of facial and manual gestures by human neonates. *Science, 198*, 74–78.

Molnar-Szakacs, I., Wu, A. D., Robles, F. J., & Iacoboni, M. (2007). Do you see what I mean? Corticospinal excitability during observation of culture-specific gestures. *PLoS One, 2*, e626.

Moran, J. M., Macrae, C. N., Heatherton, T. F. Wyland, C. L., & Kelley, W. M. (2006). Neuroanatomical evidence for distinct cognitive and affective components of self. *Journal of Cognitive Neuroscience, 18*, 1586–1594.

Morris, M., & Peng, K. (1994). Culture and cause: American and Chinese attributions for social and physical events. *Journal of Personality and Social Psychology, 67*, 949–971.

Ng, S. H., Han, S., Mao, L., & Lai, J. C. L. (2010). Dynamic bicultural brains: A fMRI study of their flexible neural representation of self and significant others in response to culture priming. *Asian Journal of Social Psychology, 13*, 83–91.

Nisbett, R. E., Peng, K., Choi, I., & Norenzayan, A. (2001). Culture and systems of thought: Holistic versus analytic cognition. *Psychological Review, 108*, 291–310.

Nisbett, R. E., & Masuda, T. (2003). Culture and point of view. *Proceedings of the National Academy of Science, 100*, 11163–11170.

Nishimura, H., Hashikawa, K., Doi, K., Iwaki, T., Watanabe, Y., & Kusuoka, H. (1999). Sign language "heard" in the auditory cortex. *Nature, 397*, 116.

Northoff, G., Heinzel, A., de Greck, M., Bermpohl, F., Dobrowolny, H., & Panksepp, J. (2006). Self-referential processing in our brain – a meta-analysis of imaging studies on the self. *Neuroimage, 31*, 440–457.

Pascual-Leone, A., Amedi, A., Fregni, F., & Merabet, L. B. (2005). The plastic human brain cortex. *Annual Review of Neuroscience, 28*, 377–401.

Peng, K., & Knowles, E. D. (2003). Culture, education, and the attribution of physical causality. *Personality and Social Psychology Bulletin, 29*, 1272–1284.

Rogers, T. B., Kuiper, N. A., & Kirker, W. S. (1977). Self-reference and the encoding of personal information. *Journal of Personality and Social Psychology, 35*, 677–688.

Rosenberg, M. (1965). *Society and the adolescent child.* Princeton, NJ: Princeton University Press.

Russell, J. A. (1994). Is there universal recognition of emotion from facial expression? A review of the cross-cultural studies. *Psychological Bulletin, 115*, 102–141.

Perner, J. (1991). *Understanding the representational mind.* Cambridge, MA: MIT Press.

Platek, S. M., Keenan, J. P., Gallup, G. G., Jr., & Mohamed, F. B. (2004). Where am I? The neurological correlates of self and other. *Brain Research Cognitive Brain Research, 19*, 114–222.

Platek, S. M., Wathne, K., Tierney, N. G., & Thomson, J. W. (2008). Neural correlates of self-face recognition: An effect-location meta-analysis. *Brain Research, 1232*, 173–184.

Powell, J. L., Lewis, P. A., Dunbar, R. I., García-Fiñana, M., & Roberts, N. (2010). Orbital prefrontal cortex volume correlates with social cognitive competence. *Neuropsychologia*, *48*, 3554–3562.

Qi, J., & Zhu, Y. (2002). Self-reference effect of Chinese college students. *Psychological Science (in Chinese)*, *25*, 275–278.

Ruby, P., & Decety, J. (2003). What you believe versus what you think they believe: A neuroimaging study of conceptual perspective-taking. *European Journal of Neuroscience*, *17*, 2475–2480.

Sabbagh, M. A., Xu, F., Carlson, S. M., Moses, L. J., & Lee, K. (2006). The development of executive functioning and theory of mind. *Psychological Science*, *17*, 74–81.

Schmitt, D. P., & Allik, J. (2005). Simultaneous administration of the Rosenberg self-esteem scale in 53 nations: Exploring the universal and culture-specific features of global self-esteem. *Journal of Personality and Social Psychology*, *89*, 623–642.

Singelis, T. M. (1994). The measurement of independent and interdependent self-construals. *Personality and Social Psychology Bulletin*, *20*, 580–591.

Sugiura, M., Watanabe, J., Maeda, Y., Matsue, Y., Fukuda, H., & Kawashima, R. (2005). Cortical mechanisms of visual self-recognition. *Neuroimage*, *24*, 143–149.

Sui, J., & Han, S. (2007). Self-construal priming modulates neural substrates of self-awareness. *Psychological Science*, *18*, 861–866.

Sui, J., Liu, C. H., & Han, S. (2009). Cultural difference in neural mechanisms of self-recognition. *Social Neuroscience*, *4*, 402–411.

Tong, F., & Nakayama, K. (1999). Robust representations for faces: Evidence from visual search. *Journal of Experiment Psychology: Human Perception and Performance*, *25*, 1016–1035.

Triandis, H. C. (1989). The self and social behavior in differing cultural contexts. *Psychological Review*, *96*, 506–520.

Triandis, H. C., & Gelfand, M. J. (1998). Converging measurement of horizontal and vertical individualism and collectivism. *Journal of Personality and Social Psychology*, *74*, 118–128.

Trafimow, D., Triandis, H. C., & Goto, S. G. (1991). Some tests of the distinction between the private self and the collective self. *Journal of Personality and Social Psychology*, *60*, 649–655.

Tsai, J. L., Knutson, B., & Fung, H. H. (2006). Cultural variation in affect valuation. *Journal of Personality and Social Psychology*, *90*, 288–307.

Uddin, L. Q., Kaplan, J. T., Molnar-Szakacs, I., Zaidel, E., & Iacoboni, M. (2005). Self-face recognition activates a frontoparietal "mirror" network in the right hemisphere: An event-related fMRI study. *NeuroImage*, *25*, 926–935.

Vogeley, K., May, M., Ritzl, A., Falkai, P., Zilles, K., & Fink, G. R. (2004). Neural correlates of first-person perspective as one constituent of human self-consciousness. *Journal of Cognitive Neuroscience*, *16*, 817–827.

Wang, Q., & Conway, M. A. (2004). The stories we keep: Autobiographical memory in American and Chinese middle-aged adults. *Journal of Personality*, *72*, 911–938.

Wellman, H. M., Cross, D., & Watson, J. (2001). Meta-analysis of theory-of-mind development: The truth about false belief. *Child Development*, *72*, 655–684.

Wexler, B. (2011). Neuroplasticity: Biological evolution's contribution to cultural evolution. In S. Han, & E. Pöppel (Eds.), *Culture and neural frames of cognition and communication (on thinking)* (pp. 1–17). Berlin: Springer.

Wu, S., & Keysar, B. (2007). The effect of culture on perspective taking. *Psychological Science*, *18*, 600–606.

Xu, X., Zuo, X., Wang, X., & Han, S. (2009). Do you feel my pain? Racial group membership modulates empathic neural responses. *Journal of Neuroscience, 29,* 8525–8529.

Yamaguchi, S., Kuhlman, D. M., & Sugimori, S. (1995). Personality correlates of allocentric
tendencies in individualist and collectivist cultures. *Journal of Cross-Cultural Psychology,
26,* 658–672.

Zhu, Y., & Zhang, L. (2002).An experimental study on the self-reference effect. *Sciences in
China, Series C, 45,*120–128.

Zhu, Y., Zhang, L., Fan, J., & Han. S. (2007). Neural basis of cultural influence on self representation. *Neuroimage, 34,* 1310–1317.

4

The Social Cognitive Brain

*A Review of Key Individual Difference Parameters
with Relevance to Schizophrenia*

AMY M. JIMENEZ, DYLAN G. GEE, TYRONE D. CANNON,
AND MATTHEW D. LIEBERMAN ■

Individuals with schizophrenia exhibit poor general information processing ability, which is thought to reflect a generalized disruption of neuronal connectivity in the brain (e.g., Heinrichs & Zakzanis, 1998; Hoff et al., 1999; Karlsgodt et al., 2008; Taylor & Abrams, 1984). These impairments have been shown to adversely affect functional outcomes, including social problem-solving ability and social skill acquisition (e.g., Green, 1996; Liddle, 2000). However, a critical question is whether anything particular is disrupted in how such individuals process social information. Before that question can be answered, one would need to answer the question of whether there is something special about social information processing per se. Some have argued that social intelligence is just "general intelligence applied to social situations" (Wechsler, 1958, p. 75). This chapter will review the literature illustrating a different view, that social and emotional information processing is indeed distinct from nonsocial information processing.

The chapter will primarily focus on the state of the field of basic social cognitive neuroscience to set the stage for a focus on clinical populations; namely, social cognitive neuroscience in schizophrenia. To that end, we will focus on domains that may be particularly disrupted in individuals with schizophrenia, either based on typical clinical presentation (i.e., symptomatology) or reliance of processing on distributed neural networks, which are evidently disrupted in schizophrenia (e.g., Bullmore, Frangou, & Murray, 1997; Friston & Frith, 1995). Specifically, the focus will be on self- versus other-oriented information, emotion perception, intentional and incidental emotion regulation processes, and the tendency versus capacity to engage in such processes.

THE SELF

Social cognitive neuroscience is increasingly revealing distinct networks for social types of information, differentiating between nonemotional ("cold") cognition and social-emotional ("hot") cognition. A basic premise assumed by the existence of a cohesive social cognition network is the ability to distinguish between *self* and *other*. This would include existence of an intact sense of self to allow for self-referential knowledge, as well as the ability to understand others' mental states as necessary for psychological states such as empathy, which is important for normative subsequent social interactions. Researchers have sought to reach a workable definition of *self*, operationalizing both physical aspects of the self, including a sense of ownership and agency over one's body, and psychological aspects of the self, including self-relevance of stimuli and "metarepresentation" of one's own mental states (Gillihan & Farah, 2005; Vogeley et al., 2001). Such operational definitions allow for an empirical approach to the study of self-consciousness, a burgeoning area of inquiry within the field of social cognitive neuroscience.

Sense of ownership involves recognition of being the one who is undergoing an experience, whose body is moving or responding, whether or not the movement or response is voluntary (Gallagher, 2000). On the other hand, a sense of agency has been defined as the recognition of being the cause of an action, the sense of initiating and executing one's own actions as opposed to another's actions (Blakemore & Frith, 2003; Gallagher, 2000). To illustrate the difference between the two, a sense of ownership would be intact during passive or involuntary movements (such as when one's arm is moved by someone else), whereas a sense of agency would, in this case, be violated (David, Newen, & Vogeley, 2008). Both ownership and agency contribute to the self–other distinction in the physical domain critical to the experience of self-consciousness. However, sense of agency may be of particular relevance to patient experiences in schizophrenia, especially in regards to delusions of thought, mind, and/or action control (Gillihan & Farah, 2005). In a study by Spence and colleagues (1997), patients with delusions of control or loss of agency who erroneously attributed their actions to another showed abnormally high activation in right inferior parietal cortex (Spence et al., 1997).

According to a substantive review by Gillihan and Farah (2005), some physical aspects of the sense of self fail to show conclusive evidence of specialization, according to criteria of anatomical specificity, functional uniqueness, and functional independence. Specifically, they conclude that there does not appear to be a coherent or cohesive neural network for the holistic representation of the physical self. In addition, awareness and tracking of movement and position of the spatial layout of one's body seems to be represented in common with the layout and tracking of other people's bodies. On the other hand, body part ownership shows evidence of functional independence and anatomical specificity to the right supramarginal gyrus, as demonstrated by lesion studies (Gillihan & Farah, 2005).

Imaging studies have implicated several brain areas specifically in action ownership, or the sense of agency, beyond those regions of the motor system (i.e., premotor cortex [PMC], supplementary motor area [SMA] and pre-SMA, and the cerebellum) commonly activated by planned, imagined, or actual motor activity. As demonstrated in studies utilizing imagined and actual self-action compared to imagined or actual experimenter or other action, these regions include anterior and posterior insula, posterior inferior parietal cortex, dorsolateral prefrontal cortex (dlPFC), and the posterior segment of the superior temporal sulcus (pSTS; David et al., 2008; Farrer & Frith, 2002; Jeannerod, 2004; Leube et al., 2003; Powell, Macrae, Cloutier, Metcalfe, & Mitchell, 2009; Ruby & Decety, 2001). In particular, Farrer and Frith (2002) suggest that the anterior insula plays a role in the elaboration of an image of the body in space and in time. In addition, the insula may be a site for the integration of multimodal sensory signals associated with voluntary movements, which are attended to during self-attribution. The inferior parietal cortex, in contrast, may be a site for the elaboration of internal representations of the external world and one's interactions with it, to then represent movements in an allocentric (as opposed to egocentric) coding system that can be applied to the actions of others, as well as to the self (Farrer & Frith, 2002).

More recent studies have begun to engage multiple elements thought to be involved in the construction of self-consciousness to begin to deconstruct how such elements are organized and interact in the brain. For example, David and colleagues utilized a virtual ball-tossing game to simulate agency versus observing another person as agent of action from both a first- and third-person perspective (David et al., 2006). No significant neural interactions between agency and perspective taking were observed, although there was an overlap of activity in medial prefrontal regions associated with representations of one's own perspective and actions. Finally, few studies to date have investigated the functional relationship between regions during sense of agency to identify neural networks in support of the creation of self. In one recent study, David and colleagues (2007), utilizing a psychophysiological interaction (PPI) method, found enhanced functional connectivity between posterior inferior parietal cortex and a region of occipito-temporal cortex (also known as the extrastriate body area) during judgments of agency. Both regions were more active when visual feedback was incongruent to the subjects' own executed movements, indicating involvement in distinguishing whether actions are caused by oneself or by another person (David et al., 2007).

In terms of the psychological aspects of *self*, it is easy to intuit that the manner in which individuals process self-relevant information and self-knowledge may be distinct from that of other types of information, including information about other people and their mental states. However, capturing the nature of that distinctive processing within an experimental setting has proved to be a challenge, as evidenced by the wide range of task paradigms utilized and their somewhat disparate findings (e.g., Gillihan & Farah, 2005; Lombardo et al., 2009). However, a growing body of literature continues to investigate whether a specialized neural system in the brain may support self-referential information processing. This type of information might include self-face identification, conceptual representations of self, self-evaluation, and self-referential emotions (Kircher et al., 2000; Morita et al., 2008; Platek, Keenan, Gallup, & Mohamed, 2004; Platek, Thomson, & Gallup, 2004; Powell et al., 2009; Zinck, 2008). Although overlapping in many ways with studies of the physical self, self-identification has generally been viewed as a psychological self-oriented process and has been investigated in a variety of ways. For example, studies using morphed facial images require self–other discrimination from pictures of the self morphed to varying degrees with famous, familiar, or unfamiliar faces. Neuropsychological case studies using these task paradigms have found evidence for right hemisphere specialization for self-identification (reviewed in Gillihan & Farah, 2005). A left-hand advantage in reaction time (implicating right hemisphere dominance) for self-face recognition has also been demonstrated, with the speed of recognition further facilitated by multimodal sensory self-primes (i.e., exposure to one's own body odor and seeing and hearing one's own name; Platek, Thomson, et al., 2004).

Imaging studies have sought to further localize self-identification processing. A common finding has been involvement of frontal regions, especially right inferior frontal gyrus (IFG), using morphed (e.g., Kircher et al., 2000) and passive (e.g., Kaplan, Aziz-Zadeh, Uddin, & Iacoboni, 2008; Platek, Keenan, et al., 2004) self-face identification, self-face evaluation (Morita et al., 2008), and self-voice recognition (Kaplan et al., 2008).

Conceptual knowledge of one's own personality and traits has been studied extensively, often via semantic self-labeling tasks contrasting judgments of self with judgments of famous or unknown others, and has been shown to be subserved primarily by medial PFC (mPFC; e.g., Fossati et al., 2003; Kelley et al., 2002; Powell et al., 2009). In a recent review, Lieberman (2010) noted that mPFC activity was observed in 94% of studies on self-knowledge. A comprehensive meta-analysis by Van Overwalle (2009) revealed that, more specifically, the ventral portion of mPFC (vmPFC) was engaged in 85% of studies exploring the representation, evaluation, or description of the self. The Lieberman (2010) review further revealed that the contiguous regions of the posterior cingulate cortex/precuneus (PCC/PC) were also represented in 63% of such studies on self-knowledge, and dorsal medial PFC (dmPFC) appeared in 53% of the studies.

Taken together, neuroimaging research suggests that the construction of the "self" is based on a collection of functionally independent, physically and psychologically based constituents involving distinct mental operations distributed throughout the brain, rather than on a unitary cognitive system (see Figure 4.1). Although the anterior insula seems to play a critical role in the sense of agency (e.g., Farrer & Frith, 2002), a number of other aspects of self seem to implicate mPFC, including conceptual judgments about one's personality (Lieberman, 2010), autobiographical memory (Calarge, Andreasen, & O'Leary, 2003; Maguire, 2001), and self-thought monitoring (Mason et al., 2007). Such findings may indicate a general role for mPFC (and related midline cortical regions) as subserving a unique set of cognitive operations engaged by "the self," broadly construed.

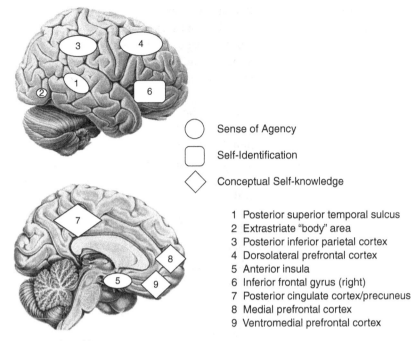

○ Sense of Agency

☐ Self-Identification

◇ Conceptual Self-knowledge

1 Posterior superior temporal sulcus
2 Extrastriate "body" area
3 Posterior inferior parietal cortex
4 Dorsolateral prefrontal cortex
5 Anterior insula
6 Inferior frontal gyrus (right)
7 Posterior cingulate cortex/precuneus
8 Medial prefrontal cortex
9 Ventromedial prefrontal cortex

Figure 4.1 The self.

UNDERSTANDING OTHERS

Many experimental investigations of the *self* rely on contrasts to conditions that reference the *other* (e.g., imagining another's actions, third-person perspective taking, and other-oriented information processing). Both self- and other processing requires the metacognitive ability to think about mental states, such as thoughts, beliefs, desires, and intentions, and make inferences about them in oneself and others. Such inferences can then be used to make predictions about the behavior of others. This is generally referred to as *theory of mind* (ToM; Premack & Woodruff, 1978) or *mentalizing*. Closely following the ability to understand other minds is the ability to relate to the mental states of others with some personal relevance or *empathy* (e.g., Derntl et al., 2010; Gallup & Platek, 2002; Keenan & Wheeler, 2002; Preston & de Waal, 2002). Clearly, these are highly intertwined abilities: By rendering the behavior of others comprehensible and predictable, both are critical for effective interpersonal relationships and normative social behavior (although see also Zahavi, 2008).

Researchers have utilized a variety of experimental paradigms to establish the neurobiological basis of ToM, largely driven by investigations of autism. Early behavioral work with children utilized false-belief tasks in which the observer knows more than the characters in a play and must model the character's perspective, which is different from their own, to answer questions about the story correctly (e.g., Baron-Cohen, Frith, & Leslie, 1985). Such a task requires awareness that different people can have different beliefs about the same situation, and this awareness can guide predictions of their subsequent behavior. Developmental psychologists have shown that children begin to successfully complete simple or "first-order" ToM tasks around age 2, and most do so reliably by age 4 (e.g., Bretherton & Beeghly, 1982; Wimmer & Perner, 1983; and see Lyons & Koenig, 2013, Chapter 1, this volume).

More developmentally advanced or "higher-order" mentalizing has also been explored behaviorally, via tasks that require attribution of more complex mental states (e.g., recursive thinking, double bluff, white lie), subtle social reasoning (e.g., recognition of irony, sarcasm, humor, or faux pas), and nuanced understanding of motivation and intention (e.g., use of pretend play, deception, and persuasion). Such studies have utilized live action plays (Baron-Cohen, 1989) and short stories or vignettes (e.g., Happé, 1994) to directly compare among different levels and types of "mind-reading" or social reasoning ability. Autistic children who successfully complete simpler ToM tasks are often severely impaired at these higher level tasks. Similar studies have been conducted with patients with damage to the orbital frontal cortex (OFC; in contrast to patients with dlPFC damage), with similar results (e.g., Stone, Baron-Cohen, & Knight, 1998).

Following this line of work, social cognitive neuroscientists have investigated the neural basis for simple and more complex ToM abilities in tasks utilizing vignettes (e.g., Fletcher et al., 1995; Saxe & Powell, 2006), cartoons (Gallagher et al., 2000), geometric shape animations depicting social interactions (e.g., Gobbini et al., 2007), and more active engagement in third-person perspective taking and mental state attribution via creation of stories about strangers (e.g., Calarge et al., 2003). Such studies have demonstrated activity in several different brain regions, including dmPFC, vmPFC, PCC/PC, temporo-parietal junction (TPJ), pSTS, and the anterior temporal cortex (aTC; see Figure 4.2) (see also Farrer & Frith, 2002; Morita et al., 2008; Platek, Keenan, et al., 2004).

In a substantive review, Carrington and Bailey (2009) considered whether task design and presentation modality (e.g., verbal vs. nonverbal; explicit vs. implicit instructions) explain the somewhat heterogeneous and widely distributed anatomical regions implicated in ToM. However, they concluded that methodological variability does not entirely account for the variation in findings. Rather, they suggest that ToM activates an integrated functional network involving several distinct core (consistently activated) and peripheral (activated depending on specifics of the task) brain regions contributing to ToM. Core regions were identified as mPFC/OFC, STS, TPJ, and PCC/PC (see also Frith & Frith, 2006; Gallagher & Frith, 2003; Siegal & Varley, 2002). Recruitment of neural systems subserving other elements of cognition, such as autobiographical memory (e.g., Calarge et al., 2003) or executive control (e.g., Saxe, Schulz, & Jiang, 2006), may also come on line as contributing but dissociable peripheral processes, depending on the specific ToM task.

Based on a meta-analysis of over 200 functional magnetic resonance imaging (fMRI) studies of social cognition, Van Overwalle (2009) further narrowed the

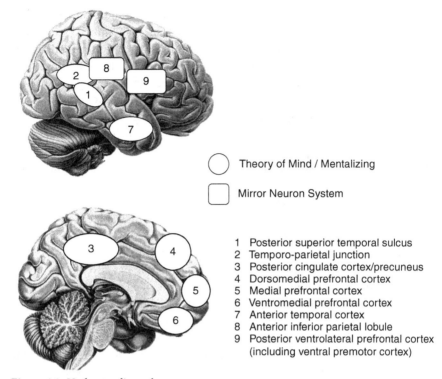

Figure 4.2 Understanding others.

core system for ToM processing to two primary regions: TPJ and mPFC. That analysis found that the primary distinction between mPFC and TPJ activation was that identification and representation of temporary mental states, such as goals, intentions, and desires of other people, engages the TPJ, especially for nonverbal material, whereas inferences about more enduring dispositions or traits of others and the self engage the mPFC. Temporary states can also activate mPFC, and this is perhaps driven by the presence of a verbal component or the necessity of spontaneous judgments of enduring states (spontaneous trait inferences).

Indeed, although the majority of studies have implicated mPFC in self-knowledge (see Lieberman, 2010; Van Overwalle, 2009), this region has also been shown to be involved in semantic judgments about personally close others (e.g., Krienen, Tu, & Buckner, 2010) and similar others (e.g., Mitchell, Banaji, & Macrae, 2005), perhaps indicating a broader role for this region in representing socially or emotionally relevant information about another person (Gallagher & Frith, 2003; Saxe & Powell, 2006). However, Mitchell and colleagues (2006) further dissociated mPFC functioning in regard to similar others with the finding that vmPFC responds to mentalizing about a similar other, whereas dmPFC was differentially involved in mentalizing about a dissimilar other (Mitchell, Macrae, & Banaji, 2006). In fact, dmPFC, in particular, is most often associated with thinking about the mental states of others (e.g., Lieberman, 2010).

Nevertheless, there is evidence of both overlapping and nonoverlapping regions of activation associated with *self* and *other* (especially similar other) processing (e.g., Frith & Frith, 2006; Rabin, Gilboa, Stuss, Mar, & Rosenbaum, 2009; Saxe, Moran, Scholz, & Gabrieli, 2006; Vogeley et al., 2001). These findings suggest that *other*-oriented processing integrally involves *self*-processing, such that neural architecture implicated in processing knowledge about the self is likewise called upon when processing knowledge about others (e.g., Platek, Keenan et al., 2004). These findings are in line with a *simulation theory* of ToM (e.g., Gallese & Goldman, 1998), which posits that perceivers use knowledge about themselves and refer to their own past experiences to infer the mental states of others (see also Apperly, 2008).

This line of thinking may implicate the putative "mirror neuron system," which is thought by some investigators to be a distributed neural system in humans for action understanding. *Mirror neurons* were so named due to findings from research in nonhuman primates that individual neurons in PMC fire not only during performance of coordinated, goal-oriented action, but also during observation of another performing these actions, suggestive of an overlap between perception and execution of action (Iacoboni, 2009). In humans, a frontal-parietal network including posterior ventrolateral PFC (comprising posterior IFG and ventral PMC) and anterior inferior parietal lobule (IPL) has been suggested as the site for a mirror neuron system (see Figure 4.2; Iacoboni et al., 1999; Lieberman, 2010; see also Jeannerod, 2004). To be sure, the research on mirror neurons is extensive, and this complex phenomenon is only briefly described here. However, the key question raised by the possibility of a mirror neuron system in humans is whether automatic imitative processes underlie biological motion detection, which may in turn underlie, at least in part, ToM processing. That is, ToM abilities may build on the capacity to recognize biological motion and goal-directed action, which appears much earlier developmentally and has been shown to be associated with pSTS activity (Lieberman, 2007). pSTS activity may thus support ToM processing via perception and representation of the intentions and goals of others implied by perceived action cues (e.g., Allison, Puce, & McCarthy, 2000; Gobbini et al., 2007).

By most accounts then, the mentalizing and mirror neuron systems are largely anatomically distinct and functionally dissociable, although they may interact in some way to aid collectively in social cognitive processes (Van Overwalle & Baetens, 2009). The precise nature of this interaction is not yet clear. Van Overwalle (2009) posits that a key component of early social information processing is the perception of goal-directed behavior, which is supported by two interactive processes. First is the perception of biological information (e.g., human faces, bodies, and movements) via specialized face (i.e., fusiform face area; FFA), body (extrastriate body area; EBA), and biological motion (pSTS) regions, followed by engagement of the mirror system, which identifies the goals behind these behaviors. A transition from the mirror to the mentalizing system may occur when mental state attributions from observation of body part and whole body motion are consciously deliberated (e.g., when participants are explicitly instructed to deliberate on the intentions of actors) and when such a focus is triggered by motions that are contextually inconsistent, implausible, or pretended. The latter may require more elaborative inferencing, perhaps beyond the purview of the mirror system (Van Overwalle & Baetens, 2009).

Spunt and Lieberman (2012) sought to directly test how these distinct systems interact in the brain during social cognition, specifically in regards to emotion recognition. They developed a paradigm requiring, in one condition, participants to identify facial expressions, hypothesized to engage the human mirror neuron system via automatic facial mimicry (Niedenthal, Mermillod, Maringer, & Hess, 2010). Another condition required mental state attributions to be made via causal emotion judgments, hypothesized to activate the mentalizing system. As predicted, explicit emotion recognition was associated with core regions of the mirror neuron system, whereas explicit mental state attribution activated areas of the mentalizing system. Furthermore, frontal mirror system regions (i.e., bilateral posterior IFG) demonstrated functional connectivity with mentalizing regions (i.e., dm/vmPFC, PCC/PC, bilateral TPJ, and left aTC), with mirror region activity preceding mentalizing region activity temporally. These findings suggest that the two systems may work in concert, with mirror activity informing mentalizing activity, to enable efficient and comprehensive emotional (and, by extension, social cognitive) processing.

The reference to emotion recognition in the preceding study highlights the fact that emotion understanding is an integral component of normal social cognition. Although effective emotional appraisals occur automatically for most of us, such judgments first require that multiple stages of complex information processing occur, several of which show evidence of disruption in individuals with schizophrenia (e.g., Karlsgodt et al., 2008) and warrant further discussion in terms of contributions from social cognitive neuroscience.

EMOTION

In a discussion of emotion within a social cognitive neuroscience framework, it is helpful to conceptualize emotion processing as occurring in a hierarchical stream, beginning with emotion perception—including perception of one's own emotions and that of others—and ending with regulation of one's emotions, which may occur intentionally with awareness or incidentally without awareness. Although a universally accepted definition of emotion may be difficult to find (e.g., Ekman, 1992; Panksepp, 2007; Russel, 2003), most researchers agree that for a stimulus to be appraised as having emotional or affective content, it must be salient and self-significant (e.g., Campos, Frankel, & Camras, 2004; LeDoux, 2000). Emotion perception cues us in to dangers and threats from our environment and those around us and facilitates the maintenance and enhancement of pleasurable or otherwise favorable experiences and relationships. Identification of emotion from facial expressions is a primary example of perception of emotion in others, which itself requires many levels of visual perceptual ability that occur on both conscious and unconscious levels, including the basic ability to process faces. Once an emotion is generated, it can be regulated through various distinct mechanisms that occur at different times in the emotion-generative process. Emotion regulation can serve many aims, including the down-regulation or up-regulation of an emotion. For example, during an altercation involving intense anger, effective emotion regulation allows one to down-regulate feelings of anger and express it in a more socially appropriate manner. In this way, such a process is adaptive and facilitates mood regulation and social interaction.

Face Perception

Human faces are essential for social interaction and communication and uniquely equipped to convey an abundance of information from person to person. As such, face perception is one of the most highly developed of human visual perceptual skills. Extensive research has been dedicated to understanding how the brain processes faces, with a focus on facial representations as distinct from other object representations, and distinct neuronal pathways involved in the perception and appraisal of various types of information conveyed by faces.

That faces are processed differently than other types of stimuli and that such processing is supported by a specialized neural system in the brain is well established. In human imaging studies, the perception of faces has been reliably associated with activity in a region of the lateral fusiform gyrus, so much so that many have come to refer to this region as the fusiform "face" area (FFA; Halgren et al., 1999; Kanwisher, McDermott, & Chun, 1997; McCarthy, Puce, Belger, & Allison, 1999). Other regions of visual extrastriate cortex that appear to be selective for faces include the inferior occipital gyrus, also known as the occipital face area (OFA; Gauthier, Skudlarski, Gore, & Anderson, 2000; Halgren et al., 1999; Rossion et al., 2003; Sergent, Ohta, & MacDonald, 1992), as well as pSTS (Engell & Haxby, 2007; Haxby, Hoffman, & Gobbini, 2000; Hooker et al., 2003). These regions of activation are usually bilateral with right hemispheric dominance (see Figure 4.3).

These three bilateral regions of occipitotemporal cortex (OFA, FFA, pSTS) may participate differentially in the different aspects of face perception (Haxby et al., 2000). Specifically, invariant aspects of faces (i.e., for identity recognition) may be processed via FFA, whereas changeable aspects (e.g., in support of expression and eye gaze detection) may be processed via pSTS, and early perception of facial features output to both of these regions occurs via OFA. Accordingly, FFA activation seems to be most prominent when comparing response to visual perception of faces to nonsense stimuli, scrambled faces, or other nonface objects utilizing passive viewing tasks or tasks in which attention is focused on the nonvariant aspects of the facial configuration (e.g., Kanwisher et al., 1997; McCarthy, Puce, Gore, & Allison, 1997; Sergent et al., 1992). Conversely, greater pSTS is elicited during tasks designed to direct attention to dynamic aspects of faces, such as direction of eye gaze or facial expression, rather than identity (Cloutier, Turk, & Macrae, 2008; Engell & Haxby, 2007; Hoffman & Haxby, 2000; Winston, Henson,

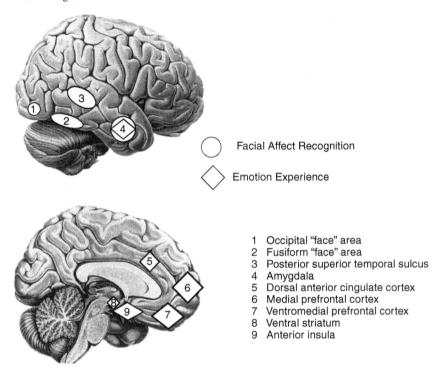

Figure 4.3 Emotion perception.

Fine-Goulden, & Dolan, 2004). Hooker et al. (2003) further demonstrated increased STS activation specifically for analysis of gaze cues that provide socially meaningful spatial information (in contrast with arrows that provide spatial information and with eye motion without spatial information; Hooker et al., 2003; see also Puce et al., 1998). Finally, support for the role of OFA as a visual processing "entry point" for face information has been supported by fMRI adaptation studies (e.g., Fox, Moon, Iara, & Barton, 2009).

   Although these areas are clearly involved in face processing, not all findings suggest the same degree of functional specificity. For example, Ganel and colleagues (2005) found significant FFA activity when subjects made judgments of facial expressions, and FFA was sensitive to variations in expression even when attention was directed to identity (Ganel, Valyear, Goshen-Gottstein, & Goodale, 2005; see also Fox et al., 2009). Other researchers have suggested that, rather than specialization only for face recognition, these face-responsive regions may be specialized for visual expertise, responding to objects perceived as unique individuals rather than category exemplars (e.g., Gauthier et al., 2000; Rhodes & McLean, 1990; Tarr & Gauthier, 2000; see also Chao, Martin, & Haxby, 1999; Spangler, Schwarzer, Korell, & Maier-Karius, 2010). In addition, as highlighted previously, right STS is usually associated with the perception of any biological movement or human action, and whether these are distinguishable to include specialty to faces is not clear (e.g., Bonda, Petrides, Ostry, & Evans, 1996). In fact, Saxe and colleagues (2004) found that right pSTS activity served a more generalized representation of observed intentional actions, not face action per se (Saxe, et al., 2004; see also Hein & Knight 2008). Finally, Rossion et al. (2003) found that, rather than receiving face-sensitive inputs from the OFA in a purely feed-forward hierarchical fashion, "feedback connections may facilitate re-entrant integration of FFA (and, presumably, STS) with OFA, allowing for normal face perception even in individuals with damages to right hemisphere inferior occipital cortex."

In summary, although advances have been made in our understanding of the neural underpinnings of face perception, more research is needed to elucidate the details of this complex system. What is clear, however, is that efficient processing of faces is reliant upon multiple interconnected brain regions acting in an orchestrated fashion. Highlighting the importance of connectivity between neuronal regions in face processing beyond a "core" system, predominantly active and perhaps selective for faces, an "extended" system may also contribute to face perception, although not exclusively involved in it (Haxby et al., 2000). These extended regions may be recruited, depending on the type of face perception, to extract meaning from faces and process the significance of the information gleaned. For example, perception of emotional facial expressions may activate the distributed neural system for emotion processing, including limbic regions such as the amygdala, dorsal anterior cingulate cortex (dACC), anterior insula, and ventral striatum (see Figure 4.3; Ishai, Schmidt, & Boesiger, 2005).

Emotional Expressions

Similar to primary face processing, the ability to display, recognize, and respond to facial expressions is a fundamental aspect of sociality in humans, critical for social information exchange (e.g., Ekman, 1993; Darwin, 1872/1998). The neural network for emotional faces has generally been investigated in imaging studies that use comparisons of blank, expressionless, or neutral faces to faces displaying an expression of emotion. A recent meta-analysis of 100 neuroimaging studies utilizing emotional face stimuli found that several brain regions were consistently activated. In addition to face-responsive regions in extrastriate occipital cortex, the amygdala was the area of greatest overlap, followed by regions of inferior temporal cortex, mPFC, and OFC (Sabatinelli et al., 2011).

Amygdala activation has most often been associated with response to fearful but also neutral faces (e.g., Kesler-West et al., 2001; Whalen et al., 2001), regardless of spatial frequency of the facial stimuli or location in the visual field (Morawetz, Baudewig, Treue, & Dechent, 2011). More generally, an abundance of literature points to the amygdala as playing a critical role in the automatic evaluation of both salient and ambiguous sensory inputs and then coordinating subsequent neurophysiological responses to these (Holland & Gallagher, 1999; LeDoux, 2000; Posner, 2001), possibly by biasing cognition toward perceived stimuli with potential emotional and social significance (Adolphs, 2003; Vuilleumier & Pourtois, 2007). For example, Critchley and colleagues (2000) compared activation to fearful and angry faces when explicitly (judging expression task) versus implicitly (judging facial gender task) attended to, and found that implicit processing involved greater amygdala activation. Similarly, Anderson and colleagues (2003) found that directing attention away from disgust and fear faces modulated regions involved in processing disgust (i.e., insula) but not amygdala; rather, amygdala activation increased. These findings suggest that when such stimuli are not attended to, amygdala processing becomes more diffuse to threat in general or attuned to the task of resolving ambiguity.

Selective involvement of other brain regions for experience of emotion in a category-specific manner has also been investigated with varying degrees of consistency. Generally, findings implicate a network of predominantly anterior limbic regions including the amygdala, ventral striatum, ACC, and anterior insula (see Figure 4.3; Kesler-West et al., 2001; Lane, Fink, Chau, & Dolan, 1997; Phillips, 2006; Sprengelmeyer, Rausch, Eysel, & Przuntek, 1998; Vytal & Hamann, 2010). In line with elements of the face processing model described above (e.g., Haxby et al., 2000; Hein & Knight, 2008), Peelen and colleagues (2010) found that mPFC and left STS activation was associated with presentation of five different emotions (fear, anger, disgust, happiness, sadness) in category-specific patterns of intensity but independent of modality of sensory input (i.e., facial expressions, body movements, or vocal intonations) or emotional intensity of the stimuli (see also Lane, Reiman, Ahern, Schwartz, & Davidson, 1997). They suggested that these "higher level" brain areas (also implicated in mental state attribution and ToM) represent emotions at an integrated, abstract, supramodal level and thus play a key role in understanding and categorizing others' emotional mental states.

Intentional Emotion Regulation

Emotions play a powerful role in both facilitating and, in some cases, hindering, individuals' experiences and social interactions. Thus, the regulation of emotion is critical to functioning. For example, effective emotion regulation may decrease experiences of negative emotion during stressful times or help to control socially inappropriate expressions of emotion during experiences of anger. Gross (1998a) defined emotion regulation as "processes by which individuals influence which emotions they have, when they have them, and how they experience and express these emotions" (p. 275). Emotion regulation can take a variety of forms, including both intentional and incidental processing. During intentional emotion regulation, individuals engage in effortful attempts to regulate their emotions. These attempts can impact experiences of emotion, expressive behavior, or physiological responding.

Emotions can be conceptualized as response tendencies that are generated after a stimulus is determined to be relevant and/or salient. Emotion regulation strategies can affect the course of the emotion-generative process at various time points. Gross (1998a) takes a process-oriented approach to describing five different types of emotion regulation: situation selection, situation modification, attention deployment, cognitive change, and response modulation. More specifically, situation selection refers to the individual's choosing of the situation in which he or she finds him- or herself. Situation modification is the process of changing that situation such that its emotional impact is changed. Of note, different situations are characterized by differences in their complexity (e.g., how many aspects of the situation can be modified) and the extent to which they can be changed. Attention deployment signifies the individual's selection of which aspect of a given situation to focus on. For example, an individual might choose to focus on a more negative or a more positive aspect of a situation. Cognitive change is the selection of which meaning is assigned to a situation. In each situation, many different meanings could exist, with each potentially leading to different emotional responses. For example, an individual might reappraise the meaning of a situation or his or her own ability to deal with the situation. Finally, response modulation is the process of altering emotional response tendencies once they have been evoked. For example, these strategies might reduce or intensify an emotional experience or expression.

Emotion regulation processes can be separated into antecedent- and response-focused strategies (Gross 1998b). Situation selection, situation modification, attention deployment, and cognitive change comprise antecedent-focused strategies, which alter the input to the emotion-generative process at an early stage. Conversely, response modulation is a type of response-focused strategy that takes place at a later stage in the process to alter the emotional response. In order to examine differential impacts of antecedent- versus response-focused strategies, Gross (1998b) compared reappraisal (antecedent-focused) and suppression (response-focused). Specifically, the study examined the effects of these strategies on emotional experience, expressive behavior, and sympathetic activation during film clips intended to elicit disgust. Participants were instructed to reappraise, suppress, or watch during the film. Reappraisal resulted in decreased self-reported subjective experience of disgust, as well as reduced behavior expressing emotion. Reappraisal had no effect on sympathetic activation. Suppression was associated with decreased expressive behavior and increased sympathetic activation. However, participants did not report changes in experience of disgust while engaging in suppression. Although both groups exhibited smaller increases in expressive behavior (disgust, emotional intensity, and activity) compared to the group that simply watched the film, ratings of disgust and emotional intensity of expressive behavior were lower in the suppression group. Interestingly, suppression failed to alter the subjective experience of emotion, despite affecting both expression and sympathetic activation.

Numerous studies have now examined neural substrates of reappraisal using fMRI. Although results vary from study to study, the most common activations associated with reappraising are in dorsolateral, ventrolateral, and dorsomedial PFC (e.g., Goldin, McRae, Ramel, & Gross, 2008; Ochsner, Bunge, Gross, & Gabrieli, 2002). Reductions in activation are commonly seen in the amygdala and other limbic regions (see Figure 4.4). Moreover, lateral PFC activations have been

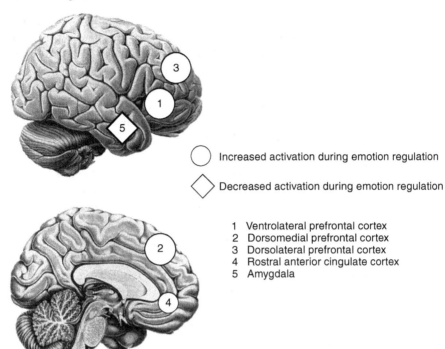

Increased activation during emotion regulation

Decreased activation during emotion regulation

1 Ventrolateral prefrontal cortex
2 Dorsomedial prefrontal cortex
3 Dorsolateral prefrontal cortex
4 Rostral anterior cingulate cortex
5 Amygdala

Figure 4.4 Emotion regulation.

seen in multiple studies to correlate inversely with both self-reported distress and with limbic activity.

One study compared the neural bases of strategies that differ in how and when they influence the emotion-generative process. Specifically, Goldin and colleagues (2008) examined activation among brain regions involved in cognitive reappraisal (early in the process) versus expressive-suppression (later in the process). In this study, participants viewed films designed to elicit negative emotion (negative) or no emotion (neutral) under the following four conditions: watch neutral, watch negative, reappraise negative, and suppress negative. Reappraisal, as compared with the watch-negative condition, was associated with early medial, dorsolateral, and ventrolateral PFC activation, along with decreased activation in amygdala and insula. However, suppression was associated with later dorsomedial, dorsolateral, and ventrolateral prefrontal responses and increased activation in the amygdala and insula. These results are consistent with the temporal dynamics evident in Gross's model (1998b) of emotion regulation strategies, as well as with the general conclusion that whereas suppression may reduce the expression of an emotion, it does little to diminish the experience.

More recently, Kanske and colleagues (2011) examined neural networks implicated in reappraisal versus distraction. Kanske et al. (2011) observed that OFC activation was uniquely activated for reappraisal. Conversely, their results demonstrated that distraction (a form of attention deployment) was associated with activation in the dorsal anterior cingulate and parietal cortex. Both reappraisal and distraction resulted in increased activation in medial and dorsolateral prefrontal and inferior parietal cortex, as well as in decreased bilateral amygdala activation. Functional connectivity analyses, intended to examine regions that significantly covaried with the amygdala, demonstrated that the amygdala covaried with different prefrontal regions for reappraisal and distraction, consistent with the distinct prefrontal regions observed to be activated during reappraisal versus distraction. Of note, participants reported decreased subjective experience of negative emotion using both strategies.

Another cognitive strategy that has been examined using neuroimaging research is *distancing* (Beauregard, Levesque, & Bourgouin, 2001; Kalisch et al., 2005). Male participants viewed erotic film clips while either passively viewing or voluntarily trying to inhibit sexual arousal. During inhibition of emotional responding, participants were encouraged to distance themselves from stimuli (i.e., to observe the scene in a detached manner). Passive viewing, which was associated with increased arousal ratings, resulted in activation in the right amygdala, right anterior temporal pole, and hypothalamus. However, attempted inhibition was associated with increased activation in right superior frontal gyrus and right anterior cingulate gyrus and was not associated with limbic activation (Beauregard et al., 2001). These results suggest that a regulatory circuit including prefrontal cortex and the amygdala are also implicated in emotion regulation associated with cognitive distancing.

In summary, intentional emotion regulation processes appear to operate by way of lateral prefrontal activations. For reappraisal, distraction, and distancing, these prefrontal activations have been accompanied by reduced amygdala activity and diminished distress responses. Suppression, however, has not been associated with reductions in either amygdala activity or distress.

Incidental Emotion Regulation and Contextual Modulation

Although often an intentional process, emotion regulation may also occur in the absence of awareness or explicit intent. Such regulation can be thought of as incidental in nature. Given that such effects have been observed in the context of processes that are effortful, but not aimed at regulation, we believe "incidental" is a more appropriate term than "automatic" or "implicit." Naturally, there is the question of whether it is appropriate to call something emotion regulation at all if it is not intentional, as emotion regulation does not seem to happen by accident.

There are several concomitants of emotion regulation, and it is reasonable to characterize a process as emotion regulation if it has all but one of these. Successful emotion regulation has been associated with changes in self-reported emotional experience, reduced physiological responses to threatening stimuli, increased lateral (usually ventrolateral) prefrontal activations, decreased limbic activity, negative correlations between prefrontal and limbic responses, and the awareness that one is trying to regulate one's emotions.

Labeling the affective component of something emotionally evocative (i.e., *affect labeling*) may be considered a form of incidental emotion regulation because all of the components of emotion regulation appear to be present, except for the awareness component. A number of studies have demonstrated the characteristic pattern of VLPFC increases, amygdala decreases, and inverse correlation between the two when people are shown an emotionally evocative image and asked to choose an affective word to characterize the picture, compared to when the same picture is shown but a nonaffect task is used (Hariri, Bookheimer, & Mazziotta, 2000; Lieberman et al., 2005, 2007; Payer, Lieberman, & London, 2011). Other studies have demonstrated physiological reductions in skin conductance associated with affect labeling (Kircanski, Lieberman, & Craske, in press; Tabibnia, Lieberman, & Craske, 2008). Finally, a recent dataset observed reliable reductions in self-reported distress associated with affect labeling (Lieberman, Inagaki, Tabibnia, & Crockett, 2011).

One recent paper (Payer, Baicy, Lieberman, & London, 2012) examined affect labeling and reappraisal within the same individuals, but on separate testing days. Using an anatomical region of interest (ROI) approach, Payer et al. found that the amygdala reductions due to affect labeling and reappraisal were highly correlated with one another (r = .77). Additionally, functional connectivity analyses were performed to identify regions that were inversely correlated with amygdala activity from moment to moment. This analysis identified a substantial cluster in right VLPFC common to both affect labeling and reappraisal. These analyses suggest that, within the same individuals, affect labeling sets in motion a similar set of processes as reappraisal. With affect labeling showing so many of the characteristics of an emotion regulation process, without awareness that labeling produces these effects (Lieberman et al., 2011), it is best characterized as incidental emotion regulation.

Other tasks have produced some of the characteristics of emotion regulation as well. For example, in a revised version of the emotional Stroop task, participants were asked to identify an emotional expression on a target emotional face (Egner, Etkin, Gale, & Hirsch, 2008; Etkin, Egner, Peraza, Kandel, & Hirsch, 2006). The faces were superimposed with irrelevant information, which was not needed to respond correctly and had the potential to be distracting. The superimposed information was either emotional or nonemotional, and either congruent or incongruent with the target emotional face. For example, a nonemotional congruent distracter would be the word "FEMALE" over a female happy face, and an emotional incongruent distracter would be the word "HAPPY" over a female fear face. Key effects were observed during incongruent trials in which participants were required to regulate their attention to incongruent distracters in order to respond correctly. The authors found that regulation of attention to emotional (as compared with nonemotional) distracters was related to increased rostral anterior cingulate cortex (rACC) activation and corresponding decreases in amygdala activity. It is not yet clear whether this constitutes a form of emotion regulation, as there have been no measures of physiological or experiential changes.

Another set of tasks is more properly characterized as *contextual modulation of affect*. In these studies, the stand-alone emotional significance of a stimulus differs as a function of the context in which it is found. In these tasks, prefrontal mechanisms seem to play a role in understanding the context, which in turn may alter limbic responses. For example, one study used surprised facial stimuli that were immediately preceded by either a positive or negative sentence that provided a context for the face (Kim et al., 2004). As demonstrated in prior work (Kim, Somerville, Johnstone, Alexander, & Whalen, 2003), surprised faces are ambiguous in nature and elicit individual differences when participants are asked to make valence judgments of them. When presented in the context of positive and negative sentences, Kim and colleagues (2004) observed increased amygdala activation to surprised faces in the context of negative compared with positive sentences and increased rACC activation for the opposite contrast (i.e., surprised faces in the context of a positive compared with negative context).

Similarly, Hare and colleagues (2005) demonstrated contextual modulation of amygdala responsivity to facial expressions in differing contexts. Specifically, an emotional go/no-go paradigm was employed, in which participants were told to press a button every time they saw a fearful face. The fearful faces were interspersed with either neutral or happy faces. The authors reported decreased amygdala activation to fearful faces in the context of happy faces (compared with neutral faces), with a simultaneous increase in VLPFC activation during fearful faces in the context of happy faces. Moreover, subsequent research using a similar emotional go/no-go paradigm demonstrated that a failure of the amygdala to habituate to emotional stimuli was associated with weaker functional connectivity between the amygdala and ventral prefrontal cortex (Hare et al., 2008).

Thus, there are a variety of ways that affect can be altered by other ongoing processes that are not deployed for the sake of regulation per se. Some of these are clearly a form of emotion regulation, and others currently fall into the category of affect modulation, but could be considered forms of emotion regulation depending on the results of future research.

CAPACITY VERSUS TENDENCY

Social cognitive neuroscience has identified the basic neural networks involved in a variety of socioemotional processes, including those reviewed here: the self, understanding others, emotion perception, emotional experience, and emotion regulation. As these are used increasingly in a translational context to probe schizophrenia and other psychopathologies, there is a critical distinction that is buried in all of this research.

All of the studies that have been conducted thus far have examined the *capacity* to perform a task and recruit particular neural regions when explicitly instructed to perform that task. In daily life, however, there are rarely experimenters inducing us to perform particular tasks, and thus our capacity, say, to engage in emotion regulation will only be useful to us to the extent that we have the *tendency* to use that ability without prompting. More critically to the study of psychopathology, deficits can affect capacities, tendencies, or both. Thus, task paradigms that exclusively focus on capacity may be unable to detect key neurocognitive deficits.

To give one example, consider empathy. In a recent study, Rameson, Morelli, and Lieberman (2012) presented individuals who were high or low in self-reported trait empathy with pictures of people in empathy-inducing situations (e.g., someone finding out they have cancer). In one condition, the capacity to enter an empathic state was tested by explicitly instructing participants to try to empathize with the targets as much as possible. Here, self-reported levels of empathic experience were the same for high- and low-trait empathy individuals. Similarly, there were no differences in neural activity—both groups showed robust activity in medial frontal regions associated with empathic processing.

In the second condition, no empathy instruction was given. Instead, participants were given a distraction task in which they had to memorize an 8-digit number while viewing the pictures. Because empathy was not explicitly induced in this condition, differential evidence of empathic processing would indicate differential tendencies to be empathic. In this condition, significant differences in experience and neural activity were observed between high- and low-trait empathy participants. Despite the distracting task and the lack of empathy instructions, high-trait empathy individuals produced just as much medial frontal activity as when they were instructed to empathize, but low-trait empathy individuals showed a dramatic drop-off in response.

Thus, these data suggest that high-trait empathy has more to do with everyday tendencies than does the capacity to be empathic. More generally, these data suggest that if paradigms include only the instructed condition, without another condition in which the participants have more freedom to respond in natural ways, important sources of variance are likely to be lost. Moreover, neuroimaging procedures that could be used to test whether an intervention has produced results might overlook successes if neurocognitive tendencies are not measured along with neurocognitive capacities.

CONCLUSION

This focused review has highlighted the distinctiveness of social and emotional information processing and demonstrated that a social cognitive neuroscience approach lends itself well to the study of key aspects of social cognition evidently disrupted in clinical populations. In particular, mapping of neural systems subserving complex social psychological phenomena, such as self-relevant and other-oriented information processing, emotion perception, and emotion regulation, reveals neural targets for investigation in schizophrenia. From basic brain mapping, the manner of inquiry in the field has begun to move forward, toward elucidating more precisely the nature of social cognition. This includes, for example, the differentiation between intentional and incidental processing and the tendency versus capacity to engage in such processes. Importantly, these more advanced lines of research allow for more accurate interpretations to be made when neural differences are seen in clinical populations. Although the field of neuroscience is clearly in nascent stage relative to other more established fields of psychology, our understanding of the social brain is rapidly advancing with this methodology. The continuous emergence of studies pushing the boundaries of which research questions we may ask with this approach ensures that our knowledge of basic science, as well as of psychopathology, will continue to advance and be further refined in years to come.

REFERENCES

Adolphs, R. (2003). Cognitive neuroscience of human social behavior. *Nature Reviews Neuroscience, 4*(3), 165–178.

Allison T., Puce A., & McCarthy, G. (2000). Social perception from visual cues: Role of the STS region. *Trends in Cognitive Science, 4*, 267–278.

Anderson, A., Christoff, K., Panitz, D., De Rosa, E., & Gabrieli, J. (2003). Neural correlates of the automatic processing of threat facial signals. *The Journal of Neuroscience, 23*(13), 5627–5633.

Apperly, I. A. (2008). Beyond Simulation–Theory and Theory–Theory: Why social cognitive neuroscience should use its own concepts to study "theory of mind". *Cognition, 107*, 266–283.

Baron-Cohen, S. (1989). The autistic child's theory of mind: A case of specific developmental delay. *The Journal of Child Psychology and Psychiatry, 30*(2), 285–297.

Baron-Cohen, S., Frith, U., & Leslie, A. M. (1985). Does the autistic child have a "theory of mind"? *Cognition, 21*, 37–46.

Beauregard, M., Levesque, J., & Bourgouin, P. (2001). Neural correlates of conscious self-regulation of emotion. *The Journal of Neuroscience, 21*, 6993–7000.

Blakemore, S. -J., & Frith, C. (2003). Self-awareness and action. *Current Opinion in Neurobiology, 13*, 219–224.

Bonda, E., Petrides, M., Ostry, D., & Evans, A. (1996). Specific involvement of human parietal systems and the amygdala in the perception of biological motion. *The Journal of Neuroscience, 16*(11), 3737–3744.

Bretherton, I., & Beeghly, M. (1982). Talking about internal states: The acquisition of an explicit theory of mind. *Developmental Psychology, 18*(6), 906–921.

Bullmore, E. T., Frangou, S., & Murray, R. M. (1997). The dysplastic net hypothesis: An integration of developmental and dysconnectivity theories of schizophrenia. *Schizophrenia Research, 28*(2–3), 143–156.

Calarge, C., Andreasen, N. C., & O'Leary, D. S. (2003). Visualizing how one brain understands another: A PET study of theory of mind. *American Journal of Psychiatry, 160*(11), 1954–1964.

Campos, J., Frankel, C., & Camras, L. (2004). On the nature of emotion regulation. *Child Development, 75*(2), 377–394.

Carrington, S. J., & Bailey, A. J. (2009). Are there theory of mind regions in the brain? A review of the neuroimaging literature. *Human Brain Mapping, 30*, 2313–2335.

Chao, L., Martin, A., & Haxby, J. (1999). Are face-responsive regions selective only for faces? *Neuroreport, 10*, 2945–2950.

Cloutier, J., Turk, D. J., & Macrae, C. N. (2008). Extracting variant and invariant information from faces: The neural substrates of gaze detection and sex categorization. *Social Neuroscience*, *3*(1), 69–78.

Critchley, H., Daly, E., Phillips, M., Brammer, M., Bullmore, E., Williams, S., et al. (2000). Explicit and implicit neural mechanisms for processing of social information from facial expressions: A functional magnetic resonance imaging study. *Human Brain Mapping*, *9*(2), 93–105.

Darwin, C. (1872/1998). *The expression of the emotions in man and animals* (pp. 55–69). Oxford, UK: Oxford University Press. (Original work published in 1872.)

David, N., Bewernick, B. H., Cohen, M. X., Newen, A., Lux, S., Fink, G. R., et al. (2006). Neural representations of self versus other: Visual–spatial perspective taking and agency in a virtual ball-tossing game. *Journal of Cognitive Neuroscience*, *18*(6), 898–910.

David, N., Cohen, M. X., Newen, A., Bewernick, B. H., Shah, N. J., Fink, G. R., et al. (2007). The extrastriate cortex distinguishes between the consequences of one's own and others' behavior. *NeuroImage*, *36*(3), 1004–1014.

David, N., Newen, A., & Vogeley, K. (2008). The "sense of agency" and its underlying cognitive and neural mechanisms. *Consciousness and Cognition*, *17*, 523–534.

Derntl, B., Finkelmeyer, A., Eickhoff, S., Kellermann, T., Falkenberg, D. I., Schneider, F., et al. (2010). Multidimensional assessment of empathic abilities: Neural correlates and gender differences. *Psychoneuroendocrinology*, *35*(1), 67–82.

Egner, T., Etkin, A., Gale, S., & Hirsch, J. (2008). Dissociable neural systems resolve conflict from emotional versus nonemotional distracters. *Cerebral Cortex*, *18*(6), 1475–1484.

Ekman, P. (1992). An argument for basic emotions. *Cognition and Emotion*, *6*, 169–200.

Ekman, P. (1993). Facial expression and emotion. *American Psychologist*, *48*, 376–379.

Engell, A., & Haxby, J. (2007). Facial expression and gaze-direction in human superior temporal sulcus. *Neuropsychologia*, *45*, 3234–3241.

Etkin, A., Egner, T., Peraza, D. M., Kandel, E. R., & Hirsch, J. (2006). Resolving emotional conflict: A role for the rostral anterior cingulated cortex in modulating activity in the amygdala. *Neuron*, *51*(6), 871–882.

Farrer, C., & Frith, C. D. (2002). Experiencing oneself vs another person as being the cause of an action: The neural correlates of the experience of agency. *NeuroImage*, *15*, 596–603.

Fletcher, P. C., Happe, F., Frith, U., Baker, S. C., Dolan, R. J., Frackowiak, R. S. J., et al. (1995). Other minds in the brain: A functional imaging study of "theory of mind" in story comprehension. *Cognition*, *57*, 109–128.

Fossati, P., Hevenor, S. J., Graham, S. J., Grady, C., Keightley, M. L., Craik, F., et al. (2003). In search of the emotional self: An fMRI study using positive and negative emotional words. *American Journal of Psychiatry*, *160*, 1938–1945.

Fox, C. J., Moon, S. Y., Iara, G., & Barton, J. J. (2009). The correlates of subjective perception of identity and expression in the face network: An fMRI adaptation study. *Neuroimage*, *44*, 569–580.

Friston, K. J., & Frith, C. D. (1995). Schizophrenia: A disconnection syndrome? *Clinical Neuroscience*, *3*(2), 89–97.

Frith, C. D., & Frith, U. (2006). The neural basis of mentalizing. *Neuron*, *50*, 531–534.

Gallagher, H. L., & Frith, C. D. (2003). Functional imaging of "theory of mind". *Trends in Cognitive Sciences 7*(2), 77–83.

Gallagher, H. L., Happe, F., Brunswick, N., Fletcher, P. C., Frith, U., & Frith, C. D. (2000). Reading the mind in cartoons and stories: An fMRI study of 'theory of mind' in verbal and nonverbal tasks. *Neuropsychologia, 38,* 11–21.

Gallagher, S. (2000). Philosophical conceptions of the self: Implications for cognitive science. *Trends in Cognitive Sciences, 4*(1), 14–21.

Gallese, V., & Goldman, A. (1998). Mirror neurons and the simulation theory of mind-reading. *Trends in Cognitive Sciences, 2*(12), 493–501.

Gallup, G. G., Jr., & Platek, S. M. (2002). Cognitive empathy presupposes self-awareness: Evidence from phylogeny, ontogeny, neuropsychology, and mental illness. *Behavioral and Brain Sciences, 25*(1), 36–37.

Ganel, T., Valyear, K., Goshen-Gottstein, Y., & Goodale, M. (2005). The involvement of the "fusiform face area" in processing facial expression. *Neuropsychologia, 43,* 1645–1654.

Gauthier, I., Skudlarski, P., Gore, J., & Anderson, A. (2000). Expertise for cars and birds recruits brain areas involved in face recognition. *Nature Neuroscience, 3*(2), 191–197.

Gillihan, S. J., & Farah, M. J. (2005). Is self special? A critical review of evidence from experimental psychology and cognitive neuroscience. *Psychological Bulletin, 131*(1), 76–97.

Gobbini, M. I., Koralek, A. C., Bryan, R. E., Montgomery, K. I., & Haxby, J. V. (2007). Two takes on the social brain: A comparison of theory of mind tasks. *Journal of Cognitive Neuroscience, 19*(11), 1803–1814.

Goldin, P. R., McRae, K., Ramel, W., & Gross, J. J. (2008). The neural bases of emotion regulation: Reappraisal and suppression of negative emotion. *Biological Psychiatry, 63*(6), 577–586.

Green, M. F. (1996). What are the functional consequences of neurocognitive deficits in schizophrenia? *American Journal of Psychiatry, 153*(3), 321–330.

Gross, J. J. (1998a). The emerging field of emotion regulation: An integrative review. *Review of General Psychology, 2,* 271–299.

Gross, J. J. (1998b). Antecedent- and response-focused emotion regulation: Divergent consequences for experience, expression, and physiology. *Journal of Personality & Social Psychology, 74,* 224–237.

Halgren, E., Dale, A., Sereno, M., Tootell, R., Marinkovic, K., et al. (1999). Location of human face-selective cortex with respect to retinotopic areas. *Human Brain Mapping, 7,* 29–37.

Happe´, F. G. E. (1994). An advanced test of theory of mind: Understanding of story characters' thoughts and feelings by able autistic, mentally handicapped, and normal children and adults. *Journal of Autism and Developmental Disorders, 24*(2), 129–154.

Hare, T. A., Tottenham, N., Davidson, M. C., Glover, G. H., & Casey, B. J. (2005). Contributions of amygdala and striatal activity in emotion regulation. *Biological Psychiatry, 57,* 624–632.

Hare, T. A., Tottenham, N., Galvan, A., Voss, H. U., Glover, G. H., & Casey, B. J. (2008). Biological substrates of emotional reactivity and regulation in adolescence during an emotional go-nogo task. *Biological Psychiatry, 63*(10), 927–934.

Hariri, A. R., Bookheimer, S. Y., & Mazziota, J. C. (2000). Modulating emotional responses: Effects of a neocortical network on the limbic system. *Neuroreport, 11,* 43–48.

Haxby, J., Hoffman, E., & Gobbini, M. (2000). The distributed human neural system for face perception. *Trends in Cognitive Sciences, 4*(6), 223–233.

Hein, G., & Knight, B. (2008). Superior temporal sulcus—It's my area: Or is it? *Journal of Cognitive Neuroscience, 20*(12), 2125–2136.

Heinrichs, R. W., & Zakzanis, K. K. (1998). Neurocognitive deficit in schizophrenia: A quantitative review of the evidence. *Neuropsychology, 12*(3), 426–445.

Hoff, A. L., Sakuma, M., Wieneke, M., Horon, R., Kushner, M., & DeLisi, L. E. (1999). Longitudinal neuropsychological follow-up study of patients with first-episode schizophrenia. *American Journal of Psychiatry, 156*(9), 1336–1341.

Hoffman, E. A., & Haxby, J. V. (2000). Distinct representations of eye gaze and identity in the distributed human neural system for face perception. *Nature Neuroscience, 3*(1), 80–84.

Holland, P., & Gallagher, M. (1999). Amygdala circuitry in attentional and representational processes. *Trends in Cognitive Sciences, 3*(2), 65–73.

Hooker, C., Paller, K., Gitelman, D., Parrish, T., Mesulam, M., et al. (2003). Brain networks for analyzing eye gaze. *Cognitive Brain Research, 17*, 406–418.

Iacoboni, M. (2009). Imitation, empathy, and mirror neurons. *Annual Review of Psychology, 60*, 653–670.

Iacoboni, M., Woods, R. P., Brass, M., Bekkering, H., Mazziotta, J. C., & Rizzolatti, G. (1999). Cortical mechanisms of human imitation. *Science, 286*, 2526–2528.

Ishai, A., Schmidt, C., & Boesiger, P. (2005). Face perception is mediated by a distributed cortical network. *Brain Research Bulletin, 67*, 87–93.

Jeannerod, M. (2004). Visual and action cues contribute to the self-other distinction. *Nature Neuroscience, 7*(5), 422–423.

Kalisch, R., Wiech, K., Critchley, H. D., Seymour, B., O'Doherty, J. P., Oakley, D. A., et al. (2005). Anxiety reduction through detachment: Subjective, physiological, and neural effects. *Journal of Cognitive Neuroscience, 17*, 874–883.

Kanske, P., Heissler, J., Schonfelder, S., Bongers, A., & Wessa, M. (2011). How to regulate emotion? Neural networks for reappraisal and distraction. *Cerebral Cortex, 21*(6), 1379–1388.

Kanwisher, N., McDermott, J., & Chun, M. (1997). The fusiform face area: A module in human extrastriate cortex specialized for face perception. *The Journal of Neuroscience, 17*, 4302–4311.

Kaplan, J. T., Aziz-Zadeh, L., Uddin, L. Q., & Iacoboni, M. (2008). The self across the senses: An fMRI study of self-face and self-voice recognition. *Social Cognitive and Affective Neuroscience, 3*, 218–223.

Karlsgodt, K. H., Sun, D., Jimenez, A. M., Lutkenhoff, E. S., Willhite, R., van Erp, T. G. M., et al. (2008). Developmental disruptions in neural connectivity in the pathophysiology of schizophrenia. *Development and Psychopathology, 20*, 1297–1327.

Keenan, J. P., & Wheeler, M. A. (2002). Elucidation of the brain correlates of cognitive empathy and self-awareness. *Behavioral and Brain Sciences, 25*(1), 40–41.

Kelley, W. M., Macrae, C. N., Wyland, C. L., Caglar, S., Inati, S., & Heatherton, T. F. (2002). Finding the self? An event-related fMRI study. *Journal of Cognitive Neuroscience, 14*(5), 785–794.

Kesler-West, M., Andersen, A., Smith, C., Avison, M., Davis, C., et al. (2001). Neural substrates of facial emotion processing using fMRI. *Cognitive Brain Research, 11*, 213–226.

Kim, H., Somerville, L. H., Johnstone, T., Alexander, A. L., & Whalen, P. J. (2003). Inverse amygdala and medial prefrontal cortex responses to surprised faces. *NeuroReport, 14*(18), 2317–2322.

Kim, H., Somerville, L. H., Johnstone, T., Polis, S., Alexander, A. L., Shin, L. M., & Whalen, P. J. (2004). Contextual modulation of amygdala responsivity to surprised faces. *Journal of Cognitive Neuroscience, 16*(10), 1730–1745.

Kircanski, K., Lieberman, M. D., & Craske, M. G. (in press). Feelings into words: Contributions of language to exposure therapy. *Psychological Science.*

Kircher, T. T. J., Senior, C., Phillips, M. L., Benson, P. J., Bullmore, E. T., Brammer, M., et al. (2000). Towards a functional neuroanatomy of self processing: Effects of faces and words. *Cognitive Brain Research, 10,* 133–144.

Krienen, F. M., Tu, P. C., & Buckner, R. L. (2010). Clan mentality: Evidence that the medial prefrontal cortex responds to close others. *The Journal of Neuroscience, 30*(41), 13906–13915.

Lane, R. D., Fink, G. R., Chau, P. M., & Dolan, R. J. (1997). Neural activation during selective attention to subjective emotional responses. *NeuroReport, 8,* 3969–3972.

Lane, R. D., Reiman, E. M., Ahern, G. L., Schwartz, G. E., & Davidson, R. J. (1997). Neuroanatomical correlates of happiness, sadness, and disgust. *American Journal of Psychiatry, 154,* 926–933.

LeDoux, J. E. (2000). Emotion circuits in the brain. *Annual Review of Neuroscience, 23,* 155–184.

Leube, D. T., Knoblich, G., Erb, M., Grodd, W., Bartels, M., & Kircher, T. T. (2003). The neural correlates of perceiving one's own movements. *NeuroImage, 20*(4), 2084–2090.

Liddle, P. F. (2000). Cognitive impairment in schizophrenia: Its impact on social functioning. *Acta Psychiatrica Scandinavica, 101,* 11–16.

Lieberman, M. D. (2007). Social cognitive neuroscience: A review of core processes. *Annual Review of Psychology, 58*(1), 259–289.

Lieberman, M. D. (2010). Social cognitive neuroscience. In S. T. Fiske, D. T. Gilbert, & G. Lindzey (Eds.), *Handbook of social psychology* (5th ed., pp. 143–193). New York: McGraw-Hill.

Lieberman, M. D., Eisenberger, N. I., Crockett, M. J., Tom, S. M., Pfeifer, J. H., & Way, B. M. (2007). Putting feelings into words: Affect labeling disrupts amygdala activity in response to affective stimuli. *Psychological Science, 18,* 421–428.

Lieberman, M. D., Hariri, A. R., Jarcho, J. M., Eisenberger, N. I., & Bookheimer, S. Y. (2005). An fMRI investigation of race-related amygdala activity in African-American and Caucasian-American individuals. *Nature Neuroscience, 8,* 720–722.

Lieberman, M. D., Inagaki, T. K., Tabibnia, G., & Crockett, M. J. (2011). Subjective responses to emotional stimuli during labeling, reappraisal, and distraction. *Emotion, 11*(3), 468–480.

Lombardo, M. V., Chakrabarti, B., Bullmore, E. T., Wheelwright, S. J., Sadek, S. A., Suckling, J., et al. (2009). Shared neural circuits for mentalizing about the self and others. *Journal of Cognitive Neuroscience, 22*(7), 1623–1635.

Lyons, K. E., & Koenig, M. A. (2013). The development of social cognition in theory and action. In D. L. Roberts & D. L. Penn (Eds.), *Social cognition in schizophrenia: From evidence to treatment* (Chapter 1). New York: Oxford University Press.

Maguire, E. A. (2001). Neuroimaging studies of autobiographical event memory. *Philosophical Transactions of the Royal Society B: Biological Sciences, 356,* 1441–1451.

Mason, M. F., Norton, M. I., Van Horn, J. D., Wegner, D. M., Grafton, S. T., & Macrae, C. N. (2007). Wandering minds: The default network and stimulus-independent thought. *Science, 315,* 393–395.

McCarthy, G., Puce, A., Belger, A., & Allison, T. (1999). Electrophysiological studies of human face perception II: Response properties of face-specific potentials generated in occipitotemporal cortex. *Cerebral Cortex, 9*(5), 431–444.

McCarthy, G., Puce, A., Gore, J. C., & Allison, T. (1997). Face-specific processing in the human fusiform gyrus. *Journal of Cognitive Neuroscience, 9*(5), 605–610.

Mitchell, J. P., Banaji, M. R., & Macrae, C. N. (2005). The link between social cognition and self-referential thought in the medial prefrontal cortex. *Journal of Cognitive Neuroscience, 17*(8), 1306–1315.

Mitchell, J. P., Macrae, C. N., & Banaji, M. R. (2006). Dissociable medial prefrontal contributions to judgments of similar and dissimilar others. *Neuron, 50*, 655–663.

Morawetz, C., Baudewig, J., Treue, S., & Dechent, P. (2011). Effects of spatial frequency and location of fearful faces on human amygdala activity. *Brain Research, 1371*, 87–99.

Morita, T., Itakura, S., Saito, D. N., Nakashita, S., Harada, T., Kochiyama, T., et al. (2008). The role of the right prefrontal cortex in self-evaluation of the face: A functional magnetic resonance imaging study. *Journal of Cognitive Neuroscience, 20*(2), 342–355.

Niedenthal, P. M., Mermillod, M., Maringer, M., & Hess, U. (2010). The Simulation of Smiles (SIMS) model: Embodied simulation and the meaning of facial expression. *Behavioral and Brain Sciences, 33*, 417–480.

Ochsner, K. N., Bunge, S. A., Gross, J. J., & Gabrieli, J. D. E. (2002). Rethinking feelings: An fMRI study of the cognitive regulation of emotion. *Journal of Cognitive Neuroscience, 14*(8), 1215–1229.

Panksepp, J. (2007). Neurologizing the psychology of affects: How appraisal-based constructivism and basic emotion theory can coexist. *Perspectives on Psychological Science, 2*, 281–296.

Payer, D. E., Baicy, K., Lieberman, M. D., & London, E.D. (2012). Overlapping neural substrates between intentional and incidental down-regulation of negative emotions. *Emotion, 12*(2), 229–235.

Payer, D. E., Lieberman, M. D., & London, E. D. (2011). Neural correlates of affect processing and aggression in methamphetamine dependence. *Archives of General Psychiatry, 68*(3), 271–282.

Peelen, M., Atkinson, A., & Vuilleumier, P. (2010). Supramodal representations of perceived emotions in the human brain. *The Journal of Neuroscience, 30*(30), 10127–10134.

Phillips, M. (2006). The neural basis of mood dysregulation in bipolar disorder. *Cognitive Neuropsychiatry, 11*(3), 233–249.

Platek, S. M., Keenan, J. P., Gallup, G. G., Jr., & Mohamed, F. B. (2004). Where am I? The neurological correlates of self and other. *Cognitive Brain Research, 19*, 114–122.

Platek, S. M., Thomson, J. W., & Gallup, G. G., Jr. (2004). Cross-modal self-recognition: The role of visual, auditory, and olfactory primes. *Consciousness and Cognition, 13*, 197–210.

Posner, M. (2001). Emotion and temperament. *Developmental Science, 4*(3), 313–329.

Powell, L. J., Macrae, C. N., Cloutier, J., Metcalfe, J., & Mitchell, J. P. (2009). Dissociable neural substrates for agentic versus conceptual representations of self. *Journal of Cognitive Neuroscience, 22*(10), 2186–2197.

Premack, D., & Woodruff, G. (1978). Does the chimpanzee have a theory of mind? *Behavioral and Brain Sciences, 4*, 515–526.

Preston, S. D., & deWaal, F. B. M. (2002). Empathy: Its ultimate and proximate bases. *Behavioral and Brain Sciences, 25*, 1–20.

Puce, A., Allison, T., Bentin, S., Gore, J. C., & McCarthy, G. (1998). Temporal cortex activation in humans viewing eye and mouth movements. *The Journal of Neuroscience, 18*(6), 2188–2199.

Rabin, J. S., Gilboa, A., Stuss, D. T., Mar, R. A., & Rosenbaum, R. S. (2009). Common and unique neural correlates of autobiographical memory and theory of mind. *Journal of Cognitive Neuroscience*, *22*(6), 1095–1111.

Rameson, L. T., Morelli, S. A., & Lieberman, M. D. (2012). The neural correlates of empathy: Experience, automaticity, and prosocial behavior. *Journal of Cognitive Neuroscience*, *24*(1), 235–245.

Rhodes, G., & McLean, I. (1990). Distinctiveness and expertise effects with homogeneous stimuli—towards a model of configural coding. *Perception*, *19*, 773–794.

Rossion, B., Caldara, R., Seghier, M., Schuller, A., Lazeyras, F., & Mayer, E. (2003). A network of occipito-temporal face-sensitive areas besides the right middle fusiform gyrus is necessary for normal face processing. *Brain*, *126*, 2381–2395.

Russell, J. A. (2003). Core affect and the psychological construction of emotion. *Psychological Review*, *110*, 145–172.

Ruby, P., & Decety, J. (2001). Effect of subjective perspective taking during simulation of action: A PET investigation of agency. *Nature Neuroscience*, *4*, 546–550.

Sabatinelli, D., Fortune, E., Li, Q., Siddiqui, A., Krafft, C., Oliver, W., et al. (2011). Emotional perception: Meta-analyses of face and natural scene processing. *Neuroimage*, *54*, 2524–2533.

Saxe, R., & Powell, L. J. (2006). It's the thought that counts: Specific brain regions for one component of theory of mind. *Psychological Science*, *17*(8), 692–699.

Saxe, R., Moran, J. M., Scholz, J., & Gabrieli, J. (2006). Overlapping and non-overlapping brain regions for theory of mind and self reflection in individual subjects. *Social Cognitive and Affective Neuroscience*, *1*, 229–234.

Saxe, R., Schulz, L. E., & Jiang, Y. V. (2006). Reading minds versus following rules: Dissociating theory of mind and executive control in the brain. *Social Neuroscience*, *1*(3–4), 284–298.

Saxe, R., Xiao, D., Kovacs, G., Perrett, D., & Kanwisher, N. (2004). A region of right posterior superior temporal sulcus responds to observed intentional actions. *Neuropsychologia*, *42*, 1435–1446.

Sergent, J., Ohta, S., & MacDonald, B. (1992). Functional neuroanatomy of face and object processing. *Brain*, *115*, 15–36.

Siegal, M., & Varley, R. (2002). Neural systems involved in 'theory of mind'. *Nature Reviews Neuroscience*, *3*, 463–471.

Spangler, S., Schwarzer, G., Korell, M., & Maier-Karius, J. (2010). The relationships between processing facial identity, emotional expression, facial speech, and gaze direction during development. *Journal of Experimental Child Psychology*, *105*, 1–19.

Spence, S. A., Brooks, D. J., Hirsch, S. R., Liddle, P. F., Meehan, J., & Grasby, P. M. (1997). A PET study of voluntary movement in schizophrenic patients experiencing passivity phenomena (delusions of alien control). *Brain*, *120*, 1997–2011.

Sprengelmeyer, R., Rausch, M., Eysel, U., & Przuntek. (1998). Neural structures associated with recognition of facial expressions of basic emotions. *Proceedings of the Royal Society of London*, *265*, 1927–1931.

Spunt, R. P., & Lieberman, M. D. (2012). An integrative model of the neural systems supporting the comprehension of observed emotional behavior. *Neuroimage*, *59*, 3050–3059.

Stone, V. E., Baron-Cohen, S., & Knight, R. T. (1998). Frontal lobe contributions to theory of mind. *Journal of Cognitive Neuroscience*, *10*(5), 640–656.

Tabibnia, G., Lieberman, M. D., & Craske, M. G. (2008). The lasting effect of words on feelings: Words may facilitate exposure effects to threatening images. *Emotion*, *8*(3), 307–317.

Tarr, M., & Gauthier, I. (2000). FFA: A flexible fusiform area for subordinate-level visual processing automatized by expertise. *Nature Neuroscience, 3*(8), 764–769.

Taylor, M. A., & Abrams, R. (1984). Cognitive impairment in schizophrenia. *American Journal of Psychiatry, 141*(2), 196–201.

Van Overwalle, F. (2009). Social cognition and the brain: A meta-analysis. *Human Brain Mapping, 30,* 829–858.

Van Overwalle, F., & Baetens, K. (2009). Understanding others' actions and goals by mirror and mentalizing systems: A meta-analysis. *NeuroImage, 48,* 564–584.

Vogeley, K., Bussfeld, P., Newen, A., Herrmann, S., Happé, F., Falkai, P., et al. (2001). Mind reading: Neural mechanisms of theory of mind and self-perspective. *NeuroImage, 14*(1), 170–181.

Vuilleumier, P., & Pourtois, G. (2007). Distributed and interactive brain mechanisms during emotion face perception: Evidence from functional neuroimaging. *Neuropsychologia, 45,* 174–194.

Vytal, K., & Hamann, S. (2010). Neuroimaging support for discrete neural correlates of basic emotions: A voxel-based meta-analysis. *Journal of Cognitive Neuroscience, 22*(12), 2864–2885.

Whalen, P., Shin, L., McInerney, S., Fischer, H., Wright, C., & Rauch, S. (2001). A functional MRI study of human amygdala responses to facial expression of fear versus anger. *Emotion, 1,* 70–83.

Wechsler, D. (1958). *The measurement and appraisal of adult intelligence* (4th ed.). Baltimore: Williams and Wilkins.

Wimmer, H., & Perner, J. (1983). Beliefs about beliefs: Representation and constraining function of wrong beliefs in young children's understanding of deception. *Cognition, 13,* 103–128.

Winston, J. S., Henson, R. N. A., Fine-Goulden, M. R., & Dolan, R. J. (2004). fMRI-adaptation reveals dissociable neural representations of identity and expression in face perception. *Journal of Neurophysiology, 92,* 1830–1839.

Zahavi, D. (2008). Simulation, projection and empathy. *Consciousness and Cognition, 17*(2), 514–522.

Zinck, A. (2008). Self-referential emotions. *Consciousness and Cognition, 17,* 496–505.

5

Social Cognitive Neuroscience

Clinical Foundations

OANA TUDUSCIUC AND RALPH ADOLPHS ■

HISTORICAL CONTEXT

The social sciences have focused on every aspect of human behavior that deal particularly with conspecifics, encompassing fields ranging from psychology to anthropology and economics. Our knowledge has evolved with time, but has taken a particular leap forward in the past several decades with the advent of modern cognitive neuroscience tools, most notably neuroimaging, thus giving rise to the field of social cognitive neuroscience. Most of the questions historically in the realm of philosophy or, more recently, psychology, are now being addressed by social cognitive neuroscience: How do we process memories of people? How do we recognize faces and their expressions? How do we make economic and political choices? And, more broadly, which of these social abilities are disproportionate or even unique to humans as compared to other animals, which are domain-specific and rely on specialized neural circuitry, which develop at what points in time, and, most pertinent to this volume, which are dysfunctional in mental illnesses such as schizophrenia?

PSYCHOLOGICAL APPROACHES

Philosophy of mind is the historical approach to understanding how we guide our interactions with other people and how we think about what is going on in their minds. Tracing its roots back to 400–500 BC, two distinct schools of philosophical thought co-existed until the 19th century, differing mainly in their view of the mind–body problem. Whereas dualists such as Plato believed the mind to be distinct from the body, with some variations, monists such as Parmenides took a position based on the unity of Nature. These initial ontological views, in turn, influenced how people thought about the relationship between the study of the mind and the study of the rest of nature: From one view, psychology should have a proprietary vocabulary and approach since its subject matter is distinct from all others; from another view, the study of the mind needed eventually to be commensurate with, or even reduced to, the study of the biological, chemical, and physical components of which it was made. Ideas such as Piaget's constructivist theory (Piaget, 1953), on the one hand, or the conditioned reflexes that Pavlov (1927) studied and that formed the basis of behaviorism (Pavlov, 1927), on the other, emerged as pioneering attempts in scientific psychology. The late 19th and early 20th centuries saw the development of behaviorism, psychoanalysis, and gestalt theory, with ideas set by B.F. Skinner (who assumed that modifying patterns of behavior was the only way to treat psychological disorders), Freud (who relied on introspection to explain them), and von Ehrenfels (who argued that the brain is a holistic entity, which perceives a more complex image of its surroundings than expected by just adding together all the components of its input). Several of these were in clear opposition: Contra behaviorism, constructivism took into account the mind's ability to filter the input from the outside world at the level of perception, and constructivists shaped the idea that internal states, feelings, and beliefs can and do influence the way we perceive the world. For instance, Piaget's genetic epistemology, which posits that knowledge is a biological function resulting from the actions of an individual (Piaget, 1953), largely fails to take into account individual filters and processing mechanisms for otherwise identical external input, thus failing to explain how we can infer new concepts based on rules and experience, but that are novel to the brain that produces them.

A more systematic and comprehensive study of the social aspect of human behavior was initiated with the so-called cognitive revolution, which argued against behaviorism in particular and was based on the idea that the brain functions and can be understood in many respects like computers, transforming inputs to outputs through rules (programs) whose elucidation was the task of the sciences of the mind (Chomsky, 1964). First articulated as a critique to Skinner's behaviorist theory, this view eventually led the way for combining evolutionary theory with psychology and was followed by the development of evolutionary psychology (Cosmides & Tooby, 1997). Taking into account innate information processing systems, along with the reverse-engineering of the psychological mechanisms that they ultimately underlie, has allowed psychologists to ask not only how a particular cognitive ability may be hard-wired in the brain, but also why and how it evolved to be so. This, in turn, holds out the promise for truly naturalizing psychology, linking the mind to the brain through a specification of how adaptive behavior and cognition evolved.

Within this framework, social psychology has focused on studying the influence of other people on our thoughts, beliefs, and behavior. As an example, after observing that children exposed to adult aggressive behavior are more likely to act aggressively (Bandura, Ross & Ross, 1961) in his famous "Bobo doll" experiments, Bandura proposed a social learning theory, which evolved into a framework for explaining the role of cognitive processes in determining human motivation and action (Ozer & Bandura, 1990). Combining social and cognitive approaches in psychology has resulted in a field that takes into account the processing of any information, external or internal, leading to the perception, thinking about, and acting toward, other people: in short, social cognition. Such social information processing can relate to the way we perceive another person and to the implicit biases we have of other people, as well as to how these are modulated by context and individual differences.

In social psychology, the term "person perception" refers to the different mental processes that we use to form impressions of other people. This includes not just a description of the cues and sensory processing on the basis of which we form these impressions, but also the varied inferences, biases, and stereotypes that come into play. The sense of being able to enter other minds and learn what they have to offer (attunement) is a ubiquitously strong and subjective conviction (Morsella, Gray et al., 2009). Perceiving someone else might give us insufficient information to get a deep evaluation of their character but enough information to form an expectation of such character based on previous experiences we might have had with people we would assign to the same category—the basis of biases and stereotypes. For instance, we might automatically assume that a painter must be eccentric, simply because we know a couple of painters, who are both rather eccentric. When making such an assumption, we are biased by our previous experience, an implicit attribution that is not necessarily true (Greenwald & Banaji, 1995) but which our past experience renders as highly probable. Finally, the way we infer other people's state of mind must take into account the context in which we find the relevant information. The notion that our perception depends on the context in which the information is presented was studied by the constructive perception theorists. For instance, if asked to look for a particular feature in a photograph, participants exhibit longer reaction times to find the target in a jumbled real-world scene than in the same, but unmodified, scene (Biederman, 1972). This introduced the idea that cognitive use of sensory information was necessary to construct a completed perception; in other words, that a previous notion of what a particular stimulus should look like has an influence on the perception of that stimulus. That is why, in a relatively dark room, even when there is not enough light to activate the cones (the color receptors on the retina) but only the rods (used for night vision, but incapable of carrying information about color), bananas will nonetheless seem yellow and cherries red (Palmer, Simone et al., 1988).

In terms of this general processing picture, the challenge for understanding mental illness is to specify the level of processing at which dysfunction may occur. The best approach here is to combine all possible sources of data: Psychological and neurobiological data should be exploited broadly, as all can give clues to the level of the deficit. Is there an abnormal input signal already at the level of the retina or early visual regions of the brain? Is there an abnormal inference based on a normal perceptual signal? Are there abnormal links to memory, abnormal control of interfering processes, or abnormal connection to decision-making and behavioral output? Of course, answers to these questions may never be clear-cut because the deficit may occur at many levels, but phrasing the questions in this way permits specific hypotheses to be tested at the process level and specific neural structures to be investigated.

NEUROSCIENCE APPROACHES

Current cognitive neuroscience tools are extremely varied in their ease of application to humans, their resolution in space and time, their cost, and the kind of conclusions they permit. At one extreme are lesion studies (see below for a classic example), which allow stronger causal inferences than do studies using electroencephalography (EEG) or functional magnetic resonance imaging (fMRI) (notably, one can say that damage to a specific structure caused the deficit, and that, therefore, this structure is normally necessary for that function; one cannot conclude, however, that the lesioned structure normally causes the function or behavior under investigation, a conclusion that requires a sort of complement to lesions, such as focal electrical stimulation). Historically, lesion studies have, without question, provided the greatest insights, ranging from Broca's patient Tan to Phineas Gage to modern cases such as patients H. M. and S. M. Each of these provided key insights into language, decision-making, declarative memory, and facial emotion recognition, respectively; each has been followed-up in much greater detail today using fMRI and other methods. What is the current state of the art? This is a hard question to answer in humans, although one should probably say that it is a combination of several methods, such as fMRI in conjunction with EEG or magnetoencephalography (MEG), permitting precise correlational mapping of structure–function relationships with the best spatial and temporal resolution possible: Where and when is a specific process implemented in the brain. Nonetheless, none of these methods permits strong causal inferences, and all lack resolution at anything close to the level of single neurons or even assemblies of neurons. However, in animals (currently primarily transgenic rodents, but to some extent also monkeys using viral vectors), the state of the art is undoubtedly optogenetics, a technique that permits precise manipulation of genetically identified populations of neurons with millisecond precision. The answer to our original question is therefore likely to be that lesion studies, EEG, fMRI, and other approaches in humans should all be carried out, and they need to be combined with optogenetic studies in animal models. Only through a combination of these varied approaches will we really be able to dissect the neural circuitry of social cognition, in both health and disease.

The classic case study of how the lesion method helped to elucidate an aspect of social cognition is that of Phineas Gage, a railroad worker, whose case was documented in detail from reports at the time (see MacMillan [2000] for a good account of this case and the complexities involved) (Figure 5.1). In September 1848, in Vermont, an explosion drove a metal rod completely through Gage's head, destroying his left frontal lobe. After this accident, his social behavior was radically altered, so that, from a man known as reliable and well mannered, he became one unable to carry out any task beyond the point of planning it and

seemed to have difficulties especially in regard to emotional and social functioning (Damasio, Grabowski et al., 1994). More recently, in patients with bilateral ventromedial prefrontal cortex lesions, overlapping in part with the lesion
that Gage suffered, severe difficulties in real-world behavior, and notably social
behavior, have been described. Whereas these patients often had an entirely
normal profile on standard neuropsychological tests of IQ, memory, language,
and perception, they are invariably impaired in social interaction. Antonio
Damasio's "somatic marker hypothesis" was one of the first theories to explain

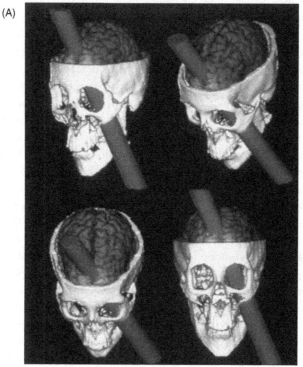

Figure 5.1 Lesions of the human orbitofrontal cortex. (A) The case of Phineas Gage, as
reconstructed by Hanna Damasio. The path of the tamping iron through Gage's brain
was reconstructed from the known dimensions of the iron, from measurements of
Gage's skull and the hole within it, and from descriptions of the accident. From Damasio,
Grabowski, Frank, Galaburda, & Damasio (1994). The return of Phineas Gage: clues
about the brain from the skull of a famous patient. The American Association for the
Advancement of Science. Reprinted with permission from AAAS. (B) Overlap representation of lesions from patients with bifrontal tumor resections who all share a behavioral
profile similar to that reported for Gage. In general, their lesions are more restricted
than Gage's, but, in all cases, they include ventral and medial regions of the prefrontal
cortex. Damage to these regions leads to a constellation of impaired emotional response,
lack of remorse, poor planning for the future, and impulsive behavior, dubbed "acquired
sociopathy." (From Bechara, Tranel, & Damasio, 2002. The somatic marker hypothesis
and decision-making. F. Boller & J. Grafman (Eds.), *Handbook of neuropsychology:
Frontal lobes* (Vol. 7, 2nd ed., pp. 117–143). Amsterdam: Elsevier.)

(B)

Subjects with acquired sociopathy (n=9)

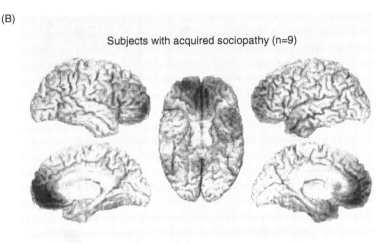

Figure 5.1 (Continued)

the constellation of impairments seen in real life with the findings from the lab: It postulated that damage to a specific sector of the prefrontal cortex, the ventromedial region, disconnected the otherwise normal perception of the patients from their ability to trigger emotional responses that would guide cognition and behavior (Damasio, 1994). The result of this disconnection was that, when confronted with complex, and perhaps especially social, situations, these patients were unable to guide the choices based on how they felt about the contemplated outcomes. The story of Phineas Gage, no doubt familiar to many readers, is a particularly compelling example of how an early (in this case, very early, even before the advent of MRI) lesion case eventually culminated in a specific theory in social neuroscience and spawned a host of other studies (using fMRI and other approaches). As with all historical cases, the actual findings have turned out to be vastly more complicated, but it nonetheless serves to illustrate a general line of approach: find a compelling and clear dissociation following a brain lesion, hypothesize the mechanism that explains this, then test the hypothesis with more refined methods.

Another, more recent, example comes from studies of a rare condition (Urbach-Wiethe disease) that causes calcification of the amygdala and can lead to bilateral amygdala damage, with affected people having difficulty recognizing fear in faces or even experiencing it, and thus being abnormally trustful of others (Adolphs, Tranel et al., 1994, 1998; Feinstein, Adolphs, Damasio, & Tranel, 2011) (Figure 5.2). In this example (discussed in more detail below), the initial lesion studies were notable for their anatomical specificity, unlike the case with Phineas Gage. Both of these examples highlight brain regions of intense interest also to those studying the neural basis of psychiatric disorders: The ventromedial prefrontal cortex and the amygdala are known to be connected, are now thought of as two components of a network that processes the value of stimuli, and have been implicated in psychopathy, depression, anxiety disorders, autism, and schizophrenia.

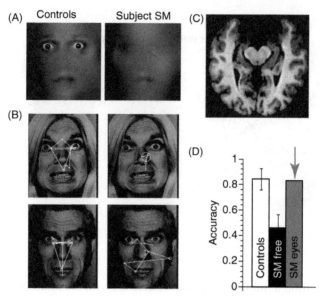

Figure 5.2 Lesions of the human amygdala. Bilateral amygdala lesions impair the use of the eyes and gaze to the eyes during emotion judgment. (A) A patient with bilateral damage to the amygdala made significantly less use of information from the eye region of faces when judging emotion. (B) While looking at whole faces, the patient (right column of images) exhibited abnormal face gaze, making far fewer fixations to the eyes than did controls (left column of images). This was observed across emotions (free viewing, emotion judgment, gender discrimination). (C) Magnetic resonance imaging scan of the patient's brain whose lesion was relatively restricted to the entire amygdala, a very rare lesion in humans. The two round black regions near the top middle of the image are the lesioned amygdalae. (D) When the subject was instructed to look at the eyes ("SM eyes," *arrow*) in a whole face, she could do this, resulting in a remarkable recovery in ability to recognize the facial expression of fear. The findings show that an apparent role for the amygdala in processing fearful facial expressions is in fact more abstract and involves the detection and attentional direction onto features that are socially informative. (Modified from Adolphs, R. et al. (2005). A mechanism for impaired fear recognition after amygdala damage. *Nature, 433,* 68–72.)

Complementing lesion studies with functional imaging in healthy individuals has revealed a network of brain areas that participate in social information processing. Returning to our initial processing outline, these can be divided into regions primarily concerned with social perception, in turn feeding into those concerned with associating those perceptions with other social knowledge, including the value of the stimuli and the possible actions toward them, to executing social behaviors toward the social stimuli. This simple perception-cognition-action scheme is, of course, importantly modulated by context and cognitive control, two modulating sets of processes in which there are large individual differences and that likely contribute importantly to psychiatric illness. A brief overview of some of the structures that come into play in such a scheme is shown in Figure 5.3.

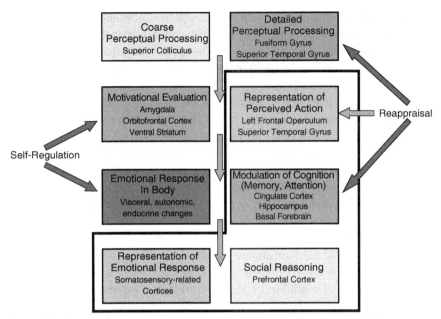

Figure 5.3 Processes and structures involved in social cognition. Several of the components contribute to social knowledge. Reappraisal and self-regulation are particular modes of feedback modulation (there will be others) whereby evaluation and emotional response to social stimuli can be volitionally influenced. (From Adolphs, R. (2003). Cognitive neuroscience of human social behavior. *Nature Reviews Neuroscience, 4*(3), 165–178.)

SOCIAL COGNITION IN THE DEVELOPING BRAIN

One way to understand the mechanisms of social cognition is to study the brains of people at the social extremes. This includes, on the one hand, autism spectrum disorders (ASD), which manifest with diminished social skills, avoidance of social contact, and high interest in nonsocial stimuli, and, on the other, Williams syndrome (WMS), which translates to overly social behavior ("hypersociability"), although it should be noted that this is certainly not merely an increase of normal social behaviors.

Autism

Autism spectrum disorders are neurodevelopmental conditions diagnosed on the basis of three major classes of behavioral impairments: social interaction (lack of social reciprocity, lack of eye-to-eye gaze, and lack of using multiple nonverbal behaviors to regulate social interaction), communication (delay or total lack of spoken language, marked impairment to initiate and sustain a conversation, lack of spontaneous and varied make-believe play), and restricted interests/repetitive behaviors (apparently inflexible adherence to specific, nonfunctional routines or rituals; motor mannerisms; persistent preoccupation with parts of objects). No single kind of abnormal behavior seems to be specific to autism, but only autism appears to have an elevated pattern of occurrence and severity of these behaviors (Bodfish, Symons et al., 2000).

Childhood ASDs include a wide range of social impairments, with some children highly functional and able to live independent lives, albeit with some awkward interaction with other people, and some children so severely impaired that they could never hope to live without substantial help from their families. However, one social skill that seems to be impaired in all of these children is the ability to attribute mental states to others (Leslie & Frith, 1987). This observation led to one of the best known theories of autism; namely, that these people have a deficit in their ability to construct a representation of other minds (Baron-Cohen, Leslie et al., 1985; Frith & Happe, 1994).

Although the basic mechanisms are still largely unknown, and the exact nature of the impairment is not yet understood, the idea that there is a domain-specific impairment in social cognition in ASD has attracted a lot of attention. There is fairly good evidence for both structural and functional abnormalities in structures thought to be concerned with processing social information, perhaps investigated most extensively in regard to face processing and structures such as the amygdala and temporal cortex (Pelphrey, Adolphs, & Morris, 2004). There is also good neuropsychological evidence that this domain of processing seems to be disproportionately impaired in otherwise high-functioning people with autism, and, indeed, in their first-degree relatives to some extent (Losh et al., 2009).

Although the hypothesis that ASD features disproportionately impaired social cognition accounts well for the social deficits in autism, it fails to explain the repetitive behaviors or restricted interests that are part of the phenotype. One attempt at linking these two domains of impairment in ASD is Baron-Cohen's "extreme male brain" hypothesis, which is based on the idea that autism features an imbalance in systematizing and empathizing, with a decrease in empathizing ability and a concomitant increase in systemizing skills (Baron-Cohen, 2002).

Another theory, coined "weak central coherence," attempts to account for the nonsocial behaviors of autism by arguing that the information processing style is different in people with ASD: They focus intensely on details, at the expense of ignoring the context and the "big picture" of the input information (Happe, 1999). In typically developing children, a strong central coherence allows them to take in information with its context, thus processing the big picture, at the expense of memory and detail. Thus, the restricted interests and obsession with detail that is seen in ASD seem to find an explanation, but the theory cannot really explain the impaired social interaction.

Another theory, although not based on a feature of the diagnostic criteria per se, is that executive dysfunction underlies many of the impairments in ASD, an idea based in part on the parallel between the impairments observed in patients with frontal lobe damage and some of the symptoms of autism, such as rigidity and perseveration. Indeed, children with autism seem to have planning deficits;

for instance, when faced with a complex planning task like the Tower of Hanoi (Bennetto, Pennington et al., 1996; Ozonoff & Jensen, 1999). They also lack cognitive flexibility, as evidenced by their inability to switch rules in the Wisconsin Card Sorting Task, when the criterion for sorting the cards suddenly changes in the game (Prior & Hoffmann, 1990), and they show dysfunctional inhibition of a prepotent response, such as not pointing to the desired reward in order to obtain it (Hughes, Russell et al., 1994). In this latter study, children with autism were presented with two boxes, one empty and the other visibly containing a reward (chocolate). In order for them to get the chocolate, they had to point to the empty box, but were unable to do so, probably due to an inability to suppress the prepotent impulse of pointing to the desired box. Additionally, children with autism seem to be impaired in self-monitoring functions, as evidenced by impaired motor estimation (Hermelin & O'Connor, 1975), error correction, and avoidance (Russell & Jarrold, 1998).

All in all, each of these hypotheses about the nature of the fundamental cognitive deficit that underlies autism is still alive and under investigation, although some more so than others. It seems unlikely that any of them in isolation will be able to account for the full pattern of impairments seen, thus raising important questions about the specificity of both the cognitive impairment and its underlying dysfunctional neural substrate (Happe et al., 2001).

Williams Syndrome

Entirely genetic in etiology, WMS describes children who appear very interested in social interaction, but are severely impaired in several nonsocial domains, particularly visuospatial processing. Caused by a hemizygous deletion of almost 26 genes from the long arm of chromosome 7 that occurs during meiosis (del7q11.23), WMS is a rare disorder, affecting about 1 in 10,000 children. The deletion includes the gene for elastin, a protein that contributes to the elasticity of blood vessels and connective tissue, which results in the particular appearance of affected individuals: long philtrum, sunken nasal bridge, and small and widely spaced teeth, as well as in some of their frequently associated complications, such as high blood pressure, cardiac disease, and hypercalcemia. In contrast to their cheerfulness and "cocktail party" personality, children with WMS are developmentally delayed, have mild to moderate mental retardation, and are impaired in their spatial skills. Showing an almost opposite social behavioral pattern to children with ASD, children with WMS offer a research path toward understanding the apparent modularity of social cognition (Karmiloff-Smith, 1995). Similar to patients with bilateral amygdala damage, they also seem to judge other people as much more approachable than do normally developing controls (Bellugi, Adolphs et al., 1999). Furthermore, it seems that their surprisingly good verbal skills are driven by a genetically determined hypersociability, complemented by an apparent lack of social fear, as suggested by studies showing that even preverbal infants with WMS display an uncharacteristic attraction toward any and all individuals,

in contrast to the stranger anxiety that keeps typically developing children cling-
ing to their mothers in the presence of strangers (Korenberg, Chen et al., 2000;
Doyle, Bellugi et al., 2004).

Williams syndrome is associated with a relative increase in amygdala volume
relative to intracranial volume as compared to age-matched controls (Capitao,
Sampaio et al., 2011) and a decreased volume of parietal regions involved in spatial cognition (Meyer-Lindenberg et al., 2004). Functional imaging studies show
that normally developing children activate the amygdala when inferring the mental states of people from photographs of their eyes (Baron-Cohen, Ring et al.,
1999), a task that is easily mastered by children with WMS, but difficult or impossible for children with ASD (Baron-Cohen, Jolliffe et al., 1997; Tager-Flusberg,
Boshart et al., 1998). Regions of the temporal lobe involved in face processing also
show clear functional abnormalities in both ASD and WMS (Meyer-Lindenberg
et al., 2005).

Comparing disorders at the two extremes of the social spectrum has provided
insights into the mechanisms and brain structures involved in the processing of
social information, while at the same time opening up questions about the heterogeneity of the social impairments and the need to consider the triad of behavioral
impairments that define autism as separate entities that may arise dissociably of
each other (Happe, Ronald, & Plomin, 2006). Given the strictly genetic etiology
and well-defined behavioral characteristics of WMS, in contrast to the continuum
of impairments that define ASD, it seems reasonable that a varied and heterogeneous etiological background (combining identified genetic variants with environmental stressors) would have an equally varied and heterogeneous behavioral
profile that might produce repetitive behaviors in the presence of normal communication and social interaction skills, or isolated impairments in social interaction
in the absence of a communication disorder. Indeed, a twin study on a large population suggests that there may be many individuals with isolated impairments in
one aspect of the triad who show difficulties of comparable severity to people with
autism although they do not meet diagnostic criteria for any recognized disorder
(Ronald, Happe et al., 2006).

One intriguing possibility suggested by developmental disorders such as autism
and WMS is that the origin of an impaired profile of putatively "cognitive" abilities
may, in fact, better be thought of as motivational rather than cognitive. In ASD,
this idea has been discussed for some time (Dawson, Meltzoff, Osterling, Rinaldi,
& Brown, 1998; Klin, Jones, Schultz, Volkmar, & Cohen, 2002). The basic picture
is that an early failure to find social stimuli rewarding in turn results in reduced
motivation to attend to social stimuli and to engage in reciprocal social behaviors
with other people. This would then result in an abnormal developmental exposure
to social stimuli, and hence an abnormal ability for social cognition due to this
reduced experience. Disentangling such motivational accounts from more purely
cognitive ones is an important future challenge for neuropsychiatry, and one that
is now being facilitated by sophisticated models and tools from reward learning
and neuroeconomics used to investigate the distinction. This issue also connects
back to what we mentioned earlier: Understanding aspects of social dysfunction

will require specifying the stage of information processing that is dysfunctional. Detailed dissection of this sort has helped to distinguish some disorders; for instance, schizophrenia and autism were found to be distinguishable in aspects of social orienting (measured using eye tracking) to complex stimuli, depending on whether faces were present in the stimuli (Sasson et al., 2007).

BRAIN AREAS INVOLVED IN SOCIAL COGNITION

The Social Brain

Comparative anatomy shows that primates have larger brains than those of all other mammals relative to their body size (Allman, McLaughlin et al., 1993), thus raising the question of what evolutionary pressure and adaptations might account for this. Possibilities range from general complex problem solving to more domain-specific abilities such as tool use, language, and social cognition. The evolution of large brains seems poorly justified by general ecological strategies for more complex problem solving, and tool use and language appear too narrowly present. The theory that emerged in the late 1980s to answer this question was that large brains evolved in primates to reflect the complexity of social interactions faced and, in particular, their competitive nature (Whiten, Byrne et al., 1991). The bigger groups that primates lived in provided protection from predators; through more eyes to keep watch and safety in numbers, these large groups provided for defense. At the same time, the bigger groups meant that members had to strike a balance between their individual needs and the needs of the group, and had to develop tools to understand the position, behavior, and intentions of other group members in order to successfully negotiate their place within the group. It is this need for understanding and navigating complex social relationships that may have endowed primates with larger brains, and there is evidence that the size of the group correlates with the size of neocortex (more specifically, the ratio of neocortex to the rest of the brain) (Dunbar, 2009). It is precisely the capacity to perceive dispositions and intentions about others that distinguishes primate behavior from that of other mammals (Brothers, 1989). Although nonsocial processing pathways can and do make sense of the direction in which another individual is moving, its size, or its speed, it is the ability of the brain to perceive socially relevant information and use this as the basis for social inferences and cognition that has prompted researchers to look for the structures that form the social brain.

The processes that allow us to infer the dispositions and intentions of others are closely related to those with which we think about ourselves and regulate our own behavior, and the brain structures involved show considerable overlap as well. Social cognition and self-relevant processing have thus been found to share considerable processes and structures in common and are frequently investigated together. These mechanisms have been proposed to draw on four psychological components that may be relatively modular: self-awareness, theory of mind (ToM), threat detection, and self-regulation (Heatherton, 2011).

The first module, self-awareness, relies on the activity of a network that includes the medial prefrontal cortex, as well as the adjacent ventral anterior cingulate cortex (Harter, Waters et al., 1998; Pfeifer, Lieberman et al., 2007). Being able to infer another individual's beliefs and judgments (ToM, the second component) relies on nearby but more dorsal regions of the medial prefrontal cortex, together with the temporoparietal junction (TPJ), temporal poles, and medial parietal cortex (Amodio & Frith, 2006; Gallagher & Frith, 2003; Mitchell, 2006; Saxe, 2006). For the third module (threat detection), the amygdala seems to play an important role (Tabbert, Stark et al., 2005), also evidenced by the difficulty of bilateral amygdala lesioned patients in discriminating facial expressions of social emotions (Adolphs, Baron-Cohen et al., 2002). There is ongoing debate about the extent to which threat detection may rely on especially fast processing through a subcortical route to the amygdala (Pessoa & Adolphs, 2010). Several of these components likely operate together and are often triggered when ongoing routine behavior needs to be interrupted. For example, the dorsal region of the anterior cingulate cortex (dACC) has been highlighted in detecting potential threat to oneself, either through physical or social pain (Shackman et al., 2011): It is activated when participants play a video game designed to elicit feelings of social rejection when the other game players suddenly stop cooperating with the research participant (Eisenberger, Lieberman et al., 2003). For the fourth component (self-regulation), there is a substantial literature linking this also to sectors of the prefrontal cortex and fractionating it into more cognitive and more emotional aspects; there are also insights from lesion studies, as patients with prefrontal cortex lesions are often impaired in self-monitoring and regulation (Eslinger & Damasio, 1985).

There are, of course, many other sets of processes relevant to human social behavior, and many different schemes for attempting to categorize them in some way. The simplest categorizations typically assume that there are two broad types, often mapping onto a classical distinction from cognitive psychology: that between controlled and automatic processing (Schneider & Shiffrin, 1977). This dichotomous scheme has spawned a host of putatively associated attributes: Automatic processing is often thought to be also emotional and nonconscious, whereas controlled processing is thought to be "cognitive" and accessible to conscious report. More closely related to social cognition, a distinction has been made between reflexive and reflective processing, emphasizing that social cognition features both relatively shallow and automatic processing, as well as processing that often requires some of the metacognitive abilities mentioned above (Lieberman, 2007).

The Prefrontal Cortex

The PFC is a collection of cortical areas in the frontal lobes, anterior to the premotor cortex. It is interconnected to virtually all cortical sensory systems, motor systems, and many subcortical structures, which allows PFC to play a major role in higher cognitive functions (Asaad, Rainer et al., 2000). The PFC is involved in short-term storage of information and "executive" control of behavior, such as attention, task management, planning, and problem solving (Miller, 1999; Smith & Jonides, 1999). In general, social and emotional skills are complex, multimodal, and highly associative tasks requiring abstract internal representation. PFC neurons reflect a variety of cognitive attributes that are necessary to code, evaluate, process, store, and retrieve social information. But the PFC is only part of a broader network of structures that includes structures such as the amygdala, the cingulate gyrus, the fusiform gyrus, the insula and other sectors of somatosensory cortex, the superior temporal sulcus, the supramarginal gyrus, and others (Adolphs, Baron-Cohen et al., 2002; Adolphs, Tranel et al., 2003).

Some broad themes have been proposed to organize the way in which the PFC contributes to cognition; for instance, more conceptually abstract, symbolic, or cognitively mediated aspects of emotion experience appear to depend on more anterior sectors of prefrontal cortex, such as the dorsal anterior cingulate cortex (Lane, Reiman et al., 1998; Ochsner & Gross, 2005), and, in general, more abstract and metacognitive aspects of cognitive control may rely on progressively more anterior regions in the frontal lobe (Koechlin, Ody, & Kouneiher, 2003). By contrast, there is some evidence that reward-driven control of behavior depends more on medial sectors of the prefrontal cortex, whereas the need to change behavior in response to changes in reward or experience of punishment may draw on more lateral sectors (Kringelbach, 2005).

The anterior cingulate gyrus plays an important role in cognitive conflict monitoring and anticipation of cognitive conflict (Botvinick, Cohen et al., 2004; Sohn, Albert et al., 2007). Macaque monkeys with bilateral lesions to the anterior cingulate cortex (ACC) exhibit deficits in social behaviors, such as fewer social interactions, reduced time near conspecifics, and fewer vocalizations (Hadland, Rushworth et al., 2003). Indeed, lesion studies in monkeys have argued that it is damage to the anterior cingulate gyrus, rather than to other sectors of the prefrontal cortex such as the orbitofrontal cortex, that may be most responsible for the social deficits seen in primates following PFC damage (Rudebeck, Buckley, Walton, & Rushworth, 2006), and it is still an important issue for further investigation to determine to what extent this also may explain the impairments seen in humans with such lesion, such as the classic case of Phineas Gage discussed earlier.

The ACC, particularly ventral ACC, has been associated with affective/emotional processing for some time (Devinsky, Morrell et al., 1995), and it shows differential activation for empathy and social intuition (Völlm, Taylor et al., 2006) and cooperation (Rilling, Gutman et al., 2002). The ACC has long been known to be involved in pain perception (its white matter connections are a target of neurosurgery for treating intractable pain). Neurosurgical recordings in humans have documented single neurons that respond to pain (Hutchison, Davis et al., 1999) and motivate behavior more generally (Vogt, 2005). All of these findings taken together argue that the involvement of the ACC in emotion processing is related to the strong motivation to behave in a certain way and the need to monitor conflict, both of which may feature more prominently, on average, in social behavior than in other aspects of behavior. Although analyses based primarily on human fMRI studies have argued for some time that more ventral sectors of the ACC are disproportionately concerned with emotion-related regulation and control, and more dorsal sectors with more purely "cognitive" aspects of control, this anatomical dichotomy has recently been called into question. There is now substantial evidence that both "emotional" and "cognitive" aspects of behavioral control are intermingled in the anteromedial cingulate cortex, and it is likely that diverse aspects of conflict monitoring and control draw on a more phylogenetic basic set of functions that have to do with the need to control emotional responses in a social setting (Shackman et al., 2011).

Temporal Lobe

One of the most important abilities in social interaction is face perception, which is crucial for the recognition of socially relevant information such as identity, basic emotions (fear, happiness, etc.), and gaze direction. Although faces are visually quite similar in appearance, we extract an impressive wealth of socially relevant information from them, information that allows us to recognize threat or approval, social status, intent, focus of attention, surprise, fear, or just a welcoming smile. There is evidence to suggest that the processing of faces and their meaning draws very substantially on both cortical and subcortical structures in the temporal lobe. Most famously, there has been a long-standing argument that face processing is, to a large extent, domain-specific, relying on innate, specialized processes that primates have evolved in order to permit rapid social cognition based on seeing conspecifics. The original studies found that faces, more so than other visual stimuli, preferentially activated sectors of the ventral temporal cortex, a region that was subsequently dubbed the "fusiform face area" (Kanwisher, McDermott et al., 1997; McCarthy, Puce, Gore, & Allison, 1997). Furthermore, regions in the superior temporal sulcus (STS) are activated when participants view movement of the eyes or mouth (Puce, Allison et al., 1998), leading to a view according to which dynamic aspects of faces (emotional expression, eye gaze, biological motion) rely disproportionately on STS and STG, whereas static aspects of faces (their individuation into identity) rely on ventral temporal cortex (Haxby, Hoffman, & Gobbini, 2000). Such a distinction between processing identity and emotion information from faces was already proposed in earlier psychological models (Bruce & Young, 1986).

The domain-specificity of face processing is not without debate. Two key arguments revolve around the question of whether face-specific processing is anatomically specific or depends on more distributed regions: Initial studies found that a spatially quite distributed set of cortical regions carried information about faces, not just the fusiform face area (Haxby et al., 2001), but recent studies still argue that the fusiform face area plays a disproportionately important role in disambiguating faces from other classes of objects (Reddy & Kanwisher, 2007). A second argument has focused on the question of whether domain specificity arises from innate mechanisms for processing faces or is derivative of a more abstract computational function of expertise-based subordinate-level categorization: Are we born with a module for face processing, or is the fusiform face area trained up to process faces because they happen to be the most frequent objects we need to identify? Some studies have linked the expertise we have at recognizing novel objects to the activity measured in the fusiform face area of the brain (Gauthier, Tarr et al., 1999), and thus these studies suggest that, in order for humans to distinguish socially relevant features in a face, they need to develop the expertise of discriminating between visually highly similar inputs that yet convey very distinct social information (Tarr & Gauthier, 2000). Such very specialized demands might give rise to apparent domain-specific modules for social processing (Grusec & Davidov, 2010), like a module for anticipating the behavior of others in a reciprocal and competitive setting, or a module for generating regulating behaviors (such as punishment for noncooperative members of the group).

The responses of single neurons in the ventral temporal cortex to faces (recorded with electrodes in the brains of macaque monkeys) provide further support for the modularity of face processing (Tsao, Freiwald et al., 2006) and have begun to sketch out an entire network of interconnected "patches" of regions in the temporal and frontal cortex that process the various aspects of faces (Moeller, Freiwald, & Tsao, 2008). Although we do not yet have equivalent detailed data from humans, there are some data now from intracranial recordings in epilepsy patients that also argue for a distributed set of cortical regions in the temporal lobe that carry information about many different aspects of faces (Tsuchiya, Kawasaki, Oya, Howard, & Adolphs, 2008), both dynamic and static, thus arguing against the strong earlier dichotomy (Haxby et al., 2000), or at least suggesting substantial cross-talk between functional processing streams. The debate about the domain specificity of face processing can be seen as an instance of a broader issue concerning a trade-off between two dimensions of stimulus information and functional specialization (Atkinson & Adolphs, 2011) (see Figure 5.4). One mechanism might apply to a restricted set of stimuli or to a large domain of different ones. Alternatively, one mechanism could contribute to several different processes, within either one restricted stimulus class or over many such classes.

Although dependent on similar visual input, face identification and recognition of the emotions expressed by faces are in many respects quite different processes. The hypothesis that face identification and facial expression processing are also based on distinct pathways is supported by two lines of evidence: (1) Neuropsychological studies of brain lesioned patients with impaired face perception and (2) lesion studies in monkeys. Some patients with face agnosia following temporal cortex lesions, as well as monkeys with STS banks ablation, are impaired in recognizing frontal eye gaze from visually presented faces (Campbell, Heywood et al., 1990). Functional imaging studies support the notion that the STS is involved in representing facial expressions and mouth and eye movements (Haxby, Hoffman et al., 2000) and also in reorienting the gaze in order to achieve joint attention (Materna, Dicke et al., 2008), but is less involved in face identification, as we reviewed earlier. In contrast, single-unit recordings in monkeys (Desimone, Albright et al., 1984; Tsao, Freiwald et al., 2003), and electrophysiology

Stimulus Information
(selectivity)

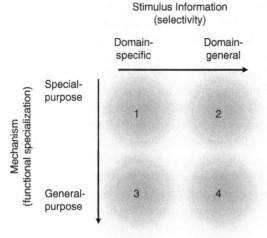

Figure 5.4 Is social cognition special? Debates about the modularity of social information processing often revolve around the two dimensions shown in this schematic: Is
the specialization at the level of processing algorithms (functional specialization), or
at the level of the type of information being processed (stimulus selectivity)? A mechanism might be functionally monolithic and apply to a restricted set of stimuli (region 1)
or applicable to a large domain of different kinds of stimuli (region 2). Alternatively, a
mechanism might contribute to several distinct processes, but, in the service of processing, be either a restricted stimulus class (region 3) or many (region 4). (Modified from
Atkinson, A. P., & Adolphs, R. (2011). The neuropsychology of face perception: beyond
simple dissociations and functional selectivity. *Philosophical Transactions of the Royal
Society of London, B, Biological Sciences, 366*(1571), 1726–1738.)

(Bentin, Allison et al., 1996) and functional imaging (Kanwisher & Yovel, 2006)
in humans, support the role of the fusiform gyrus in coding those static properties of faces needed for face identification. Remarkably, brain-damaged patients
impaired in face identification are often still able to recognize facial expressions
(Tranel & Damasio, 1988), whereas patients with impaired abilities to recognize
emotions in faces are perfectly able to identify the individuals whose faces they are
shown (Adolphs, Tranel et al., 1994). The former impairment, prosopagnosia, and
the latter, specific emotion recognition impairments (to date best documented
for the amygdala in the case of fear [Adolphs, Tranel et al., 1994] and the insula,
together with parts of the basal ganglia in the case of disgust [Calder, Keane,
Manes, Antoun, & Young, 2000; Calder, Lawrence, & Young, 2001]), constitute
a classic double-dissociation. Such a double dissociation suggests two functionally distinct pathways for the visual analysis of faces, one that involves the basic
identification of the facial features that define a particular individual, the other
a dedicated functional mechanism for the extraction of emotional information
from the face, independent of whom that face belongs to. This scheme harks back
to earlier proposals for a segregation between face identification and emotion
processing (Bruce & Young, 1986), whose details are now clearly more complex
and less dichotomous than originally thought, as we discussed above.

Amygdala

The amygdala is a key structure in the medial temporal lobe that has received considerable attention in regard to facial emotion processing and has been implicated
in a large range of psychiatric disorders. The amygdala is known to be involved
in a variety of processing related to fear, such as pavlovian fear conditioning;
recognizing fear from faces—as well as perhaps from other cues, such as body
postures and tone of voice (although the evidence is most clear for faces); and
even the conscious experience of fear (Feinstein et al., 2011). Behavioral studies on patients with amygdala lesions, as well as functional imaging studies in
neurologically healthy participants, have provided evidence that the amygdala
plays a critical role in emotion recognition from faces, and particularly negative
emotions, such as anger or fear (Adolphs, Tranel et al., 1994, 1999; Breiter, Etcoff
et al., 1996; Morris, Frith et al., 1996; Young, Bohenek et al. 1995). In general, the
impairments are disproportionate for those emotions closest to fear, although, in
other patients with bilateral amygdala lesions, the deficit is certainly not restricted
to fear (Adolphs, Tranel et al., 1999), thus highlighting an important point: Even
following complete damage to a key brain structure, the resulting dysfunction
shows individual differences that will require a broader network account of
compensatory function. A recent study investigated the conscious experience of
fear: The authors brought a patient with bilateral amygdala damage to a haunted
house, a pet store, and the lab and exposed her to various fear-eliciting stimuli,
like snakes, spiders, and unexpected threatening sounds, all of which failed to
elicit a fear experience (Feinstein et al., 2011). The amygdala has also been linked
to the regulation of social judgments and social behaviors, in particular those
having to do with approach and trust behaviors (see Adolphs [2010] for a review).
Although we rarely are aware of it, we normally keep a relatively constant social
distance to other people when we interact with them, a distance that depends on
cultural upbringing, the relationship to the person we interact with, and also the
nature of the conversation we're having with them. However, a patient with bilateral amygdala lesions shows a profound lack of such social distancing and seems
to have no sense of personal space (Kennedy & Adolphs, 2010), suggesting that
the social discomfort we normally experience when someone approaches us too
closely largely depends on social processes in the amygdala.

Amygdala responses to emotional faces are modulated by the context in which
the face occurs (Kim et al., 2004) and by the direction of eye gaze in the face
(Adams, Gordon et al., 2003). By comparing the blood oxygen level-dependent
(BOLD) signal in the amygdala of healthy volunteers when they viewed fearful
and angry faces with direct and averted gaze in the scanner, the authors found
evidence that an ambiguous threat (such as an angry face looking away or a fearful
face looking directly at the participant) elicits a more vigorous activation of the
amygdala than do clear threat situations (angry face with direct gaze and fearful
face with averted gaze). This interaction between the gaze direction and the facial
expression suggests that the amygdala is also specifically involved in detecting
threat-related ambiguity.

Table 5.1 SUMMARY OF FINDINGS FROM SUBJECT S. M.

Impaired in recognizing fear from static facial expressions
Gives abnormally low ratings of intensity to fearful faces
Impaired conditioned autonomic responses in pavlovian fear conditioning
Impaired emotional modulation of declarative memory
Abnormally positive judgments of trustworthiness and approachability from faces
Cannot judge arousal in negatively valanced stimuli
Abnormally positive preferences for abstract visual stimuli
Can discriminate between emotions normally
Can recognize fear from voice prosody but not music
Impaired in the Baron-Cohen eyes task
Less impaired in recognizing emotions in scenes when faces are erased
Mildly impaired also in recognizing sadness, but not happiness
Impaired in fixating and using information from the eye region of faces
Impaired emotional memory for gist but not details
Lack of experience of negatively valanced emotions in real life
Fixates the mouth instead of the eyes in conversations with real people
Has diminished bold signal in medial prefrontal cortex during reward expectancy
Can recognize fear from body posture and pointlight walkers
Lacks a sense of personal space
Performs normally on rapid detection and non-conscious processing of fear faces

Modified from Adolphs (2010). The list documents all the different published studies in a patient with complete bilateral amygdala lesions, highlighting the nature of the impairment found.

Taken together, all the varied impairments following amygdala lesions (cf. Table 5.1 for a summary from the famous patient S. M.) point to an important role for the amygdala in social behavior, and in particular in behaviors and judgments related to potential threat. However, recent studies indicate that the amygdala may not serve any kind of a domain-specific role for fear, or even for emotion. For one thing, neurons in the amygdala respond to a broad variety of stimuli, both aversive and appetitive (Paton, Belova, Morrison, & Salzman, 2006). For another, some BOLD-fMRI activation of the amygdala and some modulations of neuronal responses in animals seem to have nothing to do with the social or emotional nature of the stimuli but instead serve a broader role in processing any stimuli that are unpredictable (Herry et al., 2007) or ambiguous in some way (Whalen, 2007). Studies of patient S. M., who has bilateral amygdala lesions, have argued that the apparently domain-specific impairments in fear recognition from faces arise from a more abstract inability to fixate onto and process information from a particularly salient region of the face—the eyes (Adolphs et al., 2005; cf. Figure 5.2). These findings from the amygdala revisit our earlier discussion of the domain-specificity of social cognition: On the one hand, there is clear evidence for impairments that are disproportionate in the social domain and for structures that contribute more importantly to social aspects of cognition and behavior; on the other hand, in all of these cases, there is further evidence suggesting a more general and abstract information processing function, one that may underlie and explain apparently domain-specific social cognition.

Connectivity

As briefly reviewed in the previous section, many brain areas are involved in social cognitive processes, and some questions that received more attention recently focus on the mechanisms that allow them to work together and facilitate information flow between them. Surely, having a collection of clusters of neurons that become active while we assess, evaluate, and act upon social stimuli is just one piece of the puzzle. Viewed as a distributed system for social cognition, these areas reveal an intricate morphology and complex interconnectivity between the apparently distinct clusters of neurons. Understanding the processing of social information in the brain must be contingent on understanding the connectivity between—as well as the function of—each of its components, from the level of the synapse to the level of fiber pathways.

The interest in connectivity is, of course, not new, and scientists have been aware of its importance since the neuron doctrine described by Santiago Ramon y Cajal and the functional hypotheses of thinkers like Donald Hebb: Single neurons in isolation do nothing; everything comes about through their vast pattern of connectivity. But, although studying the anatomy and physiology of neurons was still possible after dissection of brain tissues, preserving and studying connectivity patterns proved a much more demanding task. With an average of about 7,000 synapses per neuron in the human brain, determining information flow between neurons, between neuronal populations, and between brain areas depends on understanding both structural and functional aspects of connectivity. There is a sense of profound progress now in some animal preparations, in particular with the advent of large-scale electron microscopic atlases, the detailed characterization of cell types and their expression patterns, and the ability to manipulate and control neuronal network activity using optogenetic techniques. Large-scale enterprises, such as the Allen Brain Atlas, are leading the way in such endeavors. Nonetheless, our ability to obtain detailed descriptions of connectivity in the human brain, let alone to manipulate it with any precision, are still a long way off.

Connectivity between brain regions has long been also a leading ingredient in neuropsychiatric models, including models of information processing in schizophrenia (Friston & Frith, 1995). For instance, Mayberg's classic model of depression (Mayberg et al., 1999), as well as more recent models of mood disorders

(Pezawas et al., 2005), has focused on the connectivity between prefrontal cortex and amygdala, in particular the idea that sectors of prefrontal cortex may provide regulatory and control components to the emotional responses implemented by the amygdala (Anand, Li et al., 2005). Focal lesion studies have also emphasized the issue: Impairments in recognizing facial emotion can arise not just from amygdala damage, but also from damage to right hemisphere white matter that may disconnect somatosensory-related cortices with structures like the amygdala and occipital regions (Adolphs, Damasio, Tranel, Cooper, & Damasio, 2000; Philippi, Mehta, Grabowski, Adolphs, & Rudrauf, 2009).

The importance of white matter integrity in cognition has been perhaps most specifically and famously studied in patients who underwent resection of the corpus callosum as a treatment for epilepsy. Such "split-brain" patients showed a pattern of impairments that offered insight into hemispheric specialization. For these patients, images shown in the left visual field have meaning, but they are not able to name them because the right hemisphere specializes in spatial and nonverbal tasks, whereas the left hemisphere dominates verbal tasks (Gazzaniga, 2005). Interestingly, in patients with developmental agenesis of the corpus callosum (AgCC), these marked split-brain symptoms are not present (Sauerwein & Lassonde, 1994), and the patients instead show a much more subtle constellation of impairments, particularly in the social domain (Paul et al., 2007). It is also striking that patients with agenesis of the corpus callosum, despite lacking the largest white matter tract in the brain, show remarkably normal functional connectivity between the hemispheres and seem to have a largely normal complement of functional networks, as revealed through an analysis of resting-state BOLD data (Tyszka et al., 2011). This latter finding may be important for understanding plasticity, reorganization, and functional compensation as well. How such normal functional networks can form without a normal structural connectivity base remains an important issue for future work.

Abnormal connectivity has been highlighted also in ASDs. In autism, high local connectivity may develop in tandem with long-range underconnectivity (Just, Cherkassky et al., 2004). This hypothesis is compatible with the weak central coherence theory and might be explained by widespread alterations in elimination and/or formation of synapses (Sporns, Tononi et al., 2000). One plausible information processing mechanism may be that the high local physical connectivity and low computational connectivity would fail to differentiate signal from noise (Rubenstein & Merzenich, 2003). Reduced connectivity between the hemispheres, consistent in particular with reduced communication through the corpus callosum, has recently been found in autism (Anderson et al., 2010).

CONCLUSION

Although studying the connections within the social cognitive neural system has improved our general understanding of the roles played by each region in processing social stimuli, the picture can only be complete when we understand the dynamics of the system, the precise timing at which each function comes into play, and the causality of each step within the network. This will require continued integration among a broad set of approaches in humans, including patient studies, as well as studies in healthy individuals, using fMRI, EEG, transcranial magnetic stimulation (TMS), and other methods, and it will continue to depend on animal models in which the questions can be addressed and causal models can be tested using methods impossible to apply in humans.

REFERENCES

Adams, R. B., Jr., Gordon, H. L., Baird, A. A., Ambady, N., & Kleck, R. E. (2003). Effects of gaze on amygdala sensitivity to anger and fear faces. *Science, 300*(5625), 1536.

Adolphs, R. (2010). What does the amygdala contribute to social cognition? Annals of the New York Academy of Sciences: The year in Cognitive Neuroscience 2010. *Annals of the New York Academy of Science, 1191,* 42–61.

Adolphs, R., Gosselin, F., Buchanan, T. W., Tranel, D., Schyns, P., & Damasio, A. R. (2005). A mechanism for impaired fear recognition after amygdala damage. *Nature, 433,* 68–72.

Adolphs, R., Damasio, H., Tranel, D., Cooper, G., & Damasio, A. R. (2000). A role for somatosensory cortices in the visual recognition of emotion as revealed by three-dimensional lesion mapping. *Journal of Neuroscience, 20*(7), 2683–2690.

Adolphs, R., Tranel, D., Damasio, H., & Damasio, A. R. (1994). Impaired recognition of emotion in facial expressions following bilateral damage to the human amygdala. *Nature, 372*(6507), 669–672.

Adolphs, R., Tranel, D., & Damasio, A. R. (1998). The human amygdala in social judgment. *Nature, 393*(6684), 470–474.

Adolphs, R., Tranel, D., Hamann, S., Young, A. W., Calder, A. J., Phelps, E. A., et al. (1999). Recognition of facial emotion in nine individuals with bilateral amygdala damage. *Neuropsychologia, 37*(10), 1111–1117.

Adolphs, R., Tranel, D., & Damasio, A. R. (2003). Dissociable neural systems for recognizing emotions. *Brain Cognition, 52*(1), 61–69.

Adolphs, R., Baron-Cohen, S., & Tranel, D. (2002). Impaired recognition of social emotions following amygdala damage. *Journal of Cognitive Neuroscience, 14*(8), 1264–1274.

Allman, J., McLaughlin, T., & Hakeem, A. (1993). Brain weight and life-span in primate species. *Proceedings of the National Academy of Science of the USA, 90*(1), 118–122.

Amodio, D. M., & Frith, C. D. (2006). Meeting of minds: The medial frontal cortex and social cognition. *Nature Reviews Neuroscience, 7*(4), 268–277.

Anand, A., Li, Y., Wang, Y., Wu, J., Gao, S., Bukhari, L., et al. (2005). Activity and connectivity of brain mood regulating circuit in depression: A functional magnetic resonance study. *Biological Psychiatry, 57*(10), 1079–1088.

Anderson, J. S., Druzgal, T. J., Froehlich, A., DuBray, M. B., Lange, N., Alexander, A. L., et al. (2010). Decreased interhemispheric functional connectivity in autism. *Cerebral Cortex, 21,* 1134–1146.

Asaad, W. F., Rainer, G., & Miller, E. K. (2000). Task-specific neural activity in the primate prefrontal cortex. *Journal of Neurophysiology, 84*(1), 451–459.

Atkinson, A. P., & Adolphs, R. (2011). The neuropsychology of face perception: Beyond simple dissociations and functional selectivity. *Philosophical Transactions of the Royal Society of London B Biological Sciences, 366*(1571), 1726–1738.

Bandura, A., Ross, D., & Ross, S. A.. (1961). Transmission of aggression through imitation of aggressive models. *Journal of Abnormal and Social Psychology, 63*, 575–582.

Baron-Cohen, S. (2002). The extreme male brain theory of autism. *Trends in Cognitive Science, 6*(6), 248–254.

Baron-Cohen, S., Jolliffe, T., Mortimore, C., & Robertson, M. (1997). Another advanced test of theory of mind: Evidence from very high functioning adults with autism or Asperger syndrome. *Journal of Child Psychology and Psychiatry, 38*(7), 813–822.

Baron-Cohen, S., Leslie, A. M., & Frith, U. (1985). Does the autistic child have a "theory of mind"? *Cognition, 21*(1), 37–46.

Baron-Cohen, S., Ring, H. A., Wheelwright, S., Bullmore, E. T., Brammer, M. J., Simmons, A., et al. (1999). Social intelligence in the normal and autistic brain: An fMRI study. *European Journal of Neuroscience, 11*(6), 1891–1898.

Bellugi, U., Adolphs, R., Cassady, C., & Chiles, M. (1999). Towards the neural basis for hypersociability in a genetic syndrome. *Neuroreport, 10*(8), 1653–1657.

Bennetto, L., Pennington, B. F., & Rogers, S. J. (1996). Intact and impaired memory functions in autism. *Child Development, 67*(4), 1816–1835.

Bentin, S., Allison, T., Puce, A., Perez, E., & McCarthy, G. (1996). Electrophysiological studies of face perception in humans. *Journal of Cognitive Neuroscience, 8*(6), 551–565.

Biederman, I. (1972). Human performance in contingent information-processing tasks. *Journal of Experimental Psychology, 93*(2), 219–238.

Bodfish, J. W., Symons, F. J., Parker, D. E., & Lewis, M. H. (2000). Varieties of repetitive behavior in autism: Comparisons to mental retardation. *Journal of Autism and Developmental Disorders, 30*(3), 237–243.

Botvinick, M. M., Cohen, J. D., & Carter, C. S. (2004). Conflict monitoring and anterior cingulate cortex: An update. *Trends in Cognitive Science, 8*(12), 539–546.

Breiter, H. C., Etcoff, N. L., Whalen, P. J., Kennedy, W. A., Rauch, S. L., Buckner, R. L., et al. (1996). Response and habituation of the human amygdala during visual processing of facial expression. *Neuron, 17*(5), 875–887.

Brothers, L. (1989). A biological perspective on empathy. *American Journal of Psychiatry, 146*(1), 10–19.

Bruce, V., & Young, A. (1986). Understanding face recognition. *British Journal of Psychology, 77*, 305–327.

Calder, A. J., Keane, J., Manes, F., Antoun, N., & Young, A. W. (2000). Impaired recognition and experience of disgust following brain injury. *Nature Neuroscience, 3*, 1077–1078.

Calder, A. J., Lawrence, A. D., & Young, A. W. (2001). Neuropsychology of fear and loathing. *Nature Reviews Neuroscience, 2*, 352–363.

Campbell, R., Heywood, C. A., Cowey, A., Regard, M., & Landis, T. (1990). Sensitivity to eye gaze in prosopagnostic patients and monkeys with superior temporal sulcus ablation. *Neuropsychologia, 28*(11), 1123–1142.

Capitão, L., Sampaio, A., Sampaio, C., Vasconcelos, C., Férnandez, M., Garayzá bal, E., et al. (2011). MRI amygdala volume in Williams Syndrome. *Research in Developmental Disabilities, 32*(6), 2767–2772.

Chomsky, N. (1964). The development of grammar in child language: Formal discussion. *Monographs of the Society for Research in Child Development, 29*, 35–39.

Cosmides, L., & Tooby, J. (1997). Dissecting the computational architecture of social inference mechanisms. *Ciba Foundation Symposium, 208*, 132–156; discussion 156–161.

Damasio, A. R. (1994). Descartes' error and the future of human life. *Scientific American, 27*(4), 144.

Damasio, H., Grabowski, T., Frank, R., Galaburda, A. M., & Damasio, A. R. (1994). The return of Phineas Gage: Clues about the brain from the skull of a famous patient. *Science, 264*(5162), 1102–1105.

Dawson, G., Meltzoff, A. N., Osterling, J., Rinaldi, J., & Brown, E. (1998). Children with autism fail to orient to naturally occurring social stimuli. *Journal of Autism and Developmental Disorders, 28,* 479–485.

Desimone, R., Albright, T. D., Gross, C. G., & Bruce, C. (1984). Stimulus-selective properties of inferior temporal neurons in the macaque. *Journal of Neuroscience, 4*(8), 2051–2062.

Devinsky, O., Morrell, M. J., & Vogt, B. A. (1995). Contributions of anterior cingulate cortex to behaviour. *Brain, 118*(Pt. 1), 279–306.

Doyle, T. F., Bellugi, U., Korenberg, J. R., & Graham, J. (2004). Everybody in the world is my friend hypersociability in young children with Williams syndrome. *American Journal of Medical Genetics A, 124A*(3), 263–273.

Dunbar, R. I. (2009). The social brain hypothesis and its implications for social evolution. *Annals of Human Biology, 36*(5), 562–572.

Eisenberger, N. I., Lieberman, M. D., & Williams, K. D. (2003). Does rejection hurt? An FMRI study of social exclusion. *Science, 302*(5643), 290–292.

Eslinger, P. J., & Damasio, A. R. (1985). Severe disturbance of higher cognition after bilateral frontal lobe ablation: Patient EVR. *Neurology, 35*(12), 1731–1741.

Feinstein, J. S., Adolphs, R., Damasio, A. R., & Tranel, D. (2011). The human amygdala and the induction and experience of fear. *Current Biology, 21,* 34–38.

Friston, K. J., & Frith, C. D. (1995). Schizophrenia: A disconnection syndrome? *Clinical Neuroscience, 3*(2), 89–97.

Frith, U., & Happe, F. (1994). Autism: Beyond "theory of mind". *Cognition, 50*(1–3), 115–132.

Gallagher, H. L., & Frith, C. D. (2003). Functional imaging of 'theory of mind'. *Trends in Cognitive Science, 7*(2), 77–83.

Gazzaniga, M. S. (2005). Forty-five years of split-brain research and still going strong. *Nature Reviews Neuroscience, 6*(8), 653–659.

Greenwald, A. G., & Banaji, M. R. (1995). Implicit social cognition: Attitudes, self-esteem, and stereotypes. *Psychological Review, 102*(1), 4–27.

Grusec, J. E., & Davidov, M. (2010). Integrating different perspectives on socialization theory and research: A domain-specific approach. *Child Development, 81*(3), 687–709.

Hadland, K. A., Rushworth, M. F., Gaffan, D., & Passingham, R. E. (2003). The effect of cingulate lesions on social behaviour and emotion. *Neuropsychologia, 41*(8), 919–931.

Happe, F. (1999). Autism: Cognitive deficit or cognitive style? *Trends in Cognitive Science, 3*(6), 216–222.

Happe, F., Malhi, G. S., & Checkley, S. (2001). Acquired mind-blindness following frontal lobe surgery? A single case study of impaired 'theory of mind' in a patient treated with stereotactic anterior capsulotomy. *Neuropsychologia, 39*(1), 83–90.

Happe, F., Ronald, A., & Plomin, R. (2006). Time to give up on a single explanation for autism. *Nature Neuroscience, 9*(10), 1218–1220.

Harter, S., Waters, P., & Whitesell, N. R. (1998). Relational self-worth: Differences in perceived worth as a person across interpersonal contexts among adolescents. *Child Development, 69*(3), 756–766.

Haxby, J. V., Hoffman, E. A., & Gobbini, M. I. (2000). The distributed human neural system for face perception. *Trends in Cognitive Science, 4*(6), 223–233.

Haxby, J. V., Gobbini, M. I., Furey, M. L., Ishai, A., Schouten, J. L., & Pietrini, P. (2001). Distributed and overlapping representation of faces and objects in ventral temporal cortex. *Science, 293,* 2425–2429.

Heatherton, T. F. (2011). Neuroscience of self and self-regulation. *Annual Review of Psychology, 62,* 363–390.

Hermelin, B., & O'Connor, N. (1975). The recall of digits by normal, deaf and autistic children. *British Journal of Psychology, 66*(2), 203–209.

Herry, C., Bach, D. R., Esposito, F., DiSalle, F., Perrig, W. J., Scheffler, K., et al. (2007). Processing of temporal unpredictability in human and animal amygdala. *The Journal of Neuroscience, 27,* 5958–5966.

Hughes, C., Russell, J., & Robbins, T. W. (1994). Evidence for executive dysfunction in autism. *Neuropsychologia, 32*(4), 477–492.

Hutchison, W. D., Davis, K. D., Lozano, A. M., Tasker, R. R., & Dostrovsky, J. O. (1999). Pain-related neurons in the human cingulate cortex. *Nature Neuroscience, 2*(5), 403–405.

Just, M. A., Cherkassky, V. L., Keller, T. A., & Minshew, N. J. (2004). Cortical activation and synchronization during sentence comprehension in high-functioning autism: Evidence of underconnectivity. *Brain, 127*(Pt. 8), 1811–1821.

Kanwisher, N., McDermott, J., & Chun, M. M. (1997). The fusiform face area: A module in human extrastriate cortex specialized for face perception. *Journal of Neuroscience, 17*(11), 4302–4311.

Kanwisher, N., & Yovel, G. (2006). The fusiform face area: A cortical region specialized for the perception of faces. *Philosophical Transactions of the Royal Society of London B Biological Sciences, 361*(1476), 2109–2128.

Karmiloff-Smith, A. (1995). Annotation: The extraordinary cognitive journey from foetus through infancy. *Journal of Child Psychology and Psychiatry, 36*(8), 1293–1313.

Kennedy, D. P., & Adolphs, R. (2010). Impaired fixation to eyes following amygdala damage arises from abnormal bottom-up attention. *Neuropsychologia, 48*(12), 3392–3398.

Kim, H., Somerville, L. H., Johnstone, T., Polis, S., Alexander, A. L., Shin, L. M., et al. (2004). Contextual modulation of amygdala responsivity to surprised faces. *Journal of Cognitive Neuroscience, 16,* 1730–1745.

Klin, A., Jones, W., Schultz, R., Volkmar, F., & Cohen, D. (2002). Defining and quantifying the social phenotype in autism. *American Journal of Psychiatry, 159*(6), 895–908.

Koechlin, E., Ody, C., & Kouneiher, F. (2003). The architecture of cognitive control in the human prefrontal cortex. *Science, 302,* 1181–1185.

Korenberg, J. R., Chen, X. N., Hirota, H., Lai, Z., Bellugi, U., Burian, D., et al. (2000). VI. Genome structure and cognitive map of Williams syndrome. *Journal of Cognitive Neuroscience, 12*(Suppl. 1), 89–107.

Kringelbach, M. L. (2005). The human orbitofrontal cortex: Linking reward to hedonic experience. *Nature Reviews Neuroscience, 6,* 691–702.

Lane, R. D., Reiman, E. M., Axelrod, B., Yun, L. S., Holmes, A., & Schwartz, G. E. (1998). Neural correlates of levels of emotional awareness. Evidence of an interaction between emotion and attention in the anterior cingulate cortex. *Journal of Cognitive Neuroscience, 10*(4), 525–535.

Leslie, A. M., & Frith, U. (1987). Metarepresentation and autism: How not to lose one's marbles. *Cognition, 27*(3), 291–294.

Lieberman, M. D. (2007). Social cognitive neuroscience: A review of core processes. *Annual Review of Psychology, 58,* 259–289.

Losh, M., Adolphs, R., Poe, M., Couture, S., Penn, D., Baranek, G., et al. (2009). Neuropsychological profile of autism and broad autism phenotype. *Archives of General Psychiatry, 66,* 518–526.

MacMillan, M. (2000). *An odd kind of fame: Stories of Phineas Gage.* Cambridge, MA: MIT Press.

Materna, S., Dicke, P. W., & Thier, P. (2008). The posterior superior temporal sulcus is involved in social communication not specific for the eyes. *Neuropsychologia, 46*(11), 2759–2765.

Mayberg, H. S., Liotti, M., Brannan, S. K., McGinnis, S., Mahurin, R. K., Jerabek, P. A., et al. (1999). Reciprocal limbic-cortical function and negative mood: Converging PET findings in depression and normal sadness. *American Journal of Psychiatry, 156,* 675–682.

McCarthy, G., Puce, A., Gore, J. C., & Allison, T. (1997). Face-specific processing in the human fusiform gyrus. *Journal of Cognitive Neuroscience, 9,* 605–610.

Meyer-Lindenberg, A., Hariri, A., Munoz, K. E., Mervis, C. B., Mattay, V. S., Morris, C. A., et al. (2005). Neural correlates of genetically abnormal social cognition in Williams syndrome. *Nature Neuroscience, 8,* 991–993.

Meyer-Lindenberg, A., Kohn, P., Mervis, C. B., Kippenhan, J. S., Olsen, R. K., Morris, C. A., et al. (2004). Neural basis of genetically determined visuospatial construction deficit in Williams Syndrome. *Neuron, 43,* 623–631.

Miller, E. K. (1999). The prefrontal cortex: Complex neural properties for complex behavior. *Neuron, 22*(1), 15–17.

Mitchell, J. P. (2006). Mentalizing and Marr: An information processing approach to the study of social cognition. *Brain Research, 1079*(1), 66–75.

Moeller, S., Freiwald, W. A., & Tsao, D. Y. (2008). Patches with links: A unified system for processing faces in the Macaque temporal lobe. *Science, 320,* 1355–1359.

Morris, J. S., Frith, C. D., Perrett, D. I., Rowland, D., Young, A. W., Calder, A. J., & Dolan, R. J. (1996). A differential neural response in the human amygdala to fearful and happy facial expressions. *Nature, 383*(6603), 812–815.

Morsella, E., Gray, J. R., Krieger, S. C., & Bargh, J. A. (2009). The essence of conscious conflict: Subjective effects of sustaining incompatible intentions. *Emotion, 9*(5), 717–728.

Ochsner, K. N., & Gross, J. J. (2005). The cognitive control of emotion. *Trends in Cognitive Science, 9*(5), 242–249.

Ozer, E. M., & Bandura, A. (1990). Mechanisms governing empowerment effects: A self-efficacy analysis. *Journal of Personality and Social Psychology, 58*(3), 472–486.

Ozonoff, S., & Jensen, J. (1999). Brief report: Specific executive function profiles in three neurodevelopmental disorders. *Journal of Autism and Developmental Disorders, 29*(2), 171–177.

Palmer, S., Simone, E., & Kube, P., (1988). Reference frame effects on shape perception in two versus three dimensions. *Perception, 17*(2), 147–163.

Paton, J. J., Belova, M. A., Morrison, S. E., & Salzman, C. D. (2006). The primate amygdala represents the positive and negative value of visual stimuli during learning. *Nature, 439,* 865–870.

Paul, L. K., Brown, W. S., Adolphs, R., Tyszka, J. M., Richards, L. J., Mukherjee, P., et al. (2007). Agenesis of the corpus callosum: Genetic, developmental and functional aspects of connectivity. *Nature Reviews Neuroscience, 8,* 28.

Pavlov, I. P. (1927). *Conditioned reflexes: An investigation of the physiological activity of the cerebral cortex* (G. V. Anrep, Trans., Ed.). London: Oxford University Press.

Pelphrey, K., Adolphs, R., & Morris, J. P. (2004). Neuroanatomical substrates of social cognition dysfunction in autism. *Mental Retardation and Developmental Disabilities Research Reviews, 10*(4), 259–271.

Pezawas, L., Meyer-Lindenberg, A., Drabant, E. M., Verchinski, B. A., Munoz, K. E., Kolachana, B. S., et al. (2005). 5-HTTLPR polymorphism impacts human cingulate-amygdala interactions: A genetic susceptibility mechanism for depression. *Nature Neuroscience, 8,* 828–834.

Pessoa, L., & Adolphs, R. (2010). Emotion processing and the amygdala: From a "low road" to "many roads" of evaluating biological significance. *Nature Reviews Neuroscience, 11,* 773–782.

Pfeifer, J. H., Lieberman, M. D., & Dapretto, M. (2007). "I know you are but what am I?!": Neural bases of self- and social knowledge retrieval in children and adults. *Journal of Cognitive Neuroscience, 19*(8), 1323–1337.

Philippi, C. L., Mehta, S., Grabowski, T., Adolphs, R., & Rudrauf, D. (2009). Damage to association fiber tracts impairs recognition of the facial expression of emotion. *The Journal of Neuroscience, 29,* 15089–15099.

Piaget, J. (1953). Structures operationelles et cybernetique (Functional structures and cybernetics). *L'année Psychologique, 53*(1), 379–388.

Prior, M., & Hoffmann, W. (1990). Brief report: Neuropsychological testing of autistic children through an exploration with frontal lobe tests. *Journal of Autism and Developmental Disorders, 20*(4), 581–590.

Puce, A., Allison, T., Bentin, A., Gore, J. C., & McCarthy, G. (1998). Temporal cortex activation in humans viewing eye and mouth movements. *Journal of Neuroscience, 18*(6), 2188–2199.

Reddy, L., & Kanwisher, N. (2007). Category selectivity in the ventral visual pathway confers robustness to clutter and diverted attention. *Current Biology, 17,* 2067–2072.

Rilling, J., Gutman, D., Zeh, T., Pagnoni, G., Berns, G., & Kilts, C. (2002). A neural basis for social cooperation. *Neuron, 35*(2), 395–405.

Ronald, A., Happé, F., Bolton, P., Butcher, L. M., Price, T. S., Wheelwright, S., et al. (2006). Genetic heterogeneity between the three components of the autism spectrum: A twin study. *Journal of the American Academy of Child and Adolescent Psychiatry, 45*(6), 691–699.

Rubenstein, J. L., & Merzenich, M. M. (2003). Model of autism: Increased ratio of excitation/inhibition in key neural systems. *Genes, Brain and Behavior, 2*(5), 255–267.

Rudebeck, P. H., Buckley, M. J., Walton, M. E., & Rushworth, M. F. (2006). A role for the macaque anterior cingulate gyrus in social valuation. *Science, 313*(5791), 1310–1312.

Russell, J., & Jarrold, C. (1998). Error-correction problems in autism: Evidence for a monitoring impairment? *Journal of Autism and Developmental Disorders, 28*(3), 177–188.

Sasson, N., Tsuchiya, N., Hurley, R., Couture, S. M., Penn, D. L., Piven, J., & Adolphs, R. (2007). Orienting to social stimuli differentiates social cognitive impairment in autism and schizophrenia. *Neuropsychologia, 45,* 2580–2588.

Sauerwein, H. C., & Lassonde, M. (1994). Cognitive and sensori-motor functioning in the absence of the corpus callosum: Neuropsychological studies in callosal agenesis and callosotomized patients. *Behavioural Brain Research, 64*(1–2), 229–240.

Saxe, R. (2006). Uniquely human social cognition. *Current Opinion in Neurobiology, 16*(2), 235–239.

Schneider, W., & Shiffrin, R. M. (1977). Controlled and automatic human information processing: 1. Detection, search, and attention. *Psychological Review, 84,* 1–66.

Shackman, A. J., Salomons, T. V., Slagter, H. A., Fox, A. S., Winter, J. J., & Davidson, R. J. (2011). The integration of negative affect, pain, and cognitive control in the cingulate cortex. *Nature Reviews Neuroscience, 12,* 154–167.

Smith, E. E., & Jonides, J. (1999). Storage and executive processes in the frontal lobes. *Science, 283*(5408), 1657–1661.

Sohn, M. H., Albert, M. V., Jung, K., Carter, C. S., & Anderson, J. R. (2007). Anticipation of conflict monitoring in the anterior cingulate cortex and the prefrontal cortex. *Proceedings of the National Academy of Science of the USA, 104*(25), 10330–10334.

Sporns, O., Tononi, G., & Edelman, G. M. (2000). Theoretical neuroanatomy: Relating anatomical and functional connectivity in graphs and cortical connection matrices. *Cerebral Cortex, 10*(2), 127–141.

Tabbert, K., Stark, R., Kirsch, P., & Vaitl, D. (2005). Hemodynamic responses of the amygdala, the orbitofrontal cortex and the visual cortex during a fear conditioning paradigm. *International Journal of Psychophysiology, 57*(1), 15–23.

Tager-Flusberg, H., J. Boshart, & Baron-Cohen, S. (1998). Reading the windows to the soul: Evidence of domain-specific sparing in Williams syndrome. *Journal of Cognitive Neuroscience, 10*(5), 631–639.

Tarr, M. J., & Gauthier, I. (2000). FFA: A flexible fusiform area for subordinate-level visual processing automatized by expertise. *Nature Neuroscience, 3*(8), 764–769.

Tranel, D., & Damasio, A. R. (1988). Non-conscious face recognition in patients with face agnosia. *Behavioural Brain Research, 30*(3), 235–249.

Tsao, D. Y., Freiwald, W. A., Knutsen, T. A., Mandeville, J. B., & Tootell, R. B. (2003). Faces and objects in macaque cerebral cortex. *Nature Neuroscience, 6*(9), 989–995.

Tsao, D. Y., Freiwald, W. A., Tootell, R. B., & Livingstone, M. S. (2006). A cortical region consisting entirely of face-selective cells. *Science, 311*(5761), 670–674.

Tsuchiya, N., Kawasaki, H., Oya, H., Howard, M. A., & Adolphs, R. (2008). Decoding face information in time, frequency and space from direct intracranial recordings of the human brain. *PLoS One, 3,* e3892.

Tyszka, J. M., Kennedy, D. P., Adolphs, R., & Paul, L. K (2011). Intact bilateral resting-state networks in the absence of the corpus callosum. *The Journal of Neurocience, 31*(42), 15154–15162.

Vogt, B. A. (2005). Pain and emotion interactions in subregions of the cingulate gyrus. *Nature Reviews Neuroscience, 6*(7), 533–544.

Völlm, B. A., Taylor, A. N., Richardson, P., Corcoran, R., Stirling, J., McKie, S., et al. (2006). Neuronal correlates of theory of mind and empathy: A functional magnetic resonance imaging study in a nonverbal task. *Neuroimage, 29*(1), 90–98.

Whalen, P. J. (2007). The uncertainty of it all. *Trends in Cognitive Sciences, 11,* 499–500.

Whiten, A., Byrne, R. W., Barton, R. A., Waterman, P. G., & Henzi, S. P. (1991). Dietary and foraging strategies of baboons. *Philosophical Transactions of the Royal Society of London B Biological Sciences, 334*(1270), 187–195; discussion 195–187.

Young, S. L., Bohenek, D. L., & Fanselow, M. S. (1995). Scopolamine impairs acquisition and facilitates consolidation of fear conditioning: Differential effects for tone vs context conditioning. *Neurobiology of Learning and Memory, 63*(2), 174–180.

Descriptive and Experimental Research

Social Cognition and Functional Outcome in Schizophrenia

WILLIAM P. HORAN, JUNGHEE LEE, AND
MICHAEL F. GREEN ■

If I see someone talking in a friendly way and smiling, but they have their arms crossed in front of them, that confuses me. It throws me off—like a mixed message. I'm stuck, and I don't know how that person feels—how do you break that down?

48-YEAR-OLD MAN WITH SCHIZOPHRENIA

Among the diverse signs and symptoms that comprise the American Psychiatric Association's *Diagnostic and Statistical Manual of Mental Disorders* (DSM-IV) criteria for schizophrenia, functional impairment is the only characteristic shared by every person who is diagnosed with this disorder. Most patients experience marked impairment across multiple aspects of daily life functioning, including social relations, vocational pursuits, and independent living (Marder & Fenton, 2004; Murray & Lopez, 1996). As is evident in the quote above, dysfunction in the social domain can have far-reaching consequences across many aspects of functioning, contributing to fractured family relationships, conflict with peers and coworkers, and social isolation. In addition to their associated emotional and financial burdens for affected individuals and those who care for them, functional impairments are a major public health concern—schizophrenia ranks as the sixth leading cause of disability in men and the fifth leading cause of disability in women worldwide (WHO, 2004), and the costs to society are enormous (Murray & Lopez, 1997; Nicholl, Akhras, Diels, & Schadrack, 2010).

Unfortunately, functional impairments are refractory to current pharmacological interventions (Harvey, 2009) and only partially responsive to rehabilitation (Cook et al., 2005; Kurtz & Mueser, 2008). Despite major advances in treating the acute psychotic symptoms of schizophrenia, most patients continue to function poorly between episodes, and the long-term outcome of schizophrenia has changed little over the past 100 years (Hegarty, Baldessarini, Tohen, Waternaux, & Oepen, 1994). It has become clear that residual clinical symptoms are rather weak predictors of functional outcome, indicating that further improvements are unlikely to come about through better symptom management alone. Instead, new treatments are needed that address the key determinants of poor functional outcome. This recognition is central to prevailing recovery-oriented approaches to treatment (Kern, Glynn, Horan, & Marder, 2009), which reflect a fundamental shift from a focus on symptom reduction to a focus on functional recovery and pursuit of personally meaningful goals and aspirations.

In the context of recovery-oriented treatment development, there has been a great deal of interest in identifying key determinants of poor outcome that can be targeted through novel intervention approaches. Over the past three decades, considerable evidence has shown that impairments in neurocognition, including attention/vigilance, speed of processing, working memory, verbal learning, visual learning, reasoning, and problem-solving, are among the most important determinants of how well people with schizophrenia function in the community (Green, 1996; Green, Kern, Braff, & Mintz, 2000; Green, Kern, & Heaton, 2004). This has led to major initiatives by the National Institute of Mental Health (NIMH; e.g., Measurement and Treatment Research to Improve Cognition in Schizophrenia [MATRICS], Treatment Units for Research on Neurocognition in Schizophrenia [TURNS]) to stimulate and guide the development of new pharmacological treatments for cognitive deficits that impact outcome.

Despite these important developments, it is unlikely that interventions targeting only neurocognition will be sufficient as the amount of variance in outcome that is accounted for by neurocognition is typically in the range of 20% to 40%. Furthermore, there has until recently been a substantial gap in our understanding of the mechanisms through which neurocognitive deficits measured in the laboratory ultimately give rise to the functional deficits experienced by patients in their daily lives in the community. Thus, there is a critical need to identify other factors that contribute to functional disability.

Over the past decade, social cognition has emerged as a high-priority research topic that holds great promise for helping us understand and treat the causes of functional disability. As described elsewhere in this volume, social cognition refers to the mental operations underlying social interactions, and people with schizophrenia show substantial impairments across several social cognitive domains, including emotion perception/processing (EP), social perception (SP), attributional style (AS), and mentalizing or theory of mind (ToM). Because social cognition is so central to understanding and effectively interacting with other people, problems such as misperceptions and unexpected reactions to and from other people would be expected to adversely impact functioning across a variety of domains. In support of this expectation, growing evidence indicates that social cognitive impairments do indeed make important and unique contributions to poor functional outcome in schizophrenia.

This chapter provides an overview of the relationship between social cognition and functional outcome in schizophrenia. We begin by briefly reviewing how functional outcome is defined and assessed. We next review studies that examined correlations between different types of social cognition and different aspects of functional outcome. We then turn to more recent studies that have used sophisticated modeling techniques to examine how social cognition interacts with neurocognition to impact functional outcome. We conclude by discussing the important implications of these findings for developing new social cognitive intervention approaches that facilitate functional recovery.

FUNCTIONAL OUTCOME IN SCHIZOPHRENIA

Functional outcome is a multifaceted construct that has been defined in many different ways. It is assessed in schizophrenia using a variety of methods that focus on different domains of life (e.g., social, vocational), different levels of analysis (e.g., microscopic instrumental skills to macroscopic assessments of well-being), and different sources of information (e.g., laboratory-based measures to collateral informants) (Bellack et al., 2007). Each approach to assessing functional outcome has different advantages and disadvantages and, as discussed further below, the correspondence among these approaches, and their relations to functionally relevant variables (e.g., neurocognition), can vary considerably. Thus, it is important to consider how functional outcome is conceptualized and assessed in the context of social cognitive studies.

Figure 6.1 provides an overview of commonly used functional outcome assessment approaches and illustrative measures. At the broadest level, a distinction can be made between competence-based and attainment-based measures. Generally speaking, competence or "functional capacity" measures assess what a person is capable of doing in a controlled clinical research setting (Harvey, Velligan, & Bellack, 2007; Patterson & Mausbach, 2010). Measures of functional capacity are performance-based simulations or role-plays of activities required for adaptive daily living, such as holding a social conversation, social problem solving, selecting grocery items to prepare a meal, and planning a trip using public transportation. This approach has the advantages of providing a direct assessment of ability within a specific domain, standardization across assessments, and strong psychometric properties, including interrater agreement. Furthermore, functional capacity measures show consistently strong relations to neurocognitive functioning. However, as discussed further below, good performance on these measures indicates only that a person has the ability to perform the assessed skills, not that he or she will actually use these abilities in the course of daily life.

In contrast to competence-based measures, attainment-based measures focus on what one actually experiences and does in the real world. Two subcategories

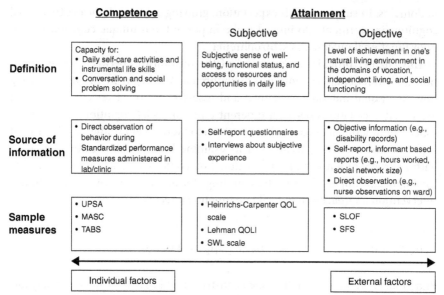

Figure 6.1 Assessment of functional outcome. MASC, Maryland Assessment of Social Competence (Bellack et al., 2007); QOL, Quality of Life scale (Heinrichs et al., 1984); QOLI, Quality of Life Inventory (Lehman, 1988); SLOF, Specific Level of Functioning Scale (Schneider & Struening, 1983); SFS, Social Functioning Scale (Birchwood, Smith, Cochran, Wetton, & Copestake, 1990); SWL, Satisfaction with Life Scale (Stein & Test, 1980); TABS, Test of Adaptive Behavior in Schizophrenia (Velligan et al., 2007); UPSA, UCSD Performance-based Skills Assessment (T. L. Patterson et al., 2001).

of attainment-based measures can be distinguished according to whether they assess: (a) a person's subjective satisfaction with or evaluation of his or her level of functioning, or (b) more objective information about level and quality of functioning. Subjective measures evaluate perceived quality of life, which refers to a person's sense of general well-being and satisfaction with his or her circumstances (Eack & Newhill, 2007; Tolman & Kurtz, 2012). These subjective appraisals are typically assessed using self-report measures that inquire about satisfaction in particular life domains, such as social, vocational, and residential, or in terms of a person's more general appraisals of overall well-being. Some measures include interview-based ratings of personal descriptions of so-called intrapsychic processes, such as motivation, interest, and empathy (Heinrichs, Hanlon, & Carpenter, 1984). Self-reports of satisfaction and well being have the virtue of simplicity and relatively low personnel/financial resource burdens, and they incorporate a person's own perception of how well he or she is functioning. However, a person's ability to accurately report on his or her own behavior can be impacted by a host of factors, such as poor insight, psychiatric symptoms, recall deficits, or mood state influences. In addition, the relation between these measures and other relevant variables, such as neurocognition and the more objective measures discussed just below, can be rather low.

Although measures in the second subcategory of "objective" attainment cover the same general domains of life as subjective measures, they can vary considerably in the type of information on which ratings are based (Harvey et al., 2011; Leifker, Patterson, Heaton, & Harvey, 2011). This ranges from relatively objective indicators (e.g., marital status, residential setting, amount of money earned), to self- or informant- (e.g., family member, clinician) reported data (e.g., number of friends and frequency of interaction), to behavioral observations of trained raters (e.g., ratings of ward behavior by psychiatric nurses). The extent to which a person benefits from enrollment in psychiatric rehabilitation is also sometimes considered within this category. Thus, these measures are intended to index relatively objective indices of a person's level of functional attainment in his or her naturalistic environment. However, information provided by different sources can vary considerably in terms of both relations to each other and to other relevant variables. For example, self-reports of functional attainment tend to provide lower correlations with neurocognitive and functional capacity measures than do informant-based assessments. However, proxy reports are often very difficult or impossible to obtain, and informants may only interact with the patient in narrowly specific life contexts. Furthermore, a host of external factors beyond an individual's control can influence actual behaviors in the community, such as the extent to which treatment or residential and social services are available.

In summary, a variety of approaches are used to define and assess functional disability in schizophrenia. It is clear that individuals with schizophrenia show substantial impairments on both competence- and achievement-based measures. These impairments are evident during the earliest phase of schizophrenia (e.g., Horan, Subotnik, Snyder, & Nuechterlein, 2006; Malla & Payne, 2005) and likely precede onset. For example, recent studies of prodromal subjects report impairments on competence and achievement measures (Addington, Penn, Woods, Addington, & Perkins, 2008a; Pinkham, Penn, Perkins, Graham, & Siege, 2007; Shim et al., 2008). Importantly, the variable correspondence among these different approaches also makes it clear that a substantial disjunction often exists between what one can do and what one actually does in the community. This likely reflects the complex, multidetermined nature of functioning, which is impacted by both individual and environmental factors. Generally speaking, functional capacity is more highly influenced by individual factors, such as neurocognitive level, whereas functional attainment is more likely to be influenced by environmental factors, such as social support, employment and housing opportunities, and treatment resources.

In light of the complex relations among different aspects of functioning and the diversity of available measures, two recent NIMH initiatives have evaluated a range of outcome measures to make empirically based recommendations about the best available measures, particularly for use in clinical trials. Regarding competence measures, the MATRICS-CT project examined several long- and short-form measures. The University of California at San Diego's (UCSD) Performance-based Skills Assessment (UPSA) (Patterson, Goldman, McKibbin, Hughs, & Jeste, 2001), which measures planning and organization, managing finances, communication, transportation, and household management skills, had the strongest overall properties for long-form measures. Among the short forms, the Test of Adaptive Behavior in Schizophrenia (TABS) (Velligan, Diamond, Glahn, Ritch, & Maples, 2007) and UPSA-Brief (Mausbach, Harvey, Goldman, Jeste, & Patterson, 2007) appeared to have the strongest features. For attainment measures, the Validation of Everyday Real-World Outcomes (VALERO) (Harvey et al., 2011) project compared a range of measures using different sources of information. The Specific Levels of Functioning (SLOF) scale (Schneider & Struening, 1983), a global measure of social, everyday living, and vocational outcomes, based on clinician ratings that combined self- and informant-reports, performed the best overall. These measures will likely be increasingly used in clinical trials for new treatments focused on neurocognition and may also be useful for bringing greater uniformity to future studies of social cognition and functional disability.

ASSOCIATION BETWEEN SOCIAL COGNITION AND FUNCTIONAL OUTCOME

A key motivation to study social cognition in schizophrenia is to explain the heterogeneity of functional outcome that is evident among people with schizophrenia. For example, misperceptions during social interactions could adversely impact how people with schizophrenia interpret the behavior of others, which may result in interpersonal conflicts and/or social withdrawal. In support of this expectation, a growing literature demonstrates associations between social cognition and various aspects of community functioning.

In 2006, Couture and colleagues (Couture, Penn, & Roberts, 2006) published the first major review of the literature in this area. This descriptive, qualitative review included 23 studies and considered four aspects of social cognition: EP, SP, AB, and ToM. Regarding outcome, two aspects of functional competence (social skills, social problem solving) and two aspects of functional attainment (social behavior within a psychiatric inpatient milieu, community functioning as assessed by various subjective and objective measures) were considered. The review documented solid initial support for cross-sectional correlations between social cognition and outcome. Results were strongest for the social cognitive domain of SP, with 10 out of 12 studies showing significant relations with competence and attainment measures. Emotion perception showed a consistent, although less robust, relationship to both types of outcome in nine out of 10 studies. The considerably smaller number of available studies for ToM ($n = 4$) and AS ($n = 2$) provided initial support for their functional relevance. The review thus documented consistent relations between social cognition and functioning, although some limitations of available studies were noted, including (a) uncertainty as to whether social cognition is more strongly related to functional capacity as compared to functional outcome, (b) nearly all studies were cross-sectional, and (3) more than half of the studies included chronically ill hospitalized patients.

The significant linkages described by Couture and colleagues were recently replicated and extended in a meta-analysis by Fett and colleagues in 2011 (Fett et al.,

2011). This review initially considered the same domains of social cognition and functional outcome as Couture et al. but used stricter criteria for inclusion in the quantitative analyses. Attributional style was ultimately excluded from the analysis because only one appropriate study was identified. For the remaining three social cognitive domains, there were sufficient numbers of studies to examine their relations to the functional outcome domain of "community functioning" (again, including various subjective and objective measures). Results indicated that community functioning was strongly related to each of the social cognitive domains, with mean correlations as follows: ToM = .48 in three studies, SP = .41 in three studies, and EP = .31 in five studies. Aside from the findings for community functioning, available studies permitted examination of only two other specific social cognition-functional outcome relationships, although both were significant. Specifically, EP had a mean correlation of .22 with social behavior in the psychiatric milieu across six studies, and SP had a mean correlation of .24 with social skills across five studies. None of the significant effects reported in this review was moderated by gender, age, or inpatient status. Although this study provides support for the general conclusions of Couture et al., it should be noted that the relatively small number of studies precludes firm conclusions about whether specific aspects of social cognition are associated with specific aspects of functional outcome.

In addition to the cross-sectional relations between social cognition and functional outcome documented in chronically ill patients in the above reviews, we are also learning more about when in the course of schizophrenia these relationships are detectable, as well as the longitudinal predictive validity of social cognition. A few studies have documented associations between aspects of social cognition and functional outcome during the early, recent-onset phase of schizophrenia in community dwelling outpatients (Addington, Saeedi, & Addington, 2006b; Williams et al., 2008) indicating that these associations are evident during the early course of schizophrenia. It remains unclear whether these relationships are detectable in vulnerable subjects prior to illness onset. Although both social cognitive impairments and functional attainment impairments have been identified in prodromal samples (Addington, Penn, Woods, Addington, & Perkins, 2008b; Green et al. in press; Pinkham et al., 2007), no published studies have demonstrated a significant linkage between these two domains prior to illness onset.

A few studies have also provided longitudinal support for social cognition prospectively predicting functional outcome (Addington et al., 2006b; Horan et al. in press; Kee, Green, Mintz, & Brekke, 2003). For example, in a recent study from our group (Horan et al., in press), 55 first-episode schizophrenia patients completed baseline and 12-month follow-up assessments of three domains of social cognition (EP, ToM, SP), as well as an objective measure of social attainment and symptom assessments. As shown in Figure 6.2, a composite score based on all three social cognitive tests demonstrated good longitudinal stability with a test–retest correlation .87. Higher baseline and 12-month social cognition scores were both robustly associated with significantly better work functioning, independent

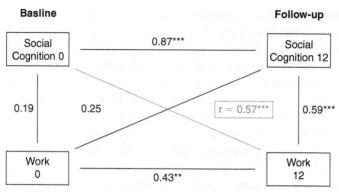

Figure 6.2 Twelve-month longitudinal prediction of functional attainment (work) in first-episode schizophrenia. Cross-lagged panel analysis revealed a significant difference (Z > 2.0) between the correlations on the two diagonals. Specifically, the correlation between baseline Social Cognition and Work Functioning at follow-up (r = .57) was significantly larger than the correlation between baseline Work Functioning and Social Cognition at follow-up (r = .25) after accounting for all other cross-sectional and longitudinal correlations in the figure. The difference between the correlations on the diagonals remained significant even after accounting for clinical symptom levels at baseline and follow-up. These results are consistent with a model in which baseline levels of social cognition drove later 12-month functional attainment in the domain of work.

living, and social functioning at the 12-month follow-up assessment. The results were particularly robust for the domain of work functioning (displayed in the figure). In line with earlier findings from our group (Kee et al., 2003), cross-lagged panel analyses were consistent with a causal model in which baseline social cognition drove later functional outcome in the domain of work, above and beyond the contribution of symptoms. These results support the notion that social cognitive impairments longitudinally predict later levels of functioning.

In summary, a solid database documents significant cross-sectional associations between social cognition and different aspects of functional outcome. The literature is not sufficiently mature to know whether particular social cognitive processes are more specifically related to functional capacity versus functional attainment, or to particular social, vocational, or independent living domains. Research is also moving beyond studies of bivariate correlations in chronically ill patients to identify both when and how social cognition influences functional outcome. In the following section, we expand on this theme by examining how social cognition interfaces with a well-established determinant of outcome—neurocognition—to impact functioning.

THE ADDED VALUE OF SOCIAL COGNITION

Because neurocognition and social cognition are both impaired and both related to poor functional outcome in schizophrenia, a fundamental question is whether neurocognition and social cognition provide uniquely informative data for understanding outcome. If a very large overlap existed between them, it would raise questions about the value of considering social cognition as an additional factor. We now turn to an overview of three lines of investigation relevant to the question of social cognition's "added value."

Neurocognitive and social cognitive tasks often share cognitive processes, such as working memory and perception, and therefore are clearly associated. Indeed, significant correlations are found between performance on measures of social cognition and neurocognition in schizophrenia (e.g., Kee, Kern, & Green, 1998; Pinkham & Penn, 2006; Sergi & Green, 2002). However, the magnitude of these relations is generally moderate. Furthermore, studies using confirmatory factor analysis in schizophrenia patients (Allen, Strauss, Donohue, & van Kammen, 2007; Bell, Tsang, Greig, & Bryson, 2009; Sergi et al., 2007) or exploratory factor analysis in participants with psychosis or heightened vulnerability to psychosis (van Hooren et al., 2008; Williams et al., 2008) indicate that models fit better when the two domains are separated, compared to when they are combined. The general conclusion from these studies is that social cognition in schizophrenia is associated with neurocognition, but is not redundant with it.

A related question is whether social cognition and neurocognition show differential correlations with functional outcome in schizophrenia. This topic was addressed in the recent meta-analyses by Fett et al. (2011), which directly compared the relative strength of correlations for social cognitive versus neurocognitive measures. Based on available studies, this issue could be most clearly evaluated with regard to the domain of "community functioning." Social cognitive measures accounted for an average of 16% of the variance in community functioning, which was significantly larger than the 6% of variance accounted for by composite measures of neurocognition (as well as by nearly all individual neurocognitive domains considered). The domain of ToM accounted for the social cognition advantage. No differential correlations for the other outcome domains were reported (despite some trends favoring social cognition), although the number of studies available for these comparisons was small. Thus, available evidence indicates that social cognition, particularly ToM, shows a stronger relation to community functioning than does neurocognition.

Along these lines, several studies have addressed the question of whether social cognition accounts for additional unique variance in outcome, above and beyond the contribution of neurocognition. Several studies using correlation and regression techniques have now evaluated this issue. It does indeed appear from several datasets that social cognition contributes incremental validity for both real-world functional attainment and functional capacity beyond that provided by neurocognition (e.g., Corrigan & Toomey, 1995; Ihnen, Penn, Corrigan, & Martin, 1998; Mancuso, Horan, Kern, & Green, 2011; Pan, Chen, Chen, & Liu, 2009; Penn, Spaulding, Reed, & Sullivan, 1996; Pinkham & Penn, 2006; Poole, Tobias, & Vinogradov, 2000; Roncone et al., 2002). Thus, neurocognition and social cognition appear to be separable domains that uniquely contribute to the prediction of functional outcome in schizophrenia.

In summary, available data support the added value of considering social cognition and neurocognition as separate domains in studies of functional outcome. In addition to showing only moderate relations to neurocognition, social cognition appears to be more strongly related to functional attainment than is neurocognition and to contribute incremental variance to various aspects of functioning. In the following section, we consider a series of modeling studies that have examined exactly how these two processes interact to impact functioning.

MODELING STUDIES: SOCIAL COGNITION AS A MEDIATOR

Linkages among neurocognition, social cognition, and functional outcome are well documented. However, the pathway(s) through which neurocognitive or social cognitive deficits ultimately lead to poor functioning are complex and likely involve a host of intervening and interacting variables. As illustrated in Figure 6.3, M.F. Green and Nuechterlein (1999) proposed that social cognition functions as a key mediator between neurocognition on the one hand and functional outcome on the other. In a mediation model, the relationship between an independent variable X (neurocognition) and a dependent variable Y (functional outcome) is explained by a third intervening, or mediating, variable M (social cognition). Consider an example of mediation from the depression literature. Neuroticism (X) is a personality trait that shows consistent relations to depression (Y). However, both neuroticism and depression are associated with rumination, and rumination (M) has been found to mediate the relation between neuroticism and depression (e.g., Roelofs, Huibers, Peeters, Arntz, & van Os, 2008). This suggests that rumination is a mechanism or route by which neuroticism ultimately leads to depression and is, therefore, an important intervention target. Using statistical modeling approaches, such as path analysis and structural equation modeling,

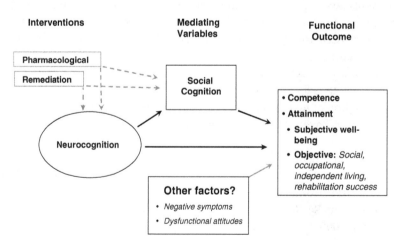

Figure 6.3 Model of relations among neurocognition, social cognition, and functional outcome

schizophrenia researchers have begun to empirically test whether social cognition mediates the link between neurocognitive impairments and functional outcome.

To our knowledge, 14 published studies from 12 independent datasets have evaluated whether social cognitive variables mediate the relation between neurocognition and one or more aspects of functional outcome in schizophrenia. These studies are summarized in Table 6.1. The sample sizes range from 26 to 178 individuals in inpatient and/or outpatient settings. Regarding functional outcome domains, eight studies evaluated aspects of attainment measures, three examined competence measures, two examined a combination of competence and attainment measures, and one focused on 12-month psychosocial rehabilitation success. Across the diverse samples, statistical methods, neurocognitive and social cognitive measures, and outcome domains reflected in these 14 studies, 13 reported support for a mediating role for social cognition. The hypothesis that social cognition serves as a mediator in explaining outcome has thus received remarkably consistent support to date.

Although the available evidence strongly supports the conceptualization of social cognition as a mediator, some methodological aspects of these studies warrant comment. First, the majority of studies were cross-sectional, which limits any inferences that can be made about causality. Second, certain subject characteristics may be relevant to consider in understanding these mechanistic relations. For example, the one study that failed to support a mediating role for social cognition used a unique inpatient forensic sample of patients who been hospitalized as an alternative to incarceration (Nienow, Docherty, Cohen, & Dinzeo, 2006). Third, the range of social cognitive variables considered has been fairly narrow, focusing largely on affect and social perception, and the role of other social cognitive variables remains to be explored. Fourth, open questions remain about the optimal modeling of functional outcome variables. For example, it remains unclear whether competence measures, which assess what one can do under ideal laboratory conditions, should be modeled either together with or separate from attainment measures of actual real-world functioning. It is also possible that different causal pathways lead to different aspects of outcome (e.g., competence measures, objective attainment measures, subjective attainment measures).

A final consideration is that these models typically leave over half the variance in outcome unaccounted for. Thus, incorporating additional variables believed to impact outcome into these models (which will require larger sample sizes) will more comprehensively account for outcome. This type of work has already begun by examining the interactive contributions of variables such as negative symptoms, motivational processes, emotional experience and reactivity, dysfunctional attitudes, and metacognition (Couture, Granholm, & Fish, 2011; Gard, Fisher, Garrett, Genevsky, & Vinogradov, 2009; Lysaker et al., 2010.; Mathews & Barch, 2010; Rassovsky, Horan, Lee, Sergi, & Green, 2011; Tso, Grove, & Taylor, 2010).

In summary, schizophrenia researchers are developing a clearer understanding of how social cognition contributes to poor functioning. Recent statistical modeling studies implicate social cognition as a key intervening step between neurocognition and functional outcome, suggesting that social cognition is more proximal

Table 6.1 STUDIES EXAMINING WHETHER SOCIAL COGNITION MEDIATES THE RELATION BETWEEN NEUROCOGNITION AND FUNCTIONAL OUTCOME IN SCHIZOPHRENIA

Study	Sample	Design	Neurocognitive and social cognitive domains	Functional outcome domain	Statistical approach	Social cognition mediates?
				Competence-based		
Nienow et al., 2006	56 schizophrenia or schizoaffective forensic inpatients	Cross-sectional	**Neurocognition function:** Vigilance; Early visual processing **Social cognition:** Affect perception	**Social Problem Solving** (AIPSS)	Regression analyses, Sobel test	No
Vaskinn et al., 2008	26 schizophrenia patients	Cross-sectional	**Neurocognition:** Verbal fluency; Processing speed; Vigilance; Working memory; Executive functions; Verbal memory; Visual memory; Problem solving; Learning Potential **Social cognition:** Affect perception	**Social Problem Solving** (AIPSS)	Regression analyses	Yes
Meyer & Kurtz, 2009	53 schizophrenia or schizoaffective outpatients	Cross-sectional	**Neurocognition:** Verbal intelligence; Vigilance; Problem-solving; Verbal memory **Social Cognition** Affect perception	**Social Problem Solving** (SSPA)	Regression analyses	Yes

				Attainment-based		
Vauth, Rusch, Wirtz, & Corrigan, 2004	133 schizophrenia inpatients	Cross-sectional	**Neurocognition:** Vigilance; Executive functions; Cognitive flexibility; Working memory; Verbal memory **Social cognition:** Social knowledge	**Objective functioning** (WPP)	Structural Equation Modeling	Yes
Brekke, Kay, Kee, & Green, 2005	139 schizophrenia or schizoaffective outpatients (100 completed the 12-month protocol)	12-month longitudinal	**Neurocognition:** Verbal fluency; Distractibility; Verbal memory; Vigilance; Executive functions **Social cognition:** Affect perception	**Objective** (CAF, RFS) **and Subjective functioning** (self-report social support scale)	Path analysis	Yes
Addington, Saeedi, & Addington, 2006a	103 outpatients: 50 first-episode psychosis, 53 multiepisode schizophrenia	12-month longitudinal	**Neurocognition:** Verbal fluency; Verbal memory; Visual memory; Working memory; Executive functions; Vigilance; Early visual processing; Visual-constructional ability; Visuomotor sequencing; Psychomotor speed **Social cognition:** Social perception; Social knowledge	**Subjective functioning** (QLS)	Regression analyses	Yes

(continued)

Table 6.1 (CONTINUED)

Study	Sample	Design	Neurocognitive and social cognitive domains	Functional outcome domain	Statistical approach	Social cognition mediates?
Sergi, Rassovsky, Nuechterlein, & Green, 2006	75 schizophrenia outpatients	Cross-sectional	**Neurocognition:** Early visual processing **Social Cognition:** Social Perception	**Objective functioning** (RFS)	Structural Equation Modeling	Yes
Horton & Silverstein, 2008	65 schizophrenia or schizoaffective outpatients (34 deaf and 31 hearing patients)	Cross-sectional	**Neurocognition:** Early visual processing; Vigilance; Verbal memory; Visual memory **Social Cognition:** Affect perception; Theory of Mind	**Objective functioning** (MCAS)	Regression analyses, Sobel test	Yes
Bell et al., 2009	151 schizophrenia or schizoaffective patients	6-month longitudinal (work therapy program)	**Neurocognition:** Executive functions; Verbal Memory; Working memory; Processing speed; Thought disorder **Social cognition:** Affect perception; Theory of Mind; BORI Egocentricity Scale; Social Discomfort on the Job	**Rehabilitation outcome:** Measures of work performance (WBI), job complexity, & consistency of working.	Path Analysis	Yes

Gard et al., 2009	91 schizophrenia outpatients	Cross-sectional	**Neurocognition:** Processing speed; Category Fluency; Working memory; Visual memory; Verbal memory. **Social Cognition:** Affect perception; Face memory; Prosody perception	**Objective functioning** (GAF scores)	Path analysis	Yes
Brittain et al, 2010	64 schizophrenia outpatients	Cross-sectional	**Neurocognition:** Early visual processing **Social Cognition:** Social perception	**Objective functioning** (RFS)	Path analysis	Yes
Rassovsky et al., In press	174 schizophrenia outpatients (Overlapping sample with Sergi et al., 2006)	Cross-sectional	**Neurocognition:** Early visual processing **Social Cognition:** Social perception	**Objective functioning** (RFS)	Structural Equation Modeling	Yes

(continued)

Table 6.1 (CONTINUED)

Study	Sample	Design	Neurocognitive and social cognitive domains	Functional outcome domain	Statistical approach	Social cognition mediates?
				Combined Competence- & Attainment-Based		
Addington, Girard, Christensen, & Addington, 2006	93 first episode and multiple-episode schizophrenia patients (Overlapping sample with Addington et al., 2006)	Cross-sectional	**Neurocognition:** Letter fluency; Verbal memory; Visual memory; Working memory; Executive functions; Attention; Early visual processing; Visual-constructional ability; Visuomotor sequencing; Psychomotor speed **Social cognition:** Affect perception; Social knowledge	**Social problem solving** (AIPPS), **Subjective & Objective functioning** (QLS, SFS)	Structural Equation Modeling	Yes
Couture et al., 2011	178 schizophrenia or schizoaffective outpatients	Cross-sectional	**Neurocognition:** Psychomotor speed; Working memory; Verbal learning; Visual learning; Executive functions **Social cognition:** Theory of mind	**Social Problem Solving** (MASC) **and Subjective functioning** (ILSS)	Path Analysis	Yes

AIPPS, Assessment of Interpersonal Problem Solving; CAF, Community Adjustment Form; GAF, Global Assessment of Functioning; ILSS, Independent Living Skills Survey; MASC, Maryland Assessment of Social Competence; MCAS, Multnomah Community Ability Scale; QLS, Quality of Life Scale; RFS, Role Functioning Scale; SAS, Social Adjustment Scale; SBS, Social Behaviour Scale; SFS, Social Functioning Scale; WBI, Work Behavior Inventory; WPP, Work Personality Profile.

to outcome than is neurocognition in the chain of causal factors that ultimately lead to poor functional outcome. Further, when social cognition is included in statistical models, the direct relationship between neurocognition and functioning is often reduced to near zero (referred to as *full mediation*).

These findings indicate that social cognition is a rational target for interventions—the proximity of social cognition to outcome suggests that improvements in this domain may generalize better to improvements in daily functioning than will improvements in neurocognition. Because social cognition serves as both an independent predictor and a mediator of outcome, it seems likely that a specific focus on neurocognition alone will not be sufficient to help patients achieve a full functional recovery. In terms of other clinical implications, these findings strongly support the importance of assessing each patient's level of social cognition. Finally, these findings support the potential value of social cognition as an important target for novel treatment development using both pharmacological and psychosocial approaches (as discussed in other chapters).

CONCLUSION

Social cognition is an important area of study in schizophrenia for several reasons, and one of them is its relationship to functioning. This chapter provides an overview of the associations between social cognition and functional outcome in schizophrenia. The studies in this area have primarily included affect and social perception, but there is increasing attention paid to other aspects of social cognition, including ToM and attributional bias. Nonetheless, some areas are largely missing altogether (e.g., empathy, emotion in biological motion). Studies of outcome have considered two distinct types of outcome; although a few have considered competence measures (i.e., simulations of daily life), most have examined self-report measures of daily functioning in the community. As research on linkages to outcome progresses, alternative functional assessment approaches, such as in-community observational methods or experience sampling methods (Bromley & Brekke, 2010), may shed further light on this issue.

At this time, a critical mass of studies have examined social cognition and functional outcome, and a large subset of these studies (14 publications based on 12 independent databases) have used sophisticated modeling techniques to evaluate pathways by which neurocognition, social cognition, and functional outcome interact. All except one of these studies demonstrated mediation by social cognition. Based on these studies, several conclusions are warranted about social cognition in schizophrenia: it is not wholly redundant with nonsocial neurocognition, but instead provides unique information; it has consistent relationships to outcome, and a meta-analysis shows these to be stronger than the relationships between neurocognition and outcome; it acts as a mediator between neurocognition and outcome, indicating that it is an important intervening variable in the pathway to recovery; and, in all of the models considered so far, it is positioned more proximal to outcome than is neurocognition. Thus, an emerging literature is helping to explain the determinants of outcome in schizophrenia and is also providing an empirical foundation and clear rationale for development of new social cognitive intervention approaches. These interventions offer strong potential for greater functional recovery in our patients.

REFERENCES

Addington, J., Girard, T. A., Christensen, B. K., & Addington, D. (2010). Social cognition mediates illness-related and cognitive influences on social function in patients with schizophrenia-spectrum disorders. *Journal of Psychiatry and Neuroscience, 35*(1), 49–54.

Addington, J., Penn, D., Woods, S. W., Addington, D., & Perkins, D. O. (2008a). Social functioning in individuals at clinical high risk for psychosis. *Schizophrenia Research, 99*, 119–124.

Addington, J., Penn, D. L., Woods, S. W., Addington, D., & Perkins, D. O. (2008b). Facial affect recognition in individuals at clinical high risk for psychosis. *British Journal of Psychiatry, 192*, 67–68.

Addington, J., Saeedi, H., & Addington, D. (2006a). Facial affect recognition: A mediator between cognitive and social functioning in psychosis? *Schizophrenia Research, 85*(1–3), 142–150.

Addington, J., Saeedi, H., & Addington, D. (2006b). Influence of social perception and social knowledge on cognitive and social functioning in early psychosis. *British Journal of Psychiatry, 189*, 373–378.

Allen, D. N., Strauss, G. P., Donohue, B., & van Kammen, D. P. (2007). Factor analytic support for social cognition as a separable cognitive domain in schizophrenia. *Schizophrenia Research, 93*(1–3), 325–333.

Bell, M., Tsang, H. W., Greig, T. C., & Bryson, G. J. (2009). Neurocognition, social cognition, perceived social discomfort, and vocational outcomes in schizophrenia. *Schizophrenia Bulletin, 35*(4), 738–747.

Bellack, A. S., Green, M. F., Cook, J. A., Fenton, W., Harvey, P. D., Heaton, R. K., et al. (2007). Assessment of community functioning in people with schizophrenia and other severe mental illnesses: A white paper based on an NIMH-sponsored workshop. *Schizophrenia Bulletin, 33*(3), 805–822.

Birchwood, M., Smith, J., Cochran, R., Wetton, S., & Copestake, S. (1990). The social functioning scale: The development and validation of a new scale of social adjustment for use in family intervention programs with schizophrenic patients. *British Journal of Psychiatry, 157*, 853–859.

Brekke, J. S., Kay, D. D., Kee, K. S., & Green, M. F. (2005). Biosocial pathways to functional outcome in schizophrenia. *Schizophrenia Research, 80*, 213–225.

Bromley, E., & Brekke, J. S. (2010). Assessing function and functional outcome in schizophrenia. *Current Topics in Behavioral Neuroscience, 4*, 3–21.

Cook, J. A., Leff, H. S., Blyler, C. R., Gold, P. B., Goldberg, R. W., Mueser, K. T., et al. (2005). Results of a multisite randomized trial of supported employment interventions for individuals with severe mental illness. *Archives of General Psychiatry, 62*(5), 505–512.

Corrigan, P. W., & Toomey, R. (1995). Interpersonal problem solving and information processing in schizophrenia. *Schizophrenia Bulletin, 21*(3), 395–403.

Couture, S. M., Granholm, E. L., & Fish, S. C. (2011). A path model investigation of neu-rocognition, theory of mind, social competence, negative symptoms and real-world functioning in schizophrenia. *Schizophrenia Research, 125,* 152–160.

Couture, S. M., Penn, D. L., & Roberts, D. L. (2006). The functional significance of social cognition in schizophrenia: A review. *Schizophrenia Bulletin, 32*(Suppl. 1), S44–S63.

Eack, S. M., & Newhill, C. E. (2007). Psychiatric symptoms and quality of life in schizo-phrenia: A meta-analysis. *Schizophrenia Bulletin, 33*(5), 1225–1237.

Fett, A. K., Viechtbauer, W., Dominguez, M. D., Penn, D. L., van Os, J., & Krabbendam, L. (2011). The relationship between neurocognition and social cognition with functional outcomes in schizophrenia: A meta-analysis. *Neuroscience and Biobehavioral Reviews, 35,* 573–588.

Gard, D. E., Fisher, M., Garrett, C., Genevsky, A., & Vinogradov, S. (2009). Motivation and its relationship to neurocognition, social cognition, and functional outcome in schizo-phrenia. *Schizophrenia Research, 115*(1), 74–81.

Green, M. F. (1996). What are the functional consequences of neurocognitive deficits in schizophrenia? *American Journal of Psychiatry, 153*(3), 321–330.

Green, M. F., Bearden, C. E., Cannon, T. D., Fiske, A. P., Hellemann, G. S., Horan, W. P., et al. (in press). Social cognition in schizophrenia, part 1: Performance across phase of illness. *Schizophrenia Bulletin.*

Green, M. F., Kern, R. S., Braff, D. L., & Mintz, J. (2000). Neurocognitive deficits and func-tional outcome in schizophrenia: Are we measuring the "right stuff"? *Schizophrenia Bulletin, 26*(1), 119–136.

Green, M. F., Kern, R. S., & Heaton, R. K. (2004). Longitudinal studies of cognition and functional outcome in schizophrenia: Implications for MATRICS. *Schizophrenia Research, 72,* 41–51.

Green, M. F., & Nuechterlein, K. H. (1999). Should schizophrenia be treated as a neurocog-nitive disorder? *Schizophrenia Bulletin, 25,* 309–319.

Greig, T. C., Bryson, G. J., & Bell, M. D. (2004). Theory of mind performance in schizo-phrenia: Diagnostic, symptom, and neuropsychological correlates. *Journal of Nervous and Mental Disease, 192,* 12–18.

Harvey, P. D. (2009). Pharmacological cognitive enhancement in schizophrenia. *Neuropsychology Review, 19,* 324–335.

Harvey, P. D., Raykov, T., Twamley, E., Vella, L., Heaton, R. K., & R.L., P. (2011). Validating the measurement of real-world functional outcomes: Phase I results of the VALERO study. *American Journal of Psychiatry, 168,* 1195–1201.

Harvey, P. D., Velligan, D. I., & Bellack, A. S. (2007). Performance-based measures of functional skills: Usefulness in clinical treatment studies. *Schizophrenia Bulletin, 33*(5), 1138–1148.

Hegarty, J. D., Baldessarini, R. J., Tohen, M., Waternaux, C., & Oepen, G. (1994). One hundred years of schizophrenia: A meta-analysis of the outcome literature. *American Journal of Psychiatry, 151,* 1409–1416.

Heinrichs, D. W., Hanlon, T. E., & Carpenter, W. T. (1984). The quality of life scale: An instrument for rating the schizophrenic deficit syndrome. *Schizophrenia Bulletin, 10,* 388–398.

Horan, W. P., Green, M. F., Degroot, M., Fiske, A., Hellemann, G., Kee, K., et al. (in press). Social cognition in schizophrenia, Part 2: 12–month stability and prediction of func-tional outcome in first-episode patients. *Schizophrenia Bulletin.*

Horan, W. P., Subotnik, K. L., Snyder, K. S., & Nuechterlein, K. H. (2006). Do recent-onset schizophrenia patients experience a "social network crisis"? *Psychiatry, 69*(2), 115–129.

Horton, H. K., & Silverstein, S. M. (2008). Social cognition as a mediator of cognition and outcome among deaf and hearing people with schizophrenia. *Schizophrenia Research, 105*(1–3), 125–137.

Ihnen, G. H., Penn, D. L., Corrigan, P. W., & Martin, J. (1998). Social perception and social skill. *Psychiatry Research, 80,* 275–286.

Kee, K. S., Green, M. F., Mintz, J., & Brekke, J. S. (2003). Is emotional processing a predictor of functional outcome in schizophrenia? *Schizophrenia Bulletin, 29,* 487–497.

Kee, K. S., Kern, R. S., & Green, M. F. (1998). Perception of emotion and neurocognitive functioning in schizophrenia: What's the link? *Psychiatry Research, 81,* 57–65.

Kern, R. S., Glynn, S. M., Horan, W. P., & Marder, S. R. (2009). Psychosocial treatments to promote functional recovery in schizophrenia. *Schizophrenia Bulletin, 35,* 347–361.

Kurtz, M. M., & Mueser, K. T. (2008). A meta-analysis of controlled research on social skills training for schizophrenia. *Journal of Consulting and Clinical Psychology, 76*(3), 491–504.

Lehman, A. F. (1988). A quality of life interview for the chronically mentally ill. *Evaluation and Program Planning, 11,* 51–62.

Leifker, F. R., Patterson, T. L., Heaton, R. K., & Harvey, P. D. (2011). Validating measures of real-world outcome: The results of the VALERO expert survey and RAND panel. *Schizophrenia Bulletin, 37*(2), 334–343.

Lysaker, P. H., Shea, A. M., Buck, K. D., Dimaggio, G., Nicolo, G., Procacci, M., et al. (2010). Metacognition as a mediator of the effects of impairments in neurocognition on social function in schizophrenia spectrum disorders. *Acta Psychiatrica Scandinavica, 122,* 405–413.

Malla, A. K., & Payne, J. (2005). First-episode psychosis: Psychopathology, quality of life, and functional outcome. *Schizophrenia Bulletin, 31,* 650–671.

Mancuso, F., Horan, W. P., Kern, R. S., & Green, M. F. (2011). Social cognition in psychosis: Multidimensional structure, clinical correlates, and relationship with functional outcome. *Schizophrenia Research, 125*(2–3), 143–151.

Marder, S. R., & Fenton, W. S. (2004). Measurement and treatment research to improve cognition in schizophrenia: NIMH MATRICS Initiative to support the development of agents for improving cognition in schizophrenia. *Schizophrenia Research, 72,* 5–10.

Mathews, J. R., & Barch, D. M. (2010). Emotion responsivity, social cognition, and functional outcome in schizophrenia. *Journal of Abnormal Psychology, 119,* 50–59.

Mausbach, B. T., Harvey, P. D., Goldman, S. R., Jeste, D. V., & Patterson, T. L. (2007). Development of a brief scale of everyday functioning in persons with serious mental illness. *Schizophrenia Bulletin, 33,* 1364–1372.

Meyer, M. B., & Kurtz, M. M. (2009). Elementary neurocognitive function, facial affect recognition and social-skills in schizophrenia. *Schizophrenia Research, 110*(1–3), 173–179.

Murray, C. J. L., & Lopez, A. D. (Eds.). (1996). *The global burden of disease.* Boston, MA: Harvard School of Public Health.

Murray, C. J. L., & Lopez, A. D. (1997). Global mortality, disability, and the contributions of risk factors: Global burden of disease study. *Lancet, 349,* 1436–1442.

Nicholl, D., Akhras, K. A., Diels, J., & Schadrack, J. (2010). Burden of schizophrenia in recent diagnosed patients: Healthcare utilisation and cost perspective. *Current Medical Research & Opinion, 26,* 943–955.

Nienow, T. M., Docherty, N. M., Cohen, A. S., & Dinzeo, T. J. (2006). Attentional dysfunction, social perception, and social competence: What is the nature of the relationship? *Journal of Abnormal Psychology, 115*(3), 408–417.

Pan, Y. J., Chen, S. H., Chen, W. J., & Liu, S. K. (2009). Affect recognition as an independent social function determinant in schizophrenia. *Comprehensive Psychiatry, 50*(5), 443–452.

Patterson, T. L., Goldman, S., McKibbin, C. L., Hughs, T., & Jeste, D. V. (2001). UCSD performance-based skills assessment: Development of a new measure of everyday functioning for severely mentally ill adults. *Schizophrenia Bulletin, 27*(2), 235–245.

Patterson, T. L., & Mausbach, B. T. (2010). Measurement of functional capacity: A new approach to understanding functional differences and real-world behavioral adaptation in those with mental illness. *Annual Review of Clinical Psychology, 6,* 139–154.

Penn, D. L., Spaulding, W. D., Reed, D., & Sullivan, M. (1996). The relationship of social cognition to ward behavior in chronic schizophrenia. *Schizophrenia Research, 20,* 327–335.

Pinkham, A. E., & Penn, D. L. (2006). Neurocognitive and social cognitive predictors of interpersonal skill in schizophrenia. *Psychiatry Research, 143*(2–3), 167–178.

Pinkham, A. E., Penn, D. L., Perkins, D. O., Graham, K. A., & Siege, M. (2007). Emotion perception and social skill over the course of psychosis: A comparison of individuals "At-risk" for psychosis and individuals with early and chronic schizophrenia spectrum illness. *Cognitive Neuropsychiatry, 12,* 198–212.

Poole, J. H., Tobias, F. C., & Vinogradov, S. (2000). The functional relevance of affect recognition errors in schizophrenia. *Journal of the International Neuropsychological Society, 6*(6), 649–658.

Rassovsky, Y., Horan, W. P., Lee, J., Sergi, M. J., & Green, M. F. (2011). Pathways between early visual processing and functional outcome in schizophrenia. *Psychological Medicine, 41,* 487–497.

Roelofs, J., Huibers, M., Peeters, F., Arntz, A., & van Os, J. (2008). Rumination and worrying as possible mediators in the relation between neuroticism and symptoms of depression and anxiety in clinically depressed individuals. *Behaviour Research and Therapy, 46*(12), 1283–1289.

Roncone, R., Falloon, I. R., Mazza, M., De Risio, A., Pollice, R., Necozione, S., et al. (2002). Is theory of mind in schizophrenia more strongly associated with clinical and social functioning than with neurocognitive deficits? *Psychopathology, 35*(5), 280–288.

Schneider, L. C., & Struening, E. L. (1983). SLOF: A behavioral rating scale for assessing the mentally ill. *Social Work Research and Abstracts, 19,* 9–21.

Sergi, M. J., & Green, M. F. (2002). Social perception and early visual processing in schizophrenia. *Schizophrenia Research, 59,* 233–241.

Sergi, M. J., Rassovsky, Y., Nuechterlein, K. H., & Green, M. F. (2006). Social perception as a mediator of the influence of early visual processing on functional status in schizophrenia. *American Journal of Psychiatry, 163,* 448–454.

Sergi, M. J., Rassovsky, Y., Widmark, C., Reist, C., Erhart, S., Braff, D. L., et al. (2007). Social cognition in schizophrenia: Relationships with neurocognition and negative symptoms. *Schizophrenia Research, 90*(1–3), 316–324.

Shim, G., Kang, D. -H., Chung, Y. S., Yoo, S. Y., Shin, N. Y., & Kwon, J. S. (2008). Social functioning deficits in young people at risk for schizophrenia. *Australian and New Zealand Journal of Psychiatry, 42,* 678–685.

Stein, L. I., & Test, M. A. (1980). Alternatives to mental hospital treatment: I. Conceptual model treatment program and clinical evaluation. *Archives of General Psychiatry, 37,* 392–397.

Tolman, A. W., & Kurtz, M. M. (2012). Neurocognitive predictors of objective and subjective quality of life in individuals with schizophrenia: A meta-analytic investigation.
Schizophrenia Bulletin, 38, 304–315.

Tso, I. F., Grove, T. B., & Taylor, S. F. (2010). Emotional experience predicts social adjustment
independent of neurocognition and social cognition in schizophrenia. *Schizophrenia
Research, 122,* 156–163.

van Hooren, S., Versmissen, D., Janssen, I., Myin- Germeys, I., Campo, J., Mengelers, R.,
et al. (2008). Social cognition and neurocognition as independent domains in psychosis.
Schizophrenia Research, 103, 257–265.

Vaskinn, A., Sundet, K., Friis, S., Simonsen, C., Birkenaes, A. B., Jonsdottir, H., et al. (2008).
Emotion perception and learning potential: Mediators between neurocognition and
social problem-solving in schizophrenia? *Journal of the International Neuropsychological
Society, 14*(2), 279–288.

Vauth, R., Rusch, N., Wirtz, M., & Corrigan, P. W. (2004). Does social cognition influence
the relation between neurocognitive deficits and vocational functioning in schizophrenia? *Psychiatry Research, 128,* 155–165.

Velligan, D. I., Diamond, P., Glahn, D. C., Ritch, J., & Maples, N. (2007). The reliability and
validity of the Test of Adaptive Behavior in Schizophrenia (TABS). *Psychiatry Research,
151,* 55–66.

WHO . (2004). *World health organization global burden of disease—2004 update.*

Williams, L. M., Whitford, T. J., Flynn, G., Wong, W., Liddell, B. J., Silverstein, S., et al.
(2008). General and social cognition in first episode schizophrenia: Identification of
separable factors and prediction of functional outcome using the IntegNeuro test battery. *Schizophrenia Research, 99*(1–3), 182–191.

7

Emotion Processing in Schizophrenia

CHRISTIAN G. KOHLER, ELIZABETH HANSON,
AND MARY E. MARCH ■

Although the majority of efforts to examine behavioral deficits in schizophrenia have focused on clinical symptoms and neurocognition, the past 25 years have seen a growing literature on *social cognition*, defined as the ability to process and apply social and interpersonal relevant information. Within this area, a primary research topic has been emotion processing. The general area of emotion processing can be separated into the different dimensions of expression, recognition, and experience. In schizophrenia, altered functions have been reported in all three dimensions to a degree not found in other psychiatric disorders. Expression and recognition of emotions are dependent on either production or reception of emotional content that is conveyed through a limited number of channels that, most importantly, include face, voice, and language. The majority of the existing literature on conveyance of emotions in healthy persons and in psychiatric disorders has focused on either facial or voice channels of communications. The use of language in schizophrenia has been the subject of a number of investigations (Covington et al., 2005) that have focused on speech morphology, syntax, and semantics; however, the use of language to convey emotional information remains to be examined. Similarly, abnormal use of motor functions for communication of emotions, including gestures and body posture, are common in schizophrenia, and these abnormalities may stem from clinical symptoms, medication side effects, or may reflect neurodevelopmental disturbances. However, the extent to which motor functions beyond facial expressions for conveyance of emotional information is affected in schizophrenia remains to be studied.

This chapter focuses on areas of emotion processing in schizophrenia that have been subject to a representative number of investigations. For emotion expression and recognition, this will include facial and speech channels, and for emotion experience, we will summarize both subjective and more objective observations that the field has relied upon to advance our understanding of hedonic experience in schizophrenia. The following sections will review how dimensions of emotion processing are affected in schizophrenia, with particular emphasis placed on the existing measurements of these functions, their relationship to stages of illness, and the potential for therapeutic interventions.

EMOTION EXPRESSION IN SCHIZOPHRENIA

Diminished expression of emotions has been recognized since the earliest descriptions of schizophrenia. Now viewed as a characteristic negative symptom of the disorder, impairment consists of prominent features that are often used in diagnosis: diminished facial and vocal expression, inappropriate affect, and paucity of expressive gestures. Although diminished vocal expression, use of expressive gestures, and inappropriate affect can be measured with widely used clinical measures of negative symptoms, diminished facial expression has received the most attention in studies of impaired emotion expression and has been found to relate to interpersonal engagement and social functioning (Bellack, Morrison, Wixted, & Mueser, 1990; Breier, Schreiber, Dyer, & Pickar, 1991). Studies have shown that blunted affect is inherent and stable throughout illness, more common among men than women, and can precede the onset of psychosis by many years (Walker, Grimes, Davis, & Smith, 1993). Notably, there has been a shift in the categorization of inappropriate affect. Once grouped in the negative symptom domain with flat affect, inappropriate affect is now viewed as independent of negative symptomatology and more closely related to the disorganization dimension of schizophrenia. Although generally most studies have supported affective flattening rather than inappropriate affect (e.g., smiling or assuming facial expressions that are incongruent with the situation or content of communication), inappropriate affect remains important when considering deficits in facial expression of emotion. If present, inappropriate affect will result in misinterpretation of emotional valence during social interactions, thus possibly contributing to poorer social outcome.

Studies that focus on vocal prosody (e.g., Hoekert, Kahn, Pijnenborg, & Aleman, 2007), or the emotional tone of voice, are limited in number and have predominantly shown that persons with schizophrenia show deficits compared to healthy controls in both spontaneous prosody (elicited through the telling of emotional stories) and prosody repetition (repeating a neutral sentence with a given emotional tone) (Leentjens et al., 1998). However, people with schizophrenia did not show deficits in stress prosody expression, as tested by reading a sentence and stressing a nominated word (Edwards, Jackson, & Pattison, 2002). The use of expressive gestures beyond the face, such as gesticulation and body posture, has not yet been systematically explored.

Assessment of Facial Affective Flattening

The major problem in assessment of flat or blunted affect has been the lack of reliable, objective, and efficient methods for quantifying facial expressions. In clinical settings, observer-based measures of negative symptoms, such as the Positive and Negative Syndrome Scale (PANSS; Kay, Fiszbein, & Opler, 1987) and the Scale for the Assessment of Negative Symptoms (SANS; Andreasen, 1982) are widely used to rate the presence and severity of affective flattening. These scales are often administered in nonstandardized, clinical settings and provide an overall measure of facial expressivity. Although such scales remain widely used, a number of efforts have been made to further elucidate and quantify facial expression measurement. Initial studies of facial affect in schizophrenia beyond standardized rating scales utilized judges who were asked to match photographs of posed affects with emotion words (happy, sad, angry, surprised, or afraid) (Gottheil, Thornton, & Exline, 1976) and identify affective themes (happy, sad, or angry) in silent film clips of subjects telling emotional stories (Gottheil, Paredes, Exline, & Winkelmayer, 1970). These studies found that posed expressions were intact whereas spontaneous expressions were decreased in schizophrenia patients compared to healthy controls.

The Facial Action Coding System (FACS), created by Ekman and Friesen in 1978, remains the gold standard for qualitative analysis of facial emotional expressions. By studying how contraction of different facial muscles changes the appearance in the face, Ekman and Friesen identified discrete facial muscle movements called *action units*, which form the basis for the scoring system. To render a score, trained human coders dissect individual facial expressions into the presence or absence of action units that produced the expression. Problems with the system are that it requires extensive training of human coders, and it may not be sensitive to subtle effects. Emotion FACS (Friesen, 1986) and Facial Expression Coding System (FACES) (Kring, Kerr, Smith, & Neale, 1993) are two measures that have been simplified from the original FACS and adapted for clinical research. Emotion FACS, or EMFACS, only identifies the presence or absence of muscle movements associated with the predicted expression of a particular emotion. FACES provides ratings of overall dynamic facial changes according to the number of positive and negative facial expressions, intensity, and duration.

Studies employing FACS ratings have generally supported the existence of impaired facial expressions in schizophrenia. Trémeau et al. (2005) examined emotional expressions in a series of experiments that utilized traditional and video-adapted FACS ratings to assess both posed and spontaneous expressions. The authors reported that schizophrenia patients exhibited deficits in both spontaneous and posed expressions; however, these deficits were similar to those exhibited by depressed patients. A study employing traditional FACS ratings of both posed and evoked expressions captured by still photography (Kohler et al., 2008a) supported clinical observations of flat and inappropriate affect, and additionally revealed specific differences involving the *Duchenne smile* for happy expressions and decreased furrowed brows in negative emotion expressions. Elements that constitute the Duchenne smile, such as eyelids tightened and cheeks raised, are necessary for a smile to appear sincere, and these movements were less common in schizophrenia. Based on FACES ratings, schizophrenia patients were shown to exhibit less expressivity as measured by the Positive and Negative Affect Schedule (PANAS), yet similar experience based on subjective ratings in response to emotion-inducing film clips (Kring, Kerr, Smith, & Neal, 1993). Based on induction by autobiographical experiences, overall duration and frequencies of emotion expressions indicated affective flattening and inappropriate affect in patients, as evidenced by neutral and non-target expressions. Separated by emotion, schizophrenia patients also exhibited impaired expression of happy, sad, and anger emotions, but not of fear or disgust (Kohler et al., 2008b).

Efforts toward a more objective measurement of facial expression include the employment of facial electromyography (EMG) and computerized algorithms for automated analysis. Facial EMG involves the placement of electrodes on two facial muscles groups, the corrugator and zygomaticus muscles. Studies utilizing facial electromyography in response to emotional films (Mattes, Schneider, Heimann, & Birbaumer, 1995; Earnst et al., 1996) and pictures (Kring, Kerr, & Earnst, 1999) have yielded mixed results, suggesting similar expressions (Earnst et al., 1996; Mattes et al., 1995), reduced zygomaticus activity during happy films (Mattes et al., 1995), and, possibly, inappropriate expressions in persons with schizophrenia (Kring et al., 1999). Limitations of facial EMG studies include possible overidentification of expressions that cannot be discerned in real-life settings and oversimplification of minute expressions resulting from measurement of only two facial muscle groups. Preliminary applications of computerized algorithms for automated analysis have been successful in developing distinct quantitative profiles for four universal emotions: happiness, sadness, anger, and fear (Verma et al., 2005). When applied to schizophrenia patients, quantitative analysis revealed distinct differences compared to controls, especially in the case of anger, and scores correlated with clinical severity of flat affect (Alvino et al., 2007). Future expansion of computerized instrumentations may have wide-ranging clinical implications in patient populations suffering affective deficits and may include, among others, examination of spontaneous emotion expression in dyadic interactions and real-life settings.

Association with Clinical Course

Many studies suggest that diminished emotion expression may precede the onset of psychosis by many years. In one such study, home movies with children who later developed schizophrenia were analyzed for facial expressivity (Walker et al., 1993). Girls who later developed schizophrenia demonstrated fewer joy expressions compared with other emotional expressions. Both boys and girls who subsequently developed schizophrenia displayed increased negative affect when compared to same-sex siblings who did not go on to develop the disorder. Studies utilizing retrospective questionnaire methods have also shown that flat affect may precede the onset of psychosis (Häfner, Maurer, & Löffler, 2003) and increase during the putative prodromal phase (Malla et al., 2002), and flat affect in persons with schizophrenia is associated with poorer premorbid adjustment from child-hood into adulthood before the onset of illness (Gur et al., 2006). Diminished facial expression has been shown to be a stable feature throughout illness, as evidenced in studies of spontaneous and posed expressions in both acute and post-acute stages (Gaebel & Wölwer 2004; Trémeau et al., 2005). Furthermore, it often continues into chronic stages following the amelioration of active psychotic symptoms, and, when compared to patients without flat affect, it has been associ-ated with lower quality of life and poor functional outcome (Gur et al., 2006; Ho, Nopoulos, Flaum, Arndt, & Andreasen, 1998; Milev, Ho, Arndt, & Andreasen, 2005).

The potential influence of extrapyramidal side effects on emotion expression remains unclear. Emotion expression can be worsened by the administration of neuroleptics with strong nigrostriatal dopaminergic blockade (Krakowski, Czobor, & Volavka, 1997; Rifkin, Quitkin, & Klein, 1975; Van Putten & May, 1978), as akinesia, or the loss of power of voluntary movement, represents a potential side effect of these medications. Although some studies have indicated an adverse effect of antipsychotic medications on facial expression (Gaebel & Wölwer, 2004); others that have examined patients both on and off antipsychotics revealed no clear effect on expressivity of emotional experience (Earnst et al., 1996; Kring et al., 1999).

Emotional Contagion

Emotional contagion is the phenomenon in verbal and nonverbal communica-tion whereby individuals automatically mirror the facial expressions and moods of others. According to Hatfield et al. (1994), the process begins with the percep-tion of others' facial expressions, which is followed by the observer's imitation in the form of covert, rapid, and involuntary movements (known as *rapid facial mimicry*). The effect of rapid facial mimicry is believed to be an afferent feedback that induces the perceived emotion in the observer, a potential requisite for the experience of empathy. This phenomenon is similar to the "chameleon effect," in which a person unconsciously mimics the postures, mannerisms, facial expres-sions, and behaviors to reflect that of others in one's current social environ-ment (Chartrand & Bargh, 1999). Chartrand and Bargh (1999) have shown that mimicry improves the quality of interpersonal interactions and increases lik-ing between interaction partners. Furthermore, they revealed that the personal characteristic of empathy increases one's likelihood to use the chameleon effect. The mirror neuron system has been linked to these aspects of social cognition. Evidence from functional magnetic resonance imaging (fMRI) investigations suggests that this process is achieved through a simulation mechanism (Carr et al., 2003). To date, studies utilizing indirect measures of mirror neuron activ-ity have yielded compelling results. In an experiment designed to assess activa-tion of mirror neurons with transcranial magnetic stimulation (TMS) in the left primary motor cortex, subjects observed arm movements while concurrent motor facilitation in thumb muscles was measured. Cortical excitability with TMS was intact in persons with schizophrenia; however, motor facilitation during the experiment was reduced (Enticott et al., 2008). In the first assessment of rapid facial mimicry in schizophrenia patients, Varcin et al. (2010) utilized electromyography to quantify activity in two major facial muscle groups while subjects viewed happy and angry expressions and found that schizophrenia patients exhibited atypical facial mimicry compared to controls. Thus, the decreased ability to appropriately perceive and mimic other's facial expressions, emotions, and behaviors may be one explanation for the social impairment commonly observed in schizophrenia.

It has been posited that schizophrenia patients' difficulties in emotional interaction may stem from a deficit in imitation abilities, which influences their ability to induce emotional contagion in others or to experience emotional contagion themselves. A number of preliminary studies lend support to the theory. In studies in which subjects were asked to imitate different facial emotion expressions, schizophrenia patients were less accurate at imitating and producing facial expressions compared to healthy controls (Park, Matthews, & Gibson, 2008; Schwartz, Mastropaolo, Rosse, Mathis, & Deutsch, 2006), and imitation accuracy strongly correlated with social competence (Park et al., 2008). In a task designed to assess emotional contagion, subjects were shown happy, sad, and neutral faces presented simultaneously with arrows, and instructed to pull their lip corners up or down according to the arrows (as in smiling or frowning) (Falkenberg, Bartels, & Wild, 2008). In healthy subjects, congruous movements (i.e., pulling lip corners up when seeing a happy face) are facilitated and dissonant movements inhibited. These tendencies, considered indicators of emotional contagion, were significantly diminished among the schizophrenia subjects.

Treatment

To date, the field lacks remediation efforts focused on improving facial expressiveness. In a small number of persons with chronic schizophrenia, Schwartz et al. (2006) found impairment in imitation of facial expressions that did not improve with real-time feedback through use of a mirror. Findings from that study also provided support that imitating and practicing emotional expressions may improve the accuracy of facial expressions. Social Cognition and Interaction Training (SCIT; Penn, Roberts, Munt, Jones, & Sheitman, 2005), an intervention with the purpose of improving social cognition and social functioning among schizophrenia patients, utilizes facial mimicry in an attempt to help participants accurately perceive the emotions of others. Although the intervention includes exercises in facial expressivity, improved expressions themselves are not a target of the intervention. Given the important role of facial expression in interpersonal communication and its implications for social functioning, improving facial expressiveness should be a key therapeutic target in future research.

EMOTION RECOGNITION

Recognition of expressions of emotion relies on abilities to analyze nonverbal and verbal communication. For nonverbal communication, this includes facial expressions, gesticulations, and body posture, and for verbal communication, the use of expressive language and speech pattern—or prosody—for conveyance of emotional content.

Facial Channel

Expression of emotions through the facial channel has been the most widely studied component of nonverbal emotion communication, based on the unique ability of the face to produce emotion expressions that are universally recogniz-able. Recognition of facial expressions of emotions are instrumental constituents of nonverbal communication, and a large number of studies have underscored the severity of impairment in schizophrenia. In a recent meta-analysis (Kohler, Walker, Martin Healey, & Moberg, 2010) that included 86 studies published between 1970 and 2007, we examined relevant methodological, demographic, and illness-related factors that moderate the severity of emotion recognition impair-ment. There appeared no difference in effect sizes for studies employing identifi-cation versus differentiation tasks, even though the two tests may be dependent on different visual and other cognitive abilities. In addition, recognition abilities are related to social competence in persons with schizophrenia (Hooker & Park, 2002; Ihnen, Penn, Corrigan, & Martin, 1998; Mueser et al., 1996; Vauth, Rüsch, Wirtz, & Corrigan, 2004) and predict later work functioning and independent liv-ing (Kee, Green, Mintz, & Brekke, 2003). Although emotion recognition impair-ment in schizophrenia has been well documented, it is questionable whether a differential deficit (Chapman & Chapman, 1978) can be demonstrated against the more general impairment in facial processing (Archer, Hay, & Young, 1994; Edwards, Pattison, Jackson, & Wales, 2001; Johnston, Katsikitis, & Carr, 2001; Kerr and Neale, 1993; Kohler, Bilker, Hagendoorn, Gur, & Gur, 2000; Novic, Luchins, & Perline, 1984; Penn et al., 2000; Salem, Kring, & Kerr, 1996). Among other reasons, impaired emotion recognition may be related to the tendency of persons with schizophrenia to visually scan features of the face that are not important in the expression of a particular emotion (Loughland, Williams, & Gordon, 2002; Sasson et al., 2007).

Speech Channel

Prosody represents the nonlexical cues in spoken language and can be divided into linguistic and emotional prosody. Although not mutually exclusive, linguis-tic prosody refers to putting emphasis on certain aspects of a sentence in order to stress the information to be conveyed, whereas emotional prosody refers to emotional tone of voice. As such, prosody contributes to the pragmatics of speech, that is, the context in which linguistic information is conveyed. The study of prosody is complex, as prosody changes considerably depending on language, culture, and even socioeconomic context, whereas for facial expressions there is agreement about a number of emotions that are universally recognized. Hoekert et al. (2007) performed a meta-analysis on more than 20 studies on prosody recognition in schizophrenia and control subjects, and they reported a very large statistical effect size that was not moderated by potential clinical moderators such as age, duration of illness, medication, and patient status, although the latter was not defined further. The authors concluded that the effect size is similar to that reported on cognitive functions in schizophrenia; therefore, prosody represents a key dysfunction that appears stable throughout different stages of the illness.

Measurement

In general, task designs within facial emotion recognition studies can be separated into those that focus on identification of specific emotions, typically choosing from a limited number of choices, and those that differentiate between differing types or intensities of emotion expressions. Although early investigations included non-standardized emotional stimuli, most subsequent studies have employed face stimuli developed by Ekman and Friesen (1978) or Gur et al. (2002). In addition, presentation of test stimuli has changed from paper to computerized administration. The black-and-white stimuli created by Ekman and Friesen consist of posed facial expressions of universally recognized emotions, including happiness, sadness, anger, fear, disgust, and surprise. Pictures are of mostly middle-aged Caucasian posers, with more recent inclusion of Asian posers. The stimuli of Gur et al. include color faces expressing happy, sad, angry, fearful, and disgusted emotions in posed and evoked conditions, across adult age groups and different ethnicities.

For prosody studies, stimuli tend to be more varied, but typically consist of audiotaped sentences or words of neutral content that are spoken aloud in an emotional intonation. Most prosody tasks are not validated, and only a few have been employed by different investigators, such as the VOICE-ID by Kerr and Neale (1993). VOICE-ID contains 21 stimuli across six emotions narrated by male and female voices and is constructed similarly to the face emotion identification by the same group, including happy, sad, anger, fear, surprise, and shame as target emotions.

Association with Clinical Course

Previous longitudinal studies in acutely ill patients and subsequent stabilization (Addington & Addington 1998, Herbener, Hill, Marvin, & Sweeney, 2005; Wölwer, Streit, Polzer, & Gaebel, 1996) indicate the potential unrelatedness of emotion recognition abilities and clinical status in schizophrenia, similar to what has been shown for neurocognition (Keefe et al., 2006). This is consistent with the above-mentioned meta-analysis (Kohler et al., 2010), in which results did not support a specific effect of illness duration on facial emotion recognition abilities. Similarly, recent meta-analysis of the relationship of prosodic abilities with illness characteristics in schizophrenia failed to find an effect of patient status, age, duration of illness, or medication status on prosody (Hoekert et al., 2007). Similar to facial recognition (Bediou et al., 2007), studies of recognition of prosody in early schizophrenia (Edwards et al., 2001; Kucharska-Pietura, David, Masiak, & Phillips, 2005) reported impairment.

Recent investigations, which are described in detail in Addington and Piskulic (2013, Chapter 10, this volume), have extended to persons at genetic or clinical risk for schizophrenia in an attempt to examine whether emotion recognition impairment represents a vulnerability marker for the illness.

Treatment

Attempts to improve emotion processing in schizophrenia have focused mainly on emotion recognition and are described in more detail in other sections of this book.

EMOTION EXPERIENCE

Long-standing observations suggest that decreased or abnormal emotion experience represent characteristic and stable dysfunction in persons with schizophrenia. Emerging evidence has underscored that deficits in emotion experience are particularly important for understanding social dysfunction and poor functional outcome in this illness. Despite the robust finding that both emotion expressivity and recognition are diminished in schizophrenia, the degree of altered experience—ranging from lack of emotion experience to depression and anxiety—is not as well elucidated. This ambiguity relates, among other things, to different methodologies for assessment and such factors as duration of illness (i.e., acute vs. chronic illness), comorbid psychopathology (i.e., depression, anxiety), cognitive deficits, and individual trait differences. Thus, formulating a better understanding of how emotion is experienced in persons with schizophrenia is of critical importance when we pursue ways to treat these seemingly insidious symptoms.

Types of Emotion Experience and Association with Clinical Course

Anhedonia, defined as a diminished capacity to experience pleasure or positive emotions, is considered a cardinal feature of the negative symptom cluster associated with schizophrenia. Importantly, anhedonia does not represent diminished capacity to experience *all* emotions, as schizophrenia patients are well known to exhibit significant clinical symptoms reflecting emotions, particularly depression and anxiety. Anhedonia itself is not specific to schizophrenia, and can be found in other disorders, such as depression, anxiety disorders, and personality disorders. In addition, it is not a ubiquitous symptom of schizophrenia, as some empirical studies report elevated levels of anhedonia in general, whereas other studies found a bimodal distribution of patients with and without anhedonia (Schürhoff et al., 2003; Silver and Shlomo, 2002; Suslow, Roestel, Ohrmann, & Arolt, 2003). Recently, Strauss and Herbener (2011) used cluster and discriminant function analyses to try to identify subgroups of patients within schizophrenia that differ in their emotional experiences. They showed that a minority of patients displayed an altered pattern of emotional responsiveness. When confronted with 131 images from the International Affective Picture System (IAPS), 40% of patients rated negative stimuli as more unpleasant and arousing compared to controls. However, the majority of patients (60%) displayed similar responses as normal controls. Furthermore, the subgroup of patients who reported increased negative emotion also displayed more severe symptoms and more functional impairment as assessed by the PANSS, Chapman Anhedonia Scales (Chapman et al., 1976), and a quality of life measurement.

In regards to clinical course, longitudinal studies generally indicate that anhedonia reflects a stable trait in schizophrenia rather than a temporary state (Herbener & Harrow, 2002; Rey et al., 1994). In most patients, anhedonia appears prominent during both acute and chronic stages of the illness (Horan, Kring, & Blanchard, 2005; Katsanis, Iacono, & Beiser, 1990; Laos, Boyer, & Legrand, 1999) and does not progress remarkably over time. Empirical evidence also suggests that anhedonia may predate the onset of illness (Erlenmeyer-Kimling et al., 1993). This evidence supports Meehl's model (1962) that posits that anhedonia is the expression of a genetic defect in the brain's limbic system, which is involved with reward.

Conceptually, anhedonia can be divided into different dimensions or types. One approach uses the nature of the pleasurable stimulus; for example, whether the hedonic experience is physical or social in nature. A study by Burbridge and Barch (2007) reported decreased arousal by negative stimuli in persons with schizophrenia, and increased social and physical anhedonia. Separating patients into deficit and non-deficit types revealed higher social and physical anhedonia associated with the deficit syndrome (Kirkpatrick & Buchanan, 1990). This finding is in contrast to Earnst and Kring (1999), who reported deficit patients to experience levels of positive and negative emotion that are equivalent to non-deficit patients and controls.

In an effort to clarify the nature of anhedonia, very recent directions in research have focused on the importance of the temporal course of emotion experience. It has been suggested that anhedonia can be divided into the temporal components of *consummatory*, *anticipatory*, and *remembered* pleasure. *Consummatory* pleasure is that pleasure experienced while "in the moment" or while participating in an activity, interaction, or event. *Anticipatory* pleasure is conceptualized as the ability to anticipate that future events will be pleasurable and, therefore, is dependent on motivation. Studies examining these constructs have yielded mixed results but prove to be a promising future direction. Some studies suggest that whereas *consummatory* pleasure is spared, patients with schizophrenia are impaired in anticipating future pleasure (Chan et al., 2010; Gard, Kring, Germans Gard, Horan, & Green, 2007), and this is seen cross-culturally (Chan et al., 2010). Subsequent studies, however, have failed to replicate these findings (Strauss, Wilbur, Warren, August, & Gold, 2011; Trémeau et al., 2010) and reported that anticipated pleasure was not impaired when compared to controls. However, despite similar levels of anticipated pleasure and motivation, patients showed a weaker relationship between motivation and consummatory pleasure (Trémeau et al., 2010). Therefore, in patients with schizophrenia, "in the moment" pleasurable experiences were less likely to induce incentive to repeat the task. In more general terms, patients may have difficulty translating their emotional experience into an appropriate goal-directed behavior (Heerey & Gold, 2007). The translation of pleasurable experiences into motivational states is referred to as "incentive salience attribution" in reward theory (Berridge & Robinson, 2003), and schizophrenia-related deficits in this capacity have also received recent support from a neuroimaging study (Waltz et al., 2009).

Empirical evidence has also suggested that people with schizophrenia have trouble maintaining an emotional experience over time, in order to guide behavior. In one study, based on startle response to transient evocative emotional stimuli (Kring, Germans Gard, & Gard, 2011), patients did not maintain the response, whereas controls did, thus indicating that the motivational system did not remain engaged in patients. This "maintenance deficit" or inability to maintain the representation of an affective or emotional experience was also shown in an fMRI study. Patients and controls did not differ in areas of brain activation when viewing emotion-eliciting pictures, but only controls maintained this pattern after the images were removed (Ursu et al., 2011), suggesting a disconnection in the prefrontal circuitry supporting the critical link between affect and goal-directed behavior. Ultimately, the inability to "hold in mind" representations of an emotional experience may interfere with a patient's pursuit of desired goals, contributing to avolition.

A second mechanism that may affect anhedonia in schizophrenia relates to the potential effect of memory impairments for emotional experiences. An inability to sufficiently remember pleasurable events may contribute to deficits in goal-directed behavior and the symptoms of avolition and anhedonia. For example, in one study, working memory deficits were found to moderate the relationship between physical anhedonia and participants' emotional experience of positive stimuli (Burbridge & Barch, 2007). Similarly, Gard et al. (2011) showed that patients' ability to recall both positive and negative stimuli decreased over time delay, even when given explicit instructions to remember their experience. Patients with schizophrenia appear to be impaired in remembering emotional experiences, particularly over delay periods, and this, in turn, may affect their motivation to engage in potentially pleasurable experiences.

Last, anhedonia may reflect impairments in reward processing (Gold, Waltz, Prentice, Morris, & Heerey, 2008). In a preference-conditioning task, Herbener (2009) found that both patients with schizophrenia and healthy controls demonstrated a greater preference for the more frequently rewarded pattern. However, following a 24-hour delay, controls continued to demonstrate this pattern but patients did not. In sum, current research in schizophrenia suggests the presences of deficits in reward processing or in memory of pleasurable events, rather than a deficit in the ability to experience pleasure during a potentially rewarding experience.

Cohen et al. (2010) have suggested a two-process theory of schizophrenia-related emotional deficits involving both ambivalence and apathy. *Ambivalence* is characterized by simultaneous activation of positive and negative emotions and reflects a dysfunction in the ability to effectively inhibit negative emotions; whereas *apathy* is characterized by anhedonia and essentially no negative emotion. Although apathy is more commonly associated with deficit syndrome patients and may be more central to the hedonic deficit in schizophrenia, both processes are central constituents of negative symptomatology and are strongly associated with functional impairment. An *affective* trait represents the stable individual tendency to experience specific emotional states. In this personality-driven view, negative affectivity (NA; i.e., the tendency to view the world as threatening, problematic, and distressing) and positive affectivity (PA; i.e., the tendency to engage in the world with energy and enthusiasm), represent two core features of emotion experience. Schizophrenia is characterized by abnormally high levels of NA and low PA throughout the illness course (Horan, Blanchard, Clark, & Green, 2008; Kring & Moran, 2008). Beyond experiencing a lack of enjoyment in pleasurable activities, it has also been shown that individuals with schizophrenia report less positive emotions (i.e., joy and happiness) and more negative emotions (i.e., fear, guilt, shame, anxiety) across a range of everyday activities (Tso, Grove, & Taylor, 2010).

Depression is common in schizophrenia, with the lifetime prevalence for a major depressive episode estimated to be 60%, much higher than the 8%-26% risk for the general population (Diwan et al., 2007; Martin et al., 1985). Anhedonia is also a common feature of depression and, therefore, unveiling the relationship among anhedonia, depression, and other clinical symptoms is critical in elucidating the nature of emotional experience in schizophrenia. Clinically, the anhedonia of depression can be viewed as a "loss of pleasure in usually enjoyed activities," whereas anhedonia of schizophrenia is a pervasive loss and diminished capacity to experience pleasure. Although overlap between depression and anhedonia may exist in schizophrenia and may be difficult to differentiate clinically (Kollias et al., 2008), there have been several factor analytic studies indicating that anhedonia and depression are separate constructs in the symptomatology of schizophrenia (Horan et al., 2005; Laos, Noisette, Legrand, & Boyer, 2000) and that they represent distinct psychopathological dimensions.

Depression is linked to suicide (Harris & Barraclough, 1997), which represents the leading cause of premature death among younger people with schizophrenia

(Caldwell & Gottesman, 1990). The rate of suicide in schizophrenia is about 10 times that of the general population and claims the lives of between 4% and 13% of sufferers (Diwan et al., 2007; Martin, Cloninger, & Guse, 1985). Persons in the acute and early stages of illness are more likely to experience suicidality (Barrett et al., 2010; Bottlender, Strauss, & Moller, 2000). In one study, the majority of schizophrenia patients who completed suicide were found to be depressed in the months preceding their death, although other factors may have contributed (Montross et al., 2008).

Anxiety disorders, although quite frequent in schizophrenia, are poorly understood and underrecognized. Anxiety symptoms and disorders can occur in any phase of the illness and may be exacerbated or triggered by unpleasant psychotic experiences, responses to adverse life events, and antipsychotics. The prevalence rate of anxiety disorders in schizophrenia has been reported to be as high as 50%, and includes posttraumatic stress disorder (PTSD), obsessive-compulsive disorder (OCD), and social anxiety disorder, with social anxiety emerging as the most common anxiety disorder (Achim et al., 2011). Preliminary evidence suggests that anxiety may be a core feature of schizophrenia unrelated to positive and negative symptoms. Social anxiety, however, may be easily misidentified as a negative symptom (e.g., social avoidance and withdrawal or low motivation and withdrawal) and therefore may go undetected and untreated. Schizophrenia with comorbid anxiety has been associated with poorer quality of life, increased lifetime suicide attempts, and increased substance abuse (Pallantini, Querciolo, & Hollander, 2004). Thus, current research directions are aimed at designing new tools for assessment of anxiety disorders in persons with schizophrenia and new treatment interventions.

The common assumption exists that emotion expression mirrors experience. Clearly, if affective flattening correlates with muted experience, this would readily identify impaired emotion experience in schizophrenia. However, findings suggest that a disjunction exists between patients' outward expression and their internal experience of emotions. Individuals with schizophrenia may show blunted affect in the form of significantly diminished expressions, but they report the same intensity of emotional experience as healthy controls. This finding has been confirmed in studies employing social interactions and nonsocial evocative stimuli (emotional film clips, tastes, cartoons) (Aghevli et al., 2003) and has been seen across laboratories independent of patients' medication status and deficit state.

It has been suggested that persons with schizophrenia may be unreliable reporters of their internal emotional states, underscoring the need for another proxy measure of emotion experience (Jaeger, Bitter, Czobor, & Volavka, 1990). Further complicating the picture is the finding that patients, despite their lack of expressivity and comparable experience to controls, show higher skin conductance reactivity to neutral, negative, and positive stimuli (i.e., film clips) (Kring & Neale, 1996). Therefore, we assume that outward displays of emotion in a person with schizophrenia may not represent an accurate reflection of his or her internal emotional experiences.

Assessment of Emotion Experience

Two main approaches exist to study emotion experience. One approach is to study mood states and more transient emotional experiences and examine whether positive or negative emotional states are related to other clinical symptoms or represent reactions to external events. Another approach focuses on more stable affective traits or individual differences in the tendency to experience emotion. Measured in this way, assessment of emotional experience requires information about the frequency and intensity of subjective experiences across a range of situations that would normally be expected to elicit changes in positive and negative emotions. A number of commonly used rating scales exist that measure emotion experience and potential effects of treatment. These scales are used to rate intensity of emotion experience, as well as symptoms of depression, anxiety, and mania. Four common approaches exist to assess emotion experience in schizophrenia, including interview-based assessment, self-report trait measures, laboratory-based assessments, and experience sampling.

INTERVIEW

In an interview-based assessment, a trained administrator uses a semi-structured interview to elicit information about daily activities and subjective emotional experiences. Some commonly used measures include the Scale for the Assessment of Negative Symptoms (SANS; Andreasen, 1982), the Positive and Negative Symptom Rating Scale (PANSS; Kay et al., 1987), the Scale for Emotional Blunting (SEB; Abrams & Taylor, 1978), and the Schedule for the Deficit Syndrome (SDS; Kirkpatrick et al., 1989). Each of these scales marginally differs in how emotional experiences are assessed. In a review by Horan et al. (2005), it was determined that anhedonia can be reliably assessed using the SANS anhedonia-asociality subscale, and this scale was deemed as the best available assessment tool at the time for measuring anhedonia.

A collaborative study is currently undergoing validation of a new negative symptom assessment scale, the Clinical Assessment Inventory of Negative Symptoms (CAINS; Forbes et al., 2010). This assessment tool is unique in that ratings are based on the person's self-reported motivation, interest, and desire, as well as on their actual behavior across social, vocational, and recreational domains. The CAINS includes measures of consummatory and anticipatory pleasure, in which persons report on pleasurable experiences they had in the past week and pleasurable experiences they think they will have in the upcoming week across all the domains.

QUESTIONNAIRES

Another way to measure hedonic ability is via self-report questionnaires; examples include the Chapman Social and Physical Anhedonia scales (Chapman et al., 1976) and the Temporal Experience of Pleasure Scale (TEPS; Gard, Germans Gard, Kring, & John, 2006). It has been questioned whether self-reports are a reliable way to measure anhedonia and experience. On one hand, self-report questionnaires limit the effects that social skills and verbal expressivity exert on measurement in an interview setting. On the other hand, it is possible that cognitive deficits associated with schizophrenia might interfere with a patient's ability to accurately remember his or her emotional experience in daily life and thus he or she may be over- or underreporting on his or her experiences. One way to overcome this obstacle is to examine emotion experience during everyday life or during emotion-induction procedures. *Experience sampling* provides a naturalistic way of assessing emotional experiences. In experience sampling, patients are cued randomly throughout the day to record their current emotions and experiences, thus eliminating the effect of memory. In laboratory-based assessments, subjects are exposed to a standard set of pleasant, neutral, and negative stimuli, such as pictures, movies, and food. Laboratory studies usually use self-report measures and/or interviews.

The type and degree of abnormal emotional experience in schizophrenia seems to differ based upon the method of assessment (i.e., self-report, experience sampling, and interview-based or laboratory-based assessments). For example, patients typically report anhedonia and deficits in emotional experience when interviews or questionnaires are used. Experience sampling studies indicate that patients report higher levels of negative emotion and lower levels of positive emotions in the course of their daily lives (Horan et al., 2005). Conversely, when patients are presented with controlled emotional stimuli (Kring & Neale, 1996), they report similar amounts of emotion experience as normal controls. *Valence* (a dimension of pleasant to unpleasant) and *arousal* (activation-deactivation) are considered two vital features of emotional experience. When fMRI is used to detect neural activity along with subjective valence and arousal ratings, blunted valence, but not arousal, was evident in response to emotional stimuli compared to controls (Dowd & Barch, 2010), thus suggesting that patients' ability to be stimulated by emotionally evocative stimuli was intact. Higher levels of anhedonia, measured by the SANS global score and Chapman scales, were associated with blunted valence within patients and controls, and this finding correlated with amygdala and right ventral striatum activity in patients and with bilateral caudate activity in controls. Past research indicates that striatal activation is associated with the anticipation of pleasurable stimuli; thus, this may represent a failure to respond to positive experiences and contribute to an inability to anticipate and desire future experiences. Therefore, decreased ability to designate stimuli as rewarding might contribute to a lack of hedonic experience in patients. In sum, interview-based measures represent a viable starting point for assessing anhedonia and in detecting possible treatment effects. However, more specific probes based on experience sampling or brain-based laboratory measure are necessary to parse elements of arousal and valence that may contribute to altered emotion experience.

Treatment Approaches

Attempts at improving emotional responding in schizophrenia include both pharmacological and psychosocial interventions. Overall, second-generation antipsychotics may allow for better patterns of emotional responsiveness than older medications (Fakra et al., 2008), and depressive symptoms in schizophrenia may respond to antidepressants. Other interventions to improve anhedonia and more generally negative symptoms have included trials with such different agents as cognitive enhancers, N-methyl-D-aspartate (NMDA) agonists, neurosteroids, and antibiotics (Hanson, Healey, Wolf, & Kohler, 2010). Nonpharmacological interventions shown to reduce anhedonia have included approaches as diverse as pet therapy (Nathans-Barel et al., 2005), paid work programs (Bryson, Lysaker, & Bell, 2002), and cognitive-behavioral therapy (Turkington, Dudley, Warman, & Beck, 2006). With increasing focus on negative symptom research, there is hope that new psychopharmacological and psychosocial interventions will be developed that specifically address different aspects of emotion experience in schizophrenia.

CONCLUSION

An extensive body of literature has documented that emotion processing is altered in schizophrenia along the different dimensions of emotion expression, recognition, and, in some cases, experience. As a central constituent of social cognition, emotion processing exerts profound influences on interpersonal functioning and quality of life. Whereas illness-related characteristics, such as age, duration of illness, clinical symptoms, and treatment, show some relationship to these abilities, there is considerable stability in emotion processing impairment following onset of illness. In addition, more recent investigations have documented that emotion processing is affected in persons at clinical and genetic or familial risk of schizophrenia, in support of the notion that emotion processing may represent a vulnerability marker for schizophrenia. Although assessment of emotion recognition is well established through the use of validated stimuli that can be reliably administered through computerized measures, assessment of emotion expression and experience have relied on diverse methods that have yielded different results with limited external validity. Future investigations of emotion expression and experience will likely benefit from administration of computerized test probes and obtaining brain-based measures that can link the observable phenotype with neurobehavioral functions.

REFERENCES

Abrams, R., & Taylor, M. A. (1978). A rating scale for emotional blunting. *American Journal of Psychiatry, 135,* 226–229.

Achim, A. M., Maziade, M., Raymond, E., Olivier, D., Merette, C., & Roy, M. A. (2011). How prevalent are anxiety disorders in schizophrenia? A meta-analysis and critical review on a significant association. *Schizophrenia Bulletin, 37,* 811–821.

Addington, J., & Addington, D. (1998). Facial affect recognition and information processing in schizophrenia and bipolar disorder. *Schizophrenia Research, 32,* 171–181.

Addington, J. , & Piskulic, D. (2013). Social cognition early in the course of the illness. In D. L. Roberts & D. L. Penn (Eds.), *Social cognition in schizophrenia: From evidence to treatment* (Chapter 10). New York: Oxford University Press.

Aghevli, M. A., Blanchard, J. J., & Horan, W. P. (2003). The expression and experience of emotion in schizophrenia: A study of social interactions. *Psychiatry Research, 119,* 261–270.

Alvino, C., Kohler, C., Barrett, F., Gur, R. E., Gur, R. C., & Verma, R. (2007). Computerized measurement of facial expression of emotions in schizophrenia. *Journal of Neuroscience Methods, 163,* 350–361.

Andreasen, N. C. (1982). Negative symptoms in schizophrenia: Definition and reliability. *Archives of General Psychiatry, 39,* 784–788.

Archer, J., Hay, D. C., & Young, A. W. (1994). Movement, face processing and schizophrenia: Evidence of a differential deficit in expression analysis. *British Journal of Clinical Psychology, 33,* 517–528.

Bargh, J. A., & Chartrand, T. (1999). The unbearable automaticity of being. *American Psychologist, 54,* 462–479.

Barrett, E. A., Sundet, K., Faerden, A., Nesvag, R., Agartz, I., Fosse, R., et al. (2010). Suicidality before and in the early phases of first episode psychosis. *Schizophrenia Research, 119,* 11–17.

Bediou, B., Asri, F., Brunelin, J., Krolak-Salmon, P., D'Amato, T., Saoud, M., et al. (2007). Emotion recognition and genetic vulnerability to schizophrenia. *British Journal of Psychiatry, 191,* 126–130.

Bellack, A. S., Morrison, R. L., Wixted, J. T., & Mueser, K. T. (1990). An analysis of social competence in schizophrenia. *British Journal of Psychiatry, 156,* 809–818.

Berridge, K. C., & Robinson, T. E. (2003). Parsing reward. *Trends in Neuroscience, 26,* 507–513.

Bottlender, R., Strauss, A., & Moller, H. J. (2000). Prevalence and background factors of depression in first admitted schizophrenic patients. *Acta Psychiatrica Scandinavica, 101,* 153–160.

Breier, A., Schreiber, J. L., Dyer, J., & Pickar, D. (1991). National Institute of Mental Health longitudinal study of chronic schizophrenia: Prognosis and predictors of outcome. *Archives of General Psychiatry, 48,* 239–246.

Bryson, G., Lysaker, P., & Bell, M. Quality of life benefits of paid work activity in schizophrenia. *Schizophrenia Bulletin, 28,* 249–257.

Burbridge, J. A., & Barch, D. M. (2007). Anhedonia and the experience of emotion in individuals with schizophrenia. *Journal of Abnormal Psychology, 116,* 30–42.

Caldwell, C. B., & Gottesman, I. I. (1990). Schizophrenics kill themselves too: A review of risk factors for suicide. *Schizophrenia Bulletin, 16,* 571–589.

Chan, R., Wang, Y., Huang, J., Shi, Y., Wang, Y., Hong, X., et al. (2010). Anticipatory and consummatory components of the experience of pleasure in schizophrenia: Cross-cultural validation and extension. *Psychiatry Research, 175,* 181–183.

Carr, L., Iacoboni, M., Dubeau, M. C., Mazziotta, J. C., & Lenzi, G. L. (2003). Neural mechanisms of empathy in humans: A relay from neural systems for imitation to limbic areas. *Proceedings of the National Academy of Sciences USA, 100,* 5497–5502.

Chapman, L. J., & Chapman, J. P. (1978). The measurement of differential deficit. *Journal of Psychiatry Research, 14,* 303–311.

Chapman, L. J., Chapman, J. P., & Raulin, M. L. (1976). Scales for physical and social anhedonia. *Journal of Abnormal Psychology, 85,* 374–382.

Cohen, A. S., Minor, K. S., & Najolia, G. M. (2010). A framework for understanding experiential deficits in schizophrenia. *Psychiatry Research, 178,* 10–16.

Covington, M. A., He, C., Brown, C., Naçi, L., McClain, J. T., Fjordbak, B. S., et al. (2005). Schizophrenia and the structure of language: The linguist's view. *Schizophrenia Research, 77,* 85–98.

Diwan, S., Cohen, C. I., Bankole, A. O., Vahia, I., Kehn, M., & Ramirez, P. M. (2007). Depression in older adults with schizophrenia spectrum disorders: Prevalence and associated factors. *American Journal Geriatric Psychiatry, 15,* 991–998.

Dowd, E. C., & Barch, D. M. (2010). Anhedonia and emotion experience in schizophrenia: Neural and behavioral indicators. *Biological Psychiatry, 67,* 902–911.

Earnst, K. S., & Kring, A. M. (1999). Emotional responding in deficit and non-deficit schizophrenia. *Psychiatry Research, 88,* 191–207.

Earnst, K. S., Kring, A. M., Kadar, M. A., Salem, J. E., Shepard, D. A., & Loosen, P. T. (1996). Facial expression in schizophrenia. *Biological Psychiatry, 40,* 556–558.

Edwards, J., Jackson, H. J., & Pattison, P. E. (2002). Emotion recognition via facial expression and affective prosody in schizophrenia: A methodological review. *Clinical Psychology Review, 22,* 789–832.

Edwards, J., Pattison, P. E., Jackson, H. J., & Wales, R. J. (2001). Facial affect and affective prosody recognition in first-episode schizophrenia. *Schizophrenia Research, 48,* 235–253.

Ekman https://face.paulekman.com/face/default.aspx, Micro Expressions

Ekman, P., & Friesen, W. V. (1978). *Manual of the Facial Action Coding System (FACS.* Palo Alto, CA: Consulting Psychologists Press.

Enticott, P. G., Hoy, K. E., Herring, S. E., Johnston, P. J., Daskalakis, Z. J., & Fitzgerald, P. B. (2008). Reduced motor facilitation during action observation in schizophrenia: A mirror neuron deficit? *Schizophrenia Research, 102,* 116–121.

Erlenmeyer-Kimling, L., Cornblatt, B. A., Rock, D., Roberts, S., Bell, M., & West, A. (1993). The New York high-risk project: Anhedonia, attentional deviance, and psychopathology. *Schizophrenia Bulletin, 19,* 141–153.

Fakra, E., Khalfa, S., Da Fonesca, S., Besnier, N., Delaveau, P., Azorin, J. M., et al. (2008). Effect of risperidone versus haloperidol on emotional responding in schizophrenic patients. *Psychopharmacology, 200,* 261–272.

Falkenberg, I., Bartels, M., & Wild, B. (2008). Keep Smiling! Facial reactions to emotional stimuli and their relationship to emotional contagion in schizophrenia. *European Archives of Psychiatry and Clinical Neuroscience, 258,* 245–253.

Forbes, C., Blanchard, J. J., Bennet, M., Horan, W. P., Kring, A., & Gur, R. (2010). Initial development and preliminary validation of a new negative symptom measure: The Clinical Assessment Interview for Negative Symptoms (CAINS). *Schizophrenia Research, 124,* 36–42.

Friesen, W. (1986). Recent developments in FACS-EMFACS. *Face value: Facial Measurement Newsletter, 1,* 1–2.

Gaebel, W., & Wölwer, W. (2004). Facial expressivity in the course of schizophrenia and depression. *European Archives of Psychiatry and Clinical Neuroscience, 254,* 335–342.

Gard, D. E., Cooper, S., Fisher, M., Genevsky, A., Mikels, J. A., & Vinogradov, S. (2011). Evidence for an emotion maintenance deficit in schizophrenia. *Psychiatry Research., 187,* 24–29

Gard, D. E., Germans Gard, M., Kring, A., & John, O. P. (2006). Anticipatory and consummatory components of the experience of pleasure: A scale development study. *Journal of Research in Personality, 40*, 1086–1102.

Gard, D. E., Kring, A. M., Germans Gard, M., Horan, W. P., & Green, M. F. (2007). Anhedonia in schizophrenia: Distinctions between anticipatory and consummatory pleasure. *Schizophrenia Research, 93*, 253–260.

Gold, J. M., Waltz, J. A., Prentice, K. J., Morris, S. E., & Heerey, E. A. (2008). Reward processing in schizophrenia: A deficit in the representation of value. *Schizophrenia Bulletin, 34*, 835–847.

Gottheil, E., Paredes, A., Exline, R. V., & Winkelmayer, R. (1970). Communication of affect in schizophrenia. *Archives of General Psychiatry, 22*, 439–444.

Gottheil, E., Thornton, C. C., & Exline, R. V. (1976). Appropriate and background affect in facial displays of emotion. *Archives of General Psychiatry, 33*, 565–568.

Gur, R. C., Sara, R., Hagendoorn, M., Marom, O., Hughett, P., Macy, L., et al. (2002). A method for obtaining 3-dimensional facial expressions and its standardization for use in neurocognitive studies. *Journal of Neuroscience Methods, 115*, 137–143.

Gur, R. E., Kohler, C. G., Ragland, J. D., Siegel, S. J., Lesko, K., Wilker, W. B., et al. (2006). Flat affect in schizophrenia: Relation to emotion processing and neurocognitive measures. *Schizophrenia Bulletin, 32*, 279–287.

Häfner, H., Maurer, K., & Löffler, W. (2003). Modeling the early course of schizophrenia. *Schizophrenia Bulletin, 29*, 325–340.

Hanson, E., Healey, K., Wolf, D., & Kohler, C. (2010). Assessment of pharmacotherapy for negative symptoms of schizophrenia. *Current Psychiatry Reports, 12*, 563–571.

Harris, E. C., & Barraclough, B. (1997). Suicide as an outcome for mental disorders. A meta-analysis. *British Journal of Psychiatry, 170*, 205–228.

Hatfield, E., Cacioppo, J. T., & Rapson, R. L. (1994). *Emotional contagion (studies in emotion & social interaction)*. New York: Cambridge University Press.

Heerey, E. A., & Gold, J. M. (2007). Patients with schizophrenia demonstrate dissociation between affective experience and motivated behavior. *Journal of Abnormal Psychology, 116*, 268–278.

Herbener, E., & Harrow, M. (2002). The course of anhedonia during 10 years of schizophrenic illness. *Journal of Abnormal Psychology, 111*, 237–248.

Herbener, E. S. (2009). Impairment in long-term retention of preference conditioning in schizophrenia. *Biological Psychiatry, 65*, 1086–1090.

Herbener, E. S., Hill, S. K., Marvin, R. W., & Sweeney, J. A. (2005). Effects of antipsychotic treatment on emotion perception deficits in first-episode schizophrenia. *American Journal of Psychiatry, 162*, 1746–1748.

Ho, B. C., Nopoulos, P., Flaum, M., Arndt, S., & Andreasen, N. C. (1998). Two-year outcome in first-episode schizophrenia: Predictive value of symptoms for quality of life. *American Journal of Psychiatry, 155*, 1196–1201.

Hoekert, M., Kahn, R. S., Pijnenborg, M., & Aleman, A. (2007). Impaired recognition and expression of emotional prosody in schizophrenia: Review and meta-analysis. *Schizophrenia Research, 96*, 135–145.

Hooker, C., & Park, S. (2002). Emotion processing and its relationship to social functioning in schizophrenia patients. *Psychiatry Research, 112*, 41–50.

Horan, W. P., Blanchard, J. J., Clark, L., & Green, M. F. (2008). Affective traits in schizophrenia and schizotypy. *Schizophrenia Bulletin, 34*, 856–874.

Horan, W. P., Kring, A. M., & Blanchard, J. J. (2005). Anhedonia in schizophrenia: A review of assessment strategies. *Schizophrenia Bulletin, 32*, 259–273.

Ihnen, G. H., Penn, D. L., Corrigan, P. W., & Martin, J. (1998). Social perception and social skill in schizophrenia. *Psychiatry Research, 80,* 275–286.

Jaeger, J., Bitter, I., Czobor, P., & Volavka, J. (1990). The measurement of subjective experience in schizophrenia: The Subjective Deficit Syndrome Scale.*Comprehensive Psychiatry, 31,* 216–226.

Johnston, P. J., Katsikitis, M., & Carr, V. J. (2001). A generalized deficit can account for problems in facial emotion recognition in schizophrenia. *Biological Psychology, 58,* 203–227.

Katsanis, J., Iacono, W., & Beiser, M. (1990). Anhedonia and perceptual aberration in first-episode psychotic patients and their relatives. *Journal of Abnormal Psychology, 99,* 202–206.

Kay, S., Fiszbein, A., & Opler, L. (1987). The positive and negative syndrome scale (PANSS) for schizophrenia. *Schizophrenia Bulletin, 13,* 261–276.

Kee, K. S., Green, M. F., Mintz, J. M., & Brekke, J. S. (2003). Is emotion processing a predictor of functional outcome in schizophrenia? *Schizophrenia Bulletin, 29,* 487–497.

Keefe, R. S., Bilder, R. M., Harvey, P. D., Davis, S. M., Palmer, B. W., Gold, J. M., et al. (2006).Baseline neurocognitive deficits in the CATIE schizophrenia trial. *Neuropsychopharmacology, 31,* 2033–2046.

Kerr, S. L., & Neale, J. M. (1993). Emotion perception in schizophrenia: Specific deficit or further evidence of generalized poor performance? *Journal of Abnormal Psychology, 102,* 312–318.

Kirkpatrick, B., & Buchanan, R. W. (1990). Anhedonia and the deficit syndrome of schizophrenia. *Psychiatry Research, 31,* 191–207.

Kirkpatrick, B., Buchanan, R. W., McKenney, P., Alphs, L. D., & Carpenter, W. R. (1989). The schedule for the deficit syndrome: An instrument for research in schizophrenia, *Psychiatry Research, 30,* 119–123.

Kohler, C. G., Bilker, W., Hagendoorn, M., Gur, R. E., & Gur, R. C. (2000). Emotion recognition deficit in schizophrenia: Association with symptomatology and cognition. *Biological Psychiatry, 48,* 127–136.

Kohler, C. G., Martin, E. A., Milonova, M., Wang, P., Verma, R., Brensinger, C. M., et al. (2008b). Dynamic evoked facial expressions of emotions in schizophrenia. *Schizophrenia Research, 105,* 30–39.

Kohler, C. G., Martin, E. A., Stolar, N., Barrett, F. S., Verma, R., Brensinger, C., et al. (2008a). Static posed and evoked facial expressions of emotions in schizophrenia. *Schizophrenia Research, 105,* 49–60.

Kohler, C. G., Walker, J. B., Martin, E. A., Healey, K., & Moberg, P. J. (2010). Facial emotion perception in schizophrenia: A meta-analytic review. *Schizophrenia Bulletin, 36,* 1009–1019.

Kollias, C. T., Kontaxakis, V. P., Havaki- Kontaxaki, B. J., Stamouli, S., Margariti, M., & Petridou, E. (2008). Association of physical and social anhedonia with depression in the acute phase of schizophrenia. *Psychopathology, 41,* 365–370.

Krakowski, M., Czobor, P., & Volavka, J. (1997). Effect of neuroleptic treatment on depressive symptoms in acute schizophrenic episodes. *Psychiatry Research, 71,* 19–26.

Kring, A., Kerr, S. L., Smith, D. A., & Neale, J. M. (1993). Flat affect in schizophrenia does not reflect diminished subjective experience of emotion. *Journal of Abnormal Psychology, 102,* 77–106.

Kring, A., & Moran, E. K. (2008). Emotional response deficits in schizophrenia: Insights from affective science. *Schizophrenia Bulletin, 34* (2008), 819–834.

Kring, A. M., Germans Gard, M., & Gard, D. E. (2011). Emotion deficits in schizophrenia: Timing matters. *Journal of Abnormal Psychology, 120*, 79–87.

Kring, A. M., Kerr, S. L., & Earnst, K. S. (1999). Schizophrenic patients show facial reactions to emotional facial expression. *Psychophysiology, 36*, 186–192.

Kring, A. M., & Neale, J. M. (1996). Do schizophrenic patients show a disjunctive relationship among expressive, experiential, and psychophysiological components of emotion? *Journal of Abnormal Psychology, 105*, 249–257.

Kucharska-Pietura, K., David, A. S., Masiak, M., & Phillips, M. L. (2005). Perception of facial and vocal affect by people with schizophrenia in early and late stages of illness. *British Journal of Psychiatry, 187*, 523–528.

Laos, G., Boyer, P., & Legrand, A. (1999). Anhedonia in the deficit syndrome of schizophrenia. *Psychopathology, 32*, 207–219.

Laos, G., Noisette, C., Legrand, A., & Boyer, P. (2000). Is anhedonia a specific dimension in chronic schizophrenia? *Schizophrenia Bulletin, 26*, 495–506.

Leentjens, A., Wielaert, S., van Harskamp, F., & Wilmink, F. (1998). Disturbances of affective prosody in patients with schizophrenia: A cross sectional study. *Journal of Neurology, Neurosurgery and Psychiatry, 64*, 375–378.

Loughland, C. M., Williams, L. M., & Gordon, E. (2002). Visual scanpaths to positive and negative facial emotions in an outpatient schizophrenia sample. *Schizophrenia Research, 55*, 159–170.

Malla, A. K., Takhar, J. J., Norman, R. M., Manchanda, R., Cortese, L., Haricharan, R., et al. (2002). Negative symptoms in first episode non-affective psychosis. *Acta Psychiatrica Scandinavica, 105*, 431–439.

Martin, R. L., Cloninger, C. R., & Guse, S. B. (1985). Frequency and differential diagnosis of depressive syndromes in schizophrenia. *Journal of Clinical Psychiatry, 46*, 9–13.

Mattes, R. M., Schneider, F., Heimann, H., & Birbaumer, N. (1995). Reduced emotional response of schizophrenic patients in remission during social interaction. *Schizophrenia Research, 17*, 249–255.

Meehl, P. E. (1962). Schizotaxia, schizotypy, schizophrenia. *American Psychologist, 17*, 827–838.

Milev, P., Ho, B. C., Arndt, S., & Andreasen, N. C. (2005). Predictive values of neurocognition and negative symptoms on functional outcome in schizophrenia: A longitudinal first-episode study with 7-year follow-up. *American Journal of Psychiatry, 162*, 495–506.

Montross, L. P., Kasckow, J., Golshan, S., Solorzano, E., Lehman, D., et al. (2008). Suicidal ideation and suicide attempts among middle-aged and older patients with schizophrenia spectrum disorders and concurrent subsyndromal depression. *The Journal of Nervous and Mental Disease, 196*, 884–890.

Mueser, K. T., Doonan, R., Penn, D. L., et al. (1996). Emotion recognition and social competence in chronic schizophrenia. *Journal of Abnormal Psychology, 105*, 271–275.

Nathans-Barel, I., Feldman, P., Berger, B., et al. (2005). Animal-assisted therapy ameliorates anhedonia in schizophrenia patients. A controlled pilot study. *Psychotherapy Psychosomatic, 74*, 31–35.

Novic, J., Luchins, D. J., & Perline, R. (1984). Facial affect recognition in schizophrenia. Is there a differential deficit? *British Journal of Psychiatry, 144*, 533–537.

Pallantini, S., Querciolo, L., & Hollander, E. (2004). Social anxiety in outpatients with schizophrenia: A relevant cause of disability. *American Journal of Psychiatry, 161*, 53–58.

Park, S., Matthews, N., & Gibson, C. (2008). Imitation, simulation, and schizophrenia. *Schizophrenia Bulletin, 34,* 698–707.

Penn, D. L., Combs, D. R., Ritchie, M. Francis, J., Cassisi, J., Morris, S., et al. (2000). Emotion recognition in schizophrenia: Further investigation of generalized versus specific deficit models. *Journal of Abnormal Psychology, 109,* 512–516.

Penn, D., Roberts, D. L., Munt, E. D., Jones, N., & Sheitman, B. (2005). Pilot study of social cognition and interaction training (SCIT) for schizophrenia. *Schizophrenia Research, 80,* 357–359.

Rey, E. R., Bailer, J., Brauer, W., et al. (1994). Stability trends and longitudinal correlations of negative and positive syndromes within a three-year follow-up of initially hospitalized schizophrenics. *Acta Psychiatrica Scandinavica, 90,* 405–412.

Rifkin, A., Quitkin, F., & Klein, D. F. (1975). Akinesia. *Archives of General Psychiatry, 332,* 672–674.

Russell, T. A., Green, M. J., Simpson, I., & Coltheart, M. (2008). Remediation of facial emotion perception in schizophrenia: Concomitant changes in visual attention. *Schizophrenia Research, 103,* 248–256.

Salem, J. E., Kring, A. M., & Kerr, S. L. (1996). More evidence for generalized poor performance in facial emotion perception in schizophrenia. *Journal of Abnormal Psychology, 105,* 480–483.

Sasson, N., Tsuchiya, N., Hurley, R., Couture S. M., Penn, D. L., Adolphs, R., et al. (2007). Orienting to social stimuli differentiates social cognitive impairment in autism and schizophrenia. *Neuropsychologia, 45,* 2580–2588.

Schneider, F., Gur, R. C., Gur, R. E., & Shtasel, D. L. (1995). Emotional processing in schizophrenia: Neurobehavioural probes in relation to psychopathology. *Schizophrenia Research, 17,* 67–75.

Schürhoff, F., Szöke, A., Bellivier, F., Turcas, C., Villemur, M., Tignol, J., et al. (2003). Anhedonia in schizophrenia: A distinct familial subtype? *Schizophrenia Research, 32,* 59–66.

Schwartz, B. L., Mastropaolo, J., Rosse, R. B., Mathis, G., & Deutsch, S. I. (2006). Imitation of facial expressions in schizophrenia. *Psychiatric Research, 145,* 87–94.

Silver, H., & Shlomo, N. (2002). Anhedonia and schizophrenia: How much is in the eye of the beholder? *Comprehensive Psychiatry, 43,* 65–68.

Strauss, G. P., & Herbener, E. S. (2011). Patterns of emotional experience in schizophrenia: Differences in emotional response to visual stimuli are associated with clinical presentation and functional outcome. *Schizophrenia Research, 128,* 117–123.

Strauss, G. P., Wilbur, R. C., Warren, K. R., August, S. M., & Gold, J. M. (2011). Anticipatory vs consummatory pleasure: What is the nature of hedonic deficits in schizophrenia. *Psychiatry Research, 187,* 36–41.

Suslow, T., Roestel, C., Ohrmann, P., & Arolt, V. (2003). The experience of basic emotions in schizophrenia with and without affective negative symptoms. *Comprehensive Psychiatry, 44,* 303–310.

Trémeau, F., Antonious, D., Cacioppo, J. T., Ziwich, R., Butler, P., et al. (2010). Anticipated, on-line and remembered positive experience in schizophrenia. *Schizophrenia Research, 122,* 199–205.

Trémeau, F., Malaspina, D., Duval, F., Corrêa, H., Hagar-Budny, M., Coin-Bariou, L., et al. (2005). Facial expressiveness in patients with schizophrenia compared to depressed patients and nonpatients comparison subjects. *American Journal of Psychiatry, 162,* 92–101.

Tso, I. F., Grove, T. B., & Taylor, S. F. (2010). Emotional experience predicts social adjustment independent of neurocognition and social cognition in schizophrenia. *Schizophrenia Research, 122,* 156–163.

Turkington, D., Dudley, R., Warman, D. M., & Beck, A. T. (2006). Cognitive-behavioral therapy for schizophrenia: A review. *American Psychological Association.*

Ursu, S., Kring, A. M., Germans Gard, M., Minzenberg, M., Yoon, J., Ragland, D., et al. (2011). Prefrontal cortical deficits and impaired cognition-emotion interactions in schizophrenia. *American Journal of Psychiatry, 168,* 276–285.

Van Putten, T., & May, P. R. (1978). Akinetic depression in schizophrenia. *Archives of General Psychiatry, 35,* 1101–1107.

Varcin, K. J., Bailey, P. E., & Henry, J. D. (2010). Empathic deficits in schizophrenia: The potential role of rapid facial mimicry. *Journal of the International Neuropsychological Society, 16,* 621–629.

Vauth, R., Rüsch, N., Wirtz, M., & Corrigan, P. W. (2004). Does social cognition influence the relation between neurocognitive deficits and vocational functioning in schizophrenia? *Psychiatry Research, 128,* 155–165.

Verma, R., Davatzikos, C., Loughead, J., Indersmitten, T., Hu, R., Kohler, C., et al. (2005). Quantification of facial expressions using high dimensional shape transformations. *Journal of Neuroscience Methods, 141,* 61–73.

Walker, E. F., Grimes, K. E., Davis, D. M., & Smith, A. J. (1993). Childhood precursors of schizophrenia: Facial expressions of emotion. *American Journal of Psychiatry, 150,* 1654–1660.

Waltz, J. A., Schweitzer, J. B., Gold, J. M., Kurup, P. K., Ross, T. J., Jo, S. B., et al. (2009). Patients with schizophrenia have a reduced neural response to both unpredictable and predictable primary reinforcers. *Neuropsychopharmacology, 34,* 1567–1577.

Wölwer, W., Frommann, N., Halfmann, S., Piaszek, A., Streit, M., & Gaebel, W. (2005). Remediation of impairments in facial affect recognition in schizophrenia: Efficacy and specificity of a new training program. *Schizophrenia Research, 80,* 295–303.

Wölwer, W., Streit, M., Polzer, U., & Gaebel, W. (1996). Facial affect recognition in the course of schizophrenia. *European Archives of Psychiatry and Clinical Neuroscience, 246,* 165–170.

8

Characteristics of Theory of Mind Impairments in Schizophrenia

AHMAD ABU-AKEL AND
SIMONE G. SHAMAY-TSOORY ■

The ability to infer mental states has been variably referred to as *mentalizing, mindreading*, and most commonly, *theory of mind* (ToM). Theory of mind, which is part of our metacognitive abilities that constitute one's knowledge of one's own cognitive processes, is essential for social and behavioral functioning in that it allows people to understand and predict behavior in terms of the state of their knowledge, intentions, beliefs, and desires. A large body of research now confirms that metacognition in general, and ToM functioning in particular, is disrupted in patients with schizophrenia, and that such impairment appears specific in schizophrenia rather than due to some executive functioning deficit, general cognitive impairment, or the presence of general psychopathology (for recent reviews and meta-analyses, see Bora, Yucel, & Pantelis, 2009; Brüne, 2005; Frith, 2004; Harrington et al., 2005a; Lee, Farrow, Spence, & Woodruff, 2004; Pickup, 2008; Sprong, Schothorst, Ellen, Hox, & Van England, 2007).

Although it appears clear that schizophrenia disrupts one's mentalizing abilities, the extent and nature to which ToM is impaired in schizophrenia remains unclear. Some report that ToM impairment in patients with schizophrenia is similar to that found in autism (e.g., Corcoran, Mercer, & Frith, 1995; Mazza, De Risio, Surian, Roncone, & Casacchia, 2001), including in individuals with high-functioning autism (Couture, Penn, Losh, Adolphs, Hurley, & Piven, 2010) and Asperger syndrome (Craig, Hatton, Craig, & Bentall, 2004). Others report that the severity of ToM impairment in schizophrenia is less severe than in autism (e.g., Pickup & Frith, 2001; Pilowsky, Yirmiya, Arbelle, & Mozes, 2000), and some even suggest the absence of any such deficits when examined in the context of conversational interactions (McCabe, Leudar, & Antaki, 2004).

Such variation in ToM performance among patients with schizophrenia is not surprising, given the heterogeneous nature of schizophrenia, the use of various ToM tasks, and the absence of a standardized ToM test (for extensive reviews, see Bora et al., 2009; Brüne, 2005; Harrington et al., 2005a). It should be noted that such variation can also be attributed to the theoretical approaches to which researchers subscribe. These can be classified into two main approaches. The first approach, which follows Frith's model (Frith, 1992) or a variation thereof (Sarfati, Harde-Bayle, Besche, & Widlocher, 1997), has attempted to assign ToM impairments in patients with schizophrenia to a specific symptom profile. According to this model, severity of ToM impairments in patients with schizophrenia is associated with specific groups of symptoms and predicts intact abilities in remitted patients (i.e., ToM impairment is a state). More specifically, ToM abilities are associated with one of the following four symptom subgroups, with decreasing level of severity: (1) behavioral signs of negative symptoms or incoherence; (2) paranoid symptoms, which include delusions of persecution and of reference, as well as third-person hallucinations; (3) passivity experiences, which include delusions of control, thought insertion, and thought broadcasting; and (4) symptoms in remission. Although there is some support for this model (e.g., Corcoran & Frith, 2003; Pickup & Frith, 2001; Stewart, Corcoran, & Drake, 2008), the exact relationship between mentalizing problems and symptoms remains unclear (Bora et al., 2009; Frith, 2004). Indeed, a major challenge to this model is the hierarchical approach to this grouping where, for example, the group of patients with behavioral signs can also have paranoid symptoms and passivity experiences. Conversely, those belonging to the paranoid group are free from any behavioral signs, but may report passivity experiences. It has been suggested that such overlap of symptom clusters across groups makes it difficult to identify which symptom or cluster of symptoms is associated with the type of impairment observed (Harrington et al., 2005a). Another potential confound is the use of inconsistent criteria for categorizing positive and negative symptoms (Harrington et al., 2005a), as well as for categorizing remitted and nonremitted patients (Pousa et al., 2008a).

The second approach suggests that severity of ToM impairment in schizophrenia is associated with abnormal ToM development, and hence is likely to be a trait (Herold, Tényi, Lénárd, & Trixler, 2002; Hollis & Taylor, 1997). This developmental approach predicts that ToM impairment, if present, exists before the onset of schizophrenia and persists over time. That ToM impairment in schizophrenia is trait-dependent is supported by findings of recent studies of individuals at high risk for and with schizophrenia. These studies have reported mentalizing problems in remitted patients (Bora, Gokcen, Kayahan, & Beznedarouglu, 2008; Herold et al., 2002; Inoue et al., 2006; Randall, Corcoran, Day, & Bentall, 2003), nonclinical high schizotypal subjects (Langdon & Coltheart, 2004), healthy delusion-prone participants (Fyfe, Williams, Mason, & Pickup, 2008), and nonpsychotic first-degree relatives of patients with schizophrenia (Irani et al., 2006; Janssen, Krabbendam, Jolles, & van Os, 2003; Mazza, Di Michele, Pollice, Casacchia, & Roncone, 2008). This evidence has been further corroborated in two recent meta-analyses of ToM performance in schizophrenia (Bora et al., 2009; Sprong et al., 2007). However, this conclusion should remain tentative as some studies did not find an association between enhanced risk of schizophrenia and ToM deficits (Couture, Penn, Addington, Woods, & Perkins, 2008; Kelemen, Keri, Must, Benedek, & Janka, 2004; Marjoram et al., 2006), and others have shown amelioration of ToM impairments in patients with schizophrenia after medication treatment (Mizrahi, Korostil, Strakstein, Zipursky, & Kapur, 2007; Savina & Beninger, 2007). Moreover, several methodological concerns suggest that much more work is needed to ascertain whether ToM impairment in schizophrenia represents a possible trait marker (for details, see Pousa, Ruiz, & David, 2008b).

Although these models are theoretically divergent, both have largely attempted to characterize ToM in schizophrenia based on the use of categorical mentalizing tasks that indicate the presence or absence of mentalizing abilities. These categorical tasks, such as the false-belief and deception tasks (e.g., Frith & Corcoran, 1996), intention-inferencing tasks (e.g., Sarfati, Hardy-Bayle, Brunet, & Widlocher, 1999), indirect speech tasks (e.g., Corcoran et al., 1995; Greig, Bryson, & Bell, 2004), and the "Reading the Mind in the Eyes Test" (e.g., Kelemen et al., 2005; Kettle, O'Brien-Simpson, & Allen, 2008) are limited in that they do not offer insight as to the nature or characteristics of this impairment other than whether patients have a functioning capacity of ToM. By using such gross pass/fail indicators of mentalizing abilities, we risk undermining the specific nature and complexity of ToM impairment in schizophrenia.

In this chapter, we propose that a fuller characterization of mentalizing abilities would require at least three levels of analyses, which include the individual's ability to *represent, attribute,* and *apply* mental states. The *representational* aspect pertains to the individual's ability to represent mental states. That is, do patients with schizophrenia suffer from a conceptual deficit in which they are unable to represent mental states at all? This would be a case of undermentalizing (Frith, 2004) or hypomentalism (Crespi & Badcock, 2008). In this context, it should be noted that ToM is not a unitary concept (e.g., Bosco et al., 2009; Lysaker et al., 2010) and is comprised of representing both cognitive (i.e., beliefs, intentions, and knowledge) and affective (i.e., emotions, desires) mental states, which are mediated by discrete neurocognitive processes and structures (Abu-Akel & Shamay-Tsoory, 2011; Kalbe et al., 2010; Shamay-Tsoory & Aharon-Peretz, 2007). Representing cognitive and affective mental states can be generated via simulation processes of mirroring and self-projection (Waytz & Mitchell, 2011) or by theorizing about the content of the mind through the use of axioms and rules of inference (Gopnik & Wellman, 1992). It is possible, however, that situations that involve affective ToM entail more self-reflection or simulation when compared with situations involving cognitive ToM (Shamay-Tsoory, 2011).

The second level of analysis pertains to the *attributional* or *agentive* aspect of mentalizing, which refers to the individual's ability to attribute mental state to self or other. That is, are patients with schizophrenia equally capable of gaining insight into their own mental states, as well as to those of others? Although the ability to represent self and other mental states and their relationship is far from straightforward (for a recent review, see Carruthers, 2009), it can be characterized by the presence of one metarepresentational mechanism that utilizes two types of information for the assignment of agency: *perception-based* information for the representation of *other* mental states, and *introspective-based* information for the representation of *self* mental states (Happé, 2003; Zinck, Lodahl, & Frith, 2009).

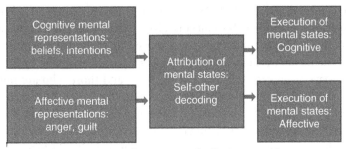

Figure 8.1 Component processes of cognitive and affective mental states.

However, both perception- and introspective-based information can be utilized while representing *self* or *other* mental states (van der Meer, Costafreda, Aleman, & David, 2010). For example, when interacting with an individual, representing her mental states may mainly rely on external cues gleaned from the environment, such as direction of eye gaze, facial expressions, and tone of voice, but it can also be computed, although not necessarily so, in consultation with internally stored information, such as autobiographical memory. Once generated, whether through simulation or theorizing, these mental states are then assigned agency (i.e., attributed to self or to another). It should be noted that we use the term *attribution* not to refer to the patient's *attributional style*, which emphasizes the patient's attributional bias of the causes of particular positive and negative events to self, other, or the situation (Green et al., 2008). Rather, it is used here to refer to the patient's ability to *attribute* or *assign* mental states to self ("these are my feelings and beliefs") or other ("these are her feelings and beliefs"). Last is the *execution/application* aspect of mentalizing, which refers to the *manner* in which the individual applies mental states. In this context, difficulties with ToM may not be related to an absence of the ability to represent mental states, but rather to an abnormality in applying (or deploying) these mental states (Abu-Akel & Bailey, 2000; Frith, 2004).

By reframing ToM abilities in terms of representation, attribution, and application of cognitive and affective mental states (see Figure 8.1), ToM impairments can be characterized along a continuum of competence and performance, and, as such, identify the various ways in which schizophrenia can affect processing of mental states. In the following section, we review evidence to demonstrate how variably schizophrenia impinges on one's ability to represent, attribute, and apply affective and cognitive mental states to self and other.

REPRESENTATION OF MENTAL STATES

In this section, we address whether patients with schizophrenia have a genuine deficit in ToM (i.e., complete conceptual loss). False-belief understanding is considered a litmus indicator for the presence of ToM. A traditional measure of false-belief understanding involves the unexpected transfer of an object from one

location to another (Wimmer & Perner, 1983), in which a patient is asked to predict where a person will say his object is, given that he first put it in one location,
and then, in his absence, the object was moved to another location by another
person. Patients answering accurately—that the person will look in the original
location—have been credited with having ToM, and those who are not able to
perform correctly are thought not to be cognizant that others have mental states.
These tests, and variations thereof, are known as *first-order ToM tasks* and have
been viewed by researchers as testing the presence or absence of the same underlying cognitive construct (however, see Harrington et al., 2005b; Tager-Flusberg &
Sullivan, 2000). This construct includes an understanding that beliefs (and other
mental states) must be represented in the mind, that beliefs may differ among
individuals who have access to different knowledge, and thus that some people's
beliefs may be falsely represented if they are based on erroneous information
(Abu-Akel & Bailey, 2001).

If passing first-order ToM demonstrates whether an individual has basic
representational abilities of mental states, and if patients with schizophrenia
have a genuine representational deficit (such as that observed in patients with
autism), then we would expect patients with schizophrenia to perform poorly
on first-order ToM tasks. In the first study addressing ToM in schizophrenia,
Corcoran et al. (1995) presented patients with short passages designed to test
one's understanding of indirect intentional speech. In this task, which requires
functional first-order representational abilities, participants are required to convey the real intended meaning of statements that include an obvious hint. On this
test, patients with negative features and incoherence scored the worst compared
to normal and psychiatric controls and schizophrenic patients with paranoid and
passivity symptoms. This finding was further replicated in subsequent studies that
employed more classic first-order ToM tasks, such as the one described above. In
a study by Frith and Corcoran (1996), for example, first-order ToM stories were
read aloud while showing a series of cartoon drawings presenting the sequence of
actions depicted in the stories. The patients with behavioral signs (which include
patients with negative features and/or incoherence) performed worst compared
to the other schizophrenic subgroups (paranoid, passivity, and remission groups)
and normal controls. In a later study, Mazza et al. (2001) categorized patients, following Liddle's (1987) three-dimensional-symptom model, into a psychomotor
poverty group, a disorganization group, and a reality distortion group. Patients
with psychomotor poverty, which to some extent corresponds to Frith's behavioral signs subgroup, performed more poorly on the first-order ToM task than did
the patients in the disorganization group and the reality distortion group. Similar
results were also reported in more recent studies in which patients with more
severe symptomatology, as assessed with instruments such as the Positive and
Negative Syndrome Scale, exhibited grave difficulties in representing first-order
mental states, similar to those difficulties observed among individuals with autism
(e.g., Marjoram et al., 2005; Stratta et al., 2010).

However, given that the results in these studies (Corcoran et al., 1995; Frith
& Corcoran, 1996; Marjoram et al., 2005; Mazza et al., 2001; Stratta et al., 2010)

were presented as relative aggregates (i.e., reported a proportion of their sub-jects as showing no impairment in such understanding) and that the tasks used are not designed along a continuum of competence and performance, it is dif-ficult to determine from these findings whether patients with negative-symptom schizophrenia truly exhibit a conceptual deficit of ToM. Moreover, none of these studies included patients with autism as controls. In fact, a series of other stud-ies seriously question whether patients with schizophrenia, including those with negative symptomatology, can be accurately described as having a conceptual ToM deficit. Pilowsky and colleagues (2000) have shown that although children with schizophrenia performed more poorly on first-order ToM tasks than typi-cally developing children, they overall had attenuated mentalizing impairments compared to children with high-functioning autism. It should be noted, however, that patients with schizophrenia, particularly those with negative symptomatol-ogy, performed similar to high-functioning autistics when tested on an advanced ToM task, the Reading the Mind in the Eyes Test (Couture et al., 2010). Moreover, confirming earlier reports (Doody, Götz, Johnstone, Frith, & Cunningham, 1998; Mitchley, Barber, Gray, Brooks, & Livingston, 1998), Pickup & Frith (2001) reported that patients with schizophrenia, including those with behavioral signs, scored perfectly on a first-order ToM task, but had discernible difficulties with a second-order ToM task in which the subject must judge whether a person has a false belief about the belief of another person. Accordingly, the authors con-clude that the mentalizing difficulties observed in patients with schizophrenia are less severe than those observed in autism. These results, in which patients with schizophrenia are able to pass basic mentalizing abilities and fail at more com-plex ones, have consistently been replicated in later studies by various research groups (Abu-Akel & Abushua'leh, 2004; Bosco et al., 2009; Brüne, 2003; Herold et al., 2002; Inoue et al., 2006; Janssen et al., 2003). In fact, when using a nondi-chotomous task, Brüne and Schaub (2011) have recently demonstrated that a sub-stantial number of patients with schizophrenia perform within the normal range. The authors suggest that this does not mean that the patients are performing like controls, but that their mentalizing abilities are not completely absent.

Weighing in on the debate concerning the extent to which ToM is impaired in schizophrenia, Langdon et al. (2006) investigated both false-belief understanding and emotion attribution. In the latter, subjects were required to think about how another person is likely to be feeling. They found that impairment in the ability to attribute emotions (happiness, sadness, shock, and anger) co-occurred with dif-ficulties in inferring false beliefs, and suggested that patients with schizophrenia have a domain-general difficulty with empathetic perspective taking. However, in more recent studies, Shamay-Tsoory and colleagues (Shamay-Tsoory et al., 2007; Shur, Shamay-Tsoory, & Levkovitz, 2008) have argued that the conflicting evi-dence concerning ToM abilities in schizophrenic patients may be a consequence of the use of various ToM tasks, which variably tap cognitive and affective compo-nents of ToM. Specifically, they proposed that the behavioral deficit of individuals with schizophrenia may be due to an impaired affective ToM (i.e., the ability to know, understand, and predict other people's *emotions*) rather than to a general

impairment in ToM. In testing this hypothesis, Shamay-Tsoory and her colleagues (2007) administered first- and second-order cognitive and affective ToM
tasks to patients with schizophrenia. Although the patients did not differ from
healthy controls on the first-order conditions (both cognitive and affective), they
were markedly impaired on the second-order affective ToM condition, but not the
second-order cognitive ToM condition. Complementing these results, Shur et al.
(2008) have demonstrated that patients with schizophrenia are also impaired on
tasks (e.g., the *faux pas* task) that require the integration of emotional and cognitive mental states (Shur et al., 2008). In this context, it should be noted that the
ability to represent emotional mental states is an important component of *empathy*, which is the ability to accurately perceive and understand the other's emotional state, and to respond to it appropriately (Leiberg & Anders, 2006). Indeed, a
number of studies have shown that patients with schizophrenia suffer from a pronounced impairment in empathic abilities (Bora et al., 2008; Derntl et al., 2009;
Haker & Rossler, 2009; Montag, Heinz, Kunz, & Gallinat, 2007). Patients with
schizophrenia have also been shown to be impaired in imitating emotional facial
expressions (Haker & Rossler, 2009), as well as in the recognition of facial expressions (Derntl et al., 2009; Hofer et al., 2009; Kosmidis et al., 2007; Pinkham, Gur,
& Gur, 2007), which could underlie their inability to successfully process affective
mental states and, consequently, their ability to empathize.

Given the evidence showing that first-order ToM processing is largely spared
in schizophrenia, and that schizophrenia seems to specifically impact the processing of affective mental states (but not cognitive mental states), a conceptual
deficit account would not accurately describe the mentalizing difficulties present in patients with schizophrenia. This suggests that the mentalizing difficulties
observed in schizophrenia are not due to an absence of representational abilities
of mental states or a general impairment in ToM abilities.

ATTRIBUTION OF MENTAL STATES

If, as suggested above, patients with schizophrenia do not suffer a deficit in
conceptual/representational abilities (i.e., they are able to represent mental
states), the second level of analysis would be to explore the extent to which
these patients are able to *attribute* or *assign* mental states to *self* and *other*.
In his original argument, Frith (1992) suggested that schizophrenia can be
understood in terms of one's ability to represent self and other mental states
in such a way that difficulties in representing self and other mental states may
result in disorders of "willed action" (e.g., negative and disorganized symptoms), disorders of self-monitoring (e.g., "passivity" phenomena), or disorders
of monitoring other people's thoughts and intentions (e.g., delusions of persecution and ideas of reference). Despite the recognition that studying the ability to attribute self mental states is important to understanding schizophrenia,
and more generally the recognition that distinguishing between self and other
mental states is fundamental to successful social interaction and understanding

interpersonal awareness, the overwhelming majority of studies have focused on patients' ability to represent and attribute mental states to *others*. As a result, the relationship between the ability to represent self and other mental states in schizophrenia has received very little attention, and this is clearly reflected by the almost exclusive use of ToM tasks that test for one's ability to attribute mental states to others.

Available evidence provides some important insights, nonetheless. Langdon et al. (1997) examined patients' ability to attribute mental state to self and others, using a recall task that required subjects to dissociate subjective mental states from objective realities to test for self mental state attribution, and picture sequencing and story-telling tasks to test for other mental state attribution. The results show that although some patients had difficulties in attributing mental states to self and other, some demonstrated a dissociation in which they were able to correctly attribute mental states to others (i.e., succeeded on the picture sequencing task) but failed in attributing mental states to self (i.e., failed on the recall of own mental state task). Findings for this latter group resonate with several studies that have consistently shown that patients with passivity experiences (alien control or thought) have intact attributional abilities of other mental states (e.g., Brüne et al., 2008; Corcoran et al., 1995; Corcoran & Frith, 2003; Frith & Corcoran, 1996; Pickup & Frith, 2001, Russell, Reynaud, Herba, Morris, & Corcoran, 2006), despite being impaired in their ability to attribute mental states to self, such as their intention to act (Daprati et al., 1997; Mlakar, Jensterle, & Frith, 1994), misattributing internally generated acts to others (Jeannerod, 1994), and have abnormal activation in brain areas involved in the evaluation of self-reference during mental state attribution (Brüne et al., 2008).

Moreover, poor ToM abilities in schizophrenia have been shown to be related to reduced insight (Bora, Sehitoglu, Aslier, Atabay, & Veznedaroglu, 2007; Gambini, Barbieri, & Scarone, 2004; Langdon & Ward, 2009; Pousa, Ruiz, & David, 2008b), and poor insight was found to be significantly associated with deficits in meta-cognitive abilities, rather than cognitive deficits per se (Koren et al., 2004). For example, in the study by Gambini et al. (2004), patients were interviewed about their delusions, followed with questions about the content of these delusions in the first-person (e.g., "Do you really think that what you just told me is real?"). Based on the patients' answers to these sets of questions, the authors concluded that patients with schizophrenia lacked insight into their delusions. However, when the questions were framed in the third-person (e.g., "If someone else told you what you just told me, would you believe him or her?"), some patients were able to modify their own mental states. That is, when patients were asked to intro-spect about their mental states, these mental states were impervious to revision. But when asked to consider these mental states from the perspective of another person, they were able to reason about the appropriateness of these mental states. Although it can be argued that these patients are able to reason about their own mental states by means of turning mindreading abilities upon themselves, one cannot rule out that these patients are using some compensatory mechanism to make sense of their behavior (Stanghellini & Ballerini, 2011). However, contrary to these studies, two recent studies suggest that attributing mental states to self is better preserved in schizophrenia than is attributing mental states to others (Bosco et al., 2009) and that disruption of other-perspective taking, rather than self-perspective inhibition, appears to more likely account for ToM impairment in schizophrenia (Bailey & Henry, 2010). Moreover, Schimansky et al. (2010) reported that abnormalities in the sense of agency among remitted or partially remitted patients with schizophrenia were unrelated to the mentalizing difficulties they exhibited when performing the Reading the Mind in the Eyes Test. Collectively, these findings suggest that self and other mental state attribution can be dissociated in schizophrenia, and that the ability to attribute mental states to others can be impaired irrespective of whether attributing mental states to the self is intact. It is interesting to note that such dissociation in self and other attribution has recently been reported for individuals with autism as well (Williams & Happé, 2009).

To our knowledge, there are no studies that have explicitly addressed the ability of patients with schizophrenia to attribute self and other mental states along the cognitive and affective dimensions. The limited evidence pertaining to the dissociability between self and other mental states in schizophrenia is inconsistent, and so it is difficult to speculate on the extent to which schizophrenia might impact agentive attribution of cognitive and affective mental states. However, we can speculate that patients with passivity phenomena will have difficulties in attributing both cognitive and affective mental states to self, but not to other. If we accept the model (as presented above) positing the presence of one metarepresentational mechanism that utilizes *perception-based* information for the representation of *other* mental states, and *introspective-based* information for the representation of *self* mental states, then we can conjecture that the inability of these patients to assign mental states to self is due to a disruption in their ability to access introspective-based information, or, as pointed to by Bedford and David (2008), due to inefficient processing of self-related material.

In all, other than the findings for the patients with passivity phenomena, the extent to which self and other mental state attribution is impaired in other types of schizophrenia warrants further research. Importantly, this research would need to introduce newly designed tests that place equal demands and appropriate similar contexts for the attribution of self and other mental states (for a promising start, see Williams & Happé, 2009). Such research is particularly important since it can inform the debate on two major theoretical issues concerning the relationship between self and other mental state attribution during mentalizing: (1) the dissociability between representing self and other cognitive and affective mental states, and its corollary, (2) the inferencing mechanism used during mindreading, such as simulation, which posits that attribution of mental states to self is a prerequisite step to gain insight into others' mental states. However, these important issues are beyond the scope of this chapter and will not be discussed further.

APPLICATION/EXECUTION OF MENTAL STATES

When patients with schizophrenia fail ToM tasks, the errors that the patients make are generally treated as evidence for the absence of a functioning capacity to represent mental states. This conclusion, as mentioned above, has been largely driven by study design in which patients are presented with a categorical task that can only reflect the absence or presence of mentalizing abilities. Abu-Akel and Bailey (2000) have argued that not all patients with schizophrenia can be correctly described as lacking an understanding of mental states, but rather they lack the ability to apply such mental states. Such abnormalities of application can manifest in two forms. On the one hand, an individual may be aware of others' mental life but fail to demonstrate this knowledge due to processing constraints. This we refer to as an *application deficit*, as opposed to a *representational deficit*. On the other hand, an individual may be able to apply mental states, albeit atypically. It has been suggested that this phenomenon, which has been described in the literature as *hyper-theory-of-mind* (Abu-Akel & Bailey, 2000), *overmentalizing* (Frith, 2004), or *hypermentalism* (Crespi & Badcock, 2008), could result from the unconstrained generation of hypotheses that can impact either the content of the mental states or the number of mental states generated. Such atypical application of mental states to one's self and to other people may result from either generating a fantastical hypothesis about the content of the mind, such as having powers of omniscience, or from difficulties in deciding among several competing hypotheses about the mind, which could result in an increase in the likelihood of choosing an erroneous hypothesis about the content of the mind.

To our knowledge, the first clue to such application deficits was presented by Bowler (1992), who demonstrated that although both patients with chronic schizophrenia and Asperger syndrome possessed knowledge about other people's minds, as measured by their success on second-order ToM tasks, they were deficient in applying this knowledge during interactions with others in everyday contexts. He concluded that "the combination of social impairment with an intact second-order theory of mind suggests that it is a failure of application rather than an absence of knowledge" (Bowler, 1992, p. 891). Although some patients with schizophrenia suffer from application deficits, other patients with disorganized, paranoid, and delusional schizophrenia are able to apply ToM, albeit atypically. By definition, ToM abilities must be available for such symptoms of delusion and paranoia to transpire. For example, schizophrenic patients with delusions of alien control who misattribute their own intentions to others (Daprati, et al., 1997) clearly represent others' minds and are capable of applying ToM, but err due to an overattribution of particular mental states to others, rather than to an inability to mentalize or apply their mentation. In a later study, Walston et al. (2000) reported that patients with "pure" persecutory delusions performed normally on ToM tasks, scoring perfectly or at a high level, and showed no evidence of any general impairment of the ability to make inferences concerning others' mental states. However, the content of these delusions suggests that these patients often attributed fantastical hypotheses about the content of the mind. A similar conclusion was presented by McCabe and collaborators (2004) when analyzing the conversations between mental health professionals and people with chronic schizophrenia. Using conversation analysis techniques, the authors showed that these patients appropriately reported first- and second-order mental states. However, their erroneous beliefs persisted despite recognizing that their interlocutor did not share their belief or accept their justifications of these beliefs as convincing. It is clear from these conversation analyses that the problems facing these patients are not due to deficit, but to management or application of their mental states.

It has been suggested that the purest evidence for overmentalizing would be to show that paranoid patients ascribe intentions to behavior that the rest of us see as mechanical or random (Blakemore, Sarfati, Bazin, & Decety, 2003; Frith, 2004). Indeed, such evidence has been observed in both healthy adults exhibiting delusion proneness (Fyfe et al., 2008) and in patients with paranoid schizophrenia (Montag et al., 2011; Russell et al., 2006; Walter et al., 2009). In the study by Fyfe and collaborators (2008), individuals were required to rate the strength of relationship between the movements of two shapes (the contingency task) and, in another, to view and then describe the movement of triangles on a computer screen in "random," "physical," and "ToM" conditions (the triangles task). In both tasks, delusion-prone individuals not only perceived meaning when the movements were random, but also tended to attribute mental states where none was indicated. The authors suggest that overmentalizing could reflect a hyperassociative cognitive style in which there is an exaggerated tendency to attribute mental states. The attribution of mental states to physical evidence has also been observed by Walter and collaborators (2009). In this neuroimaging study, patients with paranoid schizophrenia were scanned while performing one of four tasks: a physical causation condition and three intention attribution conditions. The patients performed worse than the normal controls in all conditions. Interestingly, no signal drop in putative ToM brain regions was observed for the physical causality condition, compared to the controls. This was attributed to the patients' tendency to attribute intentionality to physical objects, suggesting that patients with positive symptoms might have a hyperactive intention detector for physical events.

Most recently, Montag et al. (2011) assessed the mentalizing styles of a group of 80 patients with paranoid schizophrenia using the Movie for the Assessment of Social Cognition (MASC; (Dziobek et al., 2006), which is designed to capture whether aberrant mentalizing is due to undermentalizing (either lack of ToM or reduced ToM) or overmentalizing, and whether it is specific to cognitive or affective mental states. The authors report that although negative symptoms were associated with undermentalizing, positive symptoms, like delusions, were associated with overmentalizing. Interestingly, although Montag et al. (2011) found that undermentalizing was correlated with both cognitive and affective mental state decoding, they detected a stronger interaction between positive symptoms and a dysfunction of cognitive mentalizing than emotional mentalizing. These results largely replicate those obtained by Shamay-Tsoory and collaborators (2007), who found that affective ToM and empathy correlated with measurements of negative symptoms, whereas cognitive ToM correlated with the severity of positive symptoms. A partial confirmation of these findings can also be inferred from the study of Mehl et al. (2010), who found that schizophrenics' ability to infer intentions of others (i.e., cognitive ToM) was more strongly associated with general delusions and positive symptoms, whereas ToM abilities to infer emotions and to understand second-order false beliefs were not associated with delusions or positive symptoms. Collectively, these findings indicate that overmentalizing might apply to the cognitive dimension of ToM only, and that undermentalizing may specifically impact affective ToM (Montag et al., 2011; Shamy-Tsoory et al., 2007). However, this conclusion should remain tentative, given that patients with paranoid schizophrenia can exhibit hyperaffective mental states, such as morbid jealousy (Charlton & McClelland, 1999) and delusions of being loved or erotomania (Badcock, 2004).

Current evidence thus strongly suggests that not all schizophrenic patients can appropriately be characterized as oblivious of their own or others' minds. In fact, most patients with schizophrenia appear cognizant of mental life, but differ in their abilities to apply such knowledge. To varying degrees, the mentalizing capacity of some patients may manifest as undermentalizing due to an application deficit or processing constraints, and in others as overmentalizing, which can result either from a tendency to overattribute mental states or the unconstrained generation of mental-state hypotheses due to lack of inhibition (Abu-Akel, 2003). It has been suggested that such variation in under- and overmentalizing could be context dependent (Langdon & Brock, 2008), as there is evidence showing that the same patients can exhibit both under- and overmentalizing while performing precisely the same task (Langdon, 2005; Montag et al., 2011; Russell et al., 2006). Interestingly, in both studies by Langdon (2005), using the visual appreciation joke task, and by Russell et al. (2006), using the animated shapes task, undermentalizing was observed in the ToM condition, and overmentalizing was observed in the nonmentalistic condition, as if patients undermentalize when they are, in fact, expected to mentalize and overmentalize when they are not. Collectively, these observations raise the possibility that ToM application abilities could be highly variable within and among individuals, and are likely to be situated along a continuum of extremes of absence and excess. Therefore, it is important for future research to utilize suitable contexts in which intra- and interindividual differences in the application of ToM abilities can be examined.

CONCLUSION

Mentalizing impairments have been consistently identified in schizophrenia. However, inconsistency as to the nature and extent of these impairments abound. Our review of the literature suggests that patients with schizophrenia are largely capable of at least representing basic cognitive mental states. However, their mentalizing abilities appear to break down when performing advanced mentalizing tasks, particularly those requiring patients to infer affective mental states or the integration of cognitive and affective mental states (Shur et al., 2008). Except for patients with passivity phenomena, in which attribution of mental states to others appears intact in the face of impaired sense of self, the extent to which schizophrenia impacts one's mental-state sense of agency is unclear. Research in this domain is sorely needed to clarify the extent to which schizophrenia impacts one's mental-state sense of agency, especially along the cognitive and affective dimensions of ToM. More broadly, such research would provide important information regarding the putative relationship between self and other in processing mental states. Last, evidence suggests that the performance of patients with schizophrenia on ToM tasks vacillates along a continuum of undermentalizing, on one end, and overmentalizing, on the other. There is some evidence suggesting that undermentalizing is associated with negative symptoms and overmentalizing with positive symptoms. However, we should review this distinction with caution as there is also evidence showing that context-dependent variation could induce varying forms of mentalizing abilities within the same patient. This underscores the view that a deficit account is not appropriate to describe the mentalizing abilities of patients with schizophrenia, and, equally importantly, calls for future research to place special emphasis on the role of individual variation.

Accurate characterization of these impairments is paramount, particularly when it is becoming increasingly clear that mentalizing is a useful measure for understanding schizophrenia and psychopathology in general. In our view, separating component processes of ToM in schizophrenia is crucial to gain better insight into the nature and extent of this impairment. Here, we identified three main component processes that should be considered when characterizing ToM impairments in schizophrenia: (1) representation of cognitive and affective mental states, (2) attribution of agency to cognitive and affective mental states, and (3) the application/execution of cognitive and affective mental states. Such conceptualization allows us to characterize patients' interindividual as well as intraindividual performance along a continuum of competence and performance, and to minimize the mischaracterization of patients' ToM abilities that is often brought to bear when employing a categorical approach of presence and absence.

REFERENCES

Abu-Akel, A. (2003). A neurobiological mapping of theory of mind. *Brain Research Reviews, 43*, 29–40.

Abu-Akel, A., & Abushua'leh, K. (2004). "Theory of mind" in violent and nonviolent patients with paranoid schizophrenia. *Schizophrenia Research, 69*, 45–53.

Abu-Akel, A., & Bailey A. L. (2000). The possibility of different forms of theory of mind impairment in psychiatric and developmental disorders. *Psychological Medicine, 30*, 735–738.

Abu-Akel, A., & Bailey A. L. (2001). Indexical and symbolic referencing: What role do they play in children's success on theory of mind tasks? *Cognition, 80*, 271–281.

Abu-Akel, A., Shamay-Tsoory, S. (2011). Neuroanatomical and neurochemical bases of theory of mind. *Neuropsychologia, 49*, 2971–2984.

Badcock, C. (2004). Mentalism and mechanism: The twin models of human cognition. In C. Crawford & C. Salmon (Eds.), *Evolutionary psychology, public policy and personal decisions* (pp. 99–116). Mahwah, NJ: Lawrence Erlbaum Associates.

Bailey, P. E., & Henry, J. (2010). Separating component processes of theory of mind in schizophrenia. *The British Journal of Clinical Psychology, 49*, 43–52.

Bedford, N., & David, A. (2008). *Denial of illness in schizophrenia: Genuine or motivated?* Unpublished doctoral dissertation, Institute of Psychiatry, King's College London.

Blakemore, S. -J., Sarfati, Y., Bazin, N., & Decety, J. (2003). The detection of intentional contingencies in simple animations in patients with delusions of persecution. *Psychological Medicine, 33*, 1433–1441.

Bora, E., Gokcen, S., Kayahan, B., & Veznedaroglu, B. (2008). Deficits of social cognitive and social-perceptual aspects of theory of mind in remitted patients with schizophrenia: Effect of residual symptoms. *The Journal of Nervous and Mental Disease, 196*, 95–99.

Bora, E., Sehitoglu, G., Aslier, M., Atabay, I., & Veznedaroglu, B. (2007). Theory of mind and unawareness of illness in schizophrenia: Is poor insight a mentalizing deficit? *European Archives of Psychiatry and Clinical Neuroscience, 257*, 104–111.

Bora, B., Yucel, M., & Pantelis, C. (2009). Theory of mind impairment in schizophrenia: Meta-analysis. *Schizophrenia Research, 109*, 1–9.

Bowler, D. M. (1992). "Theory of mind" in Asperger's syndrome. *Journal of Child Psychology and Psychiatry, 33*, 877–893.

Bosco, F. M., Colle, L., De Fazio, S., Bono, A., Ruberti, S., & Tirassa, M. (2009). Th.o.m.a.s.: An exploratory assessment of theory of mind in schizophrenic subjects. *Consciousness and Cognition, 8*, 306–319.

Brüne, M. (2003). Theory of mind and the role of IQ in chronic disorganized schizophrenia. *Schizophrenia Research, 60*, 57–64.

Brüne, M. (2005). "Theory of mind" in schizophrenia: A review of the literature. *Schizophrenia Bulletin, 31*, 21–42.

Brüne, M., Lissek, S., Fuchs, N., Witthaus, H., Peters, S., Nicolas, V., et al. (2008). An fMRI study of theory of mind in schizophrenic Patients with "passivity" symptoms. *Neuropsychologia, 46*, 1992–2001.

Brüne, M., & Schaub, D. (2012). Mental state attribution in schizophrenia: What distinguishes patients with "poor" from patients with "fair" mentalizing skills? *European Psychiatry, 27*, 358–364.

Carruthers, P. (2009). How we know our own minds: The relationship between mindreading and metacognition. *Behavioral and Brain Sciences, 32*, 121–138.

Charlton, B., & McClelland, H. A. (1999). Theory of mind and the delusional disorders. *The Journal of Nervous and Mental Disease, 187*, 380–383.

Corcoran, R., & Frith, C. D. (2003). Autobiographical memory and theory of mind: Evidence of a relationship in schizophrenia. *Psychological Medicine, 33*, 897–905.

Corcoran, R., Mercer, G., & Frith, C. (1995). Schizophrenia, symptomatology and social inference: Investigating theory of mind in people with schizophrenia. *Schizophrenia Research, 17*, 5–13.

Couture, S. M., Penn, D. L., Addington, J., Woods, S. W., & Perkins, D. O. (2008). Assessment of social judgments and complex mental states in early phases of psychosis. *Schizophrenia Research, 100*, 237–241.

Couture, S. M., Penn, D. L., Losh, M., Adolphs, R., Hurley, R., & Piven, J. (2010). Comparison of social cognitive functioning in schizophrenia and high functioning autism: More convergence than divergence. *Psychological Medicine, 40*, 569–579.

Craig, J. S., Hatton, C., Craig, F. B., & Bentall, R. P. (2004). Persecutory beliefs, attributions and theory of mind: Comparison of patients with paranoid delusions, Asperger's syndrome and healthy controls. *Schizophrenia Research, 69,* 29–33.

Crespi, B., & Badcock, C. (2008). Psychosis and autism and diametrical disorders of the social brain. *Behavioral and Brain Sciences, 31,* 241–320.

Daprati, E., Franck, N., Georgieff, N., Proust, J., Pacherie, E., Dalery, J., et al. (1997). Looking for the agent: An investigation into consciousness of action and self-consciousness in schizophrenic patients. *Cognition, 65,* 71–86.

Derntl, B., Finkelmeyer, A., Toygar, T. K., Hulsmann, A., Schneider, F., Falkenberg, D. I., et al. (2009). Generalized deficit in all core components of empathy in schizophrenia. *Schizophrenia Research, 108,* 197–206.

Doody, G. A., Götz, M., Johnstone, E. C., Frith, C. D., & Cunningham Owens, D. G. (1998). Theory of mind and psychoses. *Psychological Medicine, 28,* 397–405.

Dziobek, I., Fleck, S., Kalbe, E., Rogers, K., Hassenstab, J., Brand, M., et al. (2006). Introducing MASC: A movie for the assessment of social cognition. *Journal of Autism and Developmental Disorders, 36,* 623–636.

Frith, C. (1992). *The cognitive neuropsychology of schizophrenia.* Hillsdale, NJ: LEA.

Frith, C. (2004). Schizophrenia and theory of mind. *Psychological Medicine, 34,* 385–389.

Frith, C. D., & Corcoran R. (1996). Exploring theory of mind in people with schizophrenia. *Psychological Medicine, 26,* 521–530.

Fyfe, S., Williams, C., Mason, O. J., & Pickup, G. J. (2008). Apophenia, theory of mind and schizotypy: Perceiving meaning and intentionality in randomness. *Cortex, 44,* 1316–1325.

Gambini, O., Barbieri, V., & Scarone, S. (2004). Theory of mind in schizophrenia: First person vs third person perspective. *Consciousness and Cognition, 13,* 39–46.

Gopnik, A., & Wellman, H. (1992). Why the child's theory of mind is a theory. *Mind and Language, 7,* 145–171.

Greig T. C., Bryson, G. J., & Bell, M. D. (2004). Theory of mind performance in schizophrenia: Diagnostic, symptom, and neuropsychological correlates. *Journal of Nervous and Mental Disease, 192,* 12–18.

Green, M. F., Penn, D. L., Bentall, R., Carpenter, W. T., Gaebel, W., Gur, R. C., et al. (2008). Social cognition in schizophrenia: An NIMH workshop on definitions, assessment, and research opportunities. *Schizophrenia Bulletin, 34,* 1211–1220.

Haker, H., & Rossler, W. (2009). Empathy in schizophrenia: Impaired resonance. *European Archives of Psychiatry and Clinical Neuroscience, 259,* 352–361.

Happé, F. (2003). Theory of mind and the self. *Annals of the New York Academy of Sciences, 1001,* 134–144.

Harrington, L., Langdon, R., Siegert, R. J., & McClure, J. (2005b). Schizophrenia, theory of mind, and persecutory delusions. *Cognitive Neuropsychiatry, 10,* 87–104

Harrington, L., Siegert, R., & McClure, J. (2005a). Theory of mind in schizophrenia: A critical review. *Cognitive Neuropsychiatry, 10,* 249–286.

Herold, R., Tényi, T., Lénárd, K., & Trixler, M. (2002). Theory of mind deficit in people with schizophrenia during remission. *Psychological Medicine, 32,* 1125–1129.

Hofer, A., Benecke, C., Edlinger, M., Huber, R., Kemmler, G., Rettenbacher, M. A., et al. (2009). Facial emotion recognition and its relationship to symptomatic, subjective, and functional outcomes in outpatients with chronic schizophrenia. *European Psychiatry, 24,* 27–32.

Hollis, C., & Taylor, E. (1997). Schizophrenia: A critique from the developmental perspective. In M.S. Keshavan & R. M. Murray (Eds.), *Neurodevelopment and adult psychopathology* (pp. 213–233). Cambridge, UK: Cambridge University Press.

Inoue, Y., Yamada, K., Hirano, M., Shinohara, M., Tamaoki, T., Iguchi, H., et al. (2006). Impairment of theory of mind in patients in remission following first episode of schizophrenia. *European Archives of Psychiatry and Clinical Neuroscience*, 256, 326–328.

Irani, F., Platek, S. M., Panyavin, I. S., Calkins, M. E., Kohler, C., Siegel, S. J., et al. (2006). Self-face recognition and theory of mind in patients with schizophrenia and first-degree relatives. *Schizophrenia Research*, 88, 151–160.

Janssen, I., Krabbendam, L., Jolles, J., & van Os, J. (2003). Alterations in theory of mind in patients with schizophrenia and non-psychotic relatives. *Acta Psychiatrica Scandinavica*, 108, 110–117.

Jeannerod, M. (1994). The representing brain: Neural correlates of motor intention and imagery. *Behavioral and Brain Sciences*, 17, 187–245.

Kalbe, E., Schlegel, M., Sack, A. T., Nowak, D. A., Dafotakis, M., Bangard, C., et al. (2010). Dissociating cognitive from affective theory of mind: A TMS study. *Cortex*, 46, 769–780.

Kelemen, O., Erdelyi, R., Pataki, I., Benedek, G., Janka, Z., & Keri, S. (2005). Theory of mind and motion perception in schizophrenia. *Neuropsychology*, 19, 494–500.

Kelemen, O., Keri, S., Must, A., Benedek, G., & Janka, Z. (2004). No evidence for impaired theory of mind in unaffected first-degree relatives of schizophrenia patients. *Acta Psychiatrica Scandinavica*, 110, 146–149.

Kettle, J. W. L., O'Brien-Simpson, L., & Allen, N. B. (2008). Impaired theory of mind in first-episode schizophrenia: Comparison with community, university and depressed controls. *Schizophrenia Research*, 99, 96–102.

Koren, D., Seidman, L. J., Poyurovsky, M., Goldsmith, M., Viksman, P., Zichel, S., et al. (2004). The neuropsychological basis of insight in first-episode schizophrenia: A pilot metacognitive study. *Schizophrenia Research*, 70, 195–202.

Kosmidis, M. H., Bozikas, V. P., Giannakou, M., Anezoulaki, D., Fantie, B. D., & Karavatos, A. (2007). Impaired emotion perception in schizophrenia: A differential deficit. *Psychiatry Research*, 149, 279–284.

Langdon, R. (2005). Theory of mind in schizophrenia. In B. Malle & S. Hodges (Eds.), *Other minds: How humans bridge the divide between self and others* (pp. 333–342). New York: Guilford Press.

Langdon, R., & Brock, J. (2008). Hypo- or hyper-mentalizing: It all depends upon what one means by "mentalizing". *Behavioral and Brain Sciences*, 31, 274–275.

Langdon, R., & Coltheart, M. (2004). Recognition of metaphor and irony in young adults: The impact of schizotypal traits. *Psychiatry Research*, 125, 9–20.

Langdon, R., Coltheart, M., & Ward, P. B. (2006). Empathetic perspective-taking is impaired in schizophrenia: Evidence from a study of emotion attribution and theory of mind. *Cognitive Neuropsychiatry*, 11, 133–155.

Langdon, R., Michie, P., Ward, P. B., McConaghy, N., Catts, S. V., & Coltheart, M. (1997). Defective self and/or other mentalising in schizophrenia: A cognitive neuropsychological approach. *Cognitive Neuropsychiatry*, 2, 167–193.

Langdon, R., & Ward, P. (2009). Taking the perspective of the other contributes to awareness of illness in schizophrenia. *Schizophrenia Bulletin*, 35, 1003–1011.

Lee, K. H., Farrow, T. F. D., Spence, S. A., & Woodruff, P. W. R. (2004). Social cognition, brain networks and schizophrenia. *Psychological Medicine*, 34, 391–400.

Leiberg, S., & Anders, S. (2006). The multiple facet of empathy: A survey of theory and evidence. *Progress in Brain Research*, 156, 419–440.

Liddle, P. F. (1987). The symptoms of chronic schizophrenia: A reexamination of the positive-negative dichotomy. *British Journal of Psychiatry*, 158, 340–345.

Lysaker, P. H., Olesek, K. L., Warman, D. M., Martin, J. M., Salzman, A. K., Nicolò, G., et al. (2010). Metacognition in schizophrenia: Correlates and stability of deficits in theory of mind and self-reflectivity. *Psychiatry Research*. doi:10.1016/j.psychres.2010.07.016

Marjoram, D., Gardner, C., Burns, J., Miller, P., Lawrie, S. M., & Johnstone, E. C. (2005). Symptomatology and social inference: A theory of mind study of schizophrenia and psychotic affective disorder. *Cognitive Neuropsychiatry*, *10*, 347–359.

Marjoram, D., Miller, P., Mcintosh, A. M., Cunningham Owens, D. G., Johnstone, E. C., & Lawrie, S. (2006). A neuropsychological investigation into theory of mind and enhanced risk of schizophrenia. *Psychiatry Research*, *144*, 9–37.

Mazza, M., De Risio, A., Surian, L., Roncone, R., & Casacchia, M. (2001). Selective impairments of theory of mind in people with schizophrenia. *Schizophrenia Research*, *47*, 299–308.

Mazza, M., Di Michele, V., Pollice, R., Casacchia, M., & Roncone, R. (2008). Pragmatic language and theory of mind deficits in people with schizophrenia and their relatives. *Psychopathology*, *41*, 254–263.

McCabe, R., Leudar, I., & Antaki, C. (2004). Do people with schizophrenia display theory of mind deficits in clinical interactions? *Psychological Medicine*, *34*, 401–412.

Mehl, S., Rief, W., Lüllmann, E., Ziegler, M., Kesting, M. -L., & Lincoln, T. M. (2010). Are theory of mind deficits in understanding intentions of others associated with persecutory delusions? *The Journal of Nervous and Mental Disease*, *198*, 516–519.

Mitchley, N. J., Barber, J., Gray, Y. M., Brooks, N., & Livingston, M. G. (1998). Comprehension of irony in schizophrenia. *Cognitive Neuropsychiatry*, *3*, 127–138.

Mizrahi, R., Korostil, M., Strakstein, S. E., Zipursky, R. B., & Kapur, S. (2007). The effect of antipsychotic treatment on theory of mind. *Psychological Medicine*, *37*, 595–601.

Mlakar, J., Jensterle, J., & Frith, C. (1994). Central monitoring deficiency and schizophrenic symptoms. *Psychological Medicine*, *24*, 557–564.

Montag, C., Dziobek, I., Richter, I. S., Neuhaus, K., Lehmann, A., Sylla, R., et al. (2011). Different aspects of theory of mind in paranoid schizophrenia: Evidence from a video-based assessment. *Psychiatry Research*, *186*, 203–209.

Montag, C., Heinz, A., Kunz, D., & Gallinat, J. (2007). Self-reported empathic abilities in schizophrenia. *Schizophrenia Research*, *92*, 85–89.

Pickup, G., & Frith, C. (2001). Theory of mind impairments in schizophrenia: Symptomatology, severity and specificity. *Psychological Medicine 31*, 207–220.

Pickup, G. J. (2008). Relationship between theory of mind and executive function in schizophrenia: A systematic review. *Psychopathology*, *41*, 206–213.

Pilowsky, T., Yirmiya, N., Arbelle, S., & Mozes, T. (2000). Theory of mind abilities of children with schizophrenia, children with autism, and normally developing children. *Schizophrenia Research*, *42*, 145–155.

Pinkham, A. E., Gur, R. E., & Gur, R. C. (2007). Affect recognition deficits in schizophrenia: Neural substrates and psychopharmacological implications. *Expert Review of Neurotherapeutics*, *7*, 807–816.

Pousa, E., Duno, R., Brebion, G., David, A. S., Ruiz, A. I., & Obiols, J. E. (2008a). Theory of mind deficits in chronic schizophrenia: Evidence for state dependence. *Psychiatry Research*, *158*, 1–10.

Pousa, E., Ruiz, A. I., & David, A. S. (2008b). Mentalising impairment as a trait marker of schizophrenia? *The British Journal of Psychiatry*, *192*, 312.

Randall, F., Corcoran, R., Day, J., & Bentall, R. (2003). Attention, theory of mind and causal attributions in people with persecutory delusions: A preliminary investigation. *Cognitive Neuropsychiatry*, *8*, 287–294.

Russell, T. A., Reynaud, E., Herba, G., Morris, R., & Corcoran, R. (2006). Do you see what I see? Interpretations of intentional movement in schizophrenia. *Schizophrenia Research, 81*, 101–111.

Sarfati, Y., Harde-Bayle, M. C., Besche, C., & Widlocher, D. (1997). Attribution of intentions to others in people with schizophrenia: A non-verbal exploration with comic strips. *Schizophrenia Research, 25*, 199–209.

Sarfati, Y., Hardy-Bayle, M. C., Brunet, E., & Widlocher, D. (1999). Investigating theory of mind in schizophrenia: Influence of verbalization in disorganized and non- disorganized patients. *Schizophrenia Research, 37*, 183–190.

Savina, I., & Beninger, R. J. (2007). Schizophrenic patients treated with clozapine or olanzapine perform better on theory of mind tasks than those treated with risperidone or typical antipsychotic medications. *Schizophrenia Research, 94*, 128–138.

Schimansky, J., David, N., Rössler, W., & Hake. H. (2010). Sense of agency and mentalizing: Dissociation of subdomains of social cognition in patients with schizophrenia. *Psychiatry Research, 178*, 38–45.

Shamay-Tsoory, S. G. (2011). The neural bases for empathy. *The Neuroscientist, 17*, 18–24.

Shamay-Tsoory, S. G., & Aharon-Peretz, J. (2007). Dissociable prefrontal networks for cognitive and affective theory of mind: A lesion study. *Neuropsychologia, 45*, 3054–3067.

Shamay-Tsoory, S. G., Shur, S., Barcai-Goodman, L., Medlovich, S., Harari, H., Levkovitz, Y. (2007). Dissociation of cognitive from affective components of theory of mind in schizophrenia. *Psychiatry Research, 149*, 11–23.

Shur, S., Shamay-Tsoory, S. G., & Levkovitz, Y. (2008). Integration of emotional and cognitive aspects of theory of mind in schizophrenia and its relation to prefrontal neurocognitive performance. *Cognitive Neuropsychiatry, 13*, 472–490.

Sprong, M., Schothorst, P., Ellen, V., Hox, J., & Van England, H. (2007). Theory of mind in schizophrenia: Meta-analysis. *British Journal of Psychiatry, 191*, 5–13.

Stanghellini, G., & Ballerini, M. (2011). What is it like to be a person with schizophrenia in the social world? A first-person perspective study on schizophrenic dissociality– Part 2: Methodological issues and empirical findings. *Psychopathology, 44*, 183–192.

Stewart, S. L. K., Corcoran, R., & Drake, R. J. (2008). Alignment and theory of mind in schizophrenia. *Cognitive Neuropsychiatry, 13*, 431–448.

Stratta, P., Bustini, M., Daneluzzo, E., Riccardi, I., D' Arcangelo, M., & Rossi, A. (2011). Deconstructing theory of mind in Schizophrenia. *Psychiatry Research, 190*, 32–36.

Tager-Flusberg, H., & Sullivan, K. (2000). A componential view of theory of mind: Evidence from Williams syndrome. *Cognition, 76*, 59–89.

van der Meer, L., Costafreda, S., Aleman, A., & David, A. S. (2010). Self-reflection and the brain: A theoretical review and meta-analysis of neuroimaging studies with implications for schizophrenia. *Neuroscience and Biobehavioral Reviews, 34*, 935–946.

Walston, F., Blennerhassett, R. C., & Charlton, B. G. (2000). Theory of mind, persecutory delusions and the somatic marker mechanism. *Cognitive Neuropsychiatry, 5*, 161–174.

Walter, H., Ciaramidaro, A., Adenzato, M., Vasic, N., Ardito, R. B., Erk, S., et al. (2009). Dysfunction of the social brain in schizophrenia is modulated by intention type: An fMRI study. *Social and Affective Cognitive Neuroscience, 4*, 166–176.

Waytz, A., & Mitchell, J. P. (2011). Two mechanisms for simulating other minds: Dissociation between mirroring and self-projection. *Current Directions in Psychological Science, 20*, 197–200.

Williams, D. M., & Happé, F. (2009). "What did I say?" versus "What did I think?": Attributing false beliefs to self amongst children with and without autism. *Journal of Autism and Developmental Disorders, 39*, 865–873.

Wimmer, H., & Perner, J. (1983). Beliefs about beliefs: Representation and constraining function of wrong beliefs in young children's understanding of deception. *Cognition, 13*, 103–128.

Zinck, A., Lodahl, S., & Frith, C. D. (2009). Making a case for introspection. *Behavioral and Brain Sciences, 32*, 163–164.

9

Social Cognition and the Dynamics of Paranoid Ideation

RICHARD P. BENTALL AND ALISA UDACHINA ■

Abnormal beliefs are a common feature of severe mental illness and are often reported by patients diagnosed as suffering from schizophrenia, bipolar disorder, or major depression. However, until about two decades ago, they were rarely the focus of psychological research (Oltmanns & Maher, 1988). Since that time, however, there has been a burgeoning research literature on the topic, so that summarizing and integrating the findings is no easy task.

DEFINITIONAL ISSUES

When they are held with great conviction, are apparently incomprehensible to others, and are resistant to counterargument, these kinds of beliefs are usually termed "delusions." The *Diagnostic and Statistical Manual of Mental Disorders* (DSM-IV-TR; American Psychiatric Association, 2000) defines a delusion as:

> A false belief based on incorrect inference about external reality that is firmly sustained despite what almost everyone else believes and despite what constitutes incontrovertible and obvious proof or evidence to the contrary. The belief is not one ordinarily accepted by other members of the person's culture or subculture (e.g. it is not an article of religious faith).

This definition, along with others that have been proposed, is not entirely satisfactory. What counts as "incontrovertible and obvious proof or evidence to the contrary" for example? However, despite the tendency in psychiatry to see delusions as qualitatively different from other kinds of beliefs and attitudes (so that they are, "empty speech acts, whose informational content refers to neither world or self"; Berrios, 1991), this difficulty becomes less serious if it is assumed that they exist on a continuum with other less bizarre but nonetheless tenaciously held beliefs, such as eccentric political attitudes or beliefs about the supernatural.

As we will see, there is, with some important qualifications, empirical evidence to support this assumption.

The term "paranoia," now commonly used to specifically indicate a tendency to hold abnormal beliefs about unwarranted persecution by others, has undergone a series of subtle changes in meaning over the last 100 years or so. In modern psychiatry, the term was first introduced in 1863, by Karl Ludwig Kahlbaum, to refer to a type of persistent delusional illness characterized primarily by cognitive deficits (Munro, 1982). Kraepelin (1907) later argued that the term should be confined to an uncommon, insidious, chronic illness characterized by a fixed delusional system in the absence of hallucinations or a deterioration of personality. A variety of delusional beliefs came under this category, including persecutory, grandiose, and jealous delusions (Kraepelin, 1907; Manschreck, 1989).

The publication of DSM-III (American Psychiatric Association, 1980) marked a shift toward a more modern, restricted conception of paranoia. In DSM-IV-TR (American Psychiatric Association, 2000), a persecutory delusion is defined as the belief that the person is being tormented, followed, tricked, spied upon, maliciously maligned, harassed, or ridiculed. The manual also defines Paranoid Personality Disorder in terms of a persisting pattern of distrust and suspiciousness toward others, so that others' motives are usually interpreted as malevolent. Consistent with this last concept, in popular and literary usage, the term "paranoid" has come to mean irrationally suspicious or distrustful (Manschreck & Khan, 2006).

Paranoid or persecutory delusions are perhaps the most common kind of abnormal belief seen in patients suffering from psychosis. In a study of 160 acute psychiatric inpatients in Sydney, Australia, 80% of deluded patients reported persecutory beliefs (Brakoulias & Starcevic, 2008). High rates of persecutory beliefs have also been reported in first-episode psychotic patients in Denmark (Jorgensen & Jensen, 1994) and also the United Kingdom, where a recent analysis of data from 255 consecutively admitted schizophrenia spectrum patients reported that as many as 90% showed significant levels of paranoid ideation, according to their scores on the Positive and Negative Syndrome Schedule (Moutoussis, Williams, Dayan, & Bentall, 2007). Paranoia is also observed in patients with other diagnoses, such as major depression (Frangos, Athanassenas, Tsitourides, Psilolignos, & Katsanou, 1983; Lattuada, Serretti, Cusin, Gasperini, & Smeraldi, 1999), bipolar disorder (Goodwin & Jamison., 1990), posttraumatic stress disorder (David, Kutcher, Jackson, & Mellman, 1999; Kozarić-Kovačić & Borovečki, 2005), and neurological disorders, such as dementia (Rubin & Drevets, 1988).

These observations of a high prevalence of paranoid beliefs among psychiatric patients seem to be cross-culturally robust. Ndetei and Vadher (1984) compared the abnormal beliefs of psychiatric inpatients from Europe, the Caribbean, India, Africa, the Middle East, and the Far East, and found persecutory delusions to be the most common except in Far East, where sexual delusions were more common. In the World Health Organization study of the Determinants of Outcome of Severe Mental Disorders, involving hundreds of first-contact psychotic patients in 10 different countries, almost half of the patients presented with persecutory delusions (Jablensky et al., 1992). Of course, the exact content of paranoid delusions tends to vary with time and place. For example, Sendiony (1976) found that middle- and upper-class Egyptian patients typically report persecutory delusions that have scientific or secular themes, whereas the delusions of poorer patients often involve religious institutions. In a study conducted in the Far East, Kim, Li, Jiang, and Cui (1993) reported that the paranoid delusions of Korean patients tended to reflect fears of rape, whereas fears of vampires and poisoning were more common in Chinese patients.

THE PARANOID SPECTRUM

Despite their usual attribution to mental illness, epidemiological research suggests that paranoid beliefs can also be observed in nonclinical populations. The Netherlands Mental Health Survey and Incidence Study found that the lifetime prevalence of broadly defined persecutory beliefs, which include nondistressing experiences and experiences with plausible origin, was 10%, whereas the lifetime prevalence of narrowly defined persecutory delusions (i.e., beliefs causing distress and help-seeking behavior) was about 1% (Rutten, van Os, Dominguez, & Krabbendam, 2008). New onset of persecutory delusions over a period of 1 year was observed in 0.2% of the sample using the narrow criteria and in 1% when the broad definition was used. (Within the sample, approximately a third of individuals identified as suffering from a psychotic disorder experienced narrowly defined persecutory delusions, but this proportion increased to 65% when persecutory delusions were defined more broadly.)

A similar British study assessed several thousands of individuals from the general population using the Psychosis Screening Questionnaire; individuals with identifiable psychotic disorder were deliberately excluded from the study (Johns et al., 2004). The results showed that around 9% of individuals felt that, over the past year, others were deliberately trying to harm them or their interests, and 1.5% believed that in the past year people had been plotting against them to cause harm or injury.

Longitudinal data on paranoid beliefs in the general population are available from a Swiss study, in which a general population cohort was followed for 20 years and participants were interviewed on six separate occasions between ages of 20 and 40 (Rössler et al., 2007). Although the endorsement of paranoid beliefs varied at different time points, on average, about 5% of respondents felt that, over the week preceding their interviews, others were to blame for their troubles, 7% believed that most people could not be trusted, and nearly 9% reported feeling taken advantage of. All three types of beliefs were associated with at least moderate levels of distress.

These kinds of findings have been widely taken as indicating that paranoia exists on a continuum with less severe forms of suspiciousness toward and mistrust of others. Indeed, a number of psychological investigators have developed scales for measuring paranoid thinking within healthy populations, for example university students (Fenigstein & Vanable, 1992; Freeman, 2008; Melo, Corcoran,

& Bentall, 2009). Freeman et al. (2005) explicitly investigated the possibility of a paranoid continuum in a large sample of healthy individuals recruited over the internet. Milder beliefs such as "Strangers and friends look at me critically" (on a weekly basis, endorsed by 21% of the sample) were more common than less plausible forms of paranoid beliefs such as "There is a possibility of a conspiracy against me" (on a weekly basis, endorsed only by 1% of the sample). The results also showed that the more pathological beliefs usually occurred in tandem with more common and less implausible forms of suspiciousness. Hence, Freeman and his colleagues proposed the existence of a hierarchy of paranoid beliefs, ranging from common social evaluative concerns (e.g., fear of rejection) through less common, moderately paranoid beliefs (e.g., the belief that others are trying to cause the individual distress) to full-blown paranoid delusions.

Qualitative Differences Between Psychotic and Subclinical Paranoia

The idea of a paranoid spectrum appears compelling, not only because it seems consistent with the available epidemiological data, but also because it implies that clinical paranoia may be rooted in the kind of concerns about one's position in the social universe that are perhaps a ubiquitous feature of human life. However, there is also evidence of qualitative differences between the persecutory beliefs of psychotic patients and those experienced by ordinary people. For example, in a qualitative study in which both clinical and nonclinical individuals with paranoid beliefs were interviewed, Campbell and Morrison (2007) reported that the most striking difference between the two groups was that the clinical participants felt under the control of their paranoid thoughts whereas nonclinically paranoid individuals did not.

Collip et al. (2011) used the experience sampling method (in which individuals keep diaries of their thoughts and experiences, with frequent entries over periods of days cued by electronic devices such as especially programmed digital watches) to study the context of paranoid thinking in ordinary people, nonpatients with subclinical levels of trait paranoia, and also paranoid and nonparanoid psychiatric patients. In people with low to moderate levels of trait paranoia, paranoid thoughts typically occurred in stressful circumstances, for example, when in the presence of unfamiliar others. However, in individuals with high levels of trait paranoia, paranoid thinking, although fluctuating across time, seemed relatively unaffected by stress and the individual's social context.

As we will consider in more detail later, an important distinction between two different kinds of paranoid beliefs, first proposed by Trower and Chadwick (1995), may help to illuminate the distinction between clinical and nonclinical paranoia. According to Trower and Chadwick, patients with "poor-me" (PM) paranoia believe themselves to be innocent victims of the malign intentions of others, whereas those with "bad-me" (BM) delusions believe that they are being persecuted for good reason (that they are the sort of people who others reasonably might want to persecute). Not surprisingly, it has been reported that patients with

BM delusions typically suffer from lower self-esteem than PM patients (Chadwick, Trower, Juusti-Butler, & Maguire, 2005), although the self-esteem of PM patients is still lower than that of appropriately matched healthy controls (Melo, Taylor, & Bentall, 2006). BM patients are also typically much more depressed than PM patients (Melo et al., 2006), who are sometimes quite grandiose.

In a questionnaire study involving a large student sample and a smaller sample of psychotic patients, Melo et al. (2009) found that, in the student sample, fear of persecution was positively correlated with the belief that persecution was deserved whereas, in the patient sample, even severely paranoid patients tended to report low deservedness scores. This finding is consistent with observations from other studies that have reported that BM paranoia is rare in psychotic patients (Fornells-Ambrojo & Garety, 2005; Melo et al., 2006).

A more complex picture of the paranoid beliefs of patients emerges from three longitudinal studies in which patients were asked to make repeated deservedness judgments. In a study in which 41 patients were questioned haphazardly over a period of a month, Melo et al. (2006) found that some switched from PM to BM over the follow-up period. A further study using the same methodology revealed that these changes were accompanied by changes in self-esteem (Melo & Bentall, 2012). In a more detailed study with a smaller sample, using the more intensive experience sampling method over a week, Udachina and colleagues (2012) again found that some patients' deservedness judgements fluctuated, sometimes over quite short periods. Those patients whose deservedness ratings fluctuated were typically judged to be BM at the beginning of the study, whereas the deservedness judgments of patients initially classified as PM were relatively more stable. Overall, these findings add up to a complex, dynamic picture of paranoia, with some similarities between subclinical and clinical variants, as outlined in Table 9.1. Although this degree of complexity creates challenges for the psychopathologist, it also provides some clues about the underlying psychological processes.

PARANOIA AS A FORM OF SOCIAL ADAPTATION

Over the past 10 years, epidemiologists have reported consistent evidence that a wide range of social environmental adversities confer an increased risk of psychosis, especially if these adversities are experienced during childhood. Known social risk factors for psychosis include growing up in an urban area (Pedersen & Mortensen, 2001); being a member of an ethnic minority group (Cantor-Graae, Pedersen, McNeil, & Mortensen, 2003; Selten et al., 2001; Zolkowska, Cantor, & McNeil, 2001), particularly if living in a predominantly nonminority neighborhood (Boydell et al., 2001; Veling et al., 2007) or if suffering discrimination (Reininghaus et al., 2010; Veling et al., 2008); being separated from parents early in life (Morgan et al., 2007) or experiencing other kinds of nonoptimal relationships with parents (Goldstein, 1998; Tienari et al., 2004); being the victim of sexual assault, especially in childhood (Bebbington et al., 2004; Read, van Os, Morrison, & Ross, 2005), and being the victim of bullying by peers (Arseneault et al., 2011;

Table 9.1 MODERATE VERSUS SEVERE PARANOIA

	Moderate (subclinical) paranoia	Severe (clinical) paranoia
Type of delusion	Mostly bad-me (persecution deemed as deserved)	Mostly poor-me (persecution deemed undeserved)
Context dependency	Context dependent (worse under stress or in presence of unfamiliar people)	Context independent
Subjective appraisal	Mostly positive; paranoia seen as adaptive	Both positive and negative. Individual feels controlled by paranoid thoughts
Self-esteem	Very low; highly unstable	Better than subclinical paranoia, but still lower than healthy individuals; highly unstable
Attributional style	Normal	Negative events excessively attributed to external causes

Schreier et al., 2009). Interestingly, some of these effects have been replicated with respect to subclinical psychotic experiences (e.g., Morrison & Petersen, 2003; van Os, Hanssen, Bijl, & Vollebergh, 2001) The effect sizes reported are generally much larger, and the data are much more consistent, than the findings for any single genetic contribution to psychosis (a research area in which findings have been notoriously difficult to replicate; Crow [2008]).

These observations raise the question of whether any particular kind of social adversity leads to paranoid thinking. Most studies in psychiatric epidemiology have adopted a broad definition of psychosis, so only a small number of investigations have addressed this question. In a sociological survey of residents of El Paso, in the United States, and Juarez in Mexico, Mirowsky and Ross (1983) found that paranoid beliefs were associated with social circumstances that they characterized as involving victimization and powerlessness, and they also reported that external locus of control mediated between these experiences and paranoid thinking. In a prospective study based in Holland, Janssen et al. (2003) found that experiences of discrimination predicted the future onset of paranoid beliefs. It is possible that these kinds of effects help to explain the increased risk of psychosis in certain ethnic minority groups; studies from the United States suggest that African Americans (Combs, Penn, & Fenigstein, 2002), especially if they have experienced racial discrimination (Combs et al., 2006), experience higher levels of paranoia than other ethnic groups.

In a recent study, Bentall, Wickham, Shevlin, and Varese (2012) studied the specificity of different types of adversity for different types of psychotic symptoms using data from the 2007 U.K. Adult Psychiatric Morbidity Survey. Whereas hallucinatory experiences (once comorbidity had been controlled for) appeared to be specifically associated with childhood sexual abuse, paranoid beliefs seemed to be associated with the experience of physical abuse (being frequently beaten when a child) and being separated from parents, as indexed by being brought up in institutional care.

Physical abuse might be thought of as a kind of chronic victimization, whereas being brought up in institutional care is clearly an index of disrupted attachment relations. With respect to the latter, it is interesting to note that subclinical paranoia is associated with an insecure attachment style (MacBeth, Schwannauer, & Gumley, 2008; Pickering, Simpson, & Bentall, 2008) and that adult paranoid patients, even when their symptoms are completely in remission, often report extremely negative relationships with their parents (Rankin, Bentall, Hill, & Kinderman, 2005). Hence, although any conclusions about the social origins of paranoia must be considered tentative, given the current evidence available, it seems plausible to hypothesize that lack of secure attachment relations (leading to a difficulty in trusting others), together with the experience of chronic threats, provide the life circumstances under which a paranoid way of understanding the world is most likely to develop.

Threat Anticipation as a Central Process

Sensitization to threat cues under the circumstances just described might be thought of as adaptive. Indeed, it is clearly considered to be adaptive by people experiencing either clinical or nonclinical paranoia, who often report that their beliefs have positive consequences (e.g., by endorsing questionnaire items such as "If I were not paranoid others would take advantage of me" (Campbell & Morrison, 2007; Morrison et al., 2005, 2011). Interestingly, Morrison et al. (2011) found that clinical, as opposed to nonclinical paranoia, was also characterized by the endorsement of highly negative beliefs about paranoid thinking (e.g. "My paranoia distresses me").

All vertebrate species have mechanisms for anticipating and avoiding threatening events, which have been extensively studied in the animal learning laboratory, typically by means of the conditioned avoidance paradigm. (In this paradigm, animals are presented with a warning stimulus, such as a tone, a short time before receiving an aversive stimulus, such as an electric shock. On receipt of the shock, the animal is able to execute an escape response, for example by jumping over a barrier. Very quickly, the animal learns to anticipate the shock and avoid it on detecting the warning stimulus.) Interestingly, there is evidence that dopamine circuits in the basal ganglia play an important computational role in this kind of learning (Moutoussis, Bentall, Williams, & Dayan, 2008), an observation that may be of some significance, given the widely held view that excessive dopamine transmission is involved in psychosis (Kapur, Mizrahi, & Li, 2005). Indeed, all effective antipsychotics block avoidance behavior in animals but have no impact on escape behavior (even if an animal is in receipt of an antipsychotic, once it receives an aversive stimulus, such as an electric shock, it tries very hard to get away from it). For this reason, suppression of avoidance responding is employed as an initial

screening test by pharmaceutical companies when trying to develop new antipsychotic agents (Moutoussis, Williams, Dayan, & Bentall, 2007). The implication of
these observations is that psychosis in general, and perhaps paranoid thinking in
particular, may co-opt dopamine-mediated avoidance mechanisms that are adaptive under most circumstances (an animal that could not learn to avoid threats
would have little chance of surviving to maturity).

Human beings are highly social animals (Brothers, 1990; Dunbar, 1997), so
it is perhaps not surprising that we are often preoccupied by social threats from
those around us, as opposed to threats from natural phenomena or other species.
However, studies of *threat perception and threat-related information processing* in
paranoid patients have produced a complex picture. On Stroop tasks, paranoid
patients show evidence of increased attention to threat-related words (Bentall
& Kaney, 1989) and words relating to self-esteem (Kinderman, 1994). Paranoid
patients also show a tendency to more readily recall threat-related information
compared to neutral information (Bentall, Kaney, & Bowen-Jones, 1995; Kaney,
Wolfenden, Dewey, & Bentall, 1992). Some studies have shown that patients with
paranoia, compared with healthy controls, have an enhanced ability to identify
sham facial expressions, especially of negative emotional states (Davis & Gibson,
2000; LaRusso, 1978), whereas others have shown that people with clinical or
subclinical paranoia are poor at recognizing emotional expressions in general
(Combs, Michael & Penn, 2006), and that clinically paranoid patients are poor
at recognizing individual's emotional states from their eyes (Craig, Hatton, &
Bentall, 2004). Eye tracking studies, in which patients have been asked to look at
scenes with threatening content, have revealed that patients with paranoid delusions actually direct their gaze less toward threatening information than controls
(Phillips & David, 1997b) and spend less time focusing on facial features than
nonparanoid patients (Phillips & David, 1997a). Perhaps these apparent inconsistencies can be resolved by Phillips and David's (1997b) suggestion that paranoid
individuals, like anxious patients, rapidly identify sources of threat before avert-
ing their gaze elsewhere.

Clearer evidence of the importance of social threat *anticipation* in paranoia
comes from studies in which paranoid patients and others have been asked to
estimate the likelihood of unpleasant encounters with other people. For example, Kaney, Bowen-Jones, Dewey, and Bentall (1997) asked paranoid patients,
depressed patients, and healthy controls to estimate how often various positive,
neutral, and negative social encounters had occurred to them in the previous
month, and how often these kinds of events were likely to happen in the future.
This study found that paranoid patients, compared to controls, overestimated
the likelihood of threats from others, a result that was subsequently replicated
by Corcoran et al. (2006) and by Bentall et al. (2008). Interestingly, in these studies, judgments about the likelihood of future negative events correlated with the
participants' recall of past negative events in all groups with the exception of
depressed patients. This observation suggests that, when anticipating threats, paranoid patients, like ordinary people, base their estimates of threat likelihood on
the availability of memories of similar experiences (i.e., they used the "availability

heuristic" when predicting future events; Kahneman, Slovic, & Tversky, 1982). The paranoid patients' high estimates of future threat are therefore consistent with their preferential recall of threat-related information (Bentall et al., 1995; Kaney et al., 1992) and also with their actual experiences of victimization (Bentall et al., 2012; Janssen et al., 2003; Mirowsky & Ross, 1983).

Two further aspects of these findings are worth noting. First, the negative items used in these studies were fairly generic (e.g., "someone stares at you menacingly") and were not tied to the specific content of the patients' delusions. Hence, it can be argued that what these studies demonstrate is a quite general tendency to overestimate threats. Second, Bentall et al. (2009) found that scores on these items correlated so highly with a clinical measure of paranoia that they were difficult to distinguish from the clinical measure psychometrically. Hence, this tendency seems to be a core feature of paranoid thinking.

SOCIAL-COGNITIVE DEFICITS AND PARANOIA

A number of investigators have attempted to identify specific deficits in reasoning and information processing that might influence the paranoid individual's tendency to overestimate threat. Two processes that have received particular attention are theory of mind (ToM) deficits and the jumping to conclusions bias.

Individuals are said to have a "theory of mind" if they are able to infer the mental states (beliefs, attitudes, and emotions) of other people (Baron-Cohen, 1995). It has been known for some years that autistic children, in particular, have difficulty with tasks that measure this kind of skill, for example, by requiring the participant to identify when someone holds a false belief (Baron-Cohen, Leslie, & Frith, 1985). The idea that this kind of deficit might play a role in paranoid ideation was first put forward by Chris Frith (1994). In a series of studies with Rhiannon Corcoran, he found that patients with paranoid delusions performed poorly on ToM tasks (Corcoran, Cahill, & Frith, 1997; Corcoran, Mercer, & Frith, 1995; Frith & Corcoran, 1996), leading them to argue that, during an acute psychotic episode, patients may become cognitively compromised and lose ToM skills that were intact until the onset of illness, and that this sudden inability to read the thoughts of other people might prompt the belief that others have concealed malevolent intentions.

Following these initial findings, a considerable amount of energy has been directed toward measuring ToM skills in patients with psychosis (Brune, 2005; Harrington, Siegert, & McClure, 2005). The only unequivocal finding is that ToM skills are usually impaired during a psychotic episode but, typically, not during remission. Some studies have reported that ToM impairments are specifically associated with paranoid symptoms (Corcoran et al., 2008; Randall, Corcoran, Day, & Bentall, 2003; Shryane et al., 2008), but other studies have either suggested that the impairment is not symptom-specific (e.g., Drury, Robinson, & Birchwood, 1998) or is associated with other symptoms such as thought disorder (Sarfati & Hardy-Bayle, 1999; Sarfati, Hardy-Bayles, Brunet, & Widloecher, 1999).

A second controversy is the extent to which the effects of ToM are independent of a more general psychological impairment. It has been well documented that patients with psychosis, on average, perform poorly on cognitive tests, but it is equally clear that performance on such tests correlates with social functioning and negative symptoms rather than positive symptoms such as paranoid delusions (Green, 1998). In a systematic review, Pickup (2008) was able to identify eight studies in which both ToM and executive functioning had been measured and which the latter was controlled for when determining whether ToM predicted psychosis; in all of these studies, the effect of ToM was found to survive after controlling executive functioning. However, in a more recent transdiagnostic study, which examined depressed and schizophrenia patients both with and without paranoid beliefs, it was found that ToM scores, although contributing to paranoia, correlated very highly with a short IQ test (Bentall et al., 2009).

The second kind of cognitive deficit that has been specifically investigated in relation to delusions in general and paranoia in particular is a tendency to jump to conclusions (JTC bias), typically measured by a "beads in a jar" task, in which the individual is asked to observe a sequence of blue or red beads and is asked to decide whether the beads are drawn from a jar with a majority of red beads or a jar with a majority of blue beads. After each draw, the individual can either make a decision or ask to see another bead. The general finding, first reported by Huq, Garety, and Hemsley (1988) and Garety, Hemsley, and Wessely (1991), is that, in comparison to controls, patients with delusions ask to see fewer beads before making a decision, and this has been replicated many times, including specifically with patients suffering from paranoid delusions (e.g., Corcoran et al., 2008) and with ordinary people with high levels of paranoid conviction (Freeman, Pugh, & Garety, 2008). A recent study found that, in ordinary people, a brief anxiety induction procedure led to a temporary increase in JTC bias, with a corresponding increase in paranoid thoughts (Lincoln, Lange, Burau, Exner, & Moritz, 2010).

It is tempting to believe that the JTC bias is, as its name implies, simply a tendency to make decisions on the basis of inadequate information, and that this leads to erroneous conclusions about the world or about preexisting anomalous experiences, and hence delusional beliefs (Garety et al., 2011). However, there are good reasons for doubting whether this is the case. In a version of the beads task in which individuals are asked to report their beliefs after seeing each bead, and in which the weight of the evidence first favors one jar and then the other, deluded patients more quickly shift their beliefs (Garety et al., 1991; Young & Bentall, 1997). Although deluded patients report a high subjective need for closure (a subjective need to reach definitive conclusions in the face of uncertainty; Bentall & Swarbrick, 2003), this tendency does not seem to correlate with the JTC bias (Colbert & Peters, 2002). In a recent transdiagnostic study of both depressed and schizophrenia patients, some in each group suffering from paranoid delusions, the JTC bias correlated heavily with general tests of intellectual functioning (Bentall et al., 2009). A more detailed Bayesian analysis of the choices of the participants in that study was able to break down the behavior of the participants into three parameters: the cost of waiting for further information (the standard interpretation suggests that this should be high in deluded patients), the cost of reaching the wrong decision, and a random parameter essentially representing an inability to integrate information over the multiple trials of the task. It was this last, random parameter that differentiated the paranoid patients from the controls (Moutoussis, Bentall, El-Deredy, & Dayan, 2011). Hence, it appears that the tendency to jump to conclusions may reflect a more general intellectual impairment.

EMOTIONAL FACTORS IN PARANOIA

Human beings, like other primates, tend to organize themselves in terms of social rank, with those of high social rank being much less vulnerable to social threat than those of low rank. Indeed, it has been argued that subjective self-esteem is simply an internal representation of our social rank relative to others (Allan & Gilbert, 1995; Leary, Tambor, Terdal, & Downs, 1995). Not surprisingly, therefore, some clinicians and researchers have argued that self-esteem plays an important role in paranoid thinking. For this reason, Zigler and Glick (1988) have argued that paranoid schizophrenia should be considered a camouflaged form of depression (a condition which, they argued, was similarly characterized by problems of self-esteem and preserved cognitive functioning) and not a form of schizophrenia (in which, they assumed, impaired cognitive functioning was the main feature). However, the exact relationship between self-esteem and paranoia has proved to be a focus of some controversy.

One persistent idea, which can be traced to Bleuler (1911/1950) and certain psychoanalytic writers (Colby, 1977; Colby, Faught, & Parkinson, 1979) is that paranoia arises at least partly as a defence against low self-esteem. According to this account, the paranoid individual assumes that others have malevolent intentions because this is less painful than accepting that life's misfortunes are self-caused. The most researched version of this theory, which was originally proposed by the first author and his colleagues (Bentall, Kinderman, & Kaney, 1994) and subsequently updated several times (Bentall, Corcoran, Howard, Blackwood, & Kinderman, 2001; Kinderman & Bentall, 1997), used theoretical constructs drawn from attribution theory (which concerns the social cognitive processes involved when people construct causal explanations for salient life experiences; Weiner, 2008) and also from self-discrepancy theory (a well researched model of how multiple representations of the self—for example, the actual self and the ideal self—when discrepant, lead to negative emotional states; Higgins, 1987).

The original attributional model was inspired by an early study in which paranoid patients were asked to generate attributions (statements about the likely causes) for hypothetical positive and negative events, such as being praised at work or failing an exam (Kaney & Bentall, 1989). Whereas the depressed controls in this study made excessively internal attributions for negative events (blaming themselves), the paranoid patients made excessively external attributions (blaming other people or circumstances). Bentall et al. (1994) therefore proposed that the paranoid individual has a latent negative self-schema that is easily activated when the individual is faced with a threat to a preferred view of the self, an event that would normally lead to activation of discrepancies between the person's ideal self and actual self-perceptions and therefore to depression. According to the model, paranoid individuals escape the activation of this discrepancy and associated unpleasant feelings by making external attributions (explanations) for negative events—that is, by blaming external agents for their misfortunes. Although these kinds of explanations reduce the discrepancy between self-actual and self-ideal representations, they have the less desirable effect of activating beliefs that others view them more negatively than they view themselves. It was argued that the recurrent use of this strategy leads to progressively more elaborate suspicions about the intentions of others and ultimately to a paranoid worldview. This theory predicts that explicit self-esteem in paranoia should be relatively preserved, but that self-esteem should appear very low on implicit measures.

In the first revision of the theory (Kinderman & R. Bentall, 2000; Kinderman & Bentall, 1997), a distinction was drawn between two types of external explanations: a situational attribution in which a negative experience is blamed on circumstances or bad luck, and an external-personal attribution, in which the individual blames his or her misfortunes on the malevolent actions of others. Paranoid patients were observed to make an excessive number of external-personal attributions for negative events, and it was argued that the situational attributions made by ordinary people were, by contrast, psychologically benign. The paranoid patient's tendency to make personal attributions was believed to be related to impaired ToM skills, as the ability to infer other's mental states is often required in order to make situational attributions for negative events (e.g. if, when being ignored by a friend, we assume this is because the friend is preoccupied rather than angry toward us). Consistent with this last assumption, several studies have shown that, in ordinary people, impaired ToM skills are associated with a tendency to make personal rather than situational attributions (Kinderman, Dunbar, & Bentall, 1998; Taylor & Kinderman, 2002). It was later argued that a tendency to jump to conclusions would also lead to rapid attribution generation, and therefore excessively personal rather than situational attributions, as the latter require more cognitive effort. Consistent with this assumption, Merrin, Kinderman, and Bentall (2007) found that paranoid patients searched for less information than controls when deciding the likely causes of events.

The most recent version of the attributional model (Bentall et al., 2001) took into account evidence from healthy people that showed that the relationship between attributions and self-representations is bidirectional (Kinderman & R. P. Bentall, 2000). For example, it seems that negative beliefs about the self can provoke internal (self-blaming) attributions for negative events (a person who believes him- or herself to be stupid will attribute the failure to pass an exam to him- or herself), whereas positive beliefs about the self will prompt external attributions under these circumstances (the exam must have been unfair or situational factors made revision impossible). However, the kinds of attributions we make about our experiences modulate our beliefs about ourselves (a self-blaming or

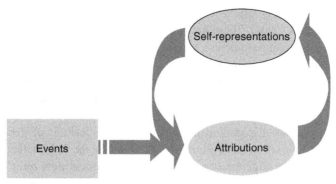

Figure 9.1 The attribution–self-representation cycle.

internal attribution for a negative event will worsen self-esteem whereas external attributions will preserve a positive view of the self, even in the face of adversity). Attributional and self-representational processes, in this model, are locked together in an attribution–self-representational cycle (see Figure 9.1). This version of the theory predicts that self-esteem will be highly unstable in paranoid patients.

A competing psychological model of paranoia has been advanced by Daniel Freeman and colleagues (Freeman, Garety, & Fowler, 2008; Freeman, Garety, Kuipers, Fowler, & Bebbington, 2002), who argue that, rather than being a form of defence, paranoid delusions are a direct extension of emotional concerns of the individual. Following an earlier suggestion by Maher (1988) that delusions reflect rational attempts to explain unusual experiences, they argue that, at the delusion formation stage, stressful life events, drug use, or a number of other factors, combined with preexisting emotional vulnerabilities, may lead to anomalous experiences that drive a search for meaning. In this search, individuals are likely to draw upon preexisting beliefs about the self, others, and the world. On this view (and consistent with the evidence on the social origins of paranoia discussed earlier), individuals will be more likely to develop a paranoid explanation if their earlier experiences (such as trauma) have provoked concerns about personal vulnerability accompanied by feelings of anxiety and depression. Preexisting anxiety is considered to be particularly relevant in this model as it reflects expectations of impeding danger. However, other emotions, such as anger and depression, may also add to the contents of the delusional system. The explanations considered in the search for meaning will also be influenced by cognitive factors, such as JTC bias and ToM deficits. Similarly to the attributional model of paranoia, this account also implicates the tendency to attribute negative events to external causes. However, the role of attributions in this case is seen as much more limited.

Freeman and colleagues further suggest that processes associated with emotion are also likely to be involved in the maintenance of delusions which, they argue, often persist because of the emotion-driven attentional and memory biases described earlier. They have also emphasized the importance of safety behaviors (avoidance behaviors designed to protect the individual from encountering their imagined threats), which are often reported by paranoid patients (Freeman, Garety, & Kuipers, 2001). These kinds of behaviors prevent the individual from testing his or her paranoid beliefs and, paradoxically, in the long run lead to an increase in distress (Freeman et al., 2007).

It is probably worth noting, before proceeding further, that these models actually have quite a lot in common. Both argue that paranoia often arises against a background of adverse social experiences. Both emphasize the importance of emotional processes in paranoid thinking, especially feelings of personal vulnerability and low self-esteem. Both also allow a role for ToM deficits and the JTC bias. The major differences are that Freeman's model puts more emphasis on anomalous experiences during the earliest stages of delusion formation, and the attributional model emphasizes defensive processes (dysfunctional attempts to repair self-esteem).

Anomalous Perceptions

There has been surprisingly little research on the role of anomalous experiences in paranoia. In an attempt to test Maher's (1988) earlier anomalous perception model of delusions, Chapman and Chapman (1988) interviewed a large sample of individuals with subclinical psychotic symptoms, finding little evidence that delusional beliefs were associated with perceptual abnormalities. In a more recent experience sampling study, Ben-Zeev, Ellington, Swendsen, and Granholm (2010) assessed psychotic patients for emotional disturbance, hallucinatory experiences, and paranoid thoughts, finding that paranoid thinking was associated with an increase in anxiety, but no evidence that these thoughts were preceded by hallucinatory experiences. However, the Freeman et al. (2002) model implies that anomalous perceptions may well be most important during the initial stage of the formation of paranoid beliefs. Consistent with this hypothesis, a study of children experiencing auditory hallucinations found that some went on to develop secondary delusional beliefs, and that those who were impaired in their performance on ToM tests were especially likely to do so (Bartels-Velthius, Blijd-Hoogwys, & van Os, 2011).

Deafness and sleep loss are two potential sources of anomalous experience that have been specifically investigated with respect to paranoia. Following clinical observations of an apparent association between the slow onset of deafness and paranoid symptoms in later life, Cooper and his colleagues suggested that elderly patients' failure to recognize that they have hearing difficulties might cause them to be mistrustful and suspicious of others (Cooper & Curry, 1976; Cooper, Garside, & Kay, 1976). In an attempt to test this hypothesis, Zimbardo, Andersen, and Kabat (1981) used hypnosis to induce a temporary state of deafness in suggestible students, allowing some to remain aware that they had been hypnotized. Those who were unaware of the source of their deafness, but not those who knew that they had been hypnotized, showed an increase in paranoia, as indicated by their responses on questionnaires and by their attitudes toward others present during the experiment. These findings are difficult to interpret because it is not clear how well hypnotic deafness simulates real hearing loss, and studies published soon afterward failed to find evidence of high rates of premorbid deafness in paranoid patients (Moore, 1981; Watt, 1985). However, more recent epidemiological investigations have found an association between hearing impairment and paranoid beliefs at the population level (Thewissen et al., 2005; van der Werf et al., 2007). This association seems to be especially strong if the hearing impairment begins early in life (Stefanis, Thewissen, Bakoula, van Os, & Myin-Germeys, 2006) and if the individual suffering from the hearing impairment grows up in a complex, inner-city environment (van der Werf, van Boxtel, & van Os, 2010).

With respect to sleep loss, Freeman, Pugh, Vorontsoya, and Southgate (2009) found that paranoid patients were especially likely to have experienced sleep difficulties, with about 50% affected. In an epidemiological study, it was found that sleep loss, along with depression and anxiety, predicted the development of paranoid symptoms at 18-month follow-up. Most impressively of all, perhaps, a pilot study of a brief psychological intervention to reduce insomnia led to a fairly rapid reduction in paranoid thinking in a small group of psychotic patients (Myers, Startup, & Freeman, 2011).

Clearly, the role of anomalous experiences in paranoia should be subjected to further investigation. The evidence that currently exists suggests that these experiences may well be important in some cases, particularly during the formation of paranoid beliefs. The findings on insomnia are particularly intriguing, although it is not clear that anomalous experiences is the mechanism behind this effect; as Freeman and his colleagues acknowledge, chronic sleep deprivation can have many effects, including cognitive impairment, depression, and anxiety, all of which may provoke paranoid thoughts.

Experiential Avoidance, Attributions, and Defensiveness in Paranoid Patients

Evidence of abnormal defensiveness in people with paranoid beliefs is more difficult to interpret. One way of construing defensiveness is in terms of the avoidance of unwanted mental contents (Moutoussis et al., 2007)—sometimes termed "experiential avoidance" (EA) by cognitive-behavior therapists (Hayes, Wilson, Gifford, Follette, & Strosahl, 1996). In two recent studies, one with students differing in scores on a paranoia questionnaire (Udachina et al., 2009), and one with psychiatric patients (Moutoussis, El-Deredy, & Bentall, in press) it was found that EA as reported by questionnaire was highly correlated with paranoia, and that this effect survived after controlling for mood. Furthermore, in the study carried out with students (Udachina et al., 2009), the experience sampling methodology was used to show that periods of self-reported paranoia were typically preceded by periods of self-reported EA. However, it is not clear to what extent self-reported EA correlates with actual, behavioral EA. In the study by Moutoussis, El-Deredy, et al. (in press), a novel experimental procedure was used that allowed participants to avoid thinking about negative aspects of the self, and no evidence of excessive avoidance was found in paranoid patients. Other evidence pertaining to this question is no clearer.

Recall that, according to the attributional model, two lines of evidence point to abnormal defensiveness. First, the model proposes that paranoid individuals show an excessive tendency to attribute negative events to external causes (the actions of others) and positive events to internal causes. This is believed to be an exaggeration of the normal "self-serving bias" that is found in ordinary people, particularly when self-esteem is threatened, and which is believed to be a method of buffering self-esteem in the face of adversity (Campbell & Sedikides, 1999). Second, the theory also suggests that, on implicit measures of self-esteem (when attributional defences are by-passed), self-esteem should be low, but that it should be relatively preserved on explicit measures.

In fact, the evidence on attributional style and paranoia is, at best, mixed. Some early studies seemed to confirm that paranoia is associated with a strong self-serving bias (Candido & Romney, 1990; Fear, Sharp, & Healy, 1996; S Kaney & Bentall, 1989), but many subsequent studies have failed to find this association. A number of factors may account for these inconsistencies in the evidence.

First, researchers have used a wide range of measures of attributional reasoning, varying from questionnaire measures such as Peterson et al's (1982) Attributional Style Questionnaire (ASQ) and Kinderman and Bentall's (1996) Internal, Personal and Situational Attributions Questionnaire (IPSAQ), through experimental procedures in which individuals have been asked to report the causes of contrived success and failure experiences (Kaney & Bentall, 1992) to naturally occurring attributions coded from interviews (Lee, Randall, Beattie, & Bentall, 2004). The ASQ, which is perhaps the most widely employed measure, has been criticized for poor reliability, especially on the crucial internality subscale (Reivich, 1995). This measure does not distinguish between external-personal and external-situational attributions, which are measured separately by the IPSAQ, which allows the calculation of an externalizing bias (the tendency to attribute positive events more than negative events to internal causes) and a personalizing bias (the tendency, when making external attributions, to assume the cause is some action of others rather than chance or situational factors).

Second, studies have involved both clinical and nonclinical participants who have varied in the severity of their paranoid beliefs. Janssen et al. (2006) reported evidence of an abnormal self-serving bias in acutely ill paranoid patients, but not in people suffering from subclinical paranoia. Combs et al. (2007) used a cluster analysis to identify groups of student participants who were maximally homogenous within each group and maximally different from each other on a range of dimensions, including depression and fear of negative evaluation. This analysis identified three discreet groups: paranoid students with high levels of depression, paranoid students with moderate depression, and paranoid students without depression. When paranoia was correlated with the externalizing and personalizing biases within the entire sample, no associations were found. However, group comparisons showed that nondepressed paranoid students and paranoid students with moderate depression showed a greater externalizing bias than the depressed paranoid students, whereas nondepressed paranoid students also showed an abnormal personalizing bias. Similar results were obtained in another study that found no association between paranoia and attributions in a large sample of students (Fornells-Ambrojo & Garety, 2009); comparisons between extreme high and extreme low scorers on paranoia revealed that paranoid students generated more external-personal attributions for negative events than their nonparanoid counterparts. Hence, attributional abnormalities seem to be associated with only the most severe levels of paranoia.

A third factor that makes the attributional data rather hard to interpret is comorbid symptoms, which have often been neglected. This limitation is particularly important with respect to depression, as it is known that low mood is associated with an attenuated or even reversed self-serving bias (Abramson, Seligman, & Teasdale, 1978; Mezulis, Abramson, Hyde, & Hankin, 2004). For example, in an apparently negative study of the association between paranoia and attributional style conducted by Humphreys and Barrowclough (2006), levels of depression were approximately twice as high in the currently paranoid patients (mean Beck Depression Index [BDI] score = 25.40) than in the nonparanoid clinical controls they were compared to (14.85). Jolley et al. (2006) estimated the relationship between paranoia and attributional style measured with the ASQ in a sample of psychotic patients while controlling for comorbid depression and grandiosity. They found that an externalizing bias for negative events but not positive events was predicted by a combination of paranoia and grandiosity, with more paranoid and more grandiose patients showing the greatest bias. In contrast, an externalizing bias for positive events was predicted by a combination of paranoia and depression. Consistent with this finding, Melo et al. (2009) reported an abnormal externalizing bias for negative events in patients with PM paranoid beliefs, but not in patients with BM beliefs.

A final complicating factor is that attributions may be better considered as *actions* than a *style*. That is, they may not be trait-like and, indeed, this is implicit in the latest version of the attributional model of paranoia and the concept of an attribution self-representation cycle (Bentall et al., 2001). Consistent with this account, Bentall and Kaney (2005) reported that paranoid patients showed an excessive externalizing bias for negative events before a contrived failure experience (participants were asked to solve a series of anagrams, some of which were unsolvable) but not afterward, when their attributional style was similar to that of depressed controls.

Self-Esteem in Paranoid Patients

A second difficulty with the attributional model of paranoia is that it seems to imply that patients, at least on explicit tests, should evidence preserved self-esteem. As Freeman et al. (1998) have pointed out, many patients suffering from paranoid delusions in fact appear to have low self-esteem. This has been confirmed in a number of studies, including a large cross-sectional study of patients with various psychiatric diagnoses conducted by the author of the attributional model (Bentall et al., 2008).

With respect to implicit measures of self-esteem, results have been very mixed. Lyon, Kaney, and Bentall (1994) administered an implicit measure of attributional style (disguised as a memory test) to paranoid patients and controls, finding that the paranoid patients made excessively self-blaming attributions for negative events (the pattern typically found in depressed patients). The results were interpreted as consistent with the defensiveness hypothesis since, it was argued, the self-derogatory attributions made by the patients on the implicit task were consistent with implicit low self-esteem. However, with the exception of one study in which paranoia was associated with low implicit and also low explicit self-esteem (Mehl et al., 2010), other researchers have not been able to replicate this finding (Diez-Alegria, Vazquez, Nieto-Moreno, Valiente, & Fuentenebro, 2006; Kristev, Jackson, & Maude, 1999; Martin & Penn, 2002).

The Implicit Attitudes Test (Greenwald & Farnham, 2000) is a more promising measure of implicit self-esteem for studies of paranoia. This well-validated measure requires individuals to sort self-relevant and self-irrelevant words, mixed with positive and negative words, into the two categories in two conditions: self or good versus other or bad and self or bad versus other or good. Greater speed when the self-relevant and positive words are sorted into the same category, as opposed to when the self-relevant and negative words are sorted into the same category, is taken as an index of positive implicit self-esteem. On this test, several research groups have reported a discrepancy between preserved explicit but impaired implicit self-esteem in paranoid patients (McKay, Langdon, & Coltheart, 2007; Moritz, Werner, & von Collani, 2006; Valliente, Cantero, Vazquez, Sanchez et al. 2011). However, once again, other studies have failed to find differences between implicit and explicit self-esteem in paranoid patients (Kesting, Mehl, Rief, Lindenmeyer, & Lincoln, 2011) and ordinary people suffering from subclinical paranoia (Cicero & Kerns, 2011). Overall, the inconsistencies in the findings are concerning and perhaps suggest that further thinking about the relationship between self-esteem and paranoia is required.

The studies considered so far have two serious limitations. First, they fail to distinguish between PM and BM paranoia. As discussed earlier, on explicit tests of self-esteem at least (appropriate studies using implicit measures have yet to be conducted), PM patients, who believe that their persecution is undeserved, show higher self-esteem than do BM patients, who believe that their persecution is deserved (Chadwick et al., 2005). Second, they have failed to address the dynamics of psychological processes, assuming that self-esteem is a relatively stable trait.

Inspired by the latest version of the attributional model of paranoia, and the concept of an attribution–self-representation cycle, Thewissen, Bentall, Lecomte, van Os, and Myin-Germeys (2008) conducted an experience sampling study, in which paranoid and nonparanoid patients, as well as healthy controls, rated their own self-esteem 10 times a day for 6 days. In this study, paranoia was associated with self-esteem that was, when averaged over the recording period, low, but also highly fluctuating. The relationship between paranoia and stability of self-esteem survived, even after average self-esteem and depression were controlled for. Using a simpler diary method, Melo and Bentall (2012) found that these shifts in self-esteem were associated with a tendency to switch between BM and PM beliefs.

In a more recent ESM study, Udachina et al. (2012) compared patients who were judged to be PM or BM at the beginning of the study period, finding again that self-esteem was unstable in relation to paranoia. Interestingly, PM and BM patients responded very differently following the onset of paranoid thoughts. In the latter group, the onset of paranoia was followed by a further reduction in self-esteem. However, as might be predicted by a defence model, in PM patients, the onset of paranoid thoughts was followed by an improvement in self-esteem.

CONCLUSION

From being a topic that was virtually neglected only two decades ago (Oltmanns & Maher, 1988), the study of delusional thinking, and paranoia in particular, has become a major focus of psychological inquiry. It might be argued that efforts so far have produced almost as much confusion as clarification and, certainly, some lines of research, particularly studies focusing on self-esteem and attributions, have generated findings that are inconsistent and sometimes contradictory. Nonetheless, there seem to be some points of consensus among researchers in the area, and it is possible to see the outlines of a dynamic, developmental model of paranoia emerging from the evidence.

First, it is now generally accepted that adverse early experiences and victimization increase the risk of paranoid beliefs in later life. Whereas previously it has not been possible to specify which kinds of adversity are associated with paranoia, the emerging evidence suggests that disturbed attachment relations and chronic victimization are particularly toxic influences. In a way, these findings are not surprising; attachment theorists argue that early relationships form a template for forming trusting relationships with others in adulthood (Holmes, 1993), so it stands to reason that disruption of these relationships, especially when combined with experiences such as discrimination, create the circumstances in which the mistrust of others is an adaptive process.

Second, the data on ToM and, especially, the JTC bias has been fairly consistent and, again, it is not hard to see why deficits in this area, especially against the kind of background we have already alluded to, might increase the tendency to assume that the world is populated by malevolent others. However, there is no agreement about the extent to which these deficits might reflect a more generalized underlying cognitive deficit, rather than deficits in specific domains (Bentall et al., 2009). If these measures are tapping into a more generalized deficit, then future research must address what this deficit is. One suggestion by Corcoran (2010) is that these tasks require an ability for "mental time travel," or to synthesize information across time. A more simple possibility is that they reflect poor executive function. An impairment of this kind might contribute to paranoid thinking by making it difficult to consider alternative, nonparanoid explanations for troubling events. As Coltheart (2007) has suggested, any account of abnormal beliefs needs to consider not only the source of the unusual ideas entertained by the patient but also why the individual is unable to reason these ideas away.

With respect to the two models of paranoia that have received most attention from researchers—the attributional account in its various forms (Bentall et al., 2001; Bentall et al., 1994; Kinderman & Bentall, 1997) and the model proposed by Freeman and his colleagues (Freeman, Garety, et al., 2008; Freeman et al., 2002)—there is no escaping the fact that the latter seems to receive more support from the available study data. If the attributional account was a viable model of the *onset* of paranoid delusions, then an abnormal attributional style should appear very early in or even before the development of paranoid thoughts. In fact, attributional abnormalities, when they have been observed, have been reported only in people with full-blown delusional systems (Janssen et al., 2006; McKay, Langdon, & Coltheart, 2005), especially those with PM or grandiose paranoia (Jolley et al., 2006; Melo et al., 2006) and not in people with subclinical paranoid ideation. Hence, attributional abnormalities tend to make a very late appearance in the evolution of the paranoid belief system. For this reason, at present, the model by Freeman and his colleagues (Freeman, Garety, et al., 2008; Freeman et al., 2002) seems to provide a better account of the processes that may be important during the emergence of paranoid beliefs which, at this stage, we have argued, tend to be of the BM variety. One feature of the Freeman et al. model that perhaps should be prioritized for future research is the role of anomalous experiences; on present evidence, it seems likely that these experiences may be important in only some patients.

Nonetheless, it may be too soon to write off the hypothesis of a paranoid defence entirely. Acute paranoid delusions, especially of the PM type, seem to be particularly associated with defensive performance on various psychological measures (McKay et al., 2007; Moritz et al., 2006; Valiente et al., 2011). Moreover, the psychological processes underlying paranoid delusions seem to be peculiarly dynamic during psychotic illness (Thewissen et al., 2008; Udachina et al., 2012), so that patients fluctuate between the PM and BM types and show corresponding changes in attributional style and self-esteem related variables (Melo et al., 2006; Melo & Bentall, in press; Udachina et al., 2012). Hence, there appears to be some evidence of defensiveness during the acute stage of a psychotic illness, and the attributional model, at least in its latest incarnation, which emphasizes dynamic, nonlinear interactions between psychological processes (Bentall et al., 2001), remains a plausible account of what may be happening at this stage. Elsewhere, we have argued that this may occur when dopamine-mediated avoidance processes are turned on self-generated cognitive processes (Moutoussis et al. 2007).

There are two important methodological implications of this review. First, future research should pay more attention to particular subtypes of paranoia. Second, and related to this, more attention should be given to the developmental precursors of paranoia. An underlying theme of this review has been the idea that paranoid beliefs emerge at the end of a long developmental pathway. A clearer understanding of the role of social cognition in paranoia is likely to emerge only following a detailed examination of the evolution of the relevant psychological processes from nascent suspiciousness, through the prodromal stage, to the acute psychotic crisis and beyond. This will require the use of sophisticated longitudinal designs that have so far been rarely applied in this field (see Peer, Kupper, Long, Brekke, & Spaulding [2007] for a discussion of these approaches).

REFERENCES

Abramson, L. Y., Seligman, M. E. P., & Teasdale, J. D. (1978). Learned helplessness in humans: Critique and reformulation. *Journal of Abnormal Psychology, 78*, 40–74.

Allan, S., & Gilbert, P. (1995). A social comparison scale: Psychometric properties and relationship to psychopathology. *Personality and Individual Differences, 19*, 293–299.

American Psychiatric Association. (1980). *Diagnostic and statistical manual of mental disorders—3rd Edition*. Washington, DC: Author.

American Psychiatric Association. (2000). *Diagnostic and statistical manual for mental disorders, 4th edition—Text revision*. Washington, DC: Author.

Arseneault, L., Cannon, M., Fisher, H. L., Polanczyk, G., Moffitt, T. E., & Caspi, A. (2011). Childhood trauma and children's emerging psychotic symptoms: A genetically sensitive longitudinal cohort study. *American Journal of Psychiatry, 168*, 65–72.

Baron-Cohen, S. (1995). *Mindblindness: An essay on autism and theory of mind*. Cambridge, MA: MIT Press.

Baron-Cohen, S., Leslie, A. M., & Frith, U. (1985). Does the autistic child have a "theory of mind"? *Cognition, 21*, 37–46.

Bartels-Velthius, A. A., Blijd-Hoogwys, E. M. A., & van Os, J. (2011). Better theory-of-mind skills in children hearing voices mitigate the risk of secondary delusion formation. *Acta Psychiatrica Scandinavica, 124*, 193–197.

Bebbington, P., Bhugra, D., Bhugra, T., Singleton, N., Farrell, M., Jenkins, R., et al. (2004). Psychosis, victimisation and childhood disadvantage: Evidence from the second British National Survey of Psychiatric Morbidity. *British Journal of Psychiatry, 185*, 220–226.

Ben-Zeev, D., Ellington, K., Swendsen, J., & Granholm, E. (2010). Examining a cognitive model of persecutory ideation in the daily life of people with schizophrenia: A computerized experience sampling study. *Schizophrenia Bulletin, 37*, 1248–1256. doi:10.1093/schbul/sbq041

Bentall, R. P., Corcoran, R., Howard, R., Blackwood, N., & Kinderman, P. (2001). Persecutory delusions: A review and theoretical integration. *Clinical Psychology Review, 21*, 1143–1192.

Bentall, R. P., & Kaney, S. (1989). Content-specific information processing and persecutory delusions: An investigation using the emotional Stroop test. *British Journal of Medical Psychology, 62*, 355–364.

Bentall, R. P., & Kaney, S. (2005). Attributional lability in depression and paranoia. *British Journal of Clinical Psychology, 44*, 475–488.

Bentall, R. P., Kaney, S., & Bowen-Jones, K. (1995). Persecutory delusions and recall of threat-related, depression-related and neutral words. *Cognitive Therapy and Research, 19*, 331–343.

Bentall, R. P., Kinderman, P., Howard, R., Blackwood, N., Cummins, S., Rowse, G., et al. (2008). Paranoid delusions in schizophrenia and depression: The transdiagnostic role of expectations of negative events and negative self-esteem. *Journal of Nervous and Mental Disease, 196,* 375–383.

Bentall, R. P., Kinderman, P., & Kaney, S. (1994). The self, attributional processes and abnormal beliefs: Towards a model of persecutory delusions. *Behaviour Research and Therapy, 32,* 331–341.

Bentall, R. P., Rowse, G., Shryane, N., Kinderman, P., Howard, R., Blackwood, N., et al. (2009). The cognitive and affective structure of paranoid delusions: A transdiagnostic investigation of patients with schizophrenia spectrum disorders and depression. *Archives of General Psychiatry, 66,* 236–247.

Bentall, R. P., & Swarbrick, R. (2003). The best laid schemas of paranoid patients: Autonomy, sociotropy and need for closure. *Psychology and Psychotherapy: Theory, Research and Practice, 76,* 163–172.

Bentall, R. P., Wickham, S., Shevlin, M., & Varese, F. (2012). Do specific early life adversities lead to specific symptoms of psychosis? A study from the 2007 The Adult Psychiatric Morbidity Survey. *Schizophrenia Bulletin, 38,* 734–740.

Berrios, G. (1991). Delusions as "wrong beliefs": A conceptual history. *British Journal of Psychiatry, 159*(Suppl. 14), 6–13.

Bleuler, E. (1950). *Dementia praecox or the group of schizophrenias* (E. Zinkin, Trans.). New York: International Universities Press. (Original work published 1911)

Boydell, J., van Os, J., McKenzie, J., Allardyce, J., Goel, R., McCreadie, R. G., et al. (2001). Incidence of schizophrenia in ethnic minorities in London: Ecological study into interactions with environment. *British Medical Journal, 323,* 1–4.

Brakoulias, V., & Starcevic, V. (2008). A cross-sectional survey of the frequency and characteristics of delusions in acute psychiatric wards. *Australasian Psychiatry, 16,* 87–91.

Brothers, L. (1990). The social brain: A project for integrating primate behavior and neurophysiology in a new domain. *Concepts in Neuroscience, 1,* 27–51.

Brune, M. (2005). "Theory of mind" in schizophrenia: A review of the literature. *Schizophrenia Bulletin, 31,* 21–42.

Campbell, M. L. C., & Morrison, A. P. (2007). The subjective experience of paranoia: Comparing the experiences of patients with psychosis and individuals with no psychiatric history. *Clinical Psychology and Psychotherapy, 14,* 63–77.

Campbell, W. K., & Sedikides, C. (1999). Self-threat magnifies the self-serving bias: A meta-analytic integration. *Review of General Psychology, 3,* 23–43.

Candido, C. L., & Romney, D. M. (1990). Attributional style in paranoid vs depressed patients. *British Journal of Medical Psychology, 63,* 355–363.

Cantor-Graae, E., Pedersen, C. B., McNeil, T. F., & Mortensen, P. B. (2003). Migration as a risk factor for schizophrenia: A Danish population-based cohort study. *British Journal of Psychiatry, 182,* 117–122.

Chadwick, P., Trower, P., Juusti-Butler, T. -M., & Maguire, N. (2005). Phenomenological evidence for two types of paranoia. *Psychopathology, 38,* 327–333.

Chapman, L. J., & Chapman, J. P. (1988). The genesis of delusions. In T. F. Oltmanns & B. A. Maher (Eds.), *Delusional beliefs* (pp. 167–183). New York: John Wiley.

Cicero, D. C., & Kerns, J. G. (2011). Is paranoia a defence against or an expression of low self-esteem? *European Journal of Personality, 25,* 326–335.

Colbert, S. M., & Peters, E. R. (2002). Need for closure and jumping-to-conclusions in delusion-prone individuals. *Journal of Nervous and Mental Disease, 190,* 27–31.

Colby, K. M. (1977). Appraisal of four psychological theories of paranoid phenomena. *Journal of Abnormal Psychology, 86,* 54–59.

Colby, K. M., Faught, W. S., & Parkinson, R. C. (1979). Cognitive therapy of paranoid conditions: Heuristic suggestions based on a computer simulation. *Cognitive Therapy and Research, 3,* 55–60.

Collip, D., Oorschot, M., Thewissen, V., van Os, J., Bentall, R. P., & Myin-Germeys, I. (2011). Social world interactions: How company connects to paranoia. *Psychological Medicine, 41,* 911–921.

Coltheart, M. (2007). The 33rd Sir Frederick Bartlett Lecture: Cognitive neuropsychiatry and delusional beliefs. *The Quarterly Journal of Experimental Psychology, 60,* 1041–1062.

Combs, D. R., Michael, C. O., & Penn, D. L. (2006). Paranoia and emotion perception across the continuum. *British Journal of Clinical Psychology, 45,* 19–31.

Combs, D. R., Penn, D. L., Cassisi, J., Michael, C., Wood, T., Wanner, J., & Adams, S. (2006). Perceived racism as a predictor of paranoia among African Americans. *Journal of Black Psychology, 32,* 87–104.

Combs, D. R., Penn, D. L., Chadwick, P., Trower, P., Michael, C. O., & Basso, M. R. (2007). Subtypes of paranoia in a nonclinical sample. *Cognitive Neuropsychiatry, 6,* 537–553.

Combs, D. R., Penn, D. L., & Fenigstein, A. (2002). Ethnic differences in subclinical paranoia: An expansion of norms of the Paranoia Scale. *Cultural Diversity and Ethnic Minority Psychology, 8,* 248–256.

Cooper, A. F., & Curry, A. R. (1976). The pathology of deafness in the paranoid and affective psychoses of later life. *Journal of Psychosomatic Medicine, 20,* 97–105.

Cooper, A. F., Garside, R. F., & Kay, D. W. (1976). A comparison of deaf and non-deaf patients with paranoid and affective psychoses. *British Journal of Psychiatry, 129,* 532–538.

Corcoran, R. (2010). The allusive cognitive deficit in paranoia: The case for mental time travel or cognitive self-projection. *Psychological Medicine, 40,* 1233–1237.

Corcoran, R., Cahill, C., & Frith, C. D. (1997). The appreciation of visual jokes in people with schizophrenia: A study of "mentalizing" ability. *Schizophrenia Research, 24,* 319–327.

Corcoran, R., Ciummins, S., Rowse, G., Moore, E., Blackwood, N., Howard, R., et al. (2006). Reasoning under uncertainty: Heuristic judgments in patients with persecutory delusions or depression. *Psychological Medicine, 36,* 1109–1118.

Corcoran, R., Mercer, G., & Frith, C. D. (1995). Schizophrenia, symptomatology and social inference: Investigating "theory of mind" in people with schizophrenia. *Schizophrenia Research, 17,* 5–13.

Corcoran, R., Rowse, G., Moore, R., Blackwood, N., Kinderman, P., Howard, R., et al. (2008). A transdiagnostic investigation of theory of mind and jumping to conclusions in paranoia: A comparison of schizophrenia and depression with and without delusions. *Psychological Medicine, 38,* 1577–1583.

Craig, J., Hatton, C., & Bentall, R. P. (2004). Persecutory beliefs, attributions and theory of mind: Comparison of patients with paranoid delusions, Asperger's syndrome and healthy controls. *Schizophrenia Research, 69,* 29–33.

Crow, T. J. (2008). The emperors of the schizophrenia polygene have no clothes. *Psychological Medicine, 38,* 1679–1680

David, D., Kutcher, G. S., Jackson, E. I., & Mellman, T. A. (1999). Psychotic symptoms in combat-related posttraumatic stress disorder. *Journal of Clinical Psychiatry, 60,* 29–32.

Davis, P. J., & Gibson, M. G. (2000). Recognition of posed and genuine facial expressions of emotion in paranoid and nonparanoid schizophrenia. *Journal of Abnormal Psychology, 109*, 445–450.

Diez-Alegria, C., Vazquez, C., Nieto-Moreno, M., Valiente, C., & Fuentenebro, F. (2006). Personalizing and externalizing biases in deluded and depressed patients: Are attributional biases a stable and specific characteristic of delusions? *British Journal of Clinical Psychology, 45*, 531–544.

Drury, V. M., Robinson, E. J., & Birchwood, M. (1998). "Theory of mind" skills during an acute episode of psychosis and following recovery. *Psychological Medicine, 28*, 1101–1112.

Dunbar., R. (1997). *Grooming, gossip and the evolution of language.* London: Faber and Faber.

Fear, C. F., Sharp, H., & Healy, D. (1996). Cognitive processes in delusional disorder. *British Journal of Psychiatry, 168*, 61–67.

Fenigstein, A., & Vanable, P. A. (1992). Paranoia and self-consciousness. *Journal of Personality and Social Psychology, 62*, 129–134.

Fornells-Ambrojo, M., & Garety, P. (2005). Bad me paranoia in early psychosis: A relatively rare phenomenon. *British Journal of Clinical Psychology, 44*, 521–528.

Fornells-Ambrojo, M., & Garety, P. A. (2009). Attributional biases in paranoia: The development and validation of the Achievement and Relationships Attributions Task (ARAT). *Cognitive Neuropsychiatry, 14*, 87–109.

Frangos, E., Athanassenas, G., Tsitourides, S., Psilolignos, P., & Katsanou, N. (1983). Psychotic depressive disorder: A separate entity? *Journal of Affective Disorders, 5*, 259–265.

Freeman, D. (2008). The assessment of persecutory ideation. In D. Freeman, R. Bentall, & P. Garety (Eds.), *Persecutory delusions: Assessment, theory, treatment* (pp. 23–52). Oxford, UK: Oxford University Press.

Freeman, D., Garety, P. A., Bebbington, P. E., Smith, B., Rollinson, R., Fowler, D., et al. (2005). Psychological investigation of the structure of paranoia in a non-clinical population. *British Journal of Psychiatry, 186*, 427–435.

Freeman, D., Garety, P., & Fowler, D. (2008). The puzzle of paranoia. In D. Freeman, R. Bentall & P. Garety (Eds.), *Persecutory delusions: Assessment, theory, treatment* (pp. 123–144). Oxford, UK: Oxford University Press.

Freeman, D., Garety, P., Fowler, D., Kuipers, E., Dunn, G., Bebbington, P., et al. (1998). The London-East Anglia randomized controlled trial of cognitive-behaviour therapy for psychosis IV: Self-esteem and persecutory delusions. *British Journal of Clinical Psychology, 37*, 415–430.

Freeman, D., Garety, P. A., & Kuipers, E. (2001). Persecutory delusions: Developing the understanding of belief maintenance and emotional distress. *Psychological Medicine, 31*, 1293–1306.

Freeman, D., Garety, P. A., Kuipers, E., Fowler, D., & Bebbington, P. E. (2002). A cognitive model of persecutory delusions. *British Journal of Clinical Psychology, 41*, 331–347.

Freeman, D., Garety, P. A., Kuipers, E., Fowler, D., Bebbington, P. E., & Dunn, G. (2007). Acting on persecutory delusions: The importance of safety seeking. *Behaviour Research and Therapy, 45*, 89–99.

Freeman, D., Pugh, K., & Garety, P. (2008). Jumping to conclusions and paranoid ideation in the general population. *Schizophrenia Research, 102*, 254–260.

Freeman, D., Pugh, K., Vorontsoya, N., & Southgate, L. (2009). Insomnia and paranoia. *Schizophrenia Research, 108*, 280–284.

Frith, C. (1994). Theory of mind in schizophrenia. In A. S. David & J. C. Cutting (Eds.), *The neuropsychology of schizophrenia* (pp. 147–161). Hove, UK: Erlbaum.

Frith, C., & Corcoran, R. (1996). Exploring "theory of mind" in people with schizophrenia. *Psychological Medicine, 26,* 521–530.

Garety, P., Freeman, D., Jolley, S., Ross, K., Waller, H., & Dunn, G. (2011). Jumping to conclusions: The psychology of delusional reasoning. *Advances in Psychiatric Treatment, 17,* 332–339.

Garety, P. A., Hemsley, D. R., & Wessely, S. (1991). Reasoning in deluded schizophrenic and paranoid patients. *Journal of Nervous and Mental Disease, 179*(4), 194–201.

Goldstein, M. J. (1998). Adolescent behavioral and intrafamilial precursors of schizophrenia spectrum disorders. *International Clinical Psychopharmacology, 13*(Suppl. 1), 101.

Goodwin, F. M., & Jamison., K. R. (1990). *Manic depressive illness.* Oxford, UK: Oxford University Press.

Green, M. F. (1998). *Schizophrenia from a neurocognitive perspective: Probing the impenetrable darkness.* Boston: Allyn and Bacon.

Greenwald, A. G., & Farnham, D. (2000). Using the implicit association test to measure self-esteem and self-concept. *Journal of Personality and Social Psychology, 79,* 1022–1038.

Harrington, L., Siegert, R., & McClure, J. N. (2005). Theory of mind in schizophrenia: A critical review. *Cognitive Neuropsychiatry, 10,* 249–286.

Hayes, S. C., Wilson, K. G., Gifford, E. V., Follette, V. M., & Strosahl, K. (1996). Experiential avoidance and behavioral disorders: A functional dimensional approach to diagnosis and treatment. *Journal of Consulting and Clinical Psychology, 64,* 1152–1168.

Higgins, E. (1987). Self-discrepancy: A theory relating self and affect. *Psychological Review, 94,* 319–340.

Holmes, J. (1993). *John Bowlby and attachment theory.* London: Routledge.

Humphreys, L., & Barrowclough, C. (2006). Attributional style, defensive functioning and persecutory delusions: Symptom-specific or general coping strategy? *British Journal of Clinical Psychology, 45,* 231–246.

Huq, S. F., Garety, P. A., & Hemsley, D. R. (1988). Probabilistic judgements in deluded and nondeluded subjects. *Quarterly Journal of Experimental Psychology, 40A,* 801–812.

Jablensky, A., Sartorius, N., Ernberg, G., Anker, M., Korten, A., Cooper, J. E., et al. (1992). Schizophrenia: Manifestations, incidence and course in different cultures. *Psychological Medicine, 20*(Suppl.), 1–97.

Janssen, I., Hanssen, M., Bak, M., Bijl, R. V., De Graaf, R., Vollenberg, W., et al. (2003). Discrimination and delusional ideation. *British Journal of Psychiatry, 182,* 71–76.

Janssen, I., Versmissen, D., Campo, J. A., Myin-Germeys, I., van OS, J., & Krabbendam, L. (2006). Attributional style and psychosis: Evidence for externalizing bias in patients but not individuals at high risk. *Psychological Medicine, 27,* 1–8.

Johns, L. C., Cannon, M., Singleton, N., Murray, R. M., Farrell, M., Brugha, T., et al. (2004). Prevalence and correlates of self-reported psychotic symptoms in the British population. *British Journal of Psychiatry, 185,* 298–305.

Jolley, S., Garety, P., Bebbington, P., Dunn, G., Freeman, D., Kuipers, E., et al. (2006). Attributional style in psychosis: The role of affect and belief type. *Behaviour Research and Therapy, 44,* 1597–1607.

Jorgensen, P., & Jensen, J. (1994). Delusional beliefs in first admitters. *Psychopathology, 27,* 100–112.

Kahneman, D., Slovic, P., & Tversky, A. (1982). *Judgement under uncertainty: Heuristics and biases.* Cambridge, UK: Cambridge University Press.

Kaney, S., & Bentall, R. P. (1989). Persecutory delusions and attributional style. *British Journal of Medical Psychology, 62,* 191–198.

Kaney, S., & Bentall, R. P. (1992). Persecutory delusions and the self-serving bias. *Journal of Nervous and Mental Disease, 180*, 773–780.

Kaney, S., Bowen-Jones, K., Dewey, M. E., & Bentall, R. P. (1997). Frequency and consensus judgements of paranoid, paranoid-depressed and depressed psychiatric patients: Subjective estimates for positive, negative and neutral events. *British Journal of Clinical Psychology, 36*, 349–364.

Kaney, S., Wolfenden, M., Dewey, M. E., & Bentall, R. P. (1992). Persecutory delusions and the recall of threatening and non-threatening propositions. *British Journal of Clinical Psychology, 31*, 85–87.

Kapur, S., Mizrahi, R., & Li, M. (2005). From dopamine to salience to psychosis—linking biology, pharmacology and phenomenology of psychosis. *Schizophrenia Research, 79*, 59–68.

Kesting, M. -L., Mehl, S., Rief, S., Lindenmeyer, J., & Lincoln, T. M. (2011). When paranoia fails to enhance self-esteem: Explicit and implicit self-esteem and its discrepancy in patients with persecutory delusions compared to depressed and healthy controls. *Psychiatry Research, 186*, 197–202.

Kim, K., Li, D., Jiang, Z., & Cui, X. (1993). Schizophrenic delusions among Koreans, Korean-Chinese and Chinese: A transcultural study. *International Journal of Social Psychiatry, 39*, 190–199.

Kinderman, P. (1994). Attentional bias, persecutory delusions and the self concept. *British Journal of Medical Psychology, 67*, 53–66.

Kinderman, P., & Bentall, R. (2000). Self-discrepancies and causal attributions: Studies of hypothesised relationships. *British Journal of Clinical Psychology, 39*, 255–273.

Kinderman, P., & Bentall, R. P. (1996). The development of a novel measure of causal attributions: The Internal Personal and Situational Attributions Questionnaire. *Personality and Individual Differences, 20*, 261–264.

Kinderman, P., & Bentall, R. P. (1997). Causal attributions in paranoia: Internal, personal and situational attributions for negative events. *Journal of Abnormal Psychology, 106*, 341–345.

Kinderman, P., & Bentall, R. P. (2000). Self-discrepancies and causal attributions: Studies of hypothesized relationships. *British Journal of Clinical Psychology, 39*, 255–273.

Kinderman, P., Dunbar, R. I. M., & Bentall, R. P. (1998). Theory of mind deficits and causal attributions. *British Journal of Psychology, 71*, 339–349.

Kozarić-Kovačić, D., & Borovečki, A. (2005). Prevalence of psychotic comorbidity in combat-related post-traumatic stress disorder. *Military Medicine, 170*, 223–226.

Kraepelin, E. (1907). *Textbook of psychiatry, 7th edition* (A. R. Diefendorf, Trans.). London: Macmillan.

Kristev, H., Jackson, H., & Maude, D. (1999). An investigation of attributional style in first-episode psychosis. *British Journal of Clinical Psychology, 88*, 181–194.

LaRusso, L. (1978). Sensitivity of paranoid patients to nonverbal cues. *Journal of Abnormal Psychology, 87*, 463–471.

Lattuada, E., Serretti, A., Cusin, C., Gasperini, M., & Smeraldi, E. (1999). Symptomatologic analysis of psychotic and non-psychotic depression. *Journal of Affective Disorders, 54*, 183–187.

Leary, M. R., Tambor, E. S., Terdal, S. K., & Downs, D. L. (1995). Self-esteem as an interpersonal monitor: The sociometer hypothesis. *Journal of Personality and Social Psychology, 68*, 518–530.

Lee, D., Randall, F., Beattie, G., & Bentall, R. P. (2004). Delusional discourse: An investigation comparing the spontaneous causal attributions of paranoid and non-paranoid individuals. *Psychology & Psychotherapy—Theory, Research, Practice, 77*, 525–540.

Lincoln, T. M., Lange, J., Burau, J., Exner, C. E., & Moritz, S. (2010). The effect of state anxiety on paranoid ideation and jumping to conclusions. An experimental investigation. *Schizophrenia Bulletin, 36*, 1140–1148.

Lyon, H. M., Kaney, S., & Bentall, R. P. (1994). The defensive function of persecutory delusions: Evidence from attribution tasks. *British Journal of Psychiatry, 164*, 637–646.

MacBeth, A., Schwannauer, M., & Gumley, A. (2008). The association between attachment style, social mentalities, and paranoid ideation: An analogue study. *Psychology and Psychotherapy: Theory, practice, research, 81*, 79–83.

Maher, B. A. (1988). Anomalous experience and delusional thinking: The logic of explanations. In T. F. Oltmanns & B. A. Maher (Eds.), *Delusional beliefs* (pp. 15–33). New York: Wiley.

Manschreck, T. C. (1989). Delusional (paranoid) disorders. In H. I. Kaplan & B. J. Sadock (Eds.), *Comprehensive textbook of psychiatry* (5th ed., pp. 816–828). Baltimore: Williams & Wilkins.

Manschreck, T. C., & Khan, N. L. (2006). Recent advances in the treatment of delusional disorder. *Canadian Journal of Psychiatry, 51*, 114–119.

Martin, J. A., & Penn, D. L. (2002). Attributional style in schizophrenia: An investigation in outpatients with and without persecutory delusions. *Schizophrenia Bulletin, 28*, 131–142.

McKay, R., Langdon, R., & Coltheart, M. (2005). Paranoia, persecutory delusions and attributional biases. *Psychiatry Research, 136*, 233–245.

McKay, R., Langdon, R., & Coltheart, M. (2007). The defensive function of persecutory delusions: An investigation using the implicit association test. *Cognitive Neuropsychiatry, 12*, 1–24.

Mehl, S., Rief, W., Lullman, E., Ziegler, M., Muller, M. J., & Lincoln, T. M. (2010). Implicit attributional style revisited: Evidence for a state-specific "self-decreasing" implicit attributional style in patients with persecutory delusions. *Cognitive Neuropsychiatry, 15*, 451–476.

Melo, S., Corcoran, R., & Bentall, R. P. (2009). The Persecution and Deservedness Scale. *Psychology and Psychotherapy: Theory, practice, research, 82*, 247–260.

Melo, S., Taylor, J., & Bentall, R. P. (2006). "Poor me" versus "bad me" paranoia and the instability of persecutory ideation. *Psychology & Psychotherapy—Theory, Research, Practice, 79*, 271–287.

Melo, S. S., & Bentall, R. P. (2012). "Poor me" vs. "bad me" paranoia: The association between self-beliefs and the instability of persecutory ideation. *Psychology & Psychotherapy: Theory, Research and Practice.* doi: 10.1111/j.2044–8341.2011.02051.x

Merrin, J., Kinderman, P., & Bentall, R. P. (2007). Jumping to conclusions and attributional style in patients with persecutory delusions. *Cognitive Therapy and Research, 31*, 741–758.

Mezulis, A. H., Abramson, L. Y., Hyde, J. S., & Hankin, B. L. (2004). Is there a universal positivity bias in attributions? A meta-analytic review of individual, developmental and cultural differences in the self-serving attributional bias. *Psychological Bulletin, 130*, 711–747.

Mirowsky, J., & Ross, C. E. (1983). Paranoia and the structure of powerlessness. *American Sociological Review, 48*, 228–239.

Moore, N. C. (1981). Is paranoid illness associated with sensory defects in the elderly? *Journal of Psychosomatic Research, 25*, 69–74.

Morgan, C., Kirkbride, J., Leff, J., Craig, T., Hutchinson, G., McKenzie, K., et al. (2007). Parental separation, loss and psychosis in different ethnic groups: A case-control study. *Psychological Medicine, 37*, 495–503.

Moritz, S., Werner, R., & von Collani, G. (2006). The inferiority complex in paranoia readdressed: A study with the Implicit Association Test. *Cognitive Neuropsychiatry, 11,* 402–415.

Morrison, A. P., Gumley, A., Schwannauer, M., Campbell, M., Gleeson, A., Griffin, E., et al. (2005). The Beliefs About Paranoia Scale: Preliminary validation of a metacognitive approach to conceptualizing paranoia. *Behavioural and Cognitive Psychotherapy, 33,* 153–164.

Morrison, A. P., Gumley, A. I., Ashcroft, K., Manousos, I. R., White, R., Gillan, K., et al. (2011). Metacognition and persecutory delusions: Tests of a metacognitive model in a clinical population and comparisons with non-patients. *British Journal of Clinical Psychology, 50,* 223–233.

Morrison, A. P., & Petersen, T. (2003). Trauma, metacognition and predisposition to hallucinations in non-patients. *Behavioural and Cognitive Psychotherapy, 31,* 235–246.

Moutoussis, M., Bentall, R. P., El-Deredy, W., & Dayan, P. (2011). Bayesian modelling of jumping-to-conclusions bias in delusional patients. *Cognitive Neuropsychiatry, 16,* 422–447.

Moutoussis, M., Bentall, R. P., Williams, J., & Dayan, P. (2008). A temporal difference account of avoidance learning. *Network: Computation in Neural Systems, 19,* 137–160.

Moutoussis, M., El-Deredy, W. & Bentall, R. P. (in press). An empirical study of defensive avoidance in paranoia. *Journal of Nervous and Mental Disease.*

Moutoussis, M., Williams, J., Dayan, P., & Bentall, R. P. (2007). Persecutory delusions and the conditioned avoidance paradigm: Towards an integration of the psychology and biology of paranoia. *Cognitive Neuropsychiatry, 12,* 495–510.

Munro, A. (1982). Paranoia revisited. *British Journal of Psychiatry, 141,* 344–349.

Myers, E., Startup, H., & Freeman, D. (2011). Cognitive behavioural treatment of insomnia in individuals with persistent persecutory delusions: A pilot trial. *Behaviour Research and Therapy, 42,* 330–336.

Ndetei, D. M., & Vadher, A. (1984). Frequency and clinical significance of delusions across cultures. *Acta Psychiatrica Scandinavica, 70,* 73–76.

Oltmanns, T. F., & Maher, B. A. (Eds.). (1988). *Delusional beliefs.* New York: John Wiley.

Pedersen, C. B., & Mortensen, P. B. (2001). Evidence of a dose-response relationship between urbanicity during upbringing and schizophrenia risk. *Archives of General Psychiatry, 58,* 1039–1046.

Peer, J. E., Kupper, Z., Long, J. D., Brekke, J. S., & Spaulding, W. D. (2007). Identifying mechanisms of treatment effects and recovery in rehabilitation of schizophrenia: Longitudinal analytic methods. *Clinical Psychology Review, 27,* 696–714.

Peterson, C., Semmel, A., Von Baeyer, C., Abramson, L., Metalsky, G. I., & Seligman, M. E. P. (1982). The Attributional Style Questionnaire. *Cognitive Therapy and Research, 6,* 287–300.

Phillips, M., & David, A. S. (1997a). Abnormal visual scan paths: A psychophysiological marker of delusions in schizophrenia. *Schizophrenia Research, 29,* 235–254.

Phillips, M., & David, A. S. (1997b). Visual scan paths are abnormal in deluded schizophrenics. *Neuropsychologia, 35,* 99–105.

Pickering, L., Simpson, J., & Bentall, R. P. (2008). Insecure attachment predicts proneness to paranoia but not hallucinations. *Personality and Individual Differences, 44,* 1212–1224.

Pickup, G. (2008). Relationship between theory of mind and executive function in schizophrenia: A systematic review. *Psychopathology, 41,* 206–213.

Randall, F., Corcoran, R., Day, J. C., & Bentall, R. P. (2003). Attention, theory of mind and causal attributions in people with paranoid delusions: A preliminary investigation. *Cognitive Neuropsychiatry, 8,* 287–294.

Rankin, P., Bentall, R. P., Hill, J., & Kinderman, P. (2005). Parental relationships and paranoid delusions: Comparisons of currently ill, remitted and healthy individuals. *Psychopathology, 38*, 16–25.

Read, J., van Os, J., Morrison, A. P., & Ross, C. A. (2005). Childhood trauma, psychosis and schizophrenia: A literature review and clinical implications. *Acta Psychiatrica Scandinavica, 112*, 330–350.

Reininghaus, U., Craig, T. K. J., Fisher, H. L., Hutchinson, G., Fearon, P., Morgan, K., et al. (2010). Ethnic identity, perceptions of disadvantage, and psychosis: Findings from the AESOP study. *Schizophrenia Research, 124*, 43–48.

Reivich, K. (1995). The measurement of explanatory style. In G. M. Buchanan & M. E. P. Seligman (Eds.), *Explanatory style* (pp. 21–48). Hillsdale, New Jersey: Lawrence Erlbaum.

Rössler, W., Reicher-Rossler, A., Angst, J., Murray, R. M., Gamma, A., Eich, D., et al. (2007). Psychotic experiences in the general population: A twenty-year prospective community study. *Schizophrenia Research, 92*, 1–14.

Rubin, E. H., & Drevets, W. C. (1988). The nature of psychotic symptoms in senile dementia of the Alzheimer type. *Journal of Geriatric Psychiatry and Neurology, 1*, 16–20.

Rutten, B. P. F., van Os, J., Dominguez, M., & Krabbendam, L. (2008). Epidemiology and social factors: Findings from the Netherlands Mental Health Survey and Incidence Study (NEMESIS). In D. Freeman, R. Bentall, & P. Garety (Eds.), *Persecutory delusions: Assessment, theory, treatment* (pp. 53–72). Oxford, UK: Oxford University Press.

Sarfati, Y., & Hardy-Bayle, M. C. (1999). How do people with schizophrenia explain the behaviour of others? A study of theory of mind and its relationship to thought and speech disorganization in schizophrenia. *Psychological Medicine, 29*, 613–620.

Sarfati, Y., Hardy-Bayles, M. C., Brunet, E., & Widloecher, D. (1999). Investigating theory of mind in schizophrenia: Influence of verbalization in disorganized and non-disorganized patients. *Schizophrenia Research, 37*, 183–190.

Schreier, A., Wolke, D., Thomas, K., Horwood, J., Hollis, C., Gunnell, D., et al. (2009). Prospective study of peer victimization in childhood and psychotic symptoms in a non-clinical population at age 12 Years. *Archives of General Psychiatry, 66*, 527–536.

Selten, J. -P., Veen, N., Feller, W., Blom, J. D., Schols, D., Camoenie, W., et al. (2001). Incidence of psychotic disorders in immigrant groups to The Netherlands. *British Journal of Psychiatry, 178*, 367–372.

Sendiony, M. F. (1976). Cultural aspects of delusions: A psychiatric study of Egypt. *Australian and New Zealand Journal of Psychiatry, 10*, 201–207.

Shryane, N. M., Corcoran, R., Rowse, G., Moore, R., Cummins, S., Blackwood, N., et al. (2008). Deception and false belief in paranoia: Modelling theory of mind stories. *Cognitive Neuropsychiatry, 13*, 8–32.

Stefanis, N., Thewissen, V., Bakoula, C., van Os, J., & Myin- Germeys, I. (2006). Hearing impairment and psychosis: A replication in a cohort of young adults. *Schizophrenia Research, 85*, 266–272.

Taylor, J., & Kinderman, P. (2002). An analogue study of attributional complexity, theory of mind deficits and paranoia. *British Journal of Psychology, 93*, 137–140.

Thewissen, V., Bentall, R. P., Lecomte, T., van Os, J., & Myin-Germeys, I. (2008). Fluctuations in self-esteem and paranoia in the context of everyday life. *Journal of Abnormal Psychology, 117*, 143–153.

Thewissen, V., Myin-Germeys, I., Bentall, R. P., de Graaf, R., Volleberghd, W., & van Os, J. (2005). Hearing impairment and psychosis revisited. *Schizophrenia Research, 76*, 99–103.

Tienari, P., Wynne, L. C., Sorri, A., Lahti, I., Laksy, K., Moring, J., et al. (2004). Long term follow-up study of Finnish adoptees. *British Journal of Psychiatry, 184*, 214–222.

Trower, P., & Chadwick, P. (1995). Pathways to defense of the self: A theory of two types of paranoia. *Clinical Psychology: Science and Practice, 2,* 263–278.

Udachina, A., Thewissen, V., Myin-Germeys, I., Fitzpatrick, S., O'Kane, A., & Bentall, R. P. (2009). Self-esteem, experiential avoidance and paranoia. *Journal of Nervous and Mental Disease, 197,* 661–668.

Udachina, A., Varese, F., Oorschot, M., Myin-Germeys, I., & Bentall, R. P. (2012). Dynamics of self-esteem in "poor-me" and "bad-me" paranoia. *Journal of Nervous and Mental Disease.* doi: 10.1097/NMD.0b013e318266ba57

Valiente, C., Cantero, D., Vazquez, C., Sanchez, A., Provencio, M., & Espinosa, R. (2011). Implicit and explicit self-esteem discrepancies in paranoia. *Journal of Abnormal Psychology, 120,* 691–699.

van der Werf, M., van Boxtel, M., & van Os, J. (2010). Evidence that the impact of hearing impairment on psychosis risk is moderated by the level of complexity of the social environment. *Schizophrenia Research, 122,* 193–198.

van der Werf, M., van Boxtel, M., Verhey, F., Jolley, J., Thewissen, V., & van Os, J. (2007). Mild hearing impairment and psychotic experiences in a normal aging population *Schizophrenia Research, 94,* 180–186.

van Os, J., Hanssen, M., Bijl, R. V., & Vollebergh, W. (2001). Prevalence of psychotic disorder and community level of psychotic symptoms: An urban-rural comparison. *Archives of General Psychiatry, 58,* 663–668.

Veling, W., Selten, J. P., Susser, E., Laan, W., Mackenbach, J. P., & Hoek, H. W. (2007). Discrimination and the incidence of psychotic disorders among ethnic minorities in the Netherlands. *International Journal of Epidemiology, 36,* 761–768.

Veling, W., Susser, E., van Os, J., Mackenbach, J. P., Selten, J. P., & Hoek, H. W. (2008). Ethnic density of neighborhoods and incidence of psychotic disorders among immigrants. *American Journal of Psychiatry, 165,* 66–73.

Watt, J. A. G. (1985). Hearing and premorbid personality in paranoid states. *American Journal of Psychiatry, 142,* 1453–1455.

Weiner, B. (2008). Reflections on the history of attribution theory and research: People, personalities, publications, problems. *Social Psychology, 39,* 151–156.

Young, H. F., & Bentall, R. P. (1997). Probabilistic reasoning in deluded, depressed and normal subjects: Effects of task difficulty and meaningful versus nonmeaningful materials. *Psychological Medicine, 27,* 455–465.

Zigler, E., & Glick, M. (1988). Is paranoid schizophrenia really camouflaged depression? *American Psychologist, 43,* 284–290.

Zimbardo, P. G., Andersen, S. M., & Kabat, L. G. (1981). Induced hearing deficit generates experimental paranoia. *Science, 212,* 1529–1531.

Zolkowska, K., Cantor, G. E., & McNeil, T. F. (2001). Increased rates of psychosis amongst immigrants to Sweden: Is migration a risk factor for psychosis? *Psychological Medicine, 31,* 669–678.

10

Social Cognition Early in the Course of the Illness

JEAN ADDINGTON AND DANIJELA PISKULIC ■

Interest and research in social cognition has experienced tremendous growth in the past 5–10 years, as is clearly presented in earlier chapters in this book. It is well established that individuals with schizophrenia have impairment on a wide range of social cognitive tasks relative to healthy controls, as well as to other diagnostic groups. What is less clear is when these impairments begin. Are they present at the start of the illness, or even before there is evidence of full-blown psychosis? Over the last 15 years, a major emphasis has been placed on early detection and intervention in the development of a psychotic illness. The goal was to detect and treat major psychotic illnesses early in their development, so that individuals could receive appropriate treatment at the earliest stage possible and have the best opportunity for recovery. This work focused on identifying young people as soon as possible after the onset of the psychotic illness (Addington et al., 2007). More recently, the focus has moved to an even earlier stage of the illness, the prodrome, since there is evidence that subclinical symptoms are present during the prepsychotic period.

In schizophrenia, the prodromal phase refers to the signs and symptoms that a person experiences prior to the onset of a full-blown syndrome (Yung, Phillips, Yuen, & McGorry, 2004). Recent developments in research have led to the development of reliable criteria to identify individuals who may be at risk of developing psychosis and thus potentially experiencing a prodrome for psychosis (McGlashan, Walsh, & Woods, 2010). The criteria for what can be thought of as a putative prodrome for psychosis was first introduced by Alison Yung and colleagues in Melbourne, Australia (Yung & McGorry, 1996) and incorporated into the Comprehensive Assessment of the At-Risk Mental State (CAARMS). These criteria were modified by McGlashan and colleagues (McGlashan et al., 2010) to form the Criteria of Psychosis-risk Syndromes (COPS). The COPS are evaluated using the Structured Interview for Prodromal Syndromes (SIPS) and the Scale of Prodromal Symptoms (SOPS) (McGlashan et al., 2010).

Both the Melbourne criteria and the COPS have three possible criteria: brief intermittent psychotic symptoms (BIPS), attenuated positive symptoms (APS) and/or genetic risk and deterioration (GRD). The BIPS state requires the presence of any one or more threshold positive psychotic symptoms that are too brief to meet diagnostic criteria for psychosis.

The APS requires the presence of at least one particular positive psychotic symptom of insufficient severity to meet diagnostic criteria for a psychotic disorder. The GRD requires having a combination of both functional decline and genetic risk; genetic risk refers to having either schizotypal personality disorder or a first-degree relative with a schizophrenia spectrum disorder (McGlashan et al., 2010).

Researchers are therefore able to prospectively follow the course of the illness, with the goal of being able to distinguish early on differences in those who go on to develop schizophrenia or another psychotic disorder from those who do not. Current evidence indicates that approximately 25% of these at-risk individuals will go on to develop a full-blown illness within 1 year and 35% in 2 years (Cannon et al., 2008). Several terms have been coined to distinguish this population from other high-risk groups, such as those with a family history risk or those with schizotypy. These individuals are considered to be at enhanced high risk and thus the Melbourne group used the term "ultra-high risk" (UHR). Since the risk is often based on the presence of clinical symptoms, these individuals have also been described as being at clinical high risk (CHR) of developing psychosis. In this chapter, the term CHR will be used to describe such samples.

First, we will review relevant literature on social cognition at the first episode, then during the period of clinical high risk, and, finally, for those who are at familial high risk of developing the illness.

SOCIAL COGNITION IN FIRST-EPISODE PSYCHOSIS

It has been well established that the performance on a range of social cognitive tests in patients with schizophrenia is reliably below that of healthy volunteers, and that it correlates with poorer functional outcomes (Fett et al., 2011). A number of reviews and meta-analytic studies have suggested a strong magnitude of impairment for social cognitive domains such as theory of mind (ToM) (Brune, 2005; Sprong, Schothorst, Vos, Hox, & van Engeland, 2007; Bora, Yucel, & Pantelis, 2009); affect recognition, both facial affect (Kohler, Walker, Martin, Healey, & Moberg, 2009) and emotional prosody (i.e., vocal emotion perception or the evaluation of emotional non-lexical cues in speech; Hoekert, Kahn, Pijnenborg, & Aleman, 2007); and social perception/knowledge (Piskulic, Addington, & Maruff, 2010). An overwhelming majority of these explorations, however, have been based on patients in the more chronic stage of the illness. It therefore remains unclear if the degree of impairment is different in earlier stages of the illness, such as at the recent onset or first episode (FE) of psychosis, and if those impairments apply to multiple domains of social cognition (Green et al., in press).

Compared to the chronic stage, FE psychosis is generally characterized by greater fluctuations in clinical presentation and can therefore be particularly informative when determining whether social cognitive deficits are state or trait phenomena, or a combination of the two (Nuechterlein et al., 1992; Horan et al., in press). It can be similarly informative when assessing if deficits in social cognition are potential vulnerability indicators while ruling out possible confounding factors such as illness chronicity and long-term medication use.

To date, evidence from cross-sectional studies suggests that FE individuals exhibit impairments on multiple domains of social cognition such as ToM, affect recognition (both facial and prosodic), social perception/knowledge, and attributional bias. In the following sections, we review findings from all studies of FE psychosis that explored deficits in those four domains of social cognition.

Affect Recognition in First-Episode Psychosis

Affect recognition is the capacity to recognize and be aware of emotional expressions in one and others. It includes identifying, facilitating, understanding, and managing emotions, either by observing body language or nonlexical cues in speech. In FE psychosis research, six studies have investigated affect perception deficits using a variety of tests. Whereas all six studies explored facial affect recognition, two studies also looked at affective prosody, making it the focus of their investigation (Edwards, Pattison, Jackson, & Wales, 2001; Kucharska-Pietura, David, Masiak, & Phillips, 2005).

All studies compared performance on affect recognition tests in groups of FE individuals with that of healthy volunteers. Changes in affect recognition across different stages of psychotic illness were examined in three studies using the cross-sectional design and comparing FE individuals with samples of participants with chronic schizophrenia (Addington, Saeedi, & Addington, 2006a; Kucharska-Pietura et al., 2005; Pinkham, Penn, Perkins, Graham, & Siegel, 2007). Temporal stability of affective processing deficits in first-episode psychosis individuals was additionally investigated by three research groups who retested their samples after a 12-month period (Addington et al., 2006a) and following a short-term antipsychotic treatment (Behere, Venkatasubramanian, Arasappa, Reddy, & Gangadhar, 2009; Herbener, Hill, Marvin, & Sweeney, 2005).

Compared to healthy volunteers, individuals with FE psychosis were reported to be impaired on multiple components of affect recognition, irrespective of modality, facial or prosodic. That is, FE individuals were reportedly performing poorer than controls on tests of affect recognition (Addington et al., 2006a; Behere et al., 2009; Edwards et al., 2001; Kucharska-Pietura et al., 2005; Pinkham et al., 2007), affective acuity (Herbener et al., 2005), and affect discrimination (Addington et al., 2006a; Herbener et al., 2005; Pinkham et al., 2007), which is in accordance with findings from studies in chronic schizophrenia (Hoekert et al., 2007; Kohler et al., 2009). Impairments in affect recognition in FE individuals were, however, of comparable (Addington et al., 2006a ; Pinkham et al., 2007) or lesser magnitude (Kucharska-Pietura et al., 2005) to those reported in chronic schizophrenia.

Furthermore, four studies have investigated the stability of deficits in affect recognition over time. Specifically, Addington and colleagues (2006a) and Horan et al. (in press) reported deficits to be stable at 12-month follow-up, which was irrespective of improvements in symptoms. Herbener et al. (2005) also reported no change in affect recognition over time. Only one study using treatment-naïve schizophrenia patients (Behere et. al., 2009) reported a reduction in affect recognition deficits, suggesting that the outcome was most likely secondary to symptom improvement following medication treatment. Thus, although there are few longitudinal studies, there is preliminary evidence of stability of affect recognition deficits in FE psychosis.

Social Perception and Social Knowledge in First-Episode Psychosis

Social perception is the awareness of cues that typically occur in social situations. Social knowledge is the awareness of what is socially expected in different situations, and it guides social interactions (Green, Olivier, Crawley, Penn, & Silverstein, 2005). Since the identification of social cues generally requires knowledge of what is expected and acceptable in social situations (Green et al., 2005), social perception and social knowledge are often considered together under the domain of social perception.

In schizophrenia research, the concept of social perception and social knowledge has not been as extensively researched as other domains, such as affect recognition and ToM, which is also true of the research in FE psychosis. To date, only two studies investigated social perception and social knowledge in FE individuals, relative to chronic schizophrenia and healthy control samples (Addington, Saeedi, & Addington, 2006b; Green et al., in press). Results of these studies demonstrated that FE individuals were as impaired as chronic schizophrenia patients in their understanding of social relationships (Green et al., in press), their ability to appraise social roles and context, and their awareness of the rules, goals, and roles that characterize social situations (Addington et al., 2006b). Longitudinal investigations of social perception and social knowledge test performance suggested persistent deficits across a 12-month study period (Horan et al., in press).

Theory of Mind in First-Episode Psychosis

Theory of mind, also referred to as *mentalizing* or *mental state attribution*, typically involves the ability to infer the intentions, dispositions, and beliefs of others (Frith & Corcoran, 1996; Green et al., 2005). To the best of our knowledge, there have been seven studies to date that examined ToM performance in FE samples. Although all studies compared FE individuals with healthy volunteers, one study additionally examined ToM performance across different stages of illness (Green et al., in press) and one study included a group of clinical controls (Kettle, O'Brien-Simpson, & Allen, 2008). Only one research group additionally examined temporal stability of ToM performance over a 12-month period (Horan et al., in press).

Findings based on comparisons with healthy volunteers from all seven studies suggest that FE individuals exhibited impaired performance on a range of ToM tests. Specifically, FE individuals were impaired in their ability to perceive complex mental states (Kettle et al., 2008), understand and describe social interactions (Koelkebeck et al., 2010), and correctly infer intentions and mental states of others (Bertrand, Sutton, Achim, Malla, & Lepage, 2007; Herold et al., 2009; Inoue et al., 2006), including understanding of irony and empathy (Green et al., in press; Williams et al., 2008). Green and colleagues (in press) compared FE individuals to patients with chronic schizophrenia using the Awareness of Social Inference Test Part III (TASIT; McDonald et al., 2003) as a measure of ToM and reported no significant group difference. Moreover, the authors reported that both clinical groups were significantly impaired on ToM compared to healthy volunteers. In a subsequent longitudinal study by the same group, FE individuals were followed up over the period of 12 months. The authors reported good longitudinal stability. Last, in the study by Kettle and colleagues (2008), in which FE individuals were compared to patients with major depressive disorder, the authors reported no difference on the "eyes task" between the two groups.

Based on the current research from FE studies, which almost exclusively comes from cross-sectional research, there is evidence that FE patients have impairments relative to controls and similar to those with a more chronic course of illness. No conclusions can be drawn regarding trait or state status of ToM impairments in psychosis, or their specificity to FE psychosis.

Attributional Style in First-Episode Psychosis

Attributional style refers to the causal explanations that individuals attribute to their own behavior and the behavior of others (Fiske & Taylor, 1991). This domain of social cognition is generally assessed in reference to patients who experience hallucinations and delusions, especially persecutory delusions, and their explanations of positive and negative life events. A tendency to internally attribute more positive than negative events to self is referred to as *self-serving bias* (SSB).

Most of what is now known about attributional style in psychosis comes from research in chronic schizophrenia. Only two studies to date investigated attributional style in FE psychosis using cross-sectional design and both overt (i.e., Pragmatic Inference Task [PIT], Winters & Neale, 1985; and Internal, Personal and Situational Attributions Questionnaire [IPSAQ], Kinderman & Bentall, 1996) and covert (i.e., Attributional Style Questionnaire [APQ], Lyon, Kaney, & Bentall, 1994) assessment methods (Humphreys & Barrowclough, 2006; Krstev, Jackson, & Maude, 1999). Based on the current evidence using overt tests of attributional style, level of paranoia did not predict SSB in FE individuals. On the covert tests, however, FE individuals reportedly showed an underlying depressive attributional style, whereby they made more external attributions for positive than for negative events and more internal attributions for negative than for positive events (Humphreys & Barrowclough, 2006; Krstev et al., 1999). Furthermore, this pattern of association in FE psychosis was the same as that reported in patients with chronic schizophrenia, although not as pronounced (Krstev et al., 1999). Given the limited evidence and lack of longitudinal research, the stability of attributional style in FE psychosis remains unclear.

Correlates of Social Cognition at the First Episode

Current findings regarding clinical, neurocognitive, and real-life functioning correlates of social cognition in FE psychosis are mixed. Results from cross-sectional studies suggest both presence and absence of association between psychopathology and performance on tests across different domains of social cognition. The same is true for longitudinal studies that reported both small reductions (Behere et al., 2009; Horan et al., in press) and no change (Addington et al., 2006a,b; Herbener et al., 2005) in social cognitive deficits following improvement in psychopathology.

Although social cognition is considered psychometrically distinguishable from neurocognition (Sergi et al., 2007), evidence from FE research suggests that there still exists a significant association between the two constructs (Addington et al., 2006a,b; Bertrand et al., 2007; Koelkebeck et al., 2010; Krstev et al., 1999). Despite the association, however, social cognitive deficits reportedly persisted even after neurocognitive performance was controlled for (Bertrand et al., 2007; Koelkebeck et al., 2010).

Finally, there is evidence to suggest that social cognition has a unique association with functional outcome in the early course of psychosis, as it was reported as a significant predictor of real-life functioning (Horan et al., in press) and a mediator of the relationship between neurocognition and poor functional outcome (Addington, Girard, Christensen, & Addington, 2010).

Summary

Overall, consistent evidence demonstrates that individuals at the first episode of psychosis not only demonstrate significant impairment in all domains of social cognition, but that this impairment is comparable to that reported in more chronic stages of illness. Although there is evidence that FE patients have deficits in all domains, relatively few studies simultaneously addressed more than one domain of social cognition and typically used one test per domain. Finally, although only a small number of studies investigated temporal stability of those impairments, there is growing evidence that these impairments are stable over time.

SOCIAL COGNITION AND CLINICAL HIGH RISK OF PSYCHOSIS

Research in the area of social cognition and the risk of psychosis is steadily growing, although only a few studies have been completed to date. There is evidence from studies examining emotion recognition both in faces and voices, and there are early studies on ToM and attributional style.

Affect Recognition in Clinical High Risk Patients

Addington and colleagues (Addington, Penn, Woods, Addington, & Perkins, 2008) examined facial affect recognition and facial affect discrimination in a sample of 86 young people who were at CHR based on the SIPS/SOPS and compared their performance to individuals with a chronic course of schizophrenia, individuals experiencing their first episode, and healthy controls. Results demonstrated that, on the identification task, the healthy controls performed significantly better than the CHR and patient groups. On the discrimination task, patient groups performed significantly more poorly than the normal controls, and the performance of the CHR group fell between that of the patient and control groups without significantly differing from either. This was in contrast to an early study by Pinkham et al. (2007), who did not find any differences between a CHR group and healthy controls on the same tasks. However, this was a very small study with 19 subjects.

A recently published study by Amminger and colleagues (in press) compared individuals at CHR based on the CAARMS with a FE psychosis group and a healthy control group. This Austrian study used a facial affect task and a measure of affective prosody designed by Edwards et al. (2001). They found deficits in the recognition of fear and sadness across both face and voice modalities for the both the CHR and the FE group compared to the healthy controls. Furthermore, in comparison to the healthy controls, both clinical groups had a significant deficit for fear and sadness recognition in faces and for anger recognition in voices. In reviewing their results, these authors suggest that this may be a trait deficit and hypothesized about amygdala involvement.

Social Perception and Social Knowledge in Clinical High Risk

Social perception is the ability to understand and appraise social roles, rules, and context. The Social Cue Recognition Test (SCRT) is one measure that has been used to assess social perception. This requires individuals to use social cues to make inferences about the situational events that generated the particular social cue or to identify interpersonal features in a given situation (Corrigan, 1997). To the best of our knowledge, no studies have addressed this in the CHR population, although one study by Couture et al. (Couture, Penn, Addington, Woods, &

Perkins 2008) used the abbreviated trustworthiness task to assess complex social judgments (Adolphs, Tranel, & Damasio, 1998) that could potentially be considered a measure of social perception. In this task, participants were shown 42 faces of unfamiliar people and were asked to imagine they had to trust the pictured person with their money or with their life. They rated how much they would trust the person on a 7-point scale, ranging from -3 (very untrustworthy) to +3 (very trustworthy). Previous work with this task has reported different biases between the two ends of the continuum in individuals with bilateral amygdala damage and in those with high-functioning autism (both groups provide more positive ratings to untrustworthy faces) (Adolphs et al., 1998; Adolphs, 2001). In Couture et al.'s study (2008), there were no differences between the CHR participants (determined by the SIPS/SOPS) and healthy controls in terms of rating the trustworthy faces, but the CHR group rated the untrustworthy faces as more positive significantly more often than did the healthy controls.

Theory of Mind in Clinical High Risk

Couture and colleagues (2008) used what is known as the "reading the mind in the eyes task." The eyes task was designed to assess adult ToM abilities (Baron-Cohen, Wheelwright, Hill, Raste, & Plumb, 2001). Participants were shown a pair of eyes and asked to choose from among four words the one that best describes what the person is thinking or feeling. The percentage of correct responses was used as a summary score for this measure, consistent with previous research. In this study with 86 CHR participants, there were no differences between the CHR group and healthy controls. The eyes task was considered by the authors to be a task of ToM, although there is some debate as to whether this is typically a task used in this domain.

Using more typical tasks of ToM, a Korean group, Chung and colleagues (Chung, Kang, Shin, Yoo, & Kwon, 2008), compared the performance of CHR group (n = 33) on the false-belief task (Perner & Wimmer, 1985), the strange story task (Happe, 1994), and a visual cartoon task (Oh et al., 2005) to that of a healthy control group. There were significant differences on the both the strange story task and the false-belief task, with the CHR group performing more poorly, but no differences were observed on the visual cartoon task.

Attributional Style in Clinical High Risk

Attributional style is the fourth domain often addressed in social cognition. One recently developed task in this area is the Ambiguous Intentions Hostility Questionnaire (AIHQ; Combs, Penn, Wicher, & Waldheter, 2007). The AIHQ is a self-report questionnaire about negative outcomes that vary intentionally or accidentally or with ambiguous intentions. Using this task, a second group of investigators from South Korea compared the attributions of 24 CHR participants to those of healthy controls ($n = 39$) and FE patients ($n = 20$) (An et al., 2010). Both the FE and CHR participants demonstrated a perceived hostility bias. In the FE group, this was related to persecutory symptoms. Similarly, in the CHR group, their attribution bias for perceiving hostility was linked to a paranoid process.

Multiple Domains

One of the issues about the prodromal studies to date is that they tended to use a single control group. As suggested by Green et al. (in press), a potentially more direct test of whether there is increasing deficits from the prodromal phase to the illness phase would include separate comparison groups that demographically matched each of the clinical groups. In this study, the tasks selected reflected three domains: the Relationships Across Domains (RAD; Sergi et al., 2009) to assess models or rules for interactions; the Awareness of Social Inference Test (Part II) (TASIT) to assess capacities to understand other minds; and the Mayer Salovey Caruso Emotional Intelligence Test 2.0 (MSCEIT; Mayer et al., 2004) to assess emotional communication. Three samples, each with their own carefully matched control group, were examined: a group of patients with a more chronic course of schizophrenia, an FE psychosis group, and a CHR group. Results of this study demonstrated impairment in schizophrenia across phase of illness. However, most interesting was a lack of evidence of progression or improvement over the three phases of the illness (i.e., from the period of high risk, to the first episode, and then to the more chronic phase of schizophrenia). Furthermore, age had a limited effect on performance for either the clinical or comparison groups. This study supports that impairment in social cognition begins in the early phases of a psychotic illness and remains stable. Although it was limited to three domains, results were consistent across all three of them.

Summary

There are, at this stage, limited studies examining social cognition in those at CHR. Studies in this area are increasing, although it is difficult to find samples, and these samples tend to be small. It appears as if those in this risk group are already demonstrating impairments in facial affect recognition that is often equivalent to that observed in individuals at their first episode of psychosis or even in those with a more chronic course of schizophrenia. Studies examining social perception and social knowledge are rare, and thus limited conclusions can be drawn. There is some evidence of impairment in tasks assessing ToM. Results from the single study on attribution fit with observation from patient populations that deficits are typically linked to paranoid or persecutory symptoms. Thus, at this stage, there is support that deficits in social cognition are already present at the prepsychotic period.

However, there are clear limitations to the current research. Longitudinal studies are rare, and there is no evidence on the longitudinal nature of these social cognitive impairments in these young people. Further work needs to be done in examining the role of such deficits in conversion from the CHR stage to that of full-blown psychosis.

Social cognition research has examined correlates of impairment such as symptoms, social functioning, and neurocognition. There is evidence that social cognition potentially mediates the relationship between neurocognition and poor functioning in both FE patients and in those with a more chronic course of schizophrenia. No such relationships have yet been explored in these CHR samples.

SOCIAL COGNITION AND FAMILY HIGH RISK OF PSYCHOSIS

Given the strong evidence for the role of genetic factors in the development of psychotic disorders, a number of studies have examined social cognitive deficits as potential markers of vulnerability to psychosis. One approach has been to investigate whether deficits identified in individuals with psychosis also occur in their unaffected biological relatives; that is, those who are at family high risk of psychosis (FHR). Such an approach is particularly useful as it evades many of the confounding factors typically associated with patient samples, such as medication side effects, prominent neurocognitive deficits, and relationships to clinical symptoms of the illness (Kee, Horan, Mintz, & Green, 2004). If social cognitive deficits are indeed enduring vulnerability indicators of psychosis, they are expected to show a substantial genetic influence and to occur with exceptionally high frequency in individuals at increased risk for schizophrenia (Nuechterlein et al., 1992).

Affect Recognition in Family High Risk Patients

Six studies have investigated affect recognition impairments in those at family high risk of psychosis. The results of these studies, however, have been somewhat varied (Alfimova et al., 2009; Bolte & Poustka, 2003; Eack, Greeno et al., 2010; Kee et al., 2004; Leppanen et al., 2006; Loughland, Williams, & Harris, 2004). In all six studies, the unaffected relatives performed significantly better on tasks of affect recognition compared to their psychotic relatives. However, four studies reported significant trends of reduced performance accuracy in unaffected relatives compared to healthy volunteers (Alfimova et al., 2009; Eack, Greeno et al., 2010; Kee et al., 2004; Leppanen et al., 2006). Specifically, Kee and colleagues (2004) and Alfimova et al. (2009) reported poorer overall performance on tests of facial affect recognition in nonpsychotic relatives compared to healthy controls. Leppanen et al. (2006) and Eack et al. (2010) reported only specific group deficits in relation to negative emotions and neutral faces, respectively. The other two studies conversely reported no significant difference in the accuracy on facial affect recognition tasks between unaffected relatives and healthy volunteers (Bolte & Poustka, 2003; Loughland et al., 2004).

The relationship of other factors, such as cognition or even the presence of psychotic-like experiences, to affect recognition in unaffected relatives has not been consistently documented. Whereas one study endorsed the relationship between attenuated psychopathology, such as schizotypal traits (Eack, Mermon et al., 2010), and affect perception, two other studies did not report any association (Alfimova et al., 2009; Kee et al., 2004). Moreover, two studies that investigated the association between neurocognitive performance and affect perception in unaffected relatives reported it to be nonsignificant (Alfimova et al., 2009; Eack, Mermon et al., 2010).

It is important to note that all reviewed investigations included tests of facial affect recognition, with the exception of Kee and colleagues (2004), who additionally examined voice affect recognition. Exploring multiple aspects of affect recognition using both visual and prosodic modalities, however, may be more effective in discerning true vulnerability indicators.

Social Perception and Social Knowledge in Family High Risk

To the best of our knowledge, only two studies to date investigated social perception and social knowledge in populations at family high risk of psychosis. In the first study, Toomey and colleagues (Toomey, Seidman, Lyons, Faraone, & Tsuang, 1999), investigated social perception of nonverbal cues using the Profile of Nonverbal Sensitivity Test (PONS), and found that unaffected relatives of people with schizophrenia demonstrated poorer test performance compared to healthy volunteers. In the second study, Baas et al. (Baas, van't Wout, Aleman, & Kahn, 2008) assessed trustworthiness evaluations about unfamiliar faces with neutral expressions in siblings of individuals with schizophrenia. Healthy siblings displayed similar, although attenuated, bias to affected siblings in judging trustworthiness, whereby they judged faces to be more trustworthy compared to healthy volunteers. Future studies, however, are required to replicate these findings using a wider battery of social perception/knowledge tests.

Theory of Mind in Family High Risk

Theory of mind deficits have been well documented in individuals with psychotic illness (Bora et al., 2009; Sprong et al., 2007), but the extent to which these deficits are aggregated in unaffected first-degree relatives has not been determined. A limited number of studies that have investigated if impaired performance on ToM tests is evidenced in those at FHR and have reported conflicting results. Two studies found no significant association between performance on ToM tests and having a family history for schizophrenia (Gibson, Penn, Prinstein, Perkins, & Belger, 2010; Kelemen et al., 2005), and two studies found a nonsignificant trend for this association (Irani et al., 2006; Marjoram et al., 2006). However, the majority of studies reported this association to be significant (Anselmetti et al., 2009;

de Achaval et al., 2010; Janssen, Krabbendam, Jolles, & van Os, 2003; Kelemen et al., 2005; Marjoram et al., 2006; Wykes, Hamid, & Wagstaff, 2001).

Some studies have addressed correlates of ToM impairments in unaffected relatives of individuals with schizophrenia. Irani et al. (2006) found that relatives with schizotypal personality traits performed significantly more poorly than relatives without such traits. In addition, Keleman and colleagues (2005) and Marjoram et al. (2006) similarly noted poorer ToM performance in relatives with past or present transient psychotic-like symptoms compared to symptom-free relatives. Some studies found an association between impairments in cognition and ToM in unaffected relatives (Janssen et al., 2003), and others did not (Anselmetti et al., 2009; de Achaval et al., 2010; Wykes, 1994).

Summary

Even though the existence of social cognitive impairments has been investigated in only a few studies to date, it is an important part of a larger effort to identify endophenotypes of psychotic disorders. Identifying possible vulnerability markers of psychosis among samples of individuals at FHR has implications for an improved understanding of schizophrenia. Based on the current research findings, individuals at FHR for psychosis demonstrate subtle impairments in most domains of social cognition. When evaluated against findings from CHR studies, however, social cognition in FHR appears to be less impaired compared to CHR individuals and more impaired compared to healthy individuals without the family risk of psychosis. Therefore, it may be that worsening of social cognitive deficits in FHR is contingent on emergence of subpsychotic symptoms and worsening in functioning, both of which are observed in CHR. However, little is known about the extent to which these attenuated deficits are associated with the transition to psychosis in individuals at FHR (Eack, Mermon et al., 2010), or with other factors, such as neurocognition. Future studies of familial risk would benefit from having a suitable design that would include FHR individuals of diverse ages and genetic loadings, comparison groups consisting of CHR individuals and those at different stages of a psychotic illness, longitudinal follow-up, and broad measures of multiple domains of social cognition (Eack et al., 2010).

CONCLUSION

Several studies have demonstrated that impairments in social cognition are present early in the course of a psychotic illness and that such impairments appear to be of a stable magnitude from the period of high risk until the more chronic phase of illness. Although all of the domains have not been examined in one study, there is evidence of impairment in the key domains of emotion perception, ToM, social perception and social knowledge, and attributional style. It is possible that this is early evidence of a vulnerability measure of illness, rather than an indicator of either the severity of the illness or of chronicity. To be a vulnerability or trait marker, the impairments need to be manifest at all stages of the disorder, including both acute and remitted periods. In addition, there needs to be evidence of the disorder in high-risk groups, such as those at FHR, those at CHR, and in those with schizotypy.

In schizotypy, some studies have supported an impairment in social cognition (Aguirre, Sergi, & Levy, 2008; Meyer & Shean, 2006; Phillips & Seidman, 2008) but other studies have not (Fernyhough, Jones, Whittle, Waterhouse, & Bentall, 2008; Jahshan & Sergi, 2007). In the present review, there is enough evidence demonstrating impaired social cognition in the risk period to warrant further work. Understanding social cognition at this early stage has clear implications for a greater understanding of the development of psychosis. It is possible that impairment that leads to distortion in perceiving and interpreting social information may have an impact on symptom development (Bentall, Kinderman, & Kaney, 1994). Attempts to understand the neural systems involved in social cognition have been addressed in other chapters (Chapters 4, 5, and 11). However, understanding the neural underpinnings of social cognition in this period of risk can only help to further our understanding of the development of the illness. With the increased interest in the role of social risk factors in the development of psychosis (van Os, Rutten, & Poulton, 2008), further research, particularly with the CHR group, can begin to explore the nature of an association between social cognitive impairments and other risk factors, such as social functioning. It remains to be determined if the emergence of social cognitive deficits precedes, coincides, or succeeds deficits in social functioning. Given that some components of social cognition, such as ToM, are suggested to be critical for effective social functioning (Roncone et al., 2002), it is possible that the early development of deficits in social cognition is secondary to social functioning deficits.

Finally, there are implications for treatment. Treatment approaches are reviewed in detail in other chapters, and, undoubtedly, the sooner one intervenes the more helpful it may be. For example, if poor social cognition is related to social functioning, there are many advantages in offering remediation of social cognitive deficits at the first episode (Eack, Mermon et al., 2010). However, treatment effectiveness studies of those at CHR are in the early stages, and there is noted improvement at least in some domains with psychosocial interventions. The impact of a social cognition remediation intervention at this high-risk stage may offer valuable insights into a range of ways to at least ameliorate the outcome.

REFERENCES

Addington, J., Cadenhead, K. S., Cannon, T. D., Cornblatt, B., McGlashan, T. H., Perkins, D. O., et al. (2007). North American prodrome longitudinal study: A collaborative multisite approach to prodromal schizophrenia research. *Schizophrenic Bulletin, 33*(3), 665–672.

Addington, J., Girard, T. A., Christensen, B. K., & Addington, D. (2010). Social cognition mediates illness-related and cognitive influences on social function in patients with schizophrenia-spectrum disorders. *Journal of Psychiatry and Neuroscience, 35*(1), 49–54.

Addington, J., Penn, D., Woods, S. W., Addington, D., & Perkins, D. O. (2008). Social functioning in individuals at clinical high risk for psychosis. *Schizophrenia Research, 99*(1–3), 119–124.

Addington, J., Saeedi, H., & Addington, D. (2006a). Facial affect recognition: A mediator between cognitive and social functioning in psychosis? *Schizophrenia Research, 85*(1–3), 142–150.

Addington, J., Saeedi, H., & Addington, D. (2006b). Influence of social perception and social knowledge on cognitive and social functioning in early psychosis. *British Journal of Psychiatry, 189*, 373–378.

Adolphs, R. (2001). The neurobiology of social cognition. *Current Opinions in Neurobiology, 11*, 231.

Adolphs, R., Tranel, D., & Damasio, A. R. (1998). The human amygdala in social judgement. *Nature, 393*, 470.

Aguirre, F., Sergi, M. J., & Levy, C. A. (2008). Emotional intelligence and social functioning in persons with schizotypy. *Schizophrenia Research, 104*(1–3), 255–264.

Alfimova, M. V., Abramova, L. I., Barhatova, A. I., Yumatova, P. E., Lyachenko, G. L., & Golimbet, V. E. (2009). Facial affect recognition deficit as a marker of genetic vulnerability to schizophrenia. *Spanish Journal of Psychology, 12*(1), 46–55.

Amminger, G. P., Schafer, M. R., Papageorgiou, K., Klier, C. M., Schlogelhofer, M., Mossaheb, N., et al. (in press). Emotion recognition in individuals at clinical high-risk for schizophrenia. *Schizophrenic Bulletin*.

An, S. K., Kang, J. I., Park, J. Y., Kim, K. R., Lee, S. Y., & Lee, E. (2010). Attribution bias in ultra-high risk for psychosis and first-episode schizophrenia. *Schizophrenia Research, 118*(1–3), 54–61.

Anselmetti, S., Bechi, M., Bosia, M., Quarticelli, C., Ermoli, E., Smeraldi, E., et al. (2009). 'Theory' of mind impairment in patients affected by schizophrenia and in their parents. *Schizophrenia Research, 115*(2–3), 278–285.

Baas, D., van't Wout, M., Aleman, A., & Kahn, R. S. (2008). Social judgement in clinically stable patients with schizophrenia and healthy relatives: Behavioural evidence of social brain dysfunction. *Psychological Medicine, 38*(5), 747.

Baron-Cohen, S., Wheelwright, S., Hill, J., Raste, Y., & Plumb, I. (2001). The "Reading the Mind in the Eyes" Test revised version: A study with normal adults, and adults with Asperger syndrome or high-functioning autism. *Journal of Child Psychology and Psychiatry, 42*(2), 241–251.

Behere, R. V., Venkatasubramanian, G., Arasappa, R., Reddy, N., & Gangadhar, B. N. (2009). Effect of risperidone on emotion recognition deficits in antipsychotic-naive schizophrenia: A short-term follow-up study. *Schizophrenia Research, 113*(1), 72–76.

Bentall, R. P., Kinderman, P., & Kaney, S. (1994). The self, attributional processes and abnormal beliefs: Towards a model of persecutory delusions. *Behaviour Research and Therapy, 32*(3), 331–341.

Bertrand, M. C., Sutton, H., Achim, A. M., Malla, A. K., & Lepage, M. (2007). Social cognitive impairments in first episode psychosis. *Schizophrenia Research, 95*, 124.

Bolte, S., & Poustka, F. (2003). The recognition of facial affect in autistic and schizophrenic subjects and their first-degree relatives. *Psychological Medicine, 33*(5), 907.

Bora, E., Yucel, M., & Pantelis, C. (2009). Theory of mind impairment in schizophrenia: Meta-analysis. *Schizophrenia Research, 109*(1–3), 1.

Brune, M. (2005). "Theory of mind" in schizophrenia: A review of the literature. *Schizophrenic Bulletin, 31*(1), 21.

Cannon, T. D., Cadenhead, K., Cornblatt, B., Woods, S. W., Addington, J., Walker, E., et al. (2008). Prediction of psychosis in youth at high clinical risk: A multisite longitudinal study in North America. *Archives of General Psychiatry, 65*(1), 28–37.

Chung, Y. S., Kang, D. H., Shin, N. Y., Yoo, S. Y., & Kwon, J. S. (2008). Deficit of theory of mind in individuals at ultra-high-risk for schizophrenia. *Schizophrenia Research, 99*(1–3), 111.

Combs, D. R., Penn, D. L., Wicher, M., & Waldheter, E. (2007). The Ambiguous Intentions Hostility Questionnaire (AIHQ): A new measure for evaluating hostile social-cognitive biases in paranoia. *Cognitive Neuropsychiatry, 12*(2), 128–143.

Corrigan, P. W. (1997). The social perceptual deficits of schizophrenia. *Psychiatry, 60*(4), 309–326.

Couture, S. M., Penn, D., Addington, J., Woods, S. W., & Perkins, D. O. (2008). Assessment of social judgements and complex mental states in the early phases of psychosis. *Schizophrenia Research, 100*, 237.

de Achaval, D., Costanzo, E. Y., Villarreal, M., Jauregui, I. O., Chiodi, A., Castro, M. N., et al. (2010). Emotion processing and theory of mind in schizophrenia patients and their unaffected first-degree relatives. *Neuropsychologia, 48*(5), 1209–1215.

Eack, S. M., Greeno, C. G., Pogue-Geile, M. F., Newhill, C. E., Hogarty, G. E., & Keshavan, M. S. (2010). Assessing social-cognitive deficits in schizophrenia with the Mayer-Salovey-Caruso Emotional Intelligence Test. *Schizophrenic Bulletin, 36*(2), 370–380.

Eack, S. M., Mermon, D. E., Montrose, D. M., Miewald, J., Gur, R. E., Gur, R. C., et al. (2010). Social cognition deficits among individuals at familial high risk for schizophrenia. *Schizophrenic Bulletin, 36*(6), 1081–1088.

Edwards, J., Pattison, P. E., Jackson, H. J., & Wales, R. J. (2001). Facial affect and affective prosody recognition in first episode schizophrenia. *Schizophrenia Research, 48*, 235.

Fernyhough, C., Jones, S. R., Whittle, C., Waterhouse, J., & Bentall, R. P. (2008). Theory of mind, schizotypy, and persecutory ideation in young adults. *Cognitive Neuropsychiatry, 13*(3), 233–249.

Fett, A. K., Viechtbauer, W., Dominguez, M. D., Penn, D. L., van Os, J., & Krabbendam, L. (2011). The relationship between neurocognition and social cognition with functional outcomes in schizophrenia: A meta-analysis. *Neuroscience and Biobehavioral Reviews, 35*(3), 573–588.

Fiske, S. T., & Taylor, S. E. (1991). *Social cognition*. New York: McGraw-Hill International.

Frith, C. D., & Corcoran, R. (1996). Exploring 'theory of mind' in people with schizophrenia. *Psychological Medicine, 26*(3), 521.

Gibson, C. M., Penn, D. L., Prinstein, M. J., Perkins, D. O., & Belger, A. (2010). Social skill and social cognition in adolescents at genetic risk for psychosis. *Schizophrenia Research, 122*(1–3), 179–184.

Green, M. F., Bearden, C. E., Cannon, T. D., Fiske, A. P., Hellemann, G. S., Horan, W. P., et al. (in press). Social cognition in schizophrenia, Part 1: Performance across phase of illness. *Schizophrenic Bulletin*.

Green, M. F., Olivier, B., Crawley, J. N., Penn, D. L., & Silverstein, S. (2005). Social cognition in schizophrenia: Recommendations from the measurement and treatment research to improve cognition in schizophrenia new approaches conference. *Schizophrenic Bulletin, 31*(4), 882.

Happe, F. G. (1994). An advanced test of theory of mind: Understanding of story characters' thoughts and feelings by able autistic, mentally handicapped, and normal children and adults. *Journal of Autism and Developmental Disorders, 24*(2), 129–154.

Herbener, E. S., Hill, S. K., Marvin, R. W., & Sweeney, J. A. (2005). Effects of antipsychotic treatment on emotion perception deficits in first-episode schizophrenia. *American Journal of Psychiatry, 162*(9), 1746–1748.

Herold, R., Feldmann, A., Simon, M., Tenyi, T., Kover, F., Nagy, F., et al. (2009). Regional gray matter reduction and theory of mind deficit in the early phase of schizophrenia: A voxel-based morphometric study. *Acta Psychiatrica Scandinavica, 119*(3), 199–208.

Hoekert, M., Kahn, R. S., Pijnenborg, M., & Aleman, A. (2007). Impaired recognition and expression of emotional prosody in schizophrenia: Review and meta-analysis. *Schizophrenia Research, 96,* 135.

Horan, W. P., Green, M. F., Degroot, M., Fiske, A., Hellemann, G., Kee, K., et al. (in press). Social cognition in schizophrenia, Part 2: 12–Month stability and prediction of functional outcome in first-episode patients. *Schizophrenic Bulletin.*

Humphreys, L., & Barrowclough, C. (2006). Attributional style, defensive functioning and persecutory delusions: Symptom-specific or general coping strategy? *British Journal of Clinical Psychology, 45*(Pt. 2), 231–246.

Inoue, Y., Yamada, K., Hirano, M., Shinohara, M., Tamaoki, T., Iguchi, H., et al. (2006). Impairment of theory of mind in patients in remission following first episode of schizophrenia. *European Archives of Psychiatry and Clinical Neuroscience, 256*(5), 326.

Irani, F., Platek, S. M., Panyavin, I. S., Calkins, M. E., Kohler, C., Siegel, S. J., et al. (2006). Self-face recognition and theory of mind in patients with schizophrenia and first-degree relatives. *Schizophrenia Research, 88*(1–3), 151.

Jahshan, C. S., & Sergi, M. J. (2007). Theory of mind, neurocognition, and functional status in schizotypy. *Schizophrenia Research, 89*(1–3), 278–286.

Janssen, I., Krabbendam, L., Jolles, J., & van Os, J. (2003). Alterations in theory of mind in patients with schizophrenia and non-psychotic relatives. *Acta Psychiatrica Scandinavica, 108*(2), 110–117.

Kee, K., Horan, W., Mintz, J., & Green, M. (2004). Do the siblings of schizophrenia patients demonstrate affect perception deficits? *Schizophrenia Bulletin, 67,* 87.

Kelemen, O., Erdelyi, R., Pataki, I., Benedek, G., Janka, Z., & Keri, S. (2005). Theory of mind and motion perception in schizophrenia. *Neuropsychology, 19*(4), 494.

Kettle, J. W., O'Brien-Simpson, L., & Allen, N. B. (2008). Impaired theory of mind in first-episode schizophrenia: Comparison with community, university and depressed controls. *Schizophrenia Research, 99*(1–3), 96.

Kinderman, P., & Bentall, R. P. (1996). A new measure of causal locus: Internal, Personal and Situational Attributions Questionnaire. *Personality and Individual Differences, 20,* 261–264.

Koelkebeck, K., Pedersen, A., Suslow, T., Kueppers, K. A., Arolt, V., & Ohrmann, P. (2010). Theory of mind in first-episode schizophrenia patients: Correlations with cognition and personality traits. *Schizophrenia Research, 119*(1–3), 115–123.

Kohler, C. G., Walker, J. B., Martin, E. A., Healey, K. M., & Moberg, P. J. (2010). Facial emotion perception in schizophrenia: A meta-analytic review. *Schizophrenic Bulletin, 36*(5),1009–1019.

Krstev, H., Jackson, H., & Maude, D. (1999). An investigation of attributional style in first-episode psychosis. *British Journal of Clinical Psychology, 38*(Pt. 2), 181–194.

Kucharska-Pietura, K., David, A. S., Masiak, M., & Phillips, M. L. (2005). Perception of facial and vocal affect by people with schizophrenia in early and late stages of illness. *British Journal of Psychiatry, 187,* 523.

Leppanen, J. M., Niehaus, D. J., Koen, L., Du Toit, E., Schoeman, R., & Emsley, R. (2006). Emotional face processing deficit in schizophrenia: A replication study in a South African Xhousa population. *Schizophrenia Research, 84,* 323.

Loughland, C. M., Williams, L. M., & Harris, A. W. (2004). Visual scanpath dysfunction in first-degree relatives of schizophrenia probands: Evidence for a vulnerability marker? *Schizophrenia Research, 67,* 11.

Lyon, H. M., Kaney, S., & Bentall, R. P. (1994). The defensive function of persecutory delusions. Evidence from attribution tasks. *British Journal of Psychiatry, 164*(5), 637–646.

Marjoram, D., Job, D. E., Whalley, H. C., Gountouna, V. E., McIntosh, A. M., Simonotto, E., et al. (2006). A visual joke fMRI investigation into theory of mind and enhanced risk of schizophrenia. *Neuroimage, 31*(4), 1850–1858.

Mayer, J. D., Salovey, P., Caruso, D. R., & Sitarenios, G. (2004). Measuring emotional intelligence with the MSCEIT V2.0. *Emotion, 3*(1), 97–105.

McDonald, S., Flanagan, S., Rollins, J., & Kinch, J. (2003). TASIT: A new clinical tool for assessing social perception after traumatic brain injury. *Journal of Head Trauma Rehabilitation, 18*(3), 219–238.

McGlashan, T., Walsh, B., & Woods, S. (2010). *The Psychosis-Risk Syndrome: Handbook for diagnosis and follow-up*. New York: Oxford University Press.

Meyer, J., & Shean, G. (2006). Social-cognitive functioning and schizotypal characteristics. *Journal of Psychology, 140*(3), 199–207.

Nuechterlein, K. H., Dawson, M. E., Gitlin, M., Ventura, J., Goldstein, M. J., Snyder, K. S., et al. (1992). Developmental processes in schizophrenic disorders: Longitudinal studies of vulnerability and stress. *Schizophrenic Bulletin, 18*(3), 387–425.

Oh, J. E., Na, M. H., Ha, T. H., Shin, Y. W., Roh, K. S., Hong, S. B., et al. (2005). Social cognition deficits of schizophrenia in cartoon task. *Journal of the Korean Neuropsychiatric Association, 44*(3), 295–302.

Perner, J., & Wimmer, H. (1985). "John thinks that Mary thinks that … ": Attribution of second-order beliefs by 5- to 10-year-old children. *Journal of Experimental Child Psychology, 39,* 437–471.

Phillips, L. K., & Seidman, L. J. (2008). Emotion processing in persons at risk for schizophrenia. *Schizophrenic Bulletin, 34*(5), 888–903.

Pinkham, A. E., Penn, D., Perkins, D. O., Graham, K., & Siegel, M. (2007). Emotion perception and social skill over the course of psychosis: A comparison of individuals at risk, and early and chronic schizophrenia spectrum illness. *Cognitive Neuropsychiatry, 12,* 198.

Piskulic, D., Addington, J., & Maruff, P. (2010). Social cognition in schizophrenia: A quantitative review of the literature. *Schizophrenia Research, 117*(2), 413.

Roncone, R., Falloon, I. R., Mazza, M., De Risio, A., Pollice, R., Necozione, S., et al. (2002). Is theory of mind in schizophrenia more strongly associated with clinical and social functioning than with neurocognitive deficits? *Psychopathology, 35*(5), 280–288.

Sergi, M. J., Rassovsky, Y., Widmark, C., Reist, C., Erhart, S., Braff, D. L., et al. (2007). Social cognition in schizophrenia: Relationships with neurocognition and negative symptoms. *Schizophrenia Research, 90*(1–3), 316–324.

Sergi, M. J., Fiske, A. P., Horan, W. P., Kern, R. S., Kee, K. S., Subotnik, K. L., et al. (2009). Development of a measure of relationship perception in schizophrenia. *Psychiatry Research, 166*(1), 54–62.

Sprong, M., Schothorst, P., Vos, E., Hox, J., & van Engeland, H. (2007). Theory of mind in schizophrenia: Meta-analysis. *British Journal of Psychiatry, 191,* 5.

Toomey, R., Seidman, L. J., Lyons, M. J., Faraone, S. V., & Tsuang, M. T. (1999). Poor perception of nonverbal social-emotional cues in relatives of schizophrenic patients. *Schizophrenia Research, 40*(2), 121–130.

van Os, J., Rutten, B. P., & Poulton, R. (2008). Gene-environment interactions in schizophrenia: Review of epidemiological findings and future directions. *Schizophrenic Bulletin, 34*(6), 1066–1082.

Williams, L. M., Whitford, T. J., Flynn, G., Wong, W., Liddell, B. J., Silverstein, S., et al. (2008). General and social cognition in first episode schizophrenia: Identification of separable factors and prediction of functional outcome using the IntegNeuro test battery. *Schizophrenia Research, 99*(1–3), 182.

Winters, K. C., & Neale, J. M. (1985). Mania and low self-esteem. *Journal of Abnormal Psychology, 94*(3), 282–290.

Wykes, T. (1994). Predicting symptomatic and behavioural outcomes of community care. *British Journal of Psychiatry, 165*(4), 486–492.

Wykes, T., Hamid, S., & Wagstaff, K. (2001). Theory of mind and executive functions in the non-psychotic siblings of patients with schizophrenia. *Schizophrenia Research, 49*((Suppl.1)), 148.

Yung, A. R., & McGorry, P. D. (1996). The prodromal phase of first-episode psychosis: Past and current conceptualizations. *Schizophrenic Bulletin, 22*(2), 353–370.

Yung, A. R., Phillips, L. J., Yuen, H. P., & McGorry, P. D. (2004). Risk factors for psychosis in an ultra high-risk group: Psychopathology and clinical features. *Schizophrenia Research, 67*(2–3), 131–142.

11

The Social Cognitive Neuroscience of Schizophrenia

AMY E. PINKHAM ■

There has long been an interest in uncovering the brain basis of dysfunction in schizophrenia, and social cognition has proved no exception. Relatively soon after the initial reports of social cognitive impairment were published, researchers began to apply the technology and methods of neuroscience to the study of social cognition in schizophrenia, and, as the availability of neuroimaging facilities increased, so too did investigations of the neural correlates of social cognitive dysfunction. To date, a large literature has accrued, and the majority of this work has focused on the key domains of social cognition identified in the previous chapters (i.e., emotion processing, theory of mind [ToM], and social cognitive bias). The current review of neuroimaging findings will therefore follow a similar structure and will discuss the neural underpinnings of each of these domains in turn. This information will then be integrated to provide support for a social cognitive neural network that functions abnormally in individuals with schizophrenia and that may subserve social cognitive impairment.

EMOTION PROCESSING

Within the schizophrenia research community, emotion processing is loosely defined as the ability to perceive and use emotions (Green et al., 2008). The majority of work in this area has focused on the perception of emotion, and, although this work has spanned multiple modalities including facial and vocal expressions of emotion, most has examined the recognition of emotion from facial displays. Several lesion and functional brain imaging studies have demonstrated that a group of neural regions are involved in face processing and emotion recognition (Adolphs, 2001; Allison, Puce, & McCarthy, 2000; Vuilleumier & Pourtois, 2007). Although these regions span the visual and temporal cortices, as well as the limbic system, the lateral fusiform gyrus (FG), posterior superior temporal sulcus (STS), and amygdala have been most consistently implicated. Both the FG and STS have been linked to face processing, with the FG showing the strongest activation in response to tasks focusing on facial identity and the STS being more strongly activated during tasks that focus on the changeable aspects of the face, such as shifts in eye gaze and mouth movements associated with emotional expression (Aylward et al., 2005; Chao, Martin, & Haxby, 1999; Haxby, Hoffman, & Gobbini, 2000; Puce, Allison, Asgari, Gore, & McCarthy, 1996; Rhodes, Byatt, Michie, & Puce, 2004; Winston, Henson, Fine-Goulden, & Dolan, 2004). In contrast, via its role in directing attention to salient stimuli (Adolphs, 2010), the amygdala has been more specifically linked to emotion recognition and may be particularly important for processing negative emotions such as fear (Adolphs, 2002, 2010; Adolphs, Baron-Cohen, & Tranel, 2002; Fusar-Poli et al., 2009; Gur, Schroeder et al., 2002; Loughead, Gur, Elliott, & Gur, 2008; Phelps, 2004; Phillips et al., 1997; Vuilleumier, 2005; Whalen et al., 2004).

Work examining these neural regions in schizophrenia has included both structural and functional investigations, and, generally speaking, has adhered well to a deficit model that would suggest that reduced volume and decreased neural activation should been seen in individuals with behavioral impairments. Although the majority of studies have focused on the amygdala, findings pertaining to the FG and STS have reinforced the potential importance of these regions for understanding face and emotion processing impairments in schizophrenia. In regard to structural differences in FG, several studies have found decreased regional gray matter in the left FG of individuals with schizophrenia as compared to healthy controls (McDonald et al., 2000; Paillere-Martinot et al., 2001; T. Takahashi et al., 2006), and these findings have been replicated in both chronic (Onitsuka et al., 2003, 2006) and first-episode samples (C. U. Lee et al., 2002; Witthaus et al., 2009; although see Pinkham et al., 2005, for failure to replicate). Abnormal functioning of the FG and face specific regions of the FG have also been extensively reported in schizophrenia, with reductions in activation evident during both basic identity processing (Quintana, Wong, Ortiz-Portillo, Marder, & Mazziotta, 2003; Walther et al., 2009) and emotion recognition (Habel et al., 2010; Seiferth et al., 2009; Williams et al., 2004). Interestingly, however, reduced FG activation during emotion recognition may be specific to only those tasks that explicitly require the recognition of emotion and may not extend to tasks that are assumed to include the implicit processing of emotion, such as determining the gender or age of emotional faces (Li, Chan, McAlonan, & Gong, 2010).

Reduced STS volumes are also apparent in individuals with schizophrenia (Cachia et al., 2008); however, there is less evidence supportive of functional impairments. First, among the numerous studies of facial emotion processing in schizophrenia, the STS has not been reported as a region showing abnormal activation (Li et al., 2010). Caution is warranted in drawing conclusions based on null findings, particularly since many of these studies utilized a region-of-interest approach wherein only regions identified a priori are investigated, and the STS was not among them; yet, it is possible that no STS differences exist between patients and controls. Second, in the earliest study to specifically examine STS activation in schizophrenia, Brunet and colleagues (2003) utilized a ToM task and found that both patients and controls showed comparable levels of activation in this region. Similarly, during a task in which participants were asked to determine the trustworthiness of pictured individuals, patients showed normative levels of STS activation as compared to controls (Pinkham, Hopfinger, Pelphrey, Piven, & Penn, 2008). Although these studies may suggest intact STS functioning in schizophrenia, it is important to consider that neither of these studies used a basic face or emotion processing task. The one study that has implemented an emotion recognition paradigm while focusing on the STS actually found *hyperactivation*, rather than underactivation, in patients (Mier, Sauer et al., 2010). The authors note that this unexpected finding could be reflective of greater compensatory brain activation in patients during a relatively easy task and therefore could still be indicative of neural impairment in basic face processing.

Due to its strong links to emotion processing, the amygdala has been a ready target for schizophrenia researchers, and a substantial body of evidence has accrued demonstrating both structural and functional abnormalities in patients. A meta-analysis of structural abnormalities published in 2000 reported a 6% volume reduction in bilateral amygdala for patients (Wright et al., 2000), and more recent studies have continued to find bilateral reductions (Namiki et al., 2007; Niu et al., 2004), even among first-episode individuals (Ellison-Wright, Glahn, Laird, Thelen, & Bullmore, 2008; Joyal et al., 2003). Despite this seeming agreement among studies, a few reports have failed to find differences between healthy individuals and individuals with schizophrenia (Sumich et al., 2002; Tanskanen et al., 2005) and suggest that volumetric reductions may not be consistent across symptom profiles or illness subtypes (Sumich et al., 2002). Specifically, Sumich and colleagues found smaller left amygdala volumes in patients with paranoid schizophrenia as compared to patients with nonparanoid subtypes. Thus, structural abnormalities may be more nuanced than generalized volumetric reductions in all patients.

Likewise, functional abnormalities of the amygdala in schizophrenia also appear to be quite nuanced and complex. Initial results from investigations of amygdala activation during emotion processing appeared to converge on hypoactivation in schizophrenia, as reductions were reported during sad mood induction (Schneider et al., 1998), viewing emotionally salient stimuli (Paradiso et al., 2003; H. Takahashi et al., 2004), and assessing facial affect (Das et al., 2007; Fakra, Salgado-Pineda, Delaveau, Hariri, & Blin, 2008; Gur, McGrath et al., 2002; Habel et al., 2004; Hempel, Hempel, Schonknecht, Stippich, & Schroder, 2003; Johnston, Stojanov, Devir, & Schall, 2005; Michalopoulou et al., 2008; Phillips et al., 1999; Williams et al., 2004). However, as more studies were conducted, the findings became mixed, with a few studies reporting increased amygdala responding (i.e., hyperactivation) during emotion recognition (Blasi et al., 2009; Fernandez-Egea et al., 2010; Hall et al., 2008; Holt, Kunkel et al., 2006; Kosaka et al., 2002). Possible explanations for these conflicting results have been a focus of recent research efforts, and three conclusions can currently be drawn.

First, as noted in a recent meta-analysis, methodological differences among studies may contribute to the varied results. Anticevic and colleagues (2012) found that, across 35 studies, hypoactivation was apparent when patients and controls were compared on a contrast between neutral and emotional conditions but not when amygdala responses to only negative emotional stimuli were directly compared. This finding suggests that patients and controls show comparable levels of amygdala activation when processing emotional stimuli but that patients actually show increased amygdala responses to neutral stimuli. An increased response to neutral stimuli would yield a small difference between neutral and emotional conditions in patients as compared to controls that could then be misinterpreted as reduced amygdala activation. Thus, the nature of amygdala dysfunction in schizophrenia may be more highly related to overattributing emotional significance to neutral stimuli rather than showing aberrant responses to overtly emotional stimuli. Such a pattern of amygdala responding would be consistent with behavioral studies demonstrating that patients tend to misattribute negative emotion to neutral stimuli (Holt, Titone et al., 2006; Pinkham, Brensinger, Kohler, Gur, & Gur, 2011) and with reports of elevated tonic (i.e., baseline) amygdala activity in schizophrenia (Aleman & Kahn, 2005; Fernandez-Egea et al., 2010; Hall et al., 2008; Scheef et al., 2010; Taylor, Phan, Britton, & Liberzon, 2005).

Second, despite tendencies to treat individuals with schizophrenia as a homogenous group, amygdala functioning may differ among patients, depending on symptom presentation. For example, studies that have considered patients' levels of paranoid ideation at the time of study participation have consistently found that patients who are highly paranoid show reduced amygdala responses as compared to healthy controls, but that nonparanoid patients show normative levels of amygdala activation (Pinkham, Hopfinger, Pelphrey et al., 2008; Russell et al., 2007; Williams et al., 2004). Likewise, studies that have created subgroups of patients based on the presence or absence of flat affect have reported differences between groups, suggesting that only patients with flat affect fail to show amygdala activation while viewing negative pictures (Fahim et al., 2005) and that flat affect is associated with abnormally increased amygdala responses to fearful expressions (Gur et al., 2007).

Finally, absolute levels of amygdala activation during a task may not be as informative as patterns of amygdala activation across different stimulus categories. Specifically, Gur and colleagues (2007) demonstrated that, during emotion recognition, incorrectly identifying fearful expressions as nonfearful was associated with hyperactivation in patients as compared to controls, but that correctly identifying anger was associated with hypoactivation. Based on these findings, the authors suggest that increased amygdala activation may interfere with later cortical, top-down processing necessary for accurate identification of fear. In a similar investigation of the effect of gaze direction on recognition of threat-related facial expressions (Pinkham, Loughead et al., 2011), amygdala responses in patients were found to differ from controls only for direct-gaze anger expressions. In all other conditions, patients were comparable to control participants, revealing that amygdala hypoactivation does not generalize to all stimulus conditions. Amygdala activation to direct-gaze anger expressions was also positively correlated with level of functioning. Likewise, an investigation of amygdala responses in paranoid and nonparanoid patients during judgments of trustworthiness indicated that paranoid patients were distinguished by a failure to show normative increases in amygdala activation when a face was judged to be untrustworthy. No differences were found between groups for faces that were judged as trustworthy (Pinkham, Hopfinger, Ruparel, & Penn, 2008). Such findings suggest that impaired modulation of amygdala responding across stimulus categories may prove more meaningful for understanding social cognitive and social functioning impairments than generalized levels of activation.

THEORY OF MIND

Theory of mind broadly refers to the ability to infer the intentions, dispositions, and beliefs of others (Frith, 1992). Across a variety of ToM tasks, performance is reliably associated with activation of a specific group of cortical regions, including the medial prefrontal cortex (MPFC), STS and surrounding superior temporal gyrus, and temporoparietal junction (TPJ) (Amodio & Frith, 2006; Saxe, 2006). Lateral prefrontal cortex and anterior cingulate cortex are also cited, but less consistently (Carrington & Bailey, 2009). Although the specific role of each region has not yet been firmly established, available evidence suggests some initial conclusions. First, MPFC may perform a decoupling function that allows one to separate a mental representation from the objective representation of reality. MPFC is also activated during tasks requiring self-reflection (Gusnard, Akbudak, Shulman, & Raichle, 2001; Ochsner et al., 2004), which may be related to ToM as either a causal factor (Gallese & Goldman, 1998) or consequence (Happe, 2003). Causally, it can be hypothesized that ToM evolved only after individuals were able to master the ability to assess their own intentions and engage in self-reflection. Alternately, a fitness advantage for predicting the actions of competitors may have prompted ToM to have evolved first, with self-reflection following. Second, the STS becomes implicated in ToM for its role in detecting biological motion (Allison et al., 2000; Pelphrey et al., 2003; Thompson, Clarke, Stewart, & Puce, 2005), particularly as an individual's movements (e.g., his or her actions or changes in body posture or facial expression) may be informative for understanding his or her mental state. Finally, the role of the TPJ in ToM may be in attributing agency to others (Decety & Lamm, 2007; Farrer & Frith, 2002).

Recent neuroanatomical investigations of the frontal cortices of individuals with schizophrenia have been consistent in demonstrating reduced gray matter volumes in MPFC (Glahn et al., 2008; Hirao et al., 2008; Honea et al., 2008; Pomarol-Clotet et al., 2010). It is important to note that reduced volume does not necessarily imply reduced functional capacity; however, one study does suggest a direct link between structural abnormalities in MPFC and impaired ToM. Specifically, Yamada and colleagues (2007) found a significant association between reduced MPFC volumes and poorer abilities to attribute affective mental states to protagonists in social situations.

In line with the structural findings, reduced activation in MPFC has also been linked to poor ToM performance. The earliest study examining neural activation during mental state reasoning in individuals with schizophrenia reported that, as compared to healthy controls, patients made more errors in mental state attribution and showed less activation of the middle frontal cortex (Russell et al., 2000). More recent studies have better localized abnormalities to the MPFC and demonstrate reduced activity in this region across a variety of nonverbal ToM tasks, including both those in which patients showed behavioral impairments (Benedetti et al., 2009; Brunet et al., 2003; Walter et al., 2009) and those in which patients showed comparable performances to controls (Brune et al., 2008, 2011; K. H. Lee et al., 2006; Taylor et al., 2005).

Despite these rather consistent findings, several subtleties are worthy of note. First, the work of Walter and colleagues (2009) suggests that the presence of reduced neural activation may depend on the type of intention represented in stimuli. In this study, the investigators included three different intentionality conditions, two of which involved social intentions (i.e., intending to interact socially with another person in the future or communicating with someone in the present to achieve a goal) and one that included only a single person's non-social intention (e.g., replacing a light bulb to read a book). Reduced activation in MPFC was only evident during the two social intention conditions, and no neural differences were seen between patients and controls for private intentions. The authors speculate that this differential activation between social and nonsocial intentions may be due to the greater demand of decoupling posed by social intentions, in which is it necessary for participants to clearly distinguish between the intentions of others and their own. It is also possible, however, that these results could simply reflect differences in difficulty between conditions and that, as ToM inferences become more complex, neural abnormalities also become more pronounced.

Second, furthering their conclusion that MPFC may not be uniformly under-active in schizophrenia, Walter et al. also noted increased MPFC activation in patients relative to controls in response to a physical causality condition that did not include intentionality. This finding, which is remarkably similar to findings of increased amygdala activation to neutral emotional stimuli, suggests that patients may overattribute intentional agency in some instances and supports hypotheses of "hyper ToM" in positive-symptom schizophrenia (Abu-Akel & Bailey, 2000; see also Abu-Akel & Shamay-Tsoory, 2013, Chapter 8, this volume). Importantly, Walter et al. examined only individuals diagnosed with the paranoid subtype, and such a finding is consistent with behavioral reports of paranoid patients showing an increased tendency to overattribute intentions to the actions of a potential agent (Blakemore, Sarfati, Bazin, & Decety, 2003; Montag et al., 2011).

Third, severity of illness may also influence neural functioning. In a longitudinal study examining patients during and after an acute exacerbation of symptoms, Lee and colleagues (2006) found reduced task-related MPFC activation in patients relative to controls only during the acute phase. In contrast, once patients achieved symptomatic improvements that warranted discharge from an inpatient facility, activation of the MPFC was significantly greater and no longer differed from control participants.

Unlike those of MPFC, investigations of STS and TPJ functioning during ToM inferences have provided less consistent results. As mentioned previously, the earliest work examining neural responses during a ToM task reported comparable activation of the STS in both patients and controls during the perception of human figures, including a condition in which characters were acting intentionally (Brunet et al., 2003). A more recent study that examined both structural and functional abnormalities, however, found increased activation of posterior superior and transverse temporal gyrus in patients relative to controls (Benedetti et al., 2009). Interestingly, higher neural responses correlated negatively with performance, and these same regions also showed volumetric reductions in the patient groups. Thus, whereas greater recruitment of neural regions may potentially be seen as adaptive, these findings demonstrate links among overactivation, poor performance, and structural abnormalities that may suggest overactivation is an inefficient means of compensating for more primary deficits.

Likewise, findings pertaining to TPJ functioning have been mixed, with some studies showing reduced activation of this region and others showing overactivation. Specifically, across two studies, Brune and colleagues reported both hyperactivation (Brune et al., 2008) and hypoactivation (Brune et al., 2011) of TPJ during the same ToM task. The authors reconcile their findings by noting that the study reporting hyperactivation examined patients with passivity symptoms (e.g., third-person auditory hallucinations or delusions of control), whereas the study reporting hypoactivation included patients with more prominent negative symptoms. They note that hyperactivation in the passivity group may be due to a failure to experience the self as an agent and a tendency of patients to perceive their own thoughts and actions as externally generated, which presumably would not apply to patients without these symptoms. Findings from Walter et al. (2009) also provide evidence for both hyper- and hypoactivation, depending on intention type. As with MPFC, TPJ showed reduced activation in patients relative to controls during social intentions but greater activation during physical causality. Despite the lack of clarity regarding the exact nature of functional impairments of TPJ, the reviewed findings do indicate that this region is likely abnormal in patients, and that both symptom presentation and intention type should be considered in future investigations.

ATTRIBUTIONAL STYLE

Relatively little work has addressed the potential neural underpinnings of the attributional biases most commonly reported in schizophrenia. At present, no work has specifically examined the *personalizing bias*—the tendency to explain negative outcomes as being due to the malevolent intentions of another individual rather than a situational context. Two studies, however, have investigated the neural processes involved in expression of a self-serving bias (i.e., taking credit for successful outcomes and denying responsibility for negative outcomes). After asking five healthy individuals to respond to items from the Internal, Personal, and Situational Attributions Questionnaire (IPSAQ; Kinderman & Bentall, 1996), Blackwood et al. (2000) first reported that left middle temporal gyrus (Brodmann area [BA] 39) and precentral gyrus (BA 6) showed greater activation for internal attributions relative to external attributions. Non–self-serving attributions (i.e., internal attributions for negative events vs. external attributions for positive events) were associated specifically with activation of the left precentral gyrus, and self-serving attributions (i.e., internal attributions for positive events vs. external attributions for negative events) were linked to activation of the left superior temporal gyrus (BA 38).

A follow-up study with a larger sample provided partial replication of these results (Blackwood et al., 2003). Here, internal attributions were again accompanied by activation of precentral gyrus (BA 4/6), but additional activations were found in left lateral cerebellar hemisphere and right lingual gyrus (BA 17). Further, the contrast of external relative to internal attributions revealed specific activation of left posterior STS, and non–self-serving attributions showed activation in right angular gyrus (BA 39), left lateral orbitofrontal cortex (BA 11), and right middle temporal gyrus (BA 39). Self-serving attributions were this time associated with activation of bilateral caudate nucleus. The authors noted that activation of the regions associated with internal attributions likely reflects the representation of the self as an intentional or responsible agent, with the precentral gyrus relating to the simulation of one's own and others actions, the cerebellum playing a role in the labeling of the consequences of one's actions as the product of one's intentions, and the lingual gyrus being responsible for the visual imagery of intentional actions. In regard to the STS, the authors point out that the activation seen for external attributions probably relates to the processing of others' internal states that might accompany a personal external attribution. Finally, Blackwood and colleagues note that dorsal striatal activations, seen here as bilateral caudate, reflect the possibility that a self-serving bias may be rewarding, particularly in supporting self-esteem, as proposed by Bentall, Kinderman, and Kaney (1994), whereas activation of the frontal cortex, seen here as lateral orbitofrontal cortex, may reflect suppression of the automatic tendency to implement a self-serving attribution. Interestingly, the latter conclusion has since gained some support from an electroencephalographic (EEG) study in which non–self-serving attributions were associated with dorsomedial frontal cortex activity that was interpreted as a mechanism for suppressing the self-serving bias (Krusemark, Campbell, & Clementz, 2008).

Conflicting reports about the presence of a true self-serving bias in schizophrenia (Bentall, Corcoran, Howard, Blackwood, & Kinderman, 2001; Garety & Freeman, 1999) render it somewhat difficult to apply these findings; however, recent behavioral work has been consistent in providing evidence of an externalizing bias in patients that may be informed by the imaging work (Janssen et al., 2006; Langdon, Corner, McLaren, Ward, & Coltheart, 2006; Langdon, Ward, & Coltheart, 2010). Such a bias includes making external attributions for negative

events but does not require concomitant internal attributions for positive outcomes. Given that activation of the precentral gyrus was associated with internal attributions in both studies, it could be hypothesized that the tendency for
individuals with schizophrenia to favor external attributions may be related to
reduced activation of this region while attempting to explain events. The single
functional magnetic resonance imaging (fMRI) study that has examined attributional style in patients provides tentative support for this hypothesis, as patients
showed decreased activation of ventral premotor cortex (BA 6) as compared to
healthy controls when attempting to infer what past event caused the current emotional state of a stimulus avatar (Park et al., 2009). This study also noted reduced
right inferior frontal gyrus activation in patients, which may provide a clue for
understanding increased expression of a self-serving bias if indeed activation of
the frontal cortex serves to suppress self-serving attributions, as noted above.

EMERGING MODELS OF SOCIAL COGNITIVE IMPAIRMENT

The literature reviewed above provides convincing evidence of neural abnormalities in social cognitive brain regions in individuals with schizophrenia; however,
it falls short of providing a comprehensive neurobiological model of social cognitive impairment. This is primarily due to the fact that previous work has largely
been descriptive, and, although this is understandable given the early state of the
field, it provides only limited information about *how* neural abnormalities contribute to social cognitive impairment. Additionally, the tendency of this work to
focus on one social cognitive ability, such as emotion recognition or ToM, renders it tempting to view social cognitive impairments in schizophrenia as separate
domains subserved by abnormal functioning of discrete groups of neural regions.
However, these groups often interact in concert and show reciprocal connections
between regions (Atkinson & Adolphs, 2011; Vuilleumier & Pourtois, 2007). The
neural basis of social cognition can therefore be better thought of as a cohesive
network that more generally subserves the processing of social stimuli. Similarly,
the fact that several of the same neural structures are implicated across social
cognitive domains (e.g., the STS shows significant activation in tasks of emotion
perception, ToM, and attributional style; also see Mier, Lis et al., 2010; Ochsner,
2008) further suggests the validity of network-based models and questions the
soundness of treating ToM, emotion perception, and attributional biases as dissociable natural categories. Thus, models are needed that emphasize interactions
between brain regions and core cognitive processes.

   An emerging model that offers particular promise for furthering our understanding of social cognitive impairment in schizophrenia capitalizes on the
dual-process (DP) framework utilized in social psychology (Chaiken & Trope,
1999; see Lundberg, 2013, Chapter 2, this volume). As elegantly formulated by
Lieberman (2007), instead of focusing on a specific domain of social cognitive
processing, the DP model invokes core processing distinctions that span the different domains of social cognition by centering on the type of brain processing

that is engaged. Both automatic versus controlled and internally focused versus externally focused processes have been described; however, as applied to schizophrenia, the core processing distinction between automatic and controlled processing may be particularly relevant.

Specifically, within this framework, automatic social cognitive processing is thought to rely on perceptual, emotional, and physiological systems and to take place outside the awareness and control of the individual. In contrast, controlled social cognitive processing relies on higher order cognitive systems and is associated with awareness, intention, and effort. As the name implies, controlled processing is also under the direction of the individual and can be interrupted, thus enabling deliberate reasoning, juxtaposition, critical evaluation, and self-correction. Both types of processing are also thought to be subserved by distinct neural regions. Automatic social cognitive processing is subserved by amygdala, lateral temporal cortex (LTC) (including posterior STS and the temporal poles), and ventromedial prefrontal cortex (vMPFC), with basal ganglia and dorsal anterior cingulate cortex (dACC) being less consistently implicated. The general roles of amygdala and LTC have already been reviewed, but vMPFC is associated with the experience of empathy and making empathic judgments (Botvinick et al., 2005; Farrow et al., 2001; Shamay-Tsoory et al., 2005; Shamay-Tsoory, Tomer, Berger, & Aharon-Peretz, 2003). Controlled social cognition, conversely, is subserved by lateral and medial prefrontal cortex (LPFC and MPFC) and lateral and medial parietal cortex (LPAC and MPAC; Ochsner & Gross, 2008). In LPFC, ventral LPFC (vLPFC) plays a role in inhibiting automatic responses, including suppressing the influence of one's own experience while one is effortfully considering others' mental states (Samson, Apperly, Kathirgamanathan, & Humphreys, 2005; Vogeley et al., 2001) and downregulating amygdala activity (Cunningham, Raye, & Johnson, 2004; Richeson et al., 2003). As noted above, MPFC is associated with the cognitive estimation of others' inner states or ToM. LPAC activation, including TPJ, broadly reflects judgment of one's own behavior and reference to one's behavior when judging another's (Lieberman, 2007). Finally, MPAC functioning is associated with self-reflection (Johnson et al., 2005; Ochsner et al., 2004), self-processing (Cavanna & Trimble, 2006), and reappraisal of negative stimuli (Ochsner et al., 2004).

According to the DP model, normative and efficient social cognition relies on the interaction between automatic and controlled systems; thus, integrating the reviewed literature with the DP model would suggest that impaired social cognition in schizophrenia is the result of aberrant automatic inputs combined with unusually weak controlled processing resources. As noted above, the most recent findings demonstrate that individuals with schizophrenia show overactivation of automatic neurocircuitry (e.g., amygdala: Anticevic et al., 2012; Fernandez-Egea et al., 2010; Gur et al., 2007; STS: Mier, Sauer et al., 2010) but underactivation of controlled processing neurocircuitry (e.g., MPFC: Brunet-Gouet & Decety, 2006; vLPFC: Pinkham, Hopfinger, Pelphrey et al., 2008; Pinkham, Hopfinger, Ruparel et al., 2008). This interaction likely yields inaccurate automatic responses that remain uncorrected due to a failure to fully engage controlled processing networks. As a basic example, activation of the amygdala to a neutral facial expression may result in the conclusion that someone is angry or intending harm. Reduced vLPFC activation and subsequent controlled processing would preclude adjustment of this initial impression for situational or contextual information (e.g., "He is reading a book and is not paying attention to me, so he's likely not a threat") and may lead to inappropriate social reactions, such as feeling fearful or acting in a hostile manner toward the stimulus individual. Thus, in this example, abnormal functioning of both automatic and controlled neural networks would play a causal role in the social cognitive and social functioning impairments displayed by individuals with schizophrenia.

CONCLUSION

As studies demonstrating a direct link between social cognition and social functioning continue to emerge (for reviews, see Couture, Penn, & Roberts, 2006; Fett et al., 2011), the necessity of investigating the underlying mechanisms of social cognitive impairments becomes greater. In doing so, utilization of theoretical models like the DP model is imperative. Application of such models provides concrete, testable hypotheses for moving forward and also has implications for both pharmacological and behavioral remediation strategies. For example, several pharmacological agents show promise for attenuating amygdala responses during emotion processing (reviewed in Pinkham, Gur, & Gur, 2007), suggesting that such agents may allow for intervention at the level of automatic processing. Similarly, recently developed social cognitive behavioral interventions such as Social Cognition and Interaction Training focus on teaching individuals to "check out" their initial impressions of a stimulus (see Combs, Torres, & Basso, 2013, Chapter 16, this volume), which is in effect an effort to increase the amount of controlled cognitive processing. Both treatment approaches should yield observable changes in patterns of neural activation that would bolster theories of causal mechanism. Future work investigating this and related hypotheses is warranted. Additionally, in moving forward, it is important to note that social cognitive impairments are not specific to schizophrenia but are also prominent in other neurodevelopmental disorders, such as autism. Comparative studies that attempt to chart the specificity of social cognitive impairments at both behavioral and neural levels are also likely to contribute valuable information to remediation efforts by specifying disorder-specific mechanisms that can be capitalized on in treatment (Sasson, Pinkham, Carpenter, & Belger, 2011). It is only after a full mechanistic understanding of social cognitive impairment is established that treatments are likely to yield optimal results.

REFERENCES

Abu-Akel, A., & Bailey, A. L. (2000). The possibility of different forms of theory of mind impairment in psychiatric and developmental disorders. *Psychological Medicine, 30*(3), 735–738.

Abu-Akel, A., & Shamay-Tsoory, S. G. (2013). Characteristics of theory of mind impairments in schizophrenia. In D. L. Roberts & D. L. Penn (Eds.), *Social cognition in schizophrenia: From evidence to treatment* (Chapter 8). New York: Oxford University Press.

Adolphs, R. (2001). The neurobiology of social cognition. *Current Opinion in Neurobiology*, *11*(2), 231–239.

Adolphs, R. (2002). Recognizing emotion from facial expressions: Psychological and neurological mechanisms. *Behavioral and Cognitive Neuroscience Reviews*, *1*(1), 21–62.

Adolphs, R. (2010). What does the amygdala contribute to social cognition? *Annals of the New York Academy of Science*, *1191*, 42–61.

Adolphs, R., Baron-Cohen, S., & Tranel, D. (2002). Impaired recognition of social emotions following amygdala damage. *Journal of Cognitive Neuroscience*, *14*(8), 1264–1274.

Aleman, A., & Kahn, R. S. (2005). Strange feelings: Do amygdala abnormalities dysregulate the emotional brain in schizophrenia? *Progress in Neurobiology*, *77*(5), 283–298.

Allison, T., Puce, A., & McCarthy, G. (2000). Social perception from visual cues: Role of the STS region. *Trends in Cognitive Sciences*, *4*(7), 267–278.

Amodio, D. M., & Frith, C. D. (2006). Meeting of minds: The medial frontal cortex and social cognition. *Nature Reviews Neuroscience*, *7*(4), 268–277.

Anticevic, A., Van Snellenberg, J. X., Cohen, R. E., Repovs, G., Dowd, E. C., & Barch, D. M. (2012). Amygdala recruitment in schizophrenia in response to aversive emotional material: A meta-analysis of neuroimaging studies. *Schizophrenia Bulletin*, *38*(3), 608–621.

Atkinson, A. P., & Adolphs, R. (2011). The neuropsychology of face perception: Beyond simple dissociations and functional selectivity. *Philosophical Transactions of the Royal Society of London B: Biological Sciences*, *366*(1571), 1726–1738.

Aylward, E. H., Park, J. E., Field, K. M., Parsons, A. C., Richards, T. L., Cramer, S. C., et al. (2005). Brain activation during face perception: Evidence of a developmental change. *Journal of Cognitive Neuroscience*, *17*(2), 308–319.

Benedetti, F., Bernasconi, A., Bosia, M., Cavallaro, R., Dallaspezia, S., Falini, A., et al. (2009). Functional and structural brain correlates of theory of mind and empathy deficits in schizophrenia. *Schizophrenia Research*, *114*(1–3), 154–160.

Bentall, R. P., Corcoran, R., Howard, R., Blackwood, N., & Kinderman, P. (2001). Persecutory delusions: A review and theoretical integration. *Clinical Psychology Review*, *21*(8), 1143–1192.

Bentall, R. P., Kinderman, P., & Kaney, S. (1994). The self, attributional processes and abnormal beliefs: Towards a model of persecutory delusions. *Behaviour Research and Therapy*, *32*(3), 331–341.

Blackwood, N. J., Bentall, R. P., Ffytche, D. H., Simmons, A., Murray, R. M., & Howard, R. J. (2003). Self-responsibility and the self-serving bias: An fMRI investigation of causal attributions. *Neuroimage*, *20*(2), 1076–1085.

Blackwood, N. J., Howard, R. J., Ffytche, D. H., Simmons, A., Bentall, R. P., & Murray, R. M. (2000). Imaging attentional and attributional bias: An fMRI approach to the paranoid delusion. *Psychological Medicine*, *30*(4), 873–883.

Blakemore, S. J., Sarfati, Y., Bazin, N., & Decety, J. (2003). The detection of intentional contingencies in simple animations in patients with delusions of persecution. *Psychological Medicine*, *33*(8), 1433–1441.

Blasi, G., Popolizio, T., Taurisano, P., Caforio, G., Romano, R., Di Giorgio, A., et al. (2009). Changes in prefrontal and amygdala activity during olanzapine treatment in schizophrenia. *Psychiatry Research*, *173*(1), 31–38.

Botvinick, M., Jha, A. P., Bylsma, L. M., Fabian, S. A., Solomon, P. E., & Prkachin, K. M. (2005). Viewing facial expressions of pain engages cortical areas involved in the direct experience of pain. *Neuroimage, 25*(1), 312–319.

Brune, M., Lissek, S., Fuchs, N., Witthaus, H., Peters, S., Nicolas, V., et al. (2008). An fMRI study of theory of mind in schizophrenic patients with "passivity" symptoms. *Neuropsychologia, 46*(7), 1992–2001.

Brune, M., Ozgurdal, S., Ansorge, N., von Reventlow, H. G., Peters, S., Nicolas, V., et al. (2011). An fMRI study of "theory of mind" in at-risk states of psychosis: Comparison with manifest schizophrenia and healthy controls. *Neuroimage, 55*(1), 329–337.

Brunet-Gouet, E., & Decety, J. (2006). Social brain dysfunctions in schizophrenia: A review of neuroimaging studies. *Psychiatry Research, 148*(2–3), 75–92.

Brunet, E., Sarfati, Y., Hardy-Bayle, M. C., & Decety, J. (2003). Abnormalities of brain function during a nonverbal theory of mind task in schizophrenia. *Neuropsychologia, 41*(12), 1574–1582.

Cachia, A., Paillere-Martinot, M. L., Galinowski, A., Januel, D., de Beaurepaire, R., Bellivier, F., et al. (2008). Cortical folding abnormalities in schizophrenia patients with resistant auditory hallucinations. *Neuroimage, 39*(3), 927–935.

Carrington, S. J., & Bailey, A. J. (2009). Are there theory of mind regions in the brain? A review of the neuroimaging literature. *Human Brain Mapping, 30*(8), 2313–2335.

Cavanna, A. E., & Trimble, M. R. (2006). The precuneus: A review of its functional anatomy and behavioural correlates. *Brain, 129*(Pt. 3), 564–583.

Chaiken, S., & Trope, Y., Eds. (1999). *Dual-process theories in social psychology*. New York: Guilford.

Chao, L. L., Martin, A., & Haxby, J. V. (1999). Are face-responsive regions selective only for faces? *Neuroreport, 10*(14), 2945–2950.

Combs, D. R., Torres, J., & Basso, M. R. (2013). Social cognition and interaction training. In D. L. Roberts & D. L. Penn (Eds.), *Social cognition in schizophrenia: From evidence to treatment* (Chapter 16). New York: Oxford University Press.

Couture, S. M., Penn, D. L., & Roberts, D. L. (2006). The functional significance of social cognition in schizophrenia: A review. *Schizophrenia Bulletin, 32*(Suppl. 1), S44–S63.

Cunningham, W. A., Raye, C. L., & Johnson, M. K. (2004). Implicit and explicit evaluation: FMRI correlates of valence, emotional intensity, and control in the processing of attitudes. *Journal of Cognitive Neuroscience, 16*(10), 1717–1729.

Das, P., Kemp, A. H., Flynn, G., Harris, A. W., Liddell, B. J., Whitford, T. J., et al. (2007). Functional disconnections in the direct and indirect amygdala pathways for fear processing in schizophrenia. *Schizophrenia Research, 90*(1–3), 284–294.

Decety, J., & Lamm, C. (2007). The role of the right temporoparietal junction in social interaction: How low-level computational processes contribute to meta-cognition. *Neuroscientist, 13*(6), 580–593.

Ellison-Wright, I., Glahn, D. C., Laird, A. R., Thelen, S. M., & Bullmore, E. (2008). The anatomy of first-episode and chronic schizophrenia: An anatomical likelihood estimation meta-analysis. *American Journal of Psychiatry, 165*(8), 1015–1023.

Fahim, C., Stip, E., Mancini-Marie, A., Mensour, B., Boulay, L. J., Leroux, J. M., et al. (2005). Brain activity during emotionally negative pictures in schizophrenia with and without flat affect: An fMRI study. *Psychiatry Research, 140*(1), 1–15.

Fakra, E., Salgado-Pineda, P., Delaveau, P., Hariri, A. R., & Blin, O. (2008). Neural bases of different cognitive strategies for facial affect processing in schizophrenia. *Schizophrenia Research, 100*(1–3), 191–205.

Farrer, C., & Frith, C. D. (2002). Experiencing oneself vs another person as being the cause of an action: The neural correlates of the experience of agency. *Neuroimage, 15*(3), 596–603.

Farrow, T. F., Zheng, Y., Wilkinson, I. D., Spence, S. A., Deakin, J. F., Tarrier, N., et al. (2001). Investigating the functional anatomy of empathy and forgiveness. *Neuroreport, 12*(11), 2433–2438.

Fernandez-Egea, E., Parellada, E., Lomena, F., Falcon, C., Pavia, J., Mane, A., et al. (2010). 18FDG PET study of amygdalar activity during facial emotion recognition in schizophrenia. *European Archives of Psychiatry and Clinical Neuroscience, 260*(1), 69–76.

Fett, A. K., Viechtbauer, W., Dominguez, M. D., Penn, D. L., van Os, J., & Krabbendam, L. (2011). The relationship between neurocognition and social cognition with functional outcomes in schizophrenia: A meta-analysis. *Neuroscience and Biobehavioral Reviews, 35*(3), 573–588.

Frith, C. D. (1992). *The cognitive neuropsychology of schizophrenia.* Hove, UK: Lawrence Elrbaum Associates.

Fusar-Poli, P., Placentino, A., Carletti, F., Landi, P., Allen, P., Surguladze, S., et al. (2009). Functional atlas of emotional faces processing: A voxel-based meta-analysis of 105 functional magnetic resonance imaging studies. *Journal of Psychiatry and Neuroscience, 34*(6), 418–432.

Gallese, V., & Goldman, A. (1998). Mirror neurons and the simulation theory of mind-reading. *Trends in Cognitive Sciences, 2*(12), 493–501.

Garety, P. A., & Freeman, D. (1999). Cognitive approaches to delusions: A critical review of theories and evidence. *British Journal of Clinical Psychology, 38*(Pt. 2), 113–154.

Glahn, D. C., Laird, A. R., Ellison- Wright, I., Thelen, S. M., Robinson, J. L., Lancaster, J. L., et al. (2008). Meta-analysis of gray matter anomalies in schizophrenia: Application of anatomic likelihood estimation and network analysis. *Biological Psychiatry, 64*(9), 774–781.

Green, M. F., Penn, D. L., Bentall, R., Carpenter, W. T., Gaebel, W., Gur, R. C., et al. (2008). Social cognition in schizophrenia: An NIMH workshop on definitions, assessment, and research opportunities. *Schizophrenia Bulletin, 34,* 1211–1220.

Gur, R. C., Schroeder, L., Turner, T., McGrath, C., Chan, R. M., Turetsky, B. I., et al. (2002). Brain activation during facial emotion processing. *Neuroimage, 16*(3 Pt. 1), 651–662.

Gur, R. E., Loughead, J., Kohler, C. G., Elliott, M. A., Lesko, K., Ruparel, K., et al. (2007). Limbic activation associated with misidentification of fearful faces and flat affect in schizophrenia. *Archives of General Psychiatry, 64*(12), 1356–1366.

Gur, R. E., McGrath, C., Chan, R. M., Schroeder, L., Turner, T., Turetsky, B. I., et al. (2002). An fMRI study of facial emotion processing in patients with schizophrenia. *American Journal of Psychiatry, 159*(12), 1992–1999.

Gusnard, D. A., Akbudak, E., Shulman, G. L., & Raichle, M. E. (2001). Medial prefrontal cortex and self-referential mental activity: Relation to a default mode of brain function. *Proceedings of the National Academy of Science of the USA, 98*(7), 4259–4264.

Habel, U., Chechko, N., Pauly, K., Koch, K., Backes, V., Seiferth, N., et al. (2010). Neural correlates of emotion recognition in schizophrenia. *Schizophrenia Research, 122*(1–3), 113–123.

Habel, U., Klein, M., Shah, N. J., Toni, I., Zilles, K., Falkai, P., et al. (2004). Genetic load on amygdala hypofunction during sadness in nonaffected brothers of schizophrenia patients. *American Journal of Psychiatry, 161*(10), 1806–1813.

Hall, J., Whalley, H. C., McKirdy, J. W., Romaniuk, L., McGonigle, D., McIntosh, A. M., et al. (2008). Overactivation of fear systems to neutral faces in schizophrenia. *Biological Psychiatry, 64*(1), 70–73.

Happe, F. (2003). Theory of mind and the self. *Annals of the New York Academy of Science*, *1001*, 134–144.

Haxby, J. V., Hoffman, E. A., & Gobbini, M. I. (2000). The distributed human neural system for face perception. *Trends in Cognitive Sciences*, *4*(6), 223–233.

Hempel, A., Hempel, E., Schonknecht, P., Stippich, C., & Schroder, J. (2003). Impairment in basal limbic function in schizophrenia during affect recognition. *Psychiatry Research*, *122*(2), 115–124.

Hirao, K., Miyata, J., Fujiwara, H., Yamada, M., Namiki, C., Shimizu, M., et al. (2008). Theory of mind and frontal lobe pathology in schizophrenia: A voxel-based morphometry study. *Schizophrenia Research*, *105*(1–3), 165–174.

Holt, D. J., Kunkel, L., Weiss, A. P., Goff, D. C., Wright, C. I., Shin, L. M., et al. (2006). Increased medial temporal lobe activation during the passive viewing of emotional and neutral facial expressions in schizophrenia. *Schizophrenia Research*, *82*(2–3), 153–162.

Holt, D. J., Titone, D., Long, L. S., Goff, D. C., Cather, C., Rauch, S. L., et al. (2006). The misattribution of salience in delusional patients with schizophrenia. *Schizophrenia Research*, *83*(2–3), 247–256.

Honea, R. A., Meyer- Lindenberg, A., Hobbs, K. B., Pezawas, L., Mattay, V. S., Egan, M. F., et al. (2008). Is gray matter volume an intermediate phenotype for schizophrenia? A voxel-based morphometry study of patients with schizophrenia and their healthy siblings. *Biological Psychiatry*, *63*(5), 465–474.

Janssen, I., Versmissen, D., Campo, J. A., Myin- Germeys, I., van Os, J., & Krabbendam, L. (2006). Attribution style and psychosis: Evidence for an externalizing bias in patients but not in individuals at high risk. *Psychological Medicine*, *36*(6), 771–778.

Johnson, S. C., Schmitz, T. W., Kawahara- Baccus, T. N., Rowley, H. A., Alexander, A. L., Lee, J., et al. (2005). The cerebral response during subjective choice with and without self-reference. *Journal of Cognitive Neuroscience*, *17*(12), 1897–1906.

Johnston, P. J., Stojanov, W., Devir, H., & Schall, U. (2005). Functional MRI of facial emotion recognition deficits in schizophrenia and their electrophysiological correlates. *European Journal of Neuroscience*, *22*(5), 1221–1232.

Joyal, C. C., Laakso, M. P., Tiihonen, J., Syvalahti, E., Vilkman, H., Laakso, A., et al. (2003). The amygdala and schizophrenia: A volumetric magnetic resonance imaging study in first-episode, neuroleptic-naive patients. *Biological Psychiatry*, *54*(11), 1302–1304.

Kinderman, P., & Bentall, R. P. (1996). The development of a novel measure of causal attributions: The Internal Personal and Situational Attributions questionnaire. *Personality and Individual Differences*, *20*, 261–264.

Kosaka, H., Omori, M., Murata, T., Iidaka, T., Yamada, H., Okada, T., et al. (2002). Differential amygdala response during facial recognition in patients with schizophrenia: An fMRI study. *Schizophrenia Research*, *57*(1), 87–95.

Krusemark, E., Campbell, W., & Clementz, B. (2008). Attributions, deception, and event-related potentials: An investigation of the self-serving bias. *Psychophysiology*, *45*, 511–515.

Langdon, R., Corner, T., McLaren, J., Ward, P. B., & Coltheart, M. (2006). Externalizing and personalizing biases in persecutory delusions: The relationship with poor insight and theory-of-mind. *Behaviour Research and Therapy*, *44*(5), 699–713.

Langdon, R., Ward, P. B., & Coltheart, M. (2010). Reasoning anomalies associated with delusions in schizophrenia. *Schizophrenia Bulletin*, *36*(2), 321–330.

Lee, C. U., Shenton, M. E., Salisbury, D. F., Kasai, K., Onitsuka, T., Dickey, C. C., et al. (2002). Fusiform gyrus volume reduction in first-episode schizophrenia: A magnetic resonance imaging study. *Archives of General Psychiatry*, *59*(9), 775–781.

Lee, K. H., Brown, W. H., Egleston, P. N., Green, R. D., Farrow, T. F., Hunter, M. D., et al. (2006). A functional magnetic resonance imaging study of social cognition in schizophrenia during an acute episode and after recovery. *American Journal of Psychiatry*, *163*(11), 1926–1933.

Li, H., Chan, R. C., McAlonan, G. M., & Gong, Q. Y. (2010). Facial emotion processing in schizophrenia: A meta-analysis of functional neuroimaging data. *Schizophrenia Bulletin*, *36*(5), 1029–1039.

Lieberman, M. D. (2007). Social cognitive neuroscience: A review of core processes. *Annual Review of Psychology*, *58*, 259–289.

Loughead, J., Gur, R. C., Elliott, M., & Gur, R. E. (2008). Neural circuitry for accurate identification of facial emotions. *Brain Research*, *1194*, 37–44.

Lundberg, K. (2013). Social cognition: Social psychological insights from normal adults. In D. L. Roberts & D. L. Penn (Eds.), *Social cognition in schizophrenia: From evidence to treatment* (Chapter 2). New York: Oxford University Press.

McDonald, B., Highley, J. R., Walker, M. A., Herron, B. M., Cooper, S. J., Esiri, M. M., et al. (2000). Anomalous asymmetry of fusiform and parahippocampal gyrus gray matter in schizophrenia: A postmortem study. *American Journal of Psychiatry*, *157*(1), 40–47.

Michalopoulou, P. G., Surguladze, S., Morley, L. A., Giampietro, V. P., Murray, R. M., & Shergill, S. S. (2008). Facial fear processing and psychotic symptoms in schizophrenia: Functional magnetic resonance imaging study. *British Journal of Psychiatry*, *192*(3), 191–196.

Mier, D., Lis, S., Neuthe, K., Sauer, C., Esslinger, C., Gallhofer, B., et al. (2010). The involvement of emotion recognition in affective theory of mind. *Psychophysiology*, *47*(6), 1028–1039.

Mier, D., Sauer, C., Lis, S., Esslinger, C., Wilhelm, J., Gallhofer, B., et al. (2010). Neuronal correlates of affective theory of mind in schizophrenia out-patients: Evidence for a baseline deficit. *Psychological Medicine*, *40*(10), 1607–1617.

Montag, C., Dziobek, I., Richter, I. S., Neuhaus, K., Lehmann, A., Sylla, R., et al. (2011). Different aspects of theory of mind in paranoid schizophrenia: Evidence from a video-based assessment. *Psychiatry Research*. *186*(2–3), 203–209.

Namiki, C., Hirao, K., Yamada, M., Hanakawa, T., Fukuyama, H., Hayashi, T., et al. (2007). Impaired facial emotion recognition and reduced amygdalar volume in schizophrenia. *Psychiatry Research*, *156*(1), 23–32.

Niu, L., Matsui, M., Zhou, S. Y., Hagino, H., Takahashi, T., Yoneyama, E., et al. (2004). Volume reduction of the amygdala in patients with schizophrenia: A magnetic resonance imaging study. *Psychiatry Research*, *132*(1), 41–51.

Ochsner, K. N. (2008). The social-emotional processing stream: Five core constructs and their translational potential for schizophrenia and beyond. *Biological Psychiatry*, *64*(1), 48–61.

Ochsner, K. N., & Gross, J. J. (2008). Cognitive emotion regulation: Insights from social cognitive and affective neuroscience. *Current Directions in Psychological Science*, *17*, 153–158.

Ochsner, K. N., Knierim, K., Ludlow, D. H., Hanelin, J., Ramachandran, T., Glover, G., et al. (2004). Reflecting upon feelings: An fMRI study of neural systems supporting the attribution of emotion to self and other. *Journal of Cognitive Neuroscience*, *16*(10), 1746–1772.

Onitsuka, T., Niznikiewicz, M. A., Spencer, K. M., Frumin, M., Kuroki, N., Lucia, L. C., et al. (2006). Functional and structural deficits in brain regions subserving face perception in schizophrenia. *American Journal of Psychiatry*, *163*(3), 455–462.

Onitsuka, T., Shenton, M. E., Kasai, K., Nestor, P. G., Toner, S. K., Kikinis, R., et al. (2003). Fusiform gyrus volume reduction and facial recognition in chronic schizophrenia. *Archives of General Psychiatry, 60*(4), 349–355.

Paillere-Martinot, M., Caclin, A., Artiges, E., Poline, J. B., Joliot, M., Mallet, L., et al. (2001). Cerebral gray and white matter reductions and clinical correlates in patients with early onset schizophrenia. *Schizophrenia Research, 50*(1–2), 19–26.

Paradiso, S., Andreasen, N. C., Crespo- Facorro, B., O' Leary, D. S., Watkins, G. L., Boles Ponto, L. L., et al. (2003). Emotions in unmedicated patients with schizophrenia during evaluation with positron emission tomography. *American Journal of Psychiatry, 160*(10), 1775–1783.

Park, K. M., Kim, J. J., Ku, J., Kim, S. Y., Lee, H. R., Kim, S. I., et al. (2009). Neural basis of attributional style in schizophrenia. *Neuroscience Letters, 459*(1), 35–40.

Pelphrey, K. A., Mitchell, T. V., McKeown, M. J., Goldstein, J., Allison, T., & McCarthy, G. (2003). Brain activity evoked by the perception of human walking: Controlling for meaningful coherent motion. *J Neurosci, 23*(17), 6819–6825.

Phelps, E. A. (2004). Human emotion and memory: Interactions of the amygdala and hippocampal complex. *Current Opinion in Neurobiology, 14*(2), 198–202.

Phillips, M. L., Williams, L., Senior, C., Bullmore, E. T., Brammer, M. J., Andrew, C., et al. (1999). A differential neural response to threatening and non-threatening negative facial expressions in paranoid and non-paranoid schizophrenics. *Psychiatry Research, 92*(1), 11–31.

Phillips, M. L., Young, A. W., Senior, C., Brammer, M., Andrew, C., Calder, A. J., et al. (1997). A specific neural substrate for perceiving facial expressions of disgust. *Nature, 389*(6650), 495–498.

Pinkham, A. E., Brensinger, C., Kohler, C., Gur, R. E., & Gur, R. C. (2011). Actively paranoid patients with schizophrenia over attribute anger to neutral faces. *Schizophrenia Research, 125*(2–3), 174–178.

Pinkham, A. E., Gur, R. E., & Gur, R. C. (2007). Affect recognition deficits in schizophrenia: Neural substrates and psychopharmacological implications. *Expert Review of Neurotherapeutics, 7*(7), 807–816.

Pinkham, A. E., Hopfinger, J. B., Pelphrey, K. A., Piven, J., & Penn, D. L. (2008). Neural bases for impaired social cognition in schizophrenia and autism spectrum disorders. *Schizophrenia Research, 99*, 164–175. doi: S0920-9964(07)00471-9

Pinkham, A. E., Hopfinger, J. B., Ruparel, K., & Penn, D. L. (2008). An investigation of the relationship between activation of a social cognitive neural network and social functioning. *Schizophrenia Bulletin, 34*(4), 688–697.

Pinkham, A. E., Loughead, J., Ruparel, K., Overton, E., Gur, R. E., & Gur, R. C. (2011). Abnormal modulation of amygdala activity in schizophrenia in response to direct- and averted-gaze threat-related facial expressions. *American Journal of Psychiatry, 168*(3), 293–301.

Pinkham, A. E., Penn, D., Wangelin, B., Perkins, D., Gerig, G., Gu, H., et al. (2005). Facial emotion perception and fusiform gyrus volume in first episode schizophrenia. *Schizophrenia Research, 79*(2–3), 341–343.

Pomarol-Clotet, E., Canales-Rodriguez, E. J., Salvador, R., Sarro, S., Gomar, J. J., Vila, F., et al. (2010). Medial prefrontal cortex pathology in schizophrenia as revealed by convergent findings from multimodal imaging. *Molecular Psychiatry, 15*(8), 823–830.

Puce, A., Allison, T., Asgari, M., Gore, J. C., & McCarthy, G. (1996). Differential sensitivity of human visual cortex to faces, letterstrings, and textures: A functional magnetic resonance imaging study. *Journal of Neuroscience, 16*(16), 5205–5215.

Quintana, J., Wong, T., Ortiz- Portillo, E., Marder, S. R., & Mazziotta, J. C. (2003). Right lateral fusiform gyrus dysfunction during facial information processing in schizophrenia. *Biological Psychiatry, 53*(12), 1099–1112.

Rhodes, G., Byatt, G., Michie, P. T., & Puce, A. (2004). Is the fusiform face area specialized for faces, individuation, or expert individuation? *Journal of Cognitive Neuroscience, 16*(2), 189–203.

Richeson, J. A., Baird, A. A., Gordon, H. L., Heatherton, T. F., Wyland, C. L., Trawalter, S., et al. (2003). An fMRI investigation of the impact of interracial contact on executive function. *Nature Neuroscience, 6*(12), 1323–1328.

Russell, T. A., Reynaud, E., Kucharska- Pietura, K., Ecker, C., Benson, P. J., Zelaya, F., et al. (2007). Neural responses to dynamic expressions of fear in schizophrenia. *Neuropsychologia, 45*(1), 107–123.

Russell, T. A., Rubia, K., Bullmore, E. T., Soni, W., Suckling, J., Brammer, M. J., et al. (2000). Exploring the social brain in schizophrenia: Left prefrontal underactivation during mental state attribution. *American Journal of Psychiatry, 157*(12), 2040–2042.

Samson, D., Apperly, I. A., Kathirgamanathan, U., & Humphreys, G. W. (2005). Seeing it my way: A case of a selective deficit in inhibiting self-perspective. *Brain, 128*(Pt. 5), 1102–1111.

Sasson, N. J., Pinkham, A. E., Carpenter, K. L., & Belger, A. (2011). The benefit of directly comparing autism and schizophrenia for revealing mechanisms of social cognitive impairment. *Journal of Neurodevelopmental Disorders, 3*(2), 87–100.

Saxe, R. (2006). Uniquely human social cognition. *Current Opinion in Neurobiology, 16*(2), 235–239.

Scheef, L., Manka, C., Daamen, M., Kuhn, K. U., Maier, W., Schild, H. H., et al. (2010). Resting-state perfusion in nonmedicated schizophrenic patients: A continuous arterial spin-labeling 3.0–T MR study. *Radiology, 256*(1), 253–260.

Schneider, F., Weiss, U., Kessler, C., Salloum, J. B., Posse, S., Grodd, W., et al. (1998). Differential amygdala activation in schizophrenia during sadness. *Schizophrenia Research, 34*(3), 133–142.

Seiferth, N. Y., Pauly, K., Kellermann, T., Shah, N. J., Ott, G., Herpertz- Dahlmann, B., et al. (2009). Neuronal correlates of facial emotion discrimination in early onset schizophrenia. *Neuropsychopharmacology, 34*(2), 477–487.

Shamay-Tsoory, S. G., Lester, H., Chisin, R., Israel, O., Bar-Shalom, R., Peretz, A., et al. (2005). The neural correlates of understanding the other's distress: A positron emission tomography investigation of accurate empathy. *Neuroimage, 27*(2), 468–472.

Shamay-Tsoory, S. G., Tomer, R., Berger, B. D., & Aharon-Peretz, J. (2003). Characterization of empathy deficits following prefrontal brain damage: The role of the right ventromedial prefrontal cortex. *Journal of Cognitive Neuroscience, 15*(3), 324–337.

Sumich, A., Chitnis, X. A., Fannon, D. G., O' Ceallaigh, S., Doku, V. C., Falrowicz, A., et al. (2002). Temporal lobe abnormalities in first-episode psychosis. *American Journal of Psychiatry, 159*(7), 1232–1235.

Takahashi, H., Koeda, M., Oda, K., Matsuda, T., Matsushima, E., Matsuura, M., et al. (2004). An fMRI study of differential neural response to affective pictures in schizophrenia. *Neuroimage, 22*(3), 1247–1254.

Takahashi, T., Suzuki, M., Zhou, S. Y., Tanino, R., Hagino, H., Niu, L., et al. (2006). Temporal lobe gray matter in schizophrenia spectrum: A volumetric MRI study of the fusiform gyrus, parahippocampal gyrus, and middle and inferior temporal gyri. *Schizophrenia Research, 87*(1–3), 116–126.

Tanskanen, P., Veijola, J. M., Piippo, U. K., Haapea, M., Miettunen, J. A., Pyhtinen, J., et al. (2005). Hippocampus and amygdala volumes in schizophrenia and other psychoses in the Northern Finland 1966 birth cohort. *Schizophrenia Research*, *75*(2–3), 283–294.

Taylor, S. F., Phan, K. L., Britton, J. C., & Liberzon, I. (2005). Neural response to emotional salience in schizophrenia. *Neuropsychopharmacology*, *30*(5), 984–995.

Thompson, J. C., Clarke, M., Stewart, T., & Puce, A. (2005). Configural processing of biological motion in human superior temporal sulcus. *Journal of Neuroscience*, *25*(39), 9059–9066.

Vogeley, K., Bussfeld, P., Newen, A., Herrmann, S., Happe, F., Falkai, P., et al. (2001). Mind reading: Neural mechanisms of theory of mind and self-perspective. *Neuroimage*, *14*(1 Pt. 1), 170–181.

Vuilleumier, P. (2005). Cognitive science: Staring fear in the face. *Nature*, *433*(7021), 22–23.

Vuilleumier, P., & Pourtois, G. (2007). Distributed and interactive brain mechanisms during emotion face perception: Evidence from functional neuroimaging. *Neuropsychologia*, *45*(1), 174–194.

Walter, H., Ciaramidaro, A., Adenzato, M., Vasic, N., Ardito, R. B., Erk, S., et al. (2009). Dysfunction of the social brain in schizophrenia is modulated by intention type: An fMRI study. *Social, Cognitive and Affective Neuroscience*, *4*(2), 166–176.

Walther, S., Federspiel, A., Horn, H., Bianchi, P., Wiest, R., Wirth, M., et al. (2009). Encoding deficit during face processing within the right fusiform face area in schizophrenia. *Psychiatry Research*, *172*(3), 184–191.

Whalen, P. J., Kagan, J., Cook, R. G., Davis, F. C., Kim, H., Polis, S., et al. (2004). Human amygdala responsivity to masked fearful eye whites. *Science*, *306*(5704), 2061.

Williams, L. M., Das, P., Harris, A. W., Liddell, B. B., Brammer, M. J., Olivieri, G., et al. (2004). Dysregulation of arousal and amygdala-prefrontal systems in paranoid schizophrenia. *American Journal of Psychiatry*, *161*(3), 480–489.

Winston, J. S., Henson, R. N., Fine-Goulden, M. R., & Dolan, R. J. (2004). fMRI-adaptation reveals dissociable neural representations of identity and expression in face perception. *Journal of Neurophysiology*, *92*(3), 1830–1839.

Witthaus, H., Kaufmann, C., Bohner, G., Ozgurdal, S., Gudlowski, Y., Gallinat, J., et al. (2009). Gray matter abnormalities in subjects at ultra-high risk for schizophrenia and first-episode schizophrenic patients compared to healthy controls. *Psychiatry Research*, *173*(3), 163–169.

Wright, I. C., Rabe- Hesketh, S., Woodruff, P. W., David, A. S., Murray, R. M., & Bullmore, E. T. (2000). Meta-analysis of regional brain volumes in schizophrenia. *American Journal of Psychiatry*, *157*(1), 16–25.

Yamada, M., Hirao, K., Namiki, C., Hanakawa, T., Fukuyama, H., Hayashi, T., et al. (2007). Social cognition and frontal lobe pathology in schizophrenia: A voxel-based morphometric study. *Neuroimage*, *35*(1), 292–298.

PART THREE

Treatment Approaches

12

Introduction to Social Cognitive Treatment Approaches for Schizophrenia

JOANNA M. FISZDON ■

ROOTS OF SOCIAL COGNITIVE TREATMENT APPROACHES

Although social cognitive treatments are relative newcomers to the field of psychosocial rehabilitation for schizophrenia, their roots can be traced back to more established interventions, including social skills training and neurocognitive remediation. Shared across all three types of treatments is a focus on improving specific domains in an effort to improve community and social functioning in schizophrenia. As noted by Kern (Kern, Glynn, Horan, & Marder, 2009), they all represent different approaches to facilitating recovery, each focusing on a different treatment target, but with the same overarching goal.

Social skills training is among the most established and widely studied of psychosocial therapies for schizophrenia (Bellack & Hersen, 1979; Heinssen, Liberman, & Kopelowicz, 2000; Kern et al., 2009; Kurtz, & Mueser, 2008; Liberman, 2008). Dating back to the 1970s, these treatments were originally developed based on social learning theory and operant conditioning techniques, and they focused on training specific motor behaviors related to social interactions, like eye contact, loudness and duration of speech, and speech content. As these treatments developed, their focus expanded to targeting not only the acquisition of specific motor skills but also social competence or social perception—one's ability to know when, where, and how to make specific behavioral responses (Bellack & Hersen, 1979). In a chapter on cognitive factors in the social skills of schizophrenic patients, Wallace and Boone (1984) note the crucial role of information processing in training social skills leading to successful social interactions. In a series of studies of skill training, they show the increasingly important role of cognitive factors such as attending, perceiving, and problem solving, in the successful training of more complex social skills. Social skills can be broadly grouped into three subsets: receiving skills, processing skills, and sending skills. Receiving skills focus on the processing of relevant verbal, nonverbal, and paralinguistic social information, including others' affective states and intentions, as well as on social norms and expectations for the particular situation (Liberman, 2008). The two other subsets of skill training—processing skills and sending skills— also entail social cognitive abilities, as they involve subjective judgments of the effects of different behavioral responses on another person and the modulation and delivery of such behaviors in a manner most likely to achieve the desired outcome (i.e., "how will the other person perceive and respond to what I do").

Another predecessor of social cognitive treatments is *neurocognitive remediation*. Although both neurocognitive remediation and skill training have as their ultimate goal improving social and community functioning, neurocognitive remediation focuses on remediating neurocognitive functions, including attention, memory, and problem solving (Krabbendam & Aleman, 2003; Kurtz, Moberg, Gur, & Gur, 2001; McGurk, Twamley, Sitzer, McHugo, & Mueser, 2007; Twamley, Jeste, & Bellack, 2003; Wykes, & Huddy, 2009). This approach is supported by a growing literature showing significant links between neurocognition and various aspects of functioning (Bowie & Harvey, 2005; Green, 1996; Green, Kern, Braff, & Mintz, 2000). Neurocognitive remediation approaches vary considerably in terms of duration, intensity, focus of training, delivery format, and, perhaps most importantly, in terms of theoretical rationale, with some basing their training on a restorative, bottom-up, drill-and-practice model in which the initial targets are the building blocks of cognition, such as processing speed and sustained attention, and others relying on a compensatory, top-down, approach in which the focus is on developing general strategies (e.g., chunking, mnemonics, overrehearsal) that can be applied to a range of cognitive processes. Although the overall success of neurocognitive remediation in improving neuropsychological test performance and other proximal measures has been clearly demonstrated (Krabbendam & Aleman, 2003; Twamley et al., 2003), newer studies indicate that these treatments have minimal to (at most) modest effects on functioning unless provided in the context of more broad-based psychosocial treatments, including interventions like vocational rehabilitation or skill training (McGurk et al., 2007; McGurk & Wykes, 2008), which arguably may also include a social training component. Combined with recent studies suggesting that social cognitive variables may mediate the effects of neurocognitive remediation on functional outcomes and may account for unique variance in predicting these functional outcomes (Brekke, Kay, Lee, & Green, 2005; Brekke, Hoe, Long, & Green, 2007; Sergi, Rassovsky, Nuechterlein, & Green, 2006), these neurocognitive remediation approaches can be conceptualized as a precursor to the newly emerging social cognitive treatments described in subsequent chapters of this book, in which the focus shifts from broadly remediating information processing deficits to remediating the deficits and biases in the processing of uniquely social information.

PROOF-OF-CONCEPT SOCIAL COGNITIVE STUDIES

Many of the current social cognitive treatments are rooted, at least in part, in laboratory-based proof-of-concept studies conducted in the 1990s and 2000s.

These studies were often single-session interventions focused on remediating specific social cognitive domains, such as affect recognition, attributional style, or theory of mind (ToM). The key contribution of these studies has been the identification of separable social cognitive deficits in schizophrenia, along with a demonstration of their malleability and, in some cases, generalization and durability of intervention effects.

For example, in a 1995 study by Corrigan and colleagues (Corrigan, Hirschbeck, & Wolfe, 1995), 40 individuals with schizophrenia were shown brief videotaped vignettes of social situations. Compared to a single-session 60-minute training in vigilance only, a similar length training that incorporated semantic elaboration memory techniques with the vigilance training led to higher recall of social cues presented on both the training materials as well as on an ancillary measure of social cue recognition, indicating that this component of social perception can be improved. These gains were maintained at a 2-day follow-up.

A number of proof-of-concept studies also indicate that affect recognition can be improved. Silver and colleagues (Silver, Goodman, Knoll, & Isakov, 2004) administered three 15-minute sessions of a computerized emotion training program, originally developed for individuals with autism, to 20 hospitalized patients with chronic schizophrenia. The computerized program targeted both the recognition and prediction of emotional responses, and was associated with improvements on two tasks of emotion recognition, although not on a task of emotion differentiation.

In another single-session study of facial identification training administered to inpatients with schizophrenia or schizoaffective disorder, Penn and Combs (2000) showed that performance on a trained emotion recognition task could be improved through the use of either facial mimicry (prior to making emotion judgments) or monetary reinforcement for correct responses, and that these improvements were evident at 1-week follow-up, although they did not generalize to a related measure of affect discrimination. This group of investigators later also showed that a single-session, computer-based attention shaping procedure, which combines computerized attentional prompts to key parts of the face (eyes, mouth) with monetary reinforcement for correct responses, was superior to practice or monetary reinforcement alone conditions in improving affect recognition (Combs et al., 2008). Significant group differences were evident during training, at end of training, and at 1-week follow-up on the trained emotion task. These improvements for the attention shaping group also generalized to an untrained affect recognition task administered at 1-week follow-up, with notable improvements on recognition of emotions that were not part of the original training (disgust, no emotion). However, support for more distal generalization was weak, with trend-level group differences (again favoring the attention shaping group) on an observer-rated social mixing subscale, administered 1 week after the end of training.

In another brief emotion training study, Russell and colleagues (Russell, Chu, & Phillips, 2006) examined the malleability of affect recognition performance in 20 outpatients with schizophrenia and 20 healthy controls. All participants completed a single session of the computerized Micro-Expressions Training Tool (METT). This training consists of a pretraining assessment phase in which participants are asked to identify emotions in 15-millisecond video clips of faces morphing from neutral to an emotion and back to neutral, followed by a training phase in which commonly confused emotions (e.g., anger and disgust) are shown, and subtle differences between them are explained and demonstrated. Next, participants practice labeling microexpressions and receive feedback on their performance. Finally, in the posttraining assessment phase, participants are presented with an alternative set of commonly confused microexpressions and asked again to correctly label them. Results of this brief intervention indicated that both individuals with schizophrenia as well as healthy controls improved on the posttraining assessment, with the posttraining performance of patients comparable to pretraining performance of healthy controls.

Finally, several proof-of-concept studies also examined the modifiability of ToM impairments. Sarfati and colleagues (Sarfati, Passerieux, & Hardy-Bayle, 2000) hypothesized that some ToM impairments may be due to difficulty in separating out relevant data from other contextual information and that, by forcing patients to verbally process contextual information, impairments in ToM may be attenuated. Participants were administered a "character intention task" consisting of three-panel nonverbal comic strips where, in the standard condition, the examinee was asked to choose the correct pictorial fourth panel that accurately characterized the intent of the portrayed character. In a modified condition, the fourth panel options contained sentences describing potential intentions. On the modified verbal answer format of the task, 40% of the schizophrenia participants normalized their performance to healthy control levels, suggesting that a deeper, verbal processing of information may decrease ToM impairments. In another test of the modifiability of ToM impairments in schizophrenia, Kayser and colleagues (Kayser, Sarfati, Besche, & Hardy-Bayle, 2006) asked eight schizophrenia patients to watch a total of 2 hours of short video clips portraying interactions between two or more people, then make attributional judgments about the portrayed characters' intentions and mental states. The therapist provided assistance by first asking the patients to provide an overview of the content of each video clip and, as necessary, followed up with specific questions about the likely intentions and mental states of the characters, as well as justification for the chosen interpretation. This method of verbal mediation and elaboration was associated with significant improvements on a pre–post ToM task.

These laboratory studies of social cognitive training have a number of limitations: In general, sample sizes were small, some reported only modest pre–post effects and no significant differences when compared to control groups, some failed to even include control groups, many lacked blind assessors, those that included follow-up periods were generally brief, and none examined change on real-world social functioning. Nevertheless, these studies do demonstrate that social cognitive impairments can be attenuated, and they serve as proof-of-concept studies for subsequent, more intensive intervention work in this area.

TARGETED, COMPREHENSIVE, AND BROAD-BASED
SOCIAL COGNITIVE TREATMENTS

Contemporary social cognitive interventions are often classified as targeted, comprehensive, or broad-based. As their name implies, targeted social cognitive interventions focus on a single social cognitive domain, such as affect recognition or ToM. Comprehensive interventions aim to ameliorate social cognitive impairments in a number of domains. Finally, broad-based interventions provide training in multiple social cognitive domains in the context of broader psychosocial treatment. Below is a summary of some of the better-known of these treatments. Cognitive Enhancement Therapy (CET), Integrated Neurocognitive Therapy (INT), Metacognitive Therapy (MCT), and Social Cognition and Interaction Training (SCIT), which can also be subsumed under these categories, are separately and more thoroughly reviewed in a subsequent section of this chapter.

Targeted Treatments

Affect Perception
The majority of targeted social cognitive treatments have focused on improving affect recognition. One such intervention is called Training in Affect Recognition (TAR). TAR is a 6-week, 12-session, manualized treatment consisting of three segments: identification of prototypical components of basic emotions, integration of facial elements to form quick decisions about affect, and application of learned information to the processing of nonprototypical, ambiguous facial expressions. The training relies on both compensatory and restorative techniques, includes both computerized stimuli and "desk work," and relies heavily on strategies like verbalization and self-instruction. In a preliminary feasibility open trial of TAR, Frommann and colleagues (Frommann, Streit, & Wolwer, 2003) reported that TAR met with good adherence and led to pre–post improvements on untrained affect recognition tasks.

In a more rigorous examination of the efficacy of TAR, Wolwer and colleagues (Wolwer et al., 2005) randomly assigned 77 post-acute schizophrenia inpatients and outpatients to TAR, cognitive remediation therapy (CRT), or treatment as usual (TAU). CRT consisted of 12 sessions of computerized training in attention, memory, and executive function, as well as dyad training in cognitive strategies. Adherence to the full course of treatment was not as good as in the original trial, with 24 participants dropping out prior to treatment completion (eight from the TAR group, ten from CRT, and six from TAU). However, in intent-to-treat analyses, the authors reported significant group differences in affect recognition and basic neurocognitive performance, with evidence of a double-dissociation— individuals in the TAR group improved significantly more than the other two groups on pre–post measures of affect recognition, whereas individuals in CRT improved significantly more than TAU on measures of memory and learning.

Examination of the impact of pre–post neurocognition and clinical symptoms on affect recognition performance indicated that attention and comprehension of social scripts (picture arrangement task) accounted for 19% of the variance in affect recognition improvement, whereas improvement in negative symptoms was associated with 7% of the explained variance. Because the authors included an active control group (CRT), they were also able to speculate that impairments in affect recognition were not simply a manifestation of a generalized cognitive deficit, since improvements on this domain were only found in the group receiving specific affect recognition training. In more recent evaluations, affect recognition improvements following TAR have also been replicated in a forensic schizophrenia sample, with evidence of durability of improvements at 4- to 6-week follow-up (Wolwer & Frommann, 2009), and were shown to be associated with increased activation in occipital, parietal, and frontal brain regions (Habel et al., 2010).

SOCIAL PERCEPTION

Several studies have shown that deficits in social perception can be ameliorated in schizophrenia. For example, Social Cognition Enhancement Training (SCET) (Choi & Kwon, 2006), which focuses on improving social context appraisal and perspective-taking abilities through practice with arranging cartoons of social situations, has been shown to lead to improvements in social perception, although the training did not generalize to affect recognition. The training was also rather intensive (35 1.5-hour sessions administered twice a week), and nearly 50% of the sample dropped out of the treatment before its end. The drop-out rate was similar in both the treatment and standard psychiatric rehabilitation control conditions, underscoring the well-known difficulties in psychosocial treatment engagement and adherence in this population.

Van der Gaag and colleagues (van der Gaag, Kern, van den Bosch, & Liberman, 2002) have also evaluated the efficacy of a social perception combined with emotion recognition training. This 22-session training consisted of manualized, individual 20-minute sessions, held twice weekly over approximately 3 months. Training progressed from focusing on visual, tactile, and auditory perception to integration of information from different modalities, to attention and listening skills, and, finally, to emotion recognition. Specific training strategies included verbal mediation, use of compensatory strategies to aid in recall of information, training in inductive reasoning, instruction on emotion identification, role-plays, repetition, and mimicry. Although the training included remediation of basic cognitive skills like attention, memory, and executive function, these skills were conceptualized as necessary building blocks for successful social perception. Evaluated in a sample of 42 inpatients with schizophrenia randomized to either the treatment or time-matched leisure activities, the training led to improvements in social perception, with a 23% reduction in errors on emotion matching and a 49% reduction in errors on emotion labeling. There was also some evidence of improvements in executive function; however, these were only observed in within-in-group paired t-tests.

THEORY OF MIND

There is also evidence that targeted training can ameliorate deficits in ToM. Roncone and colleagues (Roncone et al., 2004) randomly assigned 20 inpatients with residual schizophrenia to Instrumental Enrichment Program (IEP) or a usual treatment control condition. IEP, which the authors compare to Hogarty and colleagues' Cognitive Enhancement Therapy, focuses on exposing participants to new situations and decreasing ToM impairments by "teaching and learning how to change cognitive structure by transforming a passive dependent cognitive style to an autonomous one" (p. 426). IEP was conducted in a single 6-month weekly group, which included ten patients and five therapists. Compared to the control condition, IEP was associated with decreases in negative symptoms, improvements in ToM (both first- and second-order false beliefs), executive functions, strategic thinking, and affect recognition for two types of emotions—sadness and fear.

In another study of the malleability of ToM impairments, Mazza and colleagues (Mazza et al., 2010) compared changes in ToM performance following 12 sessions of Emotion and ToM Imitation Training (ETIT) or Problem Solving Skill Training (PST) administered to 33 outpatients with schizophrenia. ETIT is a group-based treatment consisting of four training phases: observing others' eye direction, imitating facial emotions, inferring others' mental states, and making attributions of intentions based on observations of others' actions. Compared to the active control condition, individuals randomized to ETIT evidenced improvements in several ToM measures, affect recognition, empathy, clinician-rated social functioning, and positive symptoms. Improvements in memory were observed only in the group receiving PST.

There is also evidence that ToM training may lead to symptom reduction. Lecardeur and colleagues (Lecardeur et al., 2009) pseudo-randomized 30 outpatients into one of three groups: usual treatment, ToM training, and training in mental flexibility. The ToM training consisted of education about mental state attributions and their relevance to social functioning, practice in the identification of meaningful social information, and practice in mental state attribution using cartoons, comic strips, and short stories. The mental flexibility training also included education about ToM and its relevance to social functioning, along with practice inhibiting initial attributions and practice applying different rules to language and categorization exercises. Compared to the control group, both treatment groups showed an improvement in positive, general, and overall psychiatric symptoms, with the mental flexibility group showing somewhat greater improvements. Neither of the treatments appeared to impact negative symptom severity. Unfortunately, the assessments were limited to measures of symptoms and subjective cognitive function, and did not include ToM or other social cognitive measures.

SUMMARY

In summary, targeted social cognitive treatments have been developed for affect recognition specifically and social perception more generally, as well as for ToM, which included attributional style training. All of these interventions have met with some success, at least on proximal measures of the targeted social cognitive domain, with mixed evidence of generalization to nontrained cognitive skills. As with the proof-of-concept studies described in the preceding section, the majority of targeted treatments did not evaluate the durability of treatment gains, nor the generalization of these gains to social functioning. Moreover, it is still unknown whether targeting single social cognitive domains can lead to clinically meaningful change, as the various social cognitive skills likely act in concert to create a pattern of interpersonal interactions, leading to impairments in overall social and community function. Nevertheless, these targeted studies provide an evaluation of potential methods that can (and have been) incorporated into more comprehensive treatments addressing a range of social cognitive functions.

Comprehensive Treatments

Comprehensive treatments targeting the full range of social cognitive impairments present in schizophrenia are relatively new to the group of social cognitive interventions. The first such comprehensive social cognitive treatment, SCIT, developed by Roberts and Penn at the University of North Carolina at Chapel Hill, is described in detail in a subsequent section of this chapter. A related treatment, called Social Cognitive Skill Training (SCST) was developed by Green, Horan, and colleagues at the University of California at Los Angeles (UCLA) and combines and expands on elements from other social cognitive treatments including SCIT and TAR. The 12-session intervention incorporates successful components of traditional skills training, including identifying specific skills related to individual social cognitive performance, providing gradual increases in trained task difficulty, and using practice and repetition to automate skills taught. The training is divided into two six-session phases: (1) emotion recognition and social perception, and (2) social attribution and ToM. Similar to SCIT, the attributional style and ToM training consists of avoiding jumping to conclusions by separating facts from guesses and "checking out" evidence in support of various beliefs, as well as applying the learned material to social situations in the patients' own lives. Novel to SCST is specific training in nonverbal cue perception and the identification of sarcasm and deception. The intervention also includes a number of new exercises and didactic training materials.

In the first evaluation of the feasibility and tolerability of SCST (Horan et al., 2009), 34 schizophrenia spectrum outpatients were recruited from a Veterans Administration hospital and randomly assigned to either the social cognitive skill training or a time- and structure-matched illness management and recovery skills group. Treatment adherence was good in both groups, with, on average, more than nine of the 12 sessions attended. Participants in both groups also reported high satisfaction/enjoyment and high perceived relevance to daily life for both groups. The social cognitive training was associated with significant improvements in affect recognition, with large between-group and medium to large within-group effect sizes; these improvements were independent of any change in neurocognitive function or clinical symptoms. There were also trend-level improvements on measures of attributional bias and ToM. Although the results of the initial study are encouraging, evaluations of social cognitive domains were relatively limited (one measure per social cognitive domain) and did not include measures of generalization to actual social functioning. Additionally, this was a small sample of mostly male veterans, and the generalizability of this intervention to nonveteran populations has not been evaluated to date. The authors speculated that a longer, more intensive training in attributional bias and ToM may be necessary to effect clinically meaningful change in these complex components of social cognition, and have expanded the full intervention into a 24-session format.

In a subsequent evaluation of the now-expanded SCST treatment (Horan et al., 2011), 85 individuals with psychotic disorders were randomized to receive one of four time-matched treatments: SCST, computerized neurocognitive remediation, a hybrid intervention that included both SCST and neurocognitive remediation components, and a standard illness management skills training group. Assessments were expanded somewhat to include measures of functional capacity and emotion management, along with neurocognition and symptoms. Data were analyzed for 68 individuals who completed at least one follow-up assessment. Group attendance was good, with, on average, 19 of 24 sessions attended across all conditions. As with the earlier study, differential effects favoring SCST were found for affect recognition, which generalized to emotion management; however, there were no significant between-group differences on measures of social perception, attributional bias, or ToM, nor on neurocognition or psychiatric symptoms. There was a trend-level improvement for social skill ability in both the SCST and the neurocognitive remediation group. Of note, baseline performance on the attributional bias measure across all groups was similar to that previously reported in healthy control samples, suggesting a potential ceiling effect. Because effects on emotion processing were specific to the SCST group, the authors conclude that this intervention has a specific effect on social cognition not observed for the other three treatment conditions, and they suggest that efforts at improving social cognition may be successful in stand-alone social cognitive treatments that do not require concomitant neurocognitive remediation. Lack of SCST effects on what may be considered higher order social cognitive domains, including social perception and ToM, may reflect the more complex nature of these processes, and the authors suggest further refinement and expansion of treatments to adequately target these domains.

Broad-Based Treatments

One of the best known and most researched broad-based treatments is Integrated Psychological Therapy (IPT), a manual-based, cognitive-behavioral group treatment that combines cognitive remediation, social cognitive remediation, and psychosocial rehabilitation. IPT consists of five subprograms: cognitive differentiation, social perception, verbal communication, social skills, and interpersonal problems solving, which are generally delivered sequentially, although booster sessions of the various subprograms may be administered based on patient need. This therapy has been studied in several countries, and entire books published on its methods and effectiveness (Mueller & Roder, 2010; Roder, Mueller, Brenner, & Spaulding, 2010), so a detailed summary of IPT research is beyond the confines of this chapter. A recent meta-analysis of the efficacy of IPT (Roder, Mueller, Mueser, & Brenner, 2006), however, indicates efficacy in all examined domains, including neurocognition, psychiatric symptoms, and psychosocial functioning, with within-group effect sizes in the medium range. This pattern of findings persists when only methodologically rigorous IPT studies with large samples are included, and it generalizes to a broad range of assessment types, settings, and treatment phases. There is also evidence that the effects of IPT are maintained or even enhanced during an average follow-up period of over 8 months. The only patient variable found to predict success of IPT was duration of illness, with shorter illness duration associated with greater treatment efficacy, suggesting that this treatment should be administered early in the course of illness.

Another well-studied comprehensive treatment with a social cognitive component is Neurocognitive Enhancement Therapy (NET). Developed by Bell and colleagues, this 6- to 12-month intervention consists of computerized neurocognitive remediation, along with a weekly social information processing group consisting of participant presentations on select topics (e.g., "A Day at Work") along with constructive feedback from other group participants. Several large-scale trials of NET plus vocational rehabilitation, compared to vocational rehabilitation alone (Bell, Bryson, Greig, Corcoran, & Wexler, 2001; Bell, Fiszdon, Greig, Wexler, & Bryson, 2007; Bell, Zito, Greig, & Wexler, 2008; Wexler & Bell, 2005), indicate that it has effects on both proximal as well as distal outcomes, including neurocognition, social cognition, and work outcomes, with lasting effects observed 6–12 months following the end of the active intervention. Sustained within-, but not between-group differences have also been reported on psychiatric symptoms and interviewer-rated general functioning (quality of life).

RESEARCH ON SOCIAL COGNITIVE TREATMENTS DESCRIBED IN SUBSEQUENT CHAPTERS

Cognitive Enhancement Therapy

CET is a broad-based psychosocial treatment combining neurocognitive remediation and social cognitive group training. Although from the beginning CET has been conceptualized as a social cognitive treatment, it nevertheless includes a significant neurocognitive training component, with neurocognition seen as a necessary building block for successful social behavior. As described in chapter 14 of this volume, the focus of the social cognitive training is on providing learning exercises that lead the individual to automatic, "gistful" processing of social information, with an emphasis placed on accurate context appraisal and appropriate perspective taking (Hogarty & Flesher, 1999a,b).

In the first published evaluation of CET (Hogarty et al., 2004), 121 chronically ill patients with schizophrenia were randomized to 2 years of CET or an illness self-management focused intervention called Enriched Supportive Therapy (EST). Comprehensive assessments by nonblind raters were conducted at study entry, 12 months into the treatment, and at 24 months after intake (end of treatment). Of the 121 patients randomized, only 12% terminated treatment early, and the 61 CET patients who remained in treatment for the 2-year duration attended on average over 91% of their scheduled therapy appointments, indicating good adherence. At the halfway point of the treatment (12 months), group differences favoring CET were observed on processing speed, neurocognition, and social adjustment, with trend-level improvements for social cognition and cognitive style. Here, cognitive style was defined as how patients approached social and instrumental tasks, and consisted of impoverishment, disorganization, and rigidity. There were no significant group differences on symptoms. At the end of the 2-year treatment, observed group differences remained or were enhanced, with large effect size improvements for CET on all assessed composite scores, with the exception of psychiatric symptoms. Most importantly perhaps, at the end of treatment, the groups differed significantly on measures of social functioning and social adjustment, including vocational and interpersonal effectiveness, instrumental task performance, and adjustment to disability. In an effort to disentangle relevant patient variables associated with treatment efficacy, the authors report that when the sample was divided into more versus less chronic patients (those ill for more or less than 15 years), among more chronic patients, CET participants improved more than EST participants only on measures of reaction time, whereas for the less chronic patients, group differences were observed on several of the assessed domains, including social functioning, suggesting that CET may be particularly helpful to individuals earlier in the course of illness.

In a subsequent report of the durability of CET effects 1 year after the conclusion of treatment (Hogarty, Greenwald, & Eack, 2006), follow-up data were available for close to 90% of the originally randomized sample. Posttreatment CET improvements were maintained on processing speed, cognitive style, social cognition, and social adjustment, and there was evidence that early (first year) improvements in processing speed mediated improvements in social cognition and social adjustment in the CET group. At follow-up, the two groups no longer differed significantly on neurocognition. The authors speculate that this may have been due to participants in both groups receiving stress reduction training, and thereby being better able to regulate stress and perform better on the neurocognitive assessment measures. Perhaps of most interest is that at the follow-up assessment, group differences were noted on several real-world outcomes, including participation in social, recreational, or therapeutic group activities, with 30% of the CET group (vs. only 9% of EST group) engaged in these types of activities. There were also group differences on the proportion of patients engaged in volunteer work (27% for CET and 4% for EST). The groups did not differ on proportions of patients in paid employment. The groups also did not differ on relapse rates, medication compliance, and frequency of treatment visits.

More recent evaluations of CET have examined its efficacy in early-course schizophrenia (Eack et al., 2007). Eighteen individuals who had been diagnosed with schizophrenia within the past 8 years were randomized to CET and 20 to EST. Assessments of emotional intelligence (a construct overlapping considerably with social cognition) were performed at study intake and 1 year into the treatment. Large effect size improvements for the CET group were reported on emotional intelligence, with performance approaching that of healthy control norms. Greatest improvements were noted for domains assessing the abilities to understand, manage, and use emotions to make decisions. A report on the 2-year effects of CET in the same sample (albeit now with a larger total sample size of 58; Eack et al., 2009) indicated that CET was associated with medium effect size improvements on neurocognition and large effect sizes on social cognition, cognitive style, social adjustment, and symptoms. In this early-course sample, CET was not associated with improvements in processing speed; however, the baseline performance of this sample was similar to the end-of-treatment performance of the more chronic sample evaluated in initial studies, and the authors suggest that this may represent a possible ceiling effect due to the relatively preserved processing speed of early-course patients. Similar to the initial CET evaluation with more chronic patients, the authors also report significant between-group differences on real-world outcomes, including social functioning, global adjustment, activities of daily living, instrumental task performance, and employment status.

An examination of employment outcomes in a subsample of 46 of the 58 randomized patients who completed the 2-year intervention (Eack, Hogarty, Greenwald, Hogarty, & Keshavan, 2011) indicated group differences for rates of competitive employment at end of treatment (54% for CET vs. 18% for EST), rates of part-time employment (29% for CET vs. 5% for EST), and weekly earnings ($208 for CET vs. $70 for EST), and a large differential effect size in reported satisfaction with employment, all favoring individuals in CET. An examination of potential predictors of CET effects on employment indicated that social cognitive, as well as neurocognitive, improvements during the treatment predicted likelihood of employment, with individuals who had large (1 standard deviation) improvements in either of these domains three times more likely to be employed at the end of the treatment. An additional analysis of predictors of CET effects on overall functioning (Eack, Pogue-Geile, Greenwald, Hogarty, & Keshavan, 2011) indicated that social cognitive improvements in emotion management and neurocognitive improvements in executive function predicted functional outcomes at the end of the treatment (Lewandowski, Eack, Hogarty, Greenwald, & Keshavan, 2011).

A further 1-year follow-up of this early-course sample (Eack, Greenwald et al., 2010) suggested that CET-associated functional improvements were maintained. Specifically, individuals in the CET condition continued to evidence significant differential effects on social adjustment measures, including social functioning, social leisure activities, major role adjustment, and overall global functioning. Durability of these social adjustment effects appeared to be mediated by neurocognitive improvements (but not social cognitive improvements) during the 2-year active phase of the study. Between-group differences in employment reported at the end of the 2-year treatment were no longer significant, with the rate of employment for the CET group remaining stable from end-of-treatment, and increasing during follow-up for the EST group.

CET has also been reported to be associated with changes in brain morphology (Eack, Hogarty et al., 2010). In a subsample of 53 of the 58 early-course schizophrenia patients described above, magnetic resonance imaging (MRI) assessments were conducted at baseline, 1 year, and 2 years. Comparing regional volume changes between the two groups at the end of treatment, CET seemed to provide a neuroprotective effect against gray matter loss in temporal lobe structures. This attenuated loss was reported to be a significant mediator of CET effects on neurocognitive and social cognitive outcomes at the end of treatment. Although the authors report a lack of group differences in dorsolateral prefrontal cortex volumes—structures frequently associated with neurocognition—they speculate that the lack of group differences in these areas may be due to relatively better preserved neurocognitive functions in early course, as compared to more chronic, schizophrenia samples. Results of between-group differences in gray matter loss should be interpreted with caution, as the authors note that they did not correct for multiple inferences, and no data from healthy controls were available to serve as a baseline of structural development and subsequent changes over time.

Taken together, available research on CET indicates that it is effective for both chronic and early-course schizophrenia, with perhaps some indication that it may be more effective in early-course samples. Comprehensive evaluations of CET effects indicate treatment-associated improvements in a broad range of domains, including neurocognition, social cognition, and real-world functioning, with evidence of some improvements 1 year into the treatment, and evidence that both neurocognitive and social cognitive improvements mediate the benefits of CET on real-world functional outcomes. CET-associated improvements appear durable for at least 1 year after the end of the active intervention.

As with any broad-based treatment, the specific effects of any single treatment component cannot be disentangled from the synergistic effects of combining neurocognitive and social cognitive training. To date, CET has only been evaluated by the research group that developed this treatment, so further evaluations by other groups would inform us of the replicability of these findings, as well as the feasibility of implementing this treatment in other settings. Finally, given the considerable length of the full intervention, there is a need to evaluate whether this treatment will be accepted and tolerated outside of a research setting, in community clinics.

Integrated Neurocognitive Therapy

INT is another broad-based social cognitive treatment, although a relative newcomer to the field. INT is a modification and refinement of the popular IPT, refocusing the treatment to specifically align with the National Institute of Mental Health (NIMH) Measurement and Treatment Research to Improve Cognition in Schizophrenia (MATRICS)-defined neurocognitive and social cognitive domains (Roder & Mueller, 2009; Roder et al., 2010). INT includes both computerized exercises, as well as cognitive-behavioral group sessions and homework assignments meant to promote generalization of training to real-world functioning. Neurocognitive training focuses on processing speed, learning and memory, executive functions, and working memory, whereas social cognitive training focuses on emotion perception, social perception, social schema, and attributional style. Sessions begin with a discussion of patients' individual resources and how they can be maximized, along with psychoeducation on specific module topics. In subsequent sessions, both compensatory and restorative strategies are evaluated and practiced, making this treatment a combination of bottom-up and top-down approaches (Mueller & Roder, 2010).

The feasibility and preliminary efficacy of INT is currently being evaluated in an international, eight-site randomized trial being conducted in Germany, Austria, and Switzerland. To date, 169 outpatients with schizophrenia have been randomized to INT or TAU. Forty-five hours of INT training was administered over 15 weeks. Comprehensive assessments of neurocognition, social cognition, and functioning were conducted at study intake, end of the active phase, and 1-year from study intake (37 weeks after completion of active phase). Although final study results have yet to be reported, preliminary analyses (Mueller, Schmidt, & Roder, 2011) indicate good treatment tolerability, with nearly 90% of randomized patients remaining in the treatment and attending more than 80% of INT sessions. Compared to TAU, INT led to improvements in neurocognition, symptoms, functioning, and social cognition, with some indication that treatment gains were maintained or even enhanced at the follow-up assessment. There is also evidence that social cognition and negative symptoms may mediate the relationship between neurocognition and functional outcomes in INT participants (Roder, 2010). However, the empirical evaluation of INT is still at a very early phase, and numerous other trials will need to be conducted to assess the treatment's feasibility, efficacy, durability, and generalizability before any conclusions can be reached.

Social Cognition and Interaction Training

SCIT is an example of a comprehensive, manualized, group-based treatment developed to target a full range of social cognitive deficits present in schizophrenia, including affect recognition, attributional style, and ToM (Penn et al., 2007). SCIT is a combination of cognitive-behavioral therapy and social skill training approaches, with a focus on active social processes. Techniques used throughout SCIT include psychoeducation, guided problem solving, Socratic questioning, and discussion shaping.

Initial manual development for the SCIT intervention began in 2003, followed by small, uncontrolled inpatient feasibility trials that have recently progressed to larger outpatient trials. In the first uncontrolled inpatient feasibility trial (Penn et al., 2005), seven individuals with chronic psychotic illness who were also identified as having difficulties interacting with others were referred to the study by state hospital treatment teams. Pre–post intervention analyses indicated significant, medium-large effect size improvement in ToM, trend-level medium effect size improvements in attributional bias, and no change in affect recognition. The SCIT intervention then underwent modification to increase the training components focusing on emotion training. In the second inpatient trial (Combs et al., 2007), 18 forensic inpatients self-selected to be in the SCIT group and were compared to 10 inpatients enrolled in a standard coping skills group. Adherence to both treatments was good (96% for SCIT, 90% for coping group), although that may have been at least in part due to the inpatient status of the sample. Relative to the coping skills control group, individuals in SCIT improved on all administered social cognitive measures, including affect recognition, ToM, and attributional bias. SCIT participants also improved their scores on social engagement and social interactions indices, although these were self-report measures and should be interpreted with caution. Finally, SCIT participants evidenced a decline in aggressive incidents on the ward, computed for the 3-month interval before the start of and after the end of the group. The above group differences remained significant after controlling for potential change in symptomatology over the course of the intervention, suggesting that they likely reflect the effects of the treatment, and not just concomitant symptom improvement.

The durability and generalizability of SCIT effects 6 months following the end of treatment was investigated in the same sample of 18 forensic inpatients (Combs et al., 2009). Since data were not available for the 10 inpatients from the original study who participated in the coping group, a new cohort of 18 nonpsychiatric community controls was recruited. At follow-up, although affect recognition and social engagement and interactions scores significantly decreased from end-of-treatment, they were still significantly better than at baseline and, most importantly, not meaningfully different from the scores of community controls. Data on generalization of effects at 6-month follow-up were mixed, with social skills performance similar to that of the community controls, but performance on a novel affect recognition measure was lower than that of the controls.

In the first outpatient quasi-experimental trial of SCIT (Roberts & Penn, 2009), 31 individuals with schizophrenia spectrum diagnoses were recruited from an outpatient psychiatry department. Although 20 of them were assigned to SCIT, the remainder (who either declined to be in the group, had a scheduling conflict, or had participated in other studies with this research group) were assigned to a TAU condition. Both intent-to-treat and completer analyses were conducted. Fourteen of the 20 SCIT participants were categorized as completers (attended more than 50% of sessions with at least two from each module). SCIT group attendance rate for the completers subgroup averaged 82% of the sessions, whereas for the entire SCIT sample it was 64%. For completer analyses, participants in SCIT improved significantly more on affect recognition and social skills performance, with medium to large within-group effect sizes. There was a trend-level effect for a secondary ToM measure, but no significant improvement on primary measures of ToM nor attributional style. When the analyses were repeated for the sample as a whole, as may be expected, the results were attenuated, with improvements in social skills performance dropping to trend level. It should be noted, however, that this sample had a pretreatment ceiling effect on the primary ToM measure and normal-range pretreatment attributional bias scores, making it less likely that change on the assessment battery would occur.

Recently, the transportability, feasibility, and acceptability of SCIT was evaluated in three outpatient rehabilitation centers providing services to individuals with serious and persistent mental illness (Roberts, Penn, Labate, Margolis, & Sterne, 2010). The sites were unaffiliated with the developers of SCIT. Graduate- or master's-level rehabilitation center clinicians with an average of 8 years of experience working with the study population administered the SCIT groups after having read the manual, participated in a training workshop, and consulted with treatment developers. Clinicians also participated in weekly supervision calls with treatment developers. SCIT was offered as an adjunct to existing interventions, and no effort was made to restrict group composition, resulting in a mixed sample of individuals with psychotic, affective, and other disorders. Since no research staff was available to conduct comprehensive pre–post social cognitive assessments, commonly used instruments were modified for group administration and training provided to clinicians in how to administer these measures in the context of the group sessions.

Of the 50 SCIT participants who completed baseline assessments, 38 completed the training (although only 34 completed posttreatment assessments), with 11 dropping out during the first three sessions. Available data from study completers indicate that, on average, they attended approximately 69% of the sessions. More than 90% reported that they found the group useful and that it helped them think about social situations and relate to other people. Participants who completed both pre- and post-assessments improved significantly on affect recognition and ToM, but not on a measure of attributional bias. Clinicians administering the intervention reported that they found the SCIT manual helpful, and that they believed the treatment would aid their clients in improving social cognition and subsequent social interactions. At the end of the transportability trial, two of the three rehabilitation centers elected to continue to provide the SCIT group as part of standard programming, whereas the third was unable to do so due to staffing issues.

Recently, the first randomized controlled trial of a modified SCIT intervention has also been published (Tas, Danaci, Cubukcuoglu & Brune, 2012). Although the original SCIT intervention encourages group participants to identify a "practice partner" with whom they can practice some of the skills learned in the group, in this SCIT adaptation, referred to as family-assisted SCIT (F-SCIT), a specific family member or close friend was included as a social cognition practice partner. This individual received four sessions of education and training, including an overview of social cognition and the SCIT intervention; information about the relationship among thoughts, feelings, and actions; information on how individuals learn from observation; and information on the importance of positive reinforcement and realistic goals/expectations for group participants. F-SCIT was also modified from the original by adding an individual session focusing on integration and transfer of learning material to everyday situations, and condensing the number of sessions to 14, with only three of those sessions specifically targeting emotion perception. Finally, since the study was conducted in Turkey, some of the original SCIT stimuli were modified to better apply to this population.

Data from 19 individuals who participated in F-SCIT and 29 individuals randomized to a "social stimulation" active control condition were very positive, indicating improvements on a range of proximal and distal outcomes. Significant differences, with medium to large between-group effect sizes, were observed for clinician-rated social functioning, symptoms, and quality of life. There were also medium to large between-group effects for several social cognitive tasks, including those measuring emotion perception, ToM, empathy, and reasoning. No significant between-group differences were observed for social perception or attributional bias. Although the results of this study are probably among the most encouraging of the SCIT trials to date, the generalizability of the family-assisted modification to other countries and cultures is uncertain—although the majority of patients in this Turkish study lived with their families and therefore likely had at least moderate family social support, this may not be the case in some other countries, including in the United States, where many individuals with chronic schizophrenia live alone or in supported housing and have limited contact with family members.

The efficacy of SCIT has also been evaluated in several other psychiatric populations. A 2008 feasibility trial (Turner-Brown, Perry, Dichter, Bodfish, & Penn, 2008) evaluated the efficacy of a modified SCIT intervention (SCIT-A) in improving social cognitive impairments in adults with high-functioning autism. SCIT was modified to emphasize distinctions between expressions of interest/disinterest and distinctions between relevant versus irrelevant social facts. Videotaped examples of social situations used throughout SCIT were also modified to better approximate the types of social challenges encountered by adults with high-functioning autism. Of the 13 individuals initially referred to the study, 11 were either randomized or assigned to SCIT-A or usual treatment (two individuals originally randomized to SCIT-A did not want to participate in the group, so were reassigned to the control condition). Five of the six SCIT-A participants reported that they found the groups useful, and, in general, participants reported that they liked the focus of the groups, although would have liked them to have been longer and wished they had had more occasions to practice skills taught during groups. SCIT-A participants improved significantly on a measure of affect recognition and at a trend-level on a questionnaire of social communication skills, although there were no group differences on actual social skills performance or ToM. This preliminary investigation suggests that SCIT-A may improve social cognitive performance in adults with high-functioning autism, and a larger, more rigorous evaluation of SCIT-A is currently under way.

In a 2010 report of the efficacy of SCIT in individuals with schizotypal features (Chan et al., 2010), 40 college students with high schizotypy ratings were randomly assigned to either SCIT or a no-treatment control. SCIT was again modified, this time so that examples of social situations were more appropriate for a nonpsychiatric sample of students from mainland China. Although no ratings of social cognition were administered, self-report ratings of general mental and physical health, along with social functioning, were collected at intake, end of treatment, and 3-month follow-up. There were no pre–post differences on outcome measures between groups; however, at 3-month follow-up, individuals in SCIT improved on self-reported somatic symptoms, anxiety, insomnia, and social dysfunction. This study suggests that SCIT may have an effect on general symptoms in individuals with schizotypy, but these results clearly need to be interpreted with caution, as all are based on self-report.

Finally, preliminary results of a just-completed controlled trial of SCIT in individuals with bipolar disorder suggest that the training may be associated with improvements in emotion perception in this population (Guillermo Lahera, personal communication).

A total of five studies have evaluated the efficacy of SCIT in schizophrenia spectrum, with an additional three studies examining its effects in other psychiatric populations. Overall, treatment-related gains in affect recognition are clear in the majority of studies that assessed this domain of social cognition. Effects on ToM are not as uniform across studies, and there is little indication that SCIT improves attributional bias, although this may at least in part be due to choice of assessment measures.

To date, there has been only one published randomized controlled trial evaluating the efficacy of a modified SCIT intervention in schizophrenia patients, and the quasi-experimental studies that have been conducted have been limited by small samples, relatively small assessment batteries lacking real-world outcomes, and little evaluation of the long-term maintenance of SCIT-associated improvements. Initial data on the feasibility of incorporating SCIT into community settings are promising, but require replication, with more rigorous assessments of treatment fidelity and pre–post social cognitive and functional changes.

Metacognitive Therapy

The aim of the targeted MCT treatment is to teach participants about cognitive biases, their negative consequences, and their relationship to psychotic symptoms, and to provide corrective experiences that will weaken patients' conviction in the accuracy of their sometimes faulty reasoning processes (Moritz & Woodward, 2007b). Although similar to cognitive-behavioral therapy for psychosis (CBTp) in its focus on reasoning biases, unlike CBTp, which targets conviction in individual delusions, MCT takes what has been referred to as a "backdoor approach" and instead focuses on the "metacognitive infrastructure," or general types of reasoning errors that are presumed to be related to the formation and maintenance of delusions, including attributional bias, jumping to conclusions (JTC) bias, bias against disconfirmatory evidence, ToM impairments, overconfidence in memory errors, and depressive cognitive patterns. Each of these biases is addressed in a series of eight MCT modules, offered in an open group format. To date, MCT has been evaluated by a number of different research groups in several countries.

In one of the first reports on the safety, acceptance, and feasibility of MCT (Moritz & Woodward, 2007a), 40 outpatients with schizophrenia spectrum diagnoses were randomly assigned to 4 weeks of twice-weekly MCT sessions or computerized cognitive remediation using CogPack. Adherence to MCT was high, with, on average, MCT participants missing fewer than one of the eight sessions, although this was not statistically different from adherence to the active control intervention. Acceptance of the treatment was significantly higher for the MCT group, however, who rated the treatment as more fun, more likely to be recommended to others, less boring, and more useful to daily life.

In a subsequent study, the efficacy of several of the MCT reasoning exercises was evaluated in 34 individuals with high conviction in current delusions (Ross, Freeman, Dunn, & Garety, 2011). Participants were randomly assigned to a single session of either reasoning training or an attentional control. Between-group analyses indicated that, compared to controls, individuals undergoing the reasoning training increased the amount of data they needed in order to draw conclusions, suggesting an attenuation in the JTC bias. However, the overall rate of individuals with a JTC bias in the treatment group remained the same, indicating that average group improvement was driven by individuals who did not have a severe JTC bias, and suggesting that a longer, more intensive treatment may be necessary to successfully remediate significant JTC biases.

Evaluations of the efficacy of a full eight-session course of MCT suggest that this more intensive treatment may in fact lead to some reductions in not only JTC but, in some cases, also in positive symptoms. Aghotor and colleagues (Aghotor, Pfueller, Moritz, Weisbrod, & Roesch-Ely, 2010) randomly assigned 30 inpatients with schizophrenia spectrum diagnoses and either past or current delusions to 4 weeks of twice-weekly MCT or a newspaper discussion group. Adherence to MTC was high, and participants reported that they felt they were successful in the training and that they were willing to recommend it to others. Although the sample size was too small to obtain statistically significant group differences, MCT was associated with medium between-group effect sizes on positive symptoms and small effects sizes on JTC bias. In another evaluation of the efficacy of eight sessions of MCT in improving positive symptoms, Kumar and colleagues (Kumar et al., 2010) randomly assigned 16 recently admitted inpatients to MCT or TAU. As can be expected when newly admitted patients are stabilized, both groups improved somewhat on assessed measures. Between-group analyses were underpowered to detect significant interactions; however, medium to large effect size differences were noted for improvement in positive symptoms and belief conviction, favoring the MCT group, and the degree of positive symptom reduction in the MCT group (28%) was more than twice that in the TAU group (12.9%). In a related study, Moritz Kerstan and colleagues (Moritz et al., 2011) examined

MCT efficacy in a sample of 36 stabilized although chronic patients (about half of whom met remission criteria). As can be expected from such a low symptom sample, there were no changes in symptomatology over the course of the intervention. Compared to a wait-list control, participants randomized to MCT improved significantly in delusional distress, memory, and quality of social relationships. Although not statistically significant, there was also a medium within-group effect size improvement in JTC bias for the MCT group.

There are also several anecdotal or unpublished reports evaluating MCT. These reports suggest that the treatment does in fact lead participants to become more aware of their reasoning biases, reduce their tendency to jump to conclusions, and increase the likelihood of considering alternative hypotheses (Gaweda, Moritz, & Kokoszka, 2009). They also suggest that even a single session of MCT can lead to reductions in JTC, paranoid thoughts, and delusional conviction, and improve the quality of social life (Moritz et al., 2011; Moritz & Woodward, 2007b).

Based on clinical experience with patients who deny the presence of even objectively measured cognitive biases, the authors of MCT recently developed an individualized metacognitive training program for individuals with psychosis (MCT+) that focuses on the same reasoning biases as addressed in the original MCT, but tailors content to specific individuals and adds a session on relapse prevention. A combination of MCT followed by MCT+ was recently compared to eight sessions of computerized cognitive training (Moritz, Veckenstedt, Randjbar, Vitzthum, & Woodward, 2011) in a sample of 48 inpatients with schizophrenia spectrum who were randomly assigned to one of the treatments. Compared to the active control, MCT/MCT+ participants rated the training more favorably, and indicated that they found it important and useful, and that they were more likely to apply it in everyday life. Significant group differences were reported for delusions, positive symptoms, and delusional conviction. There was also indication that, compared to the active control group, individuals in MCT/MCT+ significantly decreased in JTC bias. Effect sizes were in the medium range.

In summary, MCT has been evaluated in a number of different countries, although with mostly inpatient populations. It appears that although single-session administrations of select training materials are associated with some increase in data gathering and a reduction of the JTC bias, these improvements are strengthened when a full course of MCT is administered. There is also evidence that MCT is associated with decreases in delusional conviction and positive symptoms. Although encouraging, most of the published reports included small participant samples, and whereas medium effect size differences were reported for many of the assessed domains, these differences often failed to reach statistical significance. Future randomized trials of MCT will need to evaluate this treatment in larger, outpatient samples, in the context of a time-matched active control. Additional studies are also necessary to evaluate the generalizability of MCT to multiple social functioning measures, as well as the durability of treatment gains. Finally, mediator and moderator analyses will help us better understand MCT's mechanisms of action.

CONCLUSION

In the past two decades, much work has been done on the development of social cognitive interventions for individuals with psychosis. Although early proof-of-concept studies showed that social cognitive deficits in psychosis are malleable, more intensive treatments have attempted to address the full range of social cognitive deficits, as well as determine whether their improvement does in fact lead to better social functioning. Overall, a review of existing studies suggests that various domains of social cognition can be improved, and that these improvements may generalize to more distal outcomes. This is in part consistent with a recent meta-analysis of the efficacy of controlled social cognitive treatments, which indicates medium to large effect sizes on affect perception and small to medium effect sizes on ToM, but no significant effects on the handful of evaluated studies that targeted social perception and attributional bias (Kurtz & Richardson, 2011). Although this work is encouraging, much more remains to be done.

Of the treatments reviewed here, IPT has the largest and most rigorous evidence base supporting its efficacy. Many of the studies evaluating the other treatments were poorly controlled, had small samples, used brief and narrow assessment batteries, did not include measures of social functioning, and did not examine the durability of training effects. Assuming that the early positive results from these studies can be replicated in larger, more comprehensive and rigorous trials (performed by researchers unaffiliated with the developers of the treatments), many of these treatments may also require significant alteration to make their delivery feasible and acceptable in community treatment settings.

Additionally, although the majority of studies that target affect recognition have met with at least some success, there is much less of a research base to indicate that the relatively few existing treatments targeting "higher order" components of social cognition, including social perception, attributional style, and ToM, are efficacious. Future researchers will need to focus their efforts on modifying existing or developing new interventions to effectively target these arguably more complex components of social cognition. Potential treatment paradigms can be adapted from laboratory studies conducted outside the field of schizophrenia research. For example, Mathews and colleagues (Grey & Mathews 2000; Mathews & Mackintosh, 2000; Yiend, Mackintosh, & Mathews, 2005) have shown that negative interpretive biases can be experimentally induced in healthy controls. These types of experimental manipulations can be used to inform the design of complementary interventions aimed at reducing attributional biases in individuals with psychosis.

There is great heterogeneity in the treatments examined so far, and, to date, their mechanisms of action are poorly understood. In addition to disentangling the active ingredients of these treatments, future researchers will also need to determine the most appropriate and efficacious methods for the delivery of these treatments. Moreover, there is evidence that variables such as duration of illness, age, education, and inpatient versus outpatient status may mediate the efficacy of social cognitive treatments (Kurtz & Richardson, 2011), so these and other patient and treatment characteristics will need to be carefully assessed and examined in future evaluations of social cognitive treatments and their efficacy in order to best match treatments to individuals.

Finally, as noted by several other researchers (Green et al., 2008; Horan, Kern, Green, & Penn, 2008; Horan et al., 2011; Kurtz & Richardson, 2011), much more emphasis needs to be placed on the outcome measures used in treatment evaluation studies. Many of the measures employed have had unknown or questionable psychometric properties, and, in numerous cases, only a single measure was used as a proxy for each social cognitive domain. A more in-depth analysis of the psychometric properties of the various social cognitive measures and their appropriateness for clinical trials with psychosis may reveal that it is not only the specific treatment, but how its efficacy is assessed, that requires modification.

REFERENCES

Aghotor, J., Pfueller, U., Moritz, S., Weisbrod, M., & Roesch-Ely, D. (2010). Metacognitive training for patients with schizophrenia (MCT): Feasibility and preliminary evidence for its efficacy. *Journal of Behavior Therapy and Experimental Psychiatry, 41*, 207–211.

Bell, M., Bryson, G., Greig, T., Corcoran, C., & Wexler, B. E. (2001). Neurocognitive enhancement therapy with work therapy: Effects on neuropsychological test performance. *Archives of General Psychiatry, 58*(8), 763–768.

Bell, M., Fiszdon, J., Greig, T., Wexler, B., & Bryson, G. (2007). Neurocognitive enhancement therapy with work therapy in schizophrenia: 6-month follow-up of neuropsychological performance. *Journal of Rehabilitation Research & Development, 44*(5), 761–770.

Bell, M. D., Zito, W., Greig, T., & Wexler, B. E. (2008). Neurocognitive enhancement therapy with vocational services: Work outcomes at two-year follow-up. *Schizophrenia Research, 105*(1–3), 18–29.

Bellack, A. S., & Hersen, M. (1979). *Research and practice in social skills training.* New York: Plenum Press.

Bowie, C. R., & Harvey, P. D. (2005). Cognition in schizophrenia: Impairments, determinants, and functional importance. *Psychiatric Clinics of North America, 28*(3), 613–633.

Brekke, J., Kay, D. D., Lee, K. S., & Green, M. F. (2005). Biosocial pathways to functional outcome in schizophrenia. *Schizophrenia Research, 80*(2–3), 213–225.

Brekke, J. S., Hoe, M., Long, J., & Green, M. F. (2007). How neurocognition and social cognition influence functional change during community-based psychosocial rehabilitation for individuals with schizophrenia. *Schizophrenia Bulletin, 33*(5), 1247–1256.

Chan, R. C. K., Gao, X. -J., Li, X. -Y., Li, H. -H., Cui, J. -F., Deng, Y. -Y., et al. (2010). The Social Cognition and Interaction Training (SCIT): An extension to individuals with schizotypal personality features. *Psychiatry Research, 178*, 208–210.

Choi, K. H., & Kwon, J. H. (2006). Social cognition enhancement training for schizophrenia: A preliminary randomized controlled trial. *Community Mental Health Journal, 42*(2), 177–187.

Combs, D. R., Adams, S. D., Penn, D. L., Roberts, D., Tiegreen, J., & Stem, P. (2007). Social Cognition and Interaction Training (SCIT) for inpatients with schizophrenia spectrum disorders: Preliminary findings. *Schizophrenia Research, 91*(1–3), 112–116.

Combs, D. R., Elerson, K., Penn, D. L., Tiegreen, J. A., Nelson, A., Ledet, S. N., et al. (2009). Stability and generalization of Social Cognition and Interaction Training (SCIT) for schizophrenia: Six-month follow-up results. *Schizophrenia Research, 112*(1–3), 196–197.

Combs, D. R., Tosheva, A., Penn, D. L., Basso, M. R., Wanner, J. L., & Laib, K. (2008). Attentional-shaping as a means to improve emotion perception deficits in schizophrenia. *Schizophrenia Research, 105*(1–3), 68–77.

Corrigan, P. W., Hirschbeck, J. N., & Wolfe, M. (1995). Memory and vigilance training to improve social perception in schizophrenia. *Schizophrenia Research, 17*(3), 257–265.

Eack, S. M., Greenwald, D. P., Hogarty, S. S., Cooley, S. J., DiBarry, A. L., Montrose, D. M., et al. (2009). Cognitive enhancement therapy for early-course schizophrenia: Effects of a two-year randomized controlled trial. *Psychiatric Services, 60*(11), 1468–1476.

Eack, S. M., Greenwald, D. P., Hogarty, S. S., & Keshavan, M. S. (2010). One-year durability of the effects of cognitive enhancement therapy on functional outcome in early schizophrenia. *Schizophrenia Research, 120*(1–3), 210–216.

Eack, S. M., Hogarty, G. E., Cho, R. Y., Prasad, K. M., Greenwald, D. P., Hogarty, S. S., et al. (2010). Neuroprotective effects of cognitive enhancement therapy against gray matter loss in early schizophrenia: Results from a 2-year randomized controlled trial. *Archives of General Psychiatry, 67*(7), 674–682.

Eack, S. M., Hogarty, G. E., Greenwald, D. P., Hogarty, S. S., & Keshavan, M. S. (2011). Effects of Cognitive Enhancement Therapy on employment outcomes in early schizophrenia: Results from a 2-year randomized trial. *Research on Social Work Practice, 21*(1), 32–42.

Eack, S. M., Hogarty, G. E., Greenwald, D. P., Hogarty, S. S., & Keshavan, M. S. (2007). Cognitive enhancement therapy improves emotional intelligence in early course schizophrenia: Preliminary effects. *Schizophrenia Research, 89*(1–3), 308–311.

Eack, S. M., Pogue- Geile, M. F., Greenwald, D. P., Hogarty, S. S., & Keshavan, M. S. (2011). Mechanisms of functional improvement in a 2–year trial of cognitive enhancement therapy for early schizophrenia. *Psychological Medicine, 41*(6), 1253–1261.

Frommann, N., Streit, M., & Wolwer, W. (2003). Remediation of facial affect recognition impairments in patients with schizophrenia: A new training program. *Psychiatry Research, 117*(3), 281–284.

Gaweda, L., Moritz, S., & Kokoszka, A. (2009). [The metacognitive training for schizophrenia patients: Description of method and experiences from clinical practice]. *Psychiatria Polska, 43*(6), 683–692.

Green, M. F. (1996). What are the functional consequences of neurocognitive deficits in schizophrenia? *American Journal of Psychiatry, 153*(3), 321–330.

Green, M. F., Kern, R. S., Braff, D. L., & Mintz, J. (2000). Neurocognitive deficits and functional outcome in schizophrenia: Are we measuring the "right stuff"? *Schizophrenia Bulletin, 26*(1), 119–136.

Green, M. F., Penn, D. L., Bentall, R., Carpenter, W. T., Gaebel, W., Gur, R. C., et al. (2008). Social cognition in schizophrenia: An NIMH workshop on definitions, assessment, and research opportunities. *Schizophrenia Bulletin, 34*(6), 1211–1220.

Grey, S., & Mathews, A. (2000). Effects of training on interpretation of emotional ambiguity. *Quarterly Journal of Experimental Psychology A, 53*(4), 1143–1162.

Habel, U., Koch, K., Kellermann, T., Reske, M., Frommann, N., Wolwer, W., et al. (2010). Training of affect recognition in schizophrenia: Neurobiological correlates. *Social Neuroscience, 5*(1), 92–104.

Heinssen, R. K., Liberman, R. P., & Kopelowicz, A. (2000). Psychosocial skills training for schizophrenia: Lessons from the laboratory. *Schizophrenia Bulletin, 26*(1), 21–46.

Hogarty, G. E., & Flesher, S. (1999a). Developmental theory for a cognitive enhancement therapy of schizophrenia. *Schizophrenia Bulletin, 25*(4), 677–692.

Hogarty, G. E., & Flesher, S. (1999b). Practice principles of cognitive enhancement therapy for schizophrenia. *Schizophrenia Bulletin, 25*(4), 693–708.

Hogarty, G. E., Flesher, S., Ulrich, R., Carter, M., Greenwald, D., Pogue-Geile, M., et al. (2004). Cognitive enhancement therapy for schizophrenia: Effects of a 2-year randomized trial on cognition and behavior. *Archives of General Psychiatry, 61*(9), 866–876.

Hogarty, G. E., Greenwald, D. P., & Eack, S. M. (2006). Durability and mechanism of effects of cognitive enhancement therapy. *Psychiatric Services, 57*(12), 1751–1757.

Horan, W. P., Kern, R. S., Green, M. F., & Penn, D. L. (2008). Social cognition training for schizophrenia: Emerging evidence. *American Journal of Psychiatric Rehabilitation, 11*(3), 205–252.

Horan, W. P., Kern, R. S., Shokat-Fadai, K., Sergi, M. J., Wynn, J. K., & Green, M. F. (2009). Social cognitive skills training in schizophrenia: An initial efficacy study of stabilized outpatients. *Schizophrenia Research, 107*(1), 47–54.

Horan, W. P., Kern, R. S., Tripp, C., Hellemann, G., Wynn, J. K., Bell, M., et al. (2011). Efficacy and specificity of social cognitive skills training for outpatients with psychotic disorders. *Journal of Psychiatric Research, 45*(8), 1113–1122.

Kayser, N., Sarfati, Y., Besche, C., & Hardy-Bayle, M. C. (2006). Elaboration of a rehabilitation method based on a pathogenetic hypothesis of "theory of mind" impairment in schizophrenia. *Neuropsychological Rehabilitation, 16*(1), 83–95.

Kern, R. S., Glynn, S. M., Horan, W. P., & Marder, S. R. (2009). Psychosocial treatments to promote functional recovery in schizophrenia. *Schizophrenia Bulletin, 35*(2), 347–361.

Krabbendam, L., & Aleman, A. (2003). Cognitive rehabilitation in schizophrenia: A quantitative analysis of controlled studies. *Psychopharmacology, 169*(3–4), 376–382.

Kumar, D., Zia, U. I., Haq, M., Dubey, I., Dotiwala, K., Siddiqui, S. V., et al. (2010). Effects of meta-cognitive training in the reduction of positive symptoms in schizophrenia. *European Journal of Psychotherapy and Counseling, 12*, 149–158.

Kurtz, M. M., Moberg, P. J., Gur, R. C., & Gur, R. E. (2001). Approaches to cognitive remediation of neuropsychological deficits in schizophrenia: A review and meta-analysis. *Neuropsychology Review, 11*(4), 197–210.

Kurtz, M. M., & Mueser, K. T. (2008). A meta-analysis of controlled research on social skills training for schizophrenia. *Journal of Consulting & Clinical Psychology, 76*(3), 491–504.

Kurtz, M. M., & Richardson, C. L. (2011). Social cognitive training for schizophrenia: A meta-analytic investigation of controlled research. *Schizophrenia Bulletin* [Advance Access published April 27, 2011], doi: 10.1093/schbul/sbr036.

Lecardeur, L., Stip, E., Giguere, M., Blouin, G., Rodriguez, J. P., & Champagne-Lavau, M. (2009). Effects of cognitive remediation therapies on psychotic symptoms and cognitive complaints in patients with schizophrenia and related disorders: A randomized study. *Schizophrenia Research, 111*(1–3), 153–158.

Lewandowski, K. E., Eack, S. M., Hogarty, S. S., Greenwald, D. P., & Keshavan, M. S. (2011). Is cognitive enhancement therapy equally effective for patients with schizophrenia and schizoaffective disorder? *Schizophrenia Research, 125*, 291–294.

Liberman, R. P. (2008). *Recovery from disability: Manual of psychiatric rehabilitation.* Washington, DC: American Psychiatric Publishing, Inc.

Mathews, A., & Mackintosh, B. (2000). Induced emotional interpretation bias and anxiety. *Journal of Abnormal Psychology, 109*(4), 602–615.

Mazza, M., Lucci, G., Pacitti, F., Pino, M. C., Mariano, M., Casacchia, M., et al. (2010). Could schizophrenic subjects improve their social cognition abilities only with observation and imitation of social situations? *Neuropsychological Rehabilitation, 20*(5), 675–703.

McGurk, S. R., Twamley, E. W., Sitzer, D. I., McHugo, G. J., & Mueser, K. T. (2007). A meta-analysis of cognitive remediation in schizophrenia. *American Journal of Psychiatry, 164*(12), 1791–1802.

McGurk, S. R., & Wykes, T. (2008). Cognitive remediation and vocational rehabilitation. *Psychiatric Rehabilitation Journal, 31*(4), 350–359.

Moritz, S., Kerstan, A., Veckenstedt, R., Randjbar, S., Vitzthum, F., Schmidt, C., et al. (2011). Further evidence for the efficacy of a metacognitive group training in schizophrenia. *Behaviour Research & Therapy, 49*(3), 151–157.

Moritz, S., Veckenstedt, R., Randjbar, F., Vitzthum, F., & Woodward, T. S. (2011). Antipsychotic treatment beyond antipsychotics: Metacognitive intervention for schizophrenia patients improves delusional symptoms. *Psychological Medicine, 41*(9), 1823–1832.

Moritz, S., & Woodward, T. S. (2007a). Metacognitive Training for schizophrenia patients (MCT): A pilot study on feasibility, treatment adherence, and subjective efficacy. *German Journal of Psychiatry, 10*(3), 69–78.

Moritz, S., & Woodward, T. S. (2007b). Metacognitive training in schizophrenia: From basic research to knowledge translation and intervention. *Current Opinion in Psychiatry, 20*(6), 619–625.

Mueller, D. R., & Roder, V. (2010). Integrated Psychological Therapy (IPT) and Integrated Neurocognitive Therapy (INT). In V. Roder & A. Medalia (Eds.), *Understanding and treating neuro- and social cognition in schizophrenia patients* (pp. 118–144). Basel, CH: Karger.

Mueller, D. R., Schmidt, S. J., & Roder, V. (2011). Integrated Neurocognitive Therapy (INT): Final results of an international RCT including a 1–year follow-up. *Schizophrenia Bulletin, 37*(Suppl. 1), 316.

Penn, D., Roberts, D. L., Munt, E. D., Silverstein, E., Jones, N., & Sheitman, B. (2005). A pilot study of social cognition and interaction training (SCIT) for schizophrenia. *Schizophrenia Research, 80*(2–3), 357–359.

Penn, D. L., & Combs, D. (2000). Modification of affect perception deficits in schizophrenia. *Schizophrenia Research, 46*(2–3), 217.

Penn, D. L., Roberts, D. L., Combs, D., & Sterne, A. (2007). Best practices: The development of the social cognition and interaction training program for schizophrenia spectrum disorders. *Psychiatric Services, 58*(4), 449–451.

Roberts, D. L., & Penn, D. L. (2009). Social cognition and interaction training (SCIT) for outpatients with schizophrenia: A preliminary study. *Psychiatry Research, 166*(2–3), 141–147.

Roberts, D. L., Penn, D. L., Labate, D., Margolis, S. A., & Sterne, A. (2010). Transportability and feasibility of Social Cognition And Interaction Training (SCIT) in community settings. *Behavioural & Cognitive Psychotherapy, 38*(1), 35–47.

Roder, V. (2010). Integrated Neurocognitive Therapy: A group based approach to improve neuro- and social cognition *Schizophrenia Research, 117*, 143–144.

Roder, V., & Mueller, D. R. (2009). Remediation of neuro and social cognition: Results of an international randomized multi-cite study. *Schizophrenia Bulletin, 35*(Suppl. 1), 353–354.

Roder, V., Mueller, D. R., Brenner, H. D., & Spaulding, W. D. (2010). *Integrated Psychological Therapy (IPT) for the treatment of neurocognition, social cognition, and social competency in schizophrenia patients.* Cambridge, MA: Hogrefe Publishing.

Roder, V., Mueller, D. R., Mueser, K. T., & Brenner, H. D. (2006). Integrated Psychological Therapy (IPT) for schizophrenia: Is it effective? *Schizophrenia Bulletin, 32*(Suppl. 1), S81–S93.

Roncone, R., Mazza, M., Frangou, I., De Risio, A., Ussorio, D., Tozzini, C., et al. (2004). Rehabilitation of theory of mind deficit in schizophrenia: A pilot study of metacognitive strategies in group treatment. *Neuropsychological Rehabilitation, 14*(4), 421–435.

Ross, K., Freeman, D., Dunn, G., & Garety, P. (2011). A randomized experimental investigation of reasoning training for people with delusions. *Schizophrenia Bulletin, 37*(2), 324–333.

Russell, T. A., Chu, E., & Phillips, M. L. (2006). A pilot study to investigate the effectiveness of emotion recognition remediation in schizophrenia using the micro-expression training tool. *British Journal of Clinical Psychology, 45*(Pt. 4), 579–583.

Sarfati, Y., Passerieux, C., & Hardy-Bayle, M. (2000). Can verbalization remedy the theory of mind deficit in schizophrenia? *Psychopathology, 33*(5), 246–251.

Sergi, M. J., Rassovsky, Y., Nuechterlein, K. H., & Green, M. F. (2006). Social perception as a mediator of the influence of early visual processing on functional status in schizophrenia. *American Journal of Psychiatry, 163*(3), 448–454.

Silver, H., Goodman, C., Knoll, G., & Isakov, V. (2004). Brief emotion training improves recognition of facial emotions in chronic schizophrenia. A pilot study. *Psychiatry Research, 128*(2), 147–154.

Tas, C., Danaci, A.E., Cubukcuoglu, Z., & Brune, M. (2012). Impact of family involvement on social cognition training in clinically stable outpatients with schizophrenia—A randomized pilot study, *Psychiatry Research, 195*(1), 32–38.

Turner-Brown, L. M., Perry, T. D., Dichter, G. S., Bodfish, J. W., & Penn, D. L. (2008). Brief report: Feasibility of social cognition and interaction training for adults with high functioning autism. *Journal of Autism & Developmental Disorders, 38*(9), 1777–1784.

Twamley, E. W., Jeste, D. V., & Bellack, A. S. (2003). A review of cognitive training in schizophrenia. *Schizophrenia Bulletin, 29*(2), 359–382.

van der Gaag, M., Kern, R. S., van den Bosch, R. J., & Liberman, R. P. (2002). A controlled trial of cognitive remediation in schizophrenia. *Schizophrenia Bulletin, 28*(1), 167–176.

Wallace, C. J., & Boone, S. E. (1984). Cognitive factors in the social skills of schizophrenic patients: Implications for treatment. In W. Spaulding & J. Cole (Eds.), *Nebraska symposium on motivation* (Vol. 31). Lincoln, NE: University of Nebraska Press.

Wexler, B. E., & Bell, M. D. (2005). Cognitive remediation and vocational rehabilitation for schizophrenia. *Schizophrenia Bulletin, 31*(4), 931–941.

Wolwer, W., & Frommann, N. (2009). The training of affect recognition (TAR): Efficacy, functional specificity and generalization of effects. *Schizophrenia Bulletin, 35*(Suppl. 1), 351.

Wolwer, W., Frommann, N., Halfmann, S., Piaszek, A., Streit, M., & Gaebel, W. (2005). Remediation of impairments in facial affect recognition in schizophrenia: Efficacy and specificity of a new training program. *Schizophrenia Research, 80*(2–3), 295–303.

Wykes, T., & Huddy, V. (2009). Cognitive remediation for schizophrenia: It is even more complicated. *Current Opinion in Psychiatry, 22*(2), 161–167.

Yiend, J., Mackintosh, B., & Mathews, A. (2005). Enduring consequences of experimentally induced biases in interpretation. *Behaviour Research & Therapy, 43*(6), 779–797.

13

Integrated Neurocognitive Therapy

DANIEL R. MUELLER, STEFANIE J. SCHMIDT,
AND VOLKER RODER ■

Integrated Neurocognitive Therapy (INT) for schizophrenia patients represents a further development of Integrated Psychological Therapy (IPT). INT is a comprehensive, integrated, and "broad-based" therapy approach. Its intervention techniques and therapeutic tools were adopted from IPT and were further developed. Therefore, in order to understand the INT intervention, knowledge about IPT is needed. Thirty years ago, IPT was one of the very first comprehensive and manual-driven group therapy approaches for schizophrenia patients. During the last 30 years, it has been established as a standard approach in many countries, especially in Europe. IPT is a "bottom-up" and "top-down" approach, addressing both basic cognitive building blocks and higher order integrative processing. It consists of five subprograms, each with incremental steps. IPT starts with a subprogram addressing the neurocognitive domain, followed by a second subprogram to enhance social cognition. In a third stage, IPT focuses on interpersonal and social context using verbal communication tools, thereby bridging the gap between cognitive and social functioning. Finally, social competence is targeted with exercises to improve social skills (fourth subprogram) and to increase patients' mastery in coping with interpersonal and social problems (fifth subprogram) for more independent living.

The sixth, revised edition of the German IPT manual (Roder, Brenner, & Kienzle, 2008a) is now available, as well as a new, fully updated edition in English (Roder, Mueller, Spaulding, & Brenner, 2010). The manual has been translated into 12 languages, and IPT has been extensively researched. Thirty-six independent evaluation studies have been conducted in 12 countries in Europe, North and South America, and Asia. The data from these studies were recently summarized in a meta-analysis (Roder, Mueller, Mueser, & Brenner, 2006; Roder, Mueller, & Schmidt, 2011; Mueller & Roder, 2008). The results were promising for the proximal outcomes of neurocognition, social cognition, and psychosocial functioning, as well as for the more distal outcome of symptoms after therapy. These effects were maintained at follow-up. Using the complete IPT with all five subprograms generated stronger and longer lasting effects than did single subprograms, even after having controlled for therapy duration.

What We Have Learned from IPT

IPT represents a complete therapy program integrating interventions for many of the key rehabilitation goals of schizophrenia patients. In our opinion, the therapeutic success of IPT is based on the following conceptual and therapeutic strategies and techniques:

1. *IPT is a group therapy approach and therefore strongly supports group processes during treatment.* This seems to be an important requirement for social skills training within a behavioral therapy approach. However, group therapy has been rarely practiced in cognitive remediation therapy.
2. *IPT first targets neurocognition and social cognition before social and interpersonal skills are practiced.* The improvement of cognitive skills during the initial IPT subprograms reduces the rate-limiting impact of basic and social cognition within social skills therapy.
3. *IPT starts with simple exercises, which are clearly structured and thereby allow the patients to become familiar with the social context of the group.* This may be one reason why patients with negative symptoms especially benefit from the initial exercises on neurocognition.
4. *The IPT exercises are highly structured and progress sequentially in incremental steps, beginning with simple and emotionally neutral tasks and ending with complex and partially emotionally loaded tasks.* This didactic structure gives therapists greater flexibility in choosing an adequate level of difficulty in accordance with each patient's individual capacity and needs.

Evolution of IPT

During the last decade, a number of advances have been made in intervention technology and therapy topics associated with an improved understanding of functioning in schizophrenia. To take these advances into account, the IPT concept was expanded and modified in our laboratory in Bern, Switzerland. In two research projects supported by the Swiss National Foundation (SNF), our research group developed and evaluated two new therapy approaches for schizophrenia patients:

- Three cognitive social skills programs addressing residential, vocational, and recreational topics (WAF; [German abbreviation for *Wohnen, Arbeit, Freizeit*]; SNF-Grant No: 32–45577.95, Roder et al., 1996–2001). The three WAF programs (Mueller & Roder, 2005; Roder et al., 2002, 2006b, 2008b) address specific functional areas of patients' daily living.
- 2. Integrated Neurocognitive Therapy (INT; SNF-Grant No. 3200 B0–108133, Roder et al., 2005–2011) for the improvement of neurocognition and social cognition (Roder & Mueller, 2006).

Treatment Targets of INT

INT represents an extension of the two cognitive subprograms of IPT. Following IPT, the primary aim of the development of INT was to integrate neurocognitive and social cognitive exercises using group processes as therapeutic tools. The treatment targets strongly correspond with the definitions of the National Institute of Mental Health (NIMH) Measurement and Treatment Research to Improve Cognition in Schizophrenia (MATRICS) initiative (Green & Nuechterlein, 2004; Green, Oliver, Crawley, Penn, & Silverstein, 2005; Nuechterlein et al., 2004). Following the recommendations of this task force, six neurocognitive domains (speed of processing, attention/vigilance, verbal and visual learning and memory, reasoning and problem solving, and working memory) and five social cognitive domains (emotional processing, social perception, theory of mind [ToM], social schema, and attribution style) were operationalized for therapeutic intervention. The primary treatment goal of INT is to improve functioning in these neurocognitive and social cognitive domains. The secondary treatment goal is to transfer improved cognitive skills into daily living to minimize the impact of cognitive deficits on the acquisition and use of social and interpersonal skills. Requirements to realize this goal seem to be to improve patients' willingness for change by increased intrinsic motivation, to enhance patients' insight into their cognitive functioning by improving a realistic self-estimation of their own cognitive resources and deficits, and to reduce fear of failure. This should pave the way for improvement in social functioning and possibly for a reduction in negative symptoms (e.g., anhedonia), which could be maintained after the end of treatment.

THEORETICAL BASIS FOR THE INTERVENTION

Treatment Concept of INT

Following IPT (Roder et al., 2010), the concept of INT is based on an integrated model of functioning. This model was originally postulated by Green and Nuechterlein (1999) and confirmed by recent empirical data. It has been extended by our research group (Figure 13.1). It suggests that functional outcome ("coping with life successfully") is determined by a multiplicity of organismic factors, including neurocognitive and social cognitive domains described by the MATRICS initiative, as well as by positive and negative symptoms. All of them interact with recovery-oriented variables like a person's orientation to treatment, which includes such psychological factors as (a) a patient's knowledge and insight into his or her own functioning, (b) intrinsic motivation for therapeutic change, and (c) self-efficacy expectancies in patients' daily living.

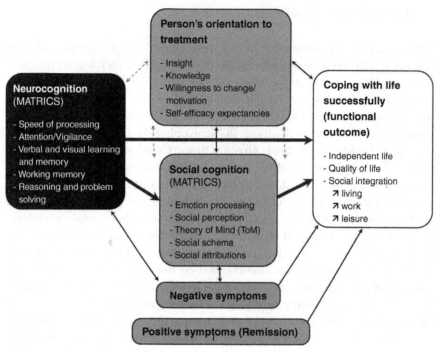

Figure 13.1 Integrative model of possible mediators between neurocognition and functional outcome.

Therapy Rationale of INT

Based on the broad clinical experience and research on IPT, INT includes the following main intervention techniques and rationales:

1. INT interventions take place in a group setting. A team of a therapist and a co-therapist support group processes, using them as a therapeutic tool. Two-thirds of the therapy sessions are held in a standard cognitive-behavioral group therapy setting and one-third use PC-based exercises. However, group interactions are not restricted to the social cognitive part of INT, as they are important for the generation of compensation strategies for addressing neurocognitive deficits in computerized exercises that allows patients to experience self-efficacy in a social context.

2. Every intervention addressing one of the various cognitive domains includes an introduction in which education in the respective cognitive domain is given. Teaching patients about cognitive functions and their relevance in real-life situations within a vulnerability-stress-coping framework of schizophrenia enhances patients' insight into the role of cognitive capacity. It also improves patients' knowledge about their own cognitive functioning and the effects of illness on cognition in general.

3. INT combines bottom-up drill and practice exercises with top-down learning of compensation strategies. Over the course of therapy, the main focus shifts from restitution to strategy learning.

4. Like in IPT, the incremental steps of INT are built sequentially. They always begin with simple, low-level, and not emotionally loaded tasks, following errorless learning principles.

5. A main goal of INT is to closely link the patient's daily living context to his or her cognitive functioning. Patients' own experiences with their cognitive functioning in the real world and the successful or unsuccessful use of strategies to cope with individual daily life demands are taken into consideration in every part of INT. This therapeutic approach should support the generalization of the acquired cognitive skills and their transfer to daily functioning.

6. This leads to a further goal of INT: generating an individual profile of resources and deficits in cognitive functioning across the addressed cognitive domains. It is particularly important to identify the cognitive resources of each patient during the therapy process as this helps to overcome the avoidance of cognitively demanding (social) situations often shown by schizophrenia patients. Additionally, it supports patients' more realistic judgment of their individual cognitive skills.

7. INT focuses on patients' intrinsic motivation during every step of treatment. This is accomplished by allowing patients to choose their degree of active participation in the group exercises and by modulating the level of difficulty, following errorless learning principles. Additionally, didactics are designed to emphasize the importance of each cognitive domain for real-life functioning.

DESCRIPTION OF THE INTERVENTION

How to Implement INT

INT includes a broad scope of interventions in neurocognitive and social cognitive domains, allowing the therapists to compose exercises according to the participants' needs. In a recently finished international evaluation study of INT, a total of 30 sessions were administered. Sessions took place biweekly, and each lasted 90 minutes, including a short break. The clinical experience clearly demonstrated that a longer lasting therapy could show more improvements. Therefore, we would recommend 50 sessions twice a week for clinical implementation.

A team of one primary therapist and one or two co-therapists lead a group of six to eight patients. At least the primary therapist should be well trained in cognitive-behavioral therapy techniques and should be familiar with group processes in groups with schizophrenia patients. In Europe, we are additionally offering INT training workshops in several languages for therapists. The main role of the primary therapist is to structure the group sessions and to support and encourage the group members by using positive reinforcement and strongly focusing on patients' resources. The function of the co-therapist(s) is formally equal to the patients' role. The co-therapist serves as a model for the patients and facilitates group processes to support and encourage weaker patients.

Infrastructural Needs

Before INT can be implemented in a clinical setting, some infrastructural needs have to be organized. Since INT includes computer-based exercises, therapy procedure requires a computer room in addition to the standard group intervention room (Figure 13.2). Each of the two rooms should provide standard equipment (therapists' PC, projector, flipchart). During a therapy session of 90 minutes, divided by a short break, PC-based exercises are limited to 30–45 minutes. Therefore, patients and therapists should be able to switch easily from the equipped PC-room to the group intervention room during each session. If an agency does not have sufficient resources to offer two rooms, the computers can be placed in the standard group room as well. However, the therapist has to make sure that there is enough space for group exercises, like role-plays. Laptops are also a good alternative. In our evaluation study, the CogPack computer program distributed by Marker Software was used. The integration of other computer programs in English seems possible.

Four Modules of INT

The bottom-up and top-down approaches of INT consists of four therapy modules. Each is separated into a neurocognitive and a social cognitive subpart, always starting with the neurocognitive part. Although INT is designed in incremental steps,

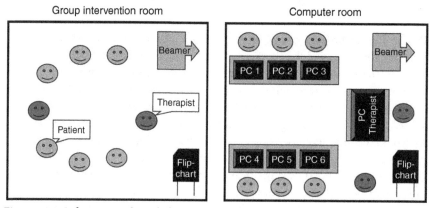

Figure 13.2 Infrastructural needs for Integrated Neurocognitive Therapy implementation.

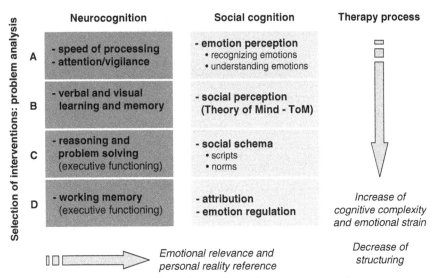

Figure 13.3 Schematic presentation of the Integrated Neurocognitive Therapy.

the content of former modules is repeated in later ones. For example, the emotion perception content of the first module is highly relevant for the attribution style of the last module, in which it is therefore repeated. A schematic presentation of INT is given in Figure 13.3. Although the first module ("A") includes tasks on basic neurocognitive functions, such as speed of processing and attention, which are treated by low-complexity interventions, the last two modules addressing executive functioning are cognitively more demanding. Besides this increase of complexity during treatment in the neurocognitive part, the emotional strain of the focused therapy topics increases in each successive module's social cognitive part, with attribution style and emotion regulation in the last module imposing the most demands on the participants. In the cross-sectional structure of each module, the emotional salience and the personal relevance is higher in the social cognitive part compared to the neurocognitive part due to the closer association of social cognition to social functioning. However, as stated above, the link to the daily living context is established in every neuro- and social cognitive intervention of INT.

Didactic Therapy Components and Therapy Materials of the Modules

It is important to keep in mind that INT uses group processes as a therapeutic tool. INT also follows cognitive-behavioral therapy principles in analyzing problems and working on solutions, such as coping techniques. Against this background, each INT module consists of *introduction* sessions followed by *consecutive* sessions, and each module uses its own set of intervention materials (Table 13.1).

INT starts with an introductory session at the beginning of every neurocognitive and social cognitive part of the four modules. The primary intervention technique of these introductory sessions is based on educational tools to support

Table 13.1 DIDACTIC THERAPY COMPONENTS AND THERAPY MATERIALS FOR
EACH OF THE FOUR INTEGRATED NEUROCOGNITIVE THERAPY MODULES

Therapy components	Materials
INTRODUCTION SESSIONS	
Perception of own resources and possibilities to optimize them in daily life Education in the focused therapy area to improve insight into problems/deficits	Worksheets Information sheets Case vignettes
CONSECUTIVE SESSIONS	
a. Compensation: looking for coping strategies (implicit learning)	Worksheets Information sheets
b. Restitution: practicing exercises (rehearsal learning, partially PC-based) following errorless learning principles	Written cards Stimulus pictures
c. In vivo exercises and homework assignments: promoting transfer and generalization	Worksheets

patients' understanding of the focused cognitive domain and its relevance in individual daily life situations. Bridging the gap between the experiences patients have during therapy and their real-world daily living context requires establishing the patients' awareness of their own resources. In addition, it requires enhancing insight into illness-specific deficits in the focused cognitive functions and their corresponding limitations in coping with daily problems. For this purpose, three kinds of psychoeducation materials are used during introduction sessions:

- *Prototypical case vignettes* (written short stories) designed for each cognitive domain. In these stories, the same fictional character has successful or unsuccessful experiences based on specific cognitive resources or deficits. The introduction of a theme through the use of these short stories gives patients an initial opportunity to discuss cognitive functioning without relation to their own often stressful, emotionally loaded experiences. In a second step, the patients are asked whether they have had experiences in daily life similar to the content of the stories.
- *Worksheets* to let patients document their individual experiences with difficulties in the respective cognitive domain during real-life daily living situations and to reflect on successful or unsuccessful coping strategies they have used to handle such situations.
- *Information sheets* to teach patients about cognitive functioning and its relevance for daily life in the focused cognitive domain, or to summarize coping strategies.

In consecutive sessions in each INT module, individual coping strategies are elaborated in the group setting. To take advantage of implicit learning in a social context, compared to lab-based drill and practice, patients have the opportunity to try out new coping strategies in the group (e.g., role plays). They compensate for cognitive deficits and optimize their individual resources for managing demands of daily life associated with cognitive functioning.

Combined with this strategy-learning approach, INT includes rehearsal-based training sessions. A broad range of materials is used in these sessions, including computerized exercises, standardized written cards, and stimulus pictures. In this approach, much of the work remains group-based, using group processes and interactions to activate patients and to simulate real-life situations. Even during computer sessions, therapists largely support group processes. For example, therapists ask patients to debate and discuss their solution and to articulate possible strategies in team competition.

Finally, in vivo exercises and homework assignments are used to promote transfer of the learned cognitive skills into practice, to support generalization of the effects to other functions, and to maintain the effects after therapy. Again, worksheets are used to document patients' experience outside of therapy.

Module A
INT starts with an introduction to the basic neurocognitive domains of speed of processing and attention, coupled with the social cognitive domain of emotion perception. In the beginning, the INT procedure is very structured and the co-therapist models each new exercise. The first exercises are simple, easy to handle, and are not affected by emotional strain.

Neurocognitive Part: Speed of Processing
Introduction session: After a short overview of the contents of INT, information-processing models and information sheets are used to educate patients regarding the impact of cognitive functioning on daily living. In this context, patients are asked for the first time about their own perceived resources and deficits in general cognitive functioning and especially in the targeted domains. To individualize the information, a worksheet including a very brief questionnaire (1 = this is a deficit; 5 = this is a resource) is used to generate a patient's personal cognitive profile.

Speed of processing: After the introduction phase, simple PC-based exercises are introduced for three reasons: to reduce schizophrenia patients' fear of the social group context and of negative expectancies through well-structured, goal-oriented exercises free of social and emotional strain; to give them confidence to be able to handle the computer; and to identify patients' individual profile of functioning in the targeted cognitive domain by comparing their performance in the PC-exercises with their personal estimation of their own resources and deficits. The level of difficulty in the PC exercises is augmented following errorless learning principles. Additionally, behavioral therapy techniques, such as positive reinforcement and positive connotation, are implemented to support patients' motivation and self-expectancies. Afterward, patients' experiences during the PC exercises are discussed in the group context. This didactic tool can be used in all of the following neurocognitive intervention parts of INT, but it will not be explicitly described in the text.

Compensation sessions: In this phase of treatment, a strong focus is given to the identification of patients' individual resources and deficits in speed of processing. The relevance of speed of processing in daily living situations is summarized for each participant. Then, patients learn coping strategies to compensate for deficits and to optimize resources by the didactic use of information sheets and work-sheets. Information sheets summarize the knowledge about the function of speed of processing in information processes and behavior. The worksheets individual-ize the information by asking patients whether they have any experience in deal-ing with such problems in work, leisure time activities, or at home. Examples of successful strategies are drinking a cup of coffee, and using self-instructions and self-reinforcement ("I know that I am able to master this task. Afterward I will enjoy a break"). All strategies are summarized first, before their probability of success is discussed in the group.

Restitution sessions: The learned compensation strategies are rehearsed in repeated PC exercises, such as reaction time tasks. Patients are encouraged to apply their own compensation strategies to the task. Therefore, the chosen strategies may differ among patients, but are practiced extensively using different exercises. For example, one patient may find self-instructions helpful to avoid distractions, whereas another patient prefers time management, including breaks.

Neurocognitive Part: Attention/Vigilance

Introduction session: A brief introduction phase complements the initial intro-ductory sessions at the beginning of the module. To introduce the new theme, the relationship between speed and attention is discussed. Thereby, alertness and vigilance are addressed separately. Both are introduced by reading prototypical short stories in the group. An excerpt of a case vignette is given in Figure 13.4. Case vignettes focus on resources and successful coping, as well as on deficits and problems.

Compensation sessions: Patients' individual experience with (un)successful coping strategies in daily living situations demanding alertness and vigilance are summarized using worksheets (Figure 13.5).

Participants receive information about alternative coping strategies, which are individualized in specific situations (e.g., work, at home, leisure time, interper-sonal situations). For example, patients learn to take a short rest during work and to focus awareness on the experience of neutral objects in the environment in order to draw attention from stressful thoughts. Finally, the individually cho-sen strategies are practiced in the group context. For example, patients learn that attention (and speed of processing) is strongly affected by one's state of mood and level of interest. Here, card-sorting exercises are introduced, which require inte-gration of emotional expression and attention to verbal stimuli.

Restitution sessions: PC-based exercises addressing attention to simulated tasks, as well as to the already described card sorting exercises, are repeatedly practiced.

Case Vignette

Once upon a morning ...

Today Peter got up earlier than usual, somehow it was easier for him. He needed a shower and two cups of coffee, but this was normal. He had slept very well and felt very alert. He noticed that he dressed himself and got ready to leave the house more quickly than usual.

Peter knew that it would be a good day for him. ......

Figure 13.4 Example of a case vignette (Module A, neurocognitive part: alertness).

In-vivo exercises and homework assignments: To promote the transfer of the learned skills into daily life and to support generalization to other areas of functioning, patients are encouraged to practice new compensation strategies in daily life. Individual goals prior to the exercise, as well as difficulties and level of success, are documented using worksheets. These documents support patients' input to the discussion in the following group session of each individual experience with coping exercises in the real-life, daily living context. In vivo exercises and homework assignments are implemented in each part of the four modules, but they will not be explicitly discussed in the following sections.

Social Cognitive Part: Emotion Perception
Introduction session: This topic has already been introduced in the neurocognitive part of Module A using the above described card sorting exercise. This is an example of the integration of neurocognitive and social cognitive intervention in INT. Patients are introduced to the discussion of perceptual processes using a filter model addressing the relationship of perception and memory and individual experience. Emotional distress and mood are identified as filters that influence perception. As an example of an information sheet, the filter model is shown in Figure 13.6. The relationship of emotional feelings to cognitive functioning, somatic reaction, and behavior is elaborated in summarizing patients' own experience.

Compensation sessions: The group identifies universal basic emotions. Patients are asked about their own or the experience of others with each of these basic emotions. The aim is to improve patients' understanding of factors

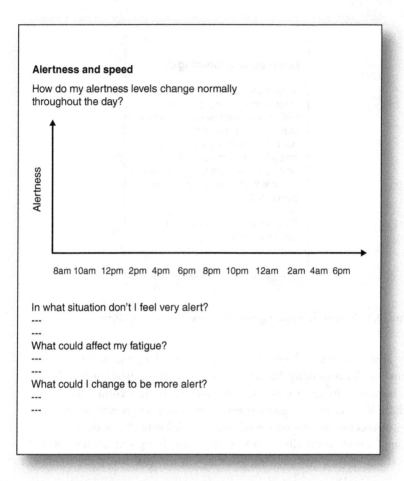

Figure 13.5 Example of a worksheet (Module A, neurocognitive part: alertness and speed).

that affect emotion and of the impact of each emotion in daily-living situations. Furthermore, patients learn facial recognition techniques and how to interpret human gestures: They are encouraged to differentiate facial affects by identifying typical features of the mouth, eyes, eyebrows, nose and facial wrinkles of each emotion. The same procedure is used for human gestures. We put special emphasis on the position of the arms, hands, and fingers, as well as of the whole body.

In complementing affect recognition exercises, a second card sorting exercise was designed to address emotional concept formation: Patients receive dark gray and light gray cards. One basic emotion is written on each of the dark gray cards. Light gray cards contain different commonly used terms, mostly referring to one basic emotion. Others are ambiguous and refer to more than one emotion (e.g., disappointment is often interpreted as anger or sadness, sometimes

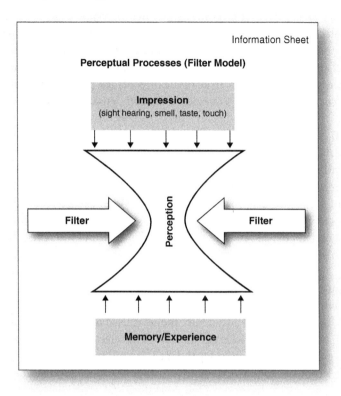

Figure 13.6 Example of an information sheet: filter model (Module A, social cognitive part, emotion recognition).

even as anxiety). Patients have to sort the cards according to the basic emotions (Figure 13.7). Each decision has to be discussed to find a group consensus. If this is not possible due to the ambiguous meaning of a word, two solutions are accepted. Finally, the impact of the emotional state on cognitive functioning in daily life is discussed in the group.

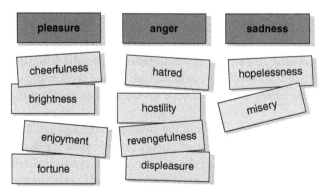

Figure 13.7 Example of a card-sorting exercise addressing emotional concept formation (Module A, social cognitive part, emotion recognition.)

Restitution sessions: A large body of pictures is available in the manual to improve affect decoding. Three difficulty levels are included: First, unambiguous pictures show simple stimuli of facial affect, followed by pictures addressing facial affect and gestures, and ending with complex pictures showing emotionally loaded interpersonal situations. In all of the three stages, patients are reinforced to use the learned interpretation strategies of the compensation sessions.

MODULE B

The two MATRICS dimensions of verbal learning and memory, as well as visual learning and memory, are dealt with separately, beginning with verbal learning and memory. The social cognitive part of this module represents a straight continuation of the perceptual process introduced in Module A. Patients learn to recognize the key information in social situations (social perception). In this context, INT works on patients' judgments about the intentions and thoughts of others in a social situation, which is defined in the literature as ToM.

Neurocognitive Part: Verbal and Visual Learning and Memory

Introduction session: Didactically, Module B is strongly related to the content of Module A. The already-introduced filter model is used to explain the relationship of perception and memory, wherein the quality of selective attention to the environment is postulated as strongly dependent on an individual's earlier experiences and mood. This neurocognitive domain is further introduced by reading two prototypical short stories in the group. One short story addresses short-term memory and the other one prospective memory. Information sheets support patients in differentiating among short-term memory, long-term memory, and prospective memory.

Compensation sessions: Again, we focus on the relevance of these abilities for successful coping with life and patients' assumptions about their own level of functioning in this area. Individual strategies of the patients used in daily life to compensate for memory deficits are summarized and completed through information sheets available for short-term memory, as well as for prospective memory. Patients then try each of the new coping strategies (e.g., chunking, immediate repetition, or external memory hook) using group exercises. Thereafter, patients' experience of their performance in the exercises is compared with their pre-exercise prediction. This allows them to identify their resources and deficits in memory domains. Having both deficits and resources is normalized using the rationale that everybody has an individual profile of cognitive functioning comprising strengths and weaknesses; it is hardly possible to have strengths in every domain of cognitive functioning.

Restitution sessions: The compensation strategies are exercised in repeated PC tasks, following errorless learning principles. Additionally, we developed group exercises addressing verbal and visual memory. These exercises simulate real-life situations, foster group processes, and are more related to interpersonal demands on memory functions than are computer exercises. For example, in a role-play in which all patients participate, every patient gets a card including the name, the hobby, the local phone number, and the favorite color of a fictional person (e.g., a politician, or a popular movie or sports star). In a highly structured exercise, each patient reads the description of the respective person on his or her card, which has to be memorized by the other group members. Such exercises, which take participants' interests of private life into account, strongly support the motivation for active participation in the program.

Social Cognitive Part: Social Perception and Theory of Mind

Introduction session: The social cognitive section of Module B is a straight continuation of the intervention on emotion perception from Module A. However, the pictures showing emotion expression are embedded in an interpersonal and social context in this module. Additionally, ToM functioning is implicitly implicated in interpersonal scenes. Patients learn about the impact of social and emotion perception and ToM functioning on interpersonal behavior using information and worksheets. The main objective is that patients learn to differentiate between facts and assumption.

Compensation sessions: The intervention in social perception is strongly based on the one used in IPT. The social pictures, which were rated for their level of difficulty, vary in visual complexity (number of presented stimuli) and emotional loading. At the beginning of the module, slides rated with a low degree of complexity and emotional loading are presented. The level of difficulty gradually increases as group members improve. Additionally, a set of more complex pictures was designed to create a higher level of difficulty. Following social learning principles, patients act out some of the pictured scenes in role-plays. This helps to activate the patients and gives them experience with key aspects of the situation. Broadly, the use of group process and role-plays is thought to stimulate ToM functioning, helping patients learn to take the perspective of others.

Didactically, patients learn social perception techniques in three steps:

1. *Gathering information*: The group members are asked to describe a slide as accurately and in as much detail as possible. At this step, the slide should not be interpreted to differ between fact and assumption.
2. *Interpretation and discussion*: Group members are asked to state their views on possible interpretations of the situation and the expressed emotions depicted on the slide. Every opinion needs justification by reference to the actual visual information gathered in the first step. All group members discuss the different possible interpretations subsequently. They learn how to judge the correctness and the likeliness of each interpretation. By comparing and substantiating various interpretations, the participants learn to evaluate the evidence for their interpretation, rather than just adopting group consensus. In addition, they learn to decode facial affect and emotional gestures and understand how and why a social situation can be interpreted in various ways.

3. *Assigning a title*: After gathering information and interpreting the
   pictures, the therapist asks the group members to choose a title for the
   picture. The title should be short and meaningful, reflecting the most
   important aspects of the social situation on the slide (summarizing the
   contents of the slide). The appropriateness of the suggested title will
   enable the therapists to verify whether the key aspects of a situation have
   been perceived and understood.

Theory of mind skills have already been improved implicitly by the interpretation of depicted interpersonal situations. Against this background, we developed
the following exercise (Figure 13.8): The group is split in two parts. While one half
leaves the room together with the co-therapist to do some alternative exercises
(called the "receiving group"), the other half (the "sending group") chooses one
picture out of a set of landscape pictures and describes it in detail, in a manner
analogous to the social perception task. The members of the sending group memorize the detailed description. The receiving group returns to the room without
knowing the targeted picture. The sending group verbalizes the description. The
members of the receiving group have to take the verbalized perspective to form
an internal picture. The receiving group then attempts to recognize the targeted
picture from a set of pictures. In further exercises, the participants have to take
over the perspective of actors in fictional written stories, movies, or comics. Some

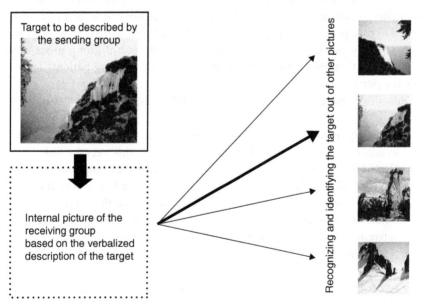

Figure 13.8 Integrated Neurocognitive Therapy Module B: example of a group exercise
using stimulus pictures addressing theory of mind (taking the perspective of other group
members). Half of the group leaves the room, the other half describes the picture in
detail; the group comes back in the room, the other group describes the picture again; the
outside group has to recognize the right picture out of others.

of the contents of these ToM exercises are also transferred into role-plays. This increases the experience of emotional impact on the actors and facilitates comparison with their individual daily-life experiences.

Restitution sessions: Social perception, emotion perception, and ToM skills are rehearsed in repeated exercises with a continuously increasing level of difficulty and emotional salience.

Module C
The neurocognitive part of Module C focuses on the MATRICS domains of reasoning and problem solving. In these domains of executive functioning, the INT procedure introduces the highest level of neurocognitive demands. The two targeted domains are dealt with separately, beginning with reasoning. The social cognitive part of this module addresses social schema, including exercises of social norms and social scripts. Therapeutically, it should be taken into consideration that many patients have negative experiences with their own inappropriate social behavior, according to general norms. Conflicts with others and emotional reactions may have been the consequences of such behavior.

Neurocognitive Part: Reasoning
Introduction session: In the educational part, the term "reasoning" is replaced by the term "thinking" in the context of daily-living situations. When reading short stories, a strong focus is given to patients' own thoughts regarding concrete social situations and their emotional impact. Information and worksheets address concept formation, cognitive flexibility, and neurobiological aspects of this cognitive domain.

Compensation sessions: Verbal concept exercises are used to enhance verbal communication skills. Patients practice finding the appropriate words during a conversation and summarizing in their own words movies they have watched or books they have read. Worksheets individualize the learned coping strategies, according to patients' daily-living situations.

Restitution sessions: Several PC exercises are used. For example, six different kinds of plants are shown on the computer screen: carnation, anemone, tulip, palm, rose, narcissus. Patients are asked which plant is different from all others (i.e., the palm). Computerized exercises are followed by group exercises concerning conceptual hierarchies and categorizing of different stimuli. For example, patients are shown a word or a phrase (e.g., "packing for a beach trip"). Afterward, brainstorming is done to gather related words. Finally, the summarized 30 to 40 related words are categorized (e.g., "toiletries," "food," "medication," "entertainment materials").

Another exercise involves the planning of specific behaviors in different situations. This is operationalized in a group exercise: The course of concrete actions well known in daily living, such as cooking spaghetti or going to a birthday party, is split apart into sequences. The therapist writes these sequences on different cards. Each patient gets one card. The group members have to put the different cards (sequences) in the right order.

Neurocognitive Part: Problem Solving

Introduction session: Patients are familiarized with problem and goal-oriented thinking (information sheet in Figure 13.9) by presenting the standard problem-solving model in seven steps commonly used in cognitive-behavioral therapy. Patients' own resources in problem solving in the context of daily living are summarized using worksheets.

Compensation sessions: The standard problem-solving techniques are applied. Didactically, the INT procedure in this part resembles an individual intervention: Each patient mentions one problem he or she actually could not solve. Problems should be rather simple, with a high probability of finding a solution during therapy (e.g., to clean the apartment, to find a friend, to stop smoking). Each patient practices the learned strategies individually, using the other group members as resources during discussion. Finally, chosen solutions are translated into action in real-life situations using homework assignments.

Restitution sessions: Patients repeat abstract lab-based computer exercises for problem solving (e.g., to find the right path out of a labyrinth or to equilibrate scales). These exercises are partly done in small groups of two or three patients to enhance group interaction and the social context of problem solving. Patients have to debate and convince the other group members of their own solution and have to find a consensus. Riddles are also used.

Social Cognitive Part: Social Schema

Introduction session: Many techniques are adopted as described in the reasoning and problem solving sections, but the emphasis is on social relations. Patients' social schema are modified in two ways: first, by the use of social action sequences (scripts), and second, by reflection on the impact of behaviors from the perspective

---

Information Sheet

Successful Problem Solving in 7 Steps

1. Identifying and analyzing the problem

2. Describing the problem

3. Generating Alternative Solutions

4. Evaluating the Alternatives

5. Deciding on a Solution

6. Translating the Solution into Action

7. Feedback sessions

Figure 13.9 Example of an information sheet: problem solving in seven steps (Module C, neurocognitive part: problem solving).

of social norms and social roles. Again, teaching is based on information and worksheets.

Compensation sessions: Patients learn and discuss which behavior is appropriate in selected social roles, according to social norms. Patients' own negative experiences, as well as personal resources, are summarized using worksheets. Furthermore, general expectancies of others and social consequences following role violation are emphasized. Movie sequences showing actors whose behavior is incompatible with general social norms and roles are analyzed sequentially. Afterward, alternative behaviors are role-played. Additionally, patients learn how to deal with social stigma (e.g., "I'm not like others"), following a normalizing approach.

Finally, patients are supported to develop goal-oriented individual planning skills, in accordance with the demands of social roles and stresses, following a strategy learning approach used in the already-described problem-solving model. These skills are repeated extensively in the restitution sessions.

Restitution sessions: In a social script exercise, cards with pictures referring to a common daily action (e.g., buying a bus ticket, ordering a meal) are presented to the group. Patients then describe the pictures on the cards and afterward try to put the cards into the right order to depict a logical sequence of events. Finally, patients find a title best describing the content of the sequence. Patients are instructed to use facts and not assumptions in discussion. Following this same procedure, an additional group exercise addressing actions of daily life is used: Patients have to assemble segments of an action into a logical sequence (e.g., repairing a bicycle).

Module D

The neurocognitive part of the last module addresses working memory. The respective interventions address cognitive flexibility and selective attention processing. Social cognitive interventions focus on the impact of individuals' attribution styles on themselves, others, and the situation. Consequently, patients' emotional strain is highest in this final part of INT treatment. Thus, strategies for coping with emotional strain associated with overstimulation are a main focus during these sessions. Patients learn to implement both emotional and behavioral coping strategies.

Neurocognitive Part: Working Memory

Introduction session: In the first educational part, patients read a short story wherein the protagonist has to shift between several actions during competitive work. The cognitive flexibility skills needed are related to the life experiences of the patients using worksheets.

In a second short story, patients learn that coping with a stress-inducing, sensory overloaded situation demands selective attention skills. Here, cognitive, emotional, behavioral, and somatic consequences of internal and external overstimulation are analyzed.

Compensation sessions: Compensation strategies are introduced using information sheets. The intervention uses worksheets, and individualizes and transfers the coping compensation strategies into concrete daily-living situations. Thereby, the impact of the environment, interpersonal and social circumstances, and individual resources are considered. Patients learn (a) how to improve cognitive flexibility, such as by using behavioral rituals to simultaneously cook and talk on the phone, and (b) how to cope with distraction, such as during work or leisure-time activities. Coping strategies addressing cognitive flexibility and selective attention are improved during role-plays in the group, focusing on interpersonal situations. For example, a patient has to communicate with another patient while all other group members are talking very loudly to simulate overstimulation in a restaurant.

Restitution sessions: By means of PC-based exercises, patients first practice the learned strategies on a highly abstract level. An example of a PC-based exercise is to identify a targeted stimulus in a bulk of similar but not identical stimuli. Additionally, patients improve their selective attention using stimuli of complex pictures. An example of a complex picture is included in Figure 13.10. While showing this picture, patients listen to a brief story; for example, that the therapist wants to send a letter. Then patients are asked whether they can help to find the post office. Finally, repeated role-plays stimulate the use of cognitive flexibility skills in social context before each patient tries to implement the learned skills in his or her personal life.

Social Cognitive Part: Attribution And Emotion Regulation

Many schizophrenia patients suffer from persistent positive symptoms associated with negative life experiences. The social cognitive domain of attribution is often

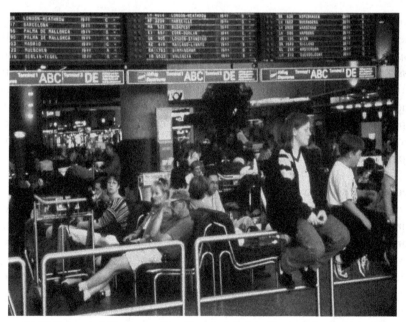

Figure 13.10 Integrated Neurocognitive Therapy Module D: example of a pictured stimuli group exercise addressing selective attention (working memory): "Where is the post office?".

strongly related to positive symptoms. In appraising a situation, schizophrenia patients often jump to conclusions without gathering all the information or show an overgeneralized attributional style. Because intervening on attributions can be stressful for the patients, INT addresses this theme at the end of treatment, when the group has established high cohesion (friendship and confidence).

Introduction session: This final part of INT starts with education about individual attributional styles that determine thinking and behavior (attributional bias). Continuing the content of the previously introduced neurocognitive part of INT, the association of attributional styles with overstimulation and emotional strain is described. Introducing a vulnerability-stress-coping model, patients learn to understand how individual stress is determined, how emotional strain reduces functional capacity, and how to manage stressful situations.

Compensation sessions: Here, INT works with standardized descriptions of concrete situations. The fictional protagonist, who is well known from the short stories previously read in the group, acts in situations taken out of real life. The probability is high that some patients have had comparable experiences. For example, "Peter (fictional protagonist) is sitting in a restaurant drinking a coffee and reading a newspaper. A man eating at another table looks at him from time to time." Patients are asked to describe the situation in detail and to generate hypotheses about why the man is looking at Peter. A typical paranoid attribution would be that the man is looking at Peter because the man is a police officer who is monitoring him. The didactic means are the same as in the social cognitive part of Module B addressing social perception: First, patients have to gather all the information available before they generate a hypothesis reflecting their interpretation of the situation. In other words, patients are taught to use facts instead of assumptions and that listing of facts has to be completed before the situation can be interpreted. This procedure diminishes patients' tendency to jump to inadequate conclusions. Afterward, all alternative hypotheses are summarized and evaluated. The cognitive, emotional, and behavioral consequences of each hypothesis are analyzed. The described situation is practiced in role-plays to stimulate patients' perception of related feelings. This represents one goal of INT: Patients experience their feelings related to a concrete situation, and they realize that a change in thinking and behavior has emotional consequences. Patients may thereby learn to make less stressful attributions.

In a final stress-inoculation training, including relaxation strategies like self-instruction and visualization techniques, patients learn to identify their own stress indicators and to cope with individual stress reactions. They learn to distinguish between behavioral and emotional coping techniques using information sheets. An example from our lab: A patient reports how he has managed to deal with a stressful situation in his daily-life context using behavioral and emotional coping strategies. He was waiting for a colleague at the stairs of the station, as he had arrived too early. However, the station security personnel told him to go away. In former times, this would have caused feelings of anger and aggressive reactions. However, he thought that they were only doing their job. Consequently, he walked away without complaining about their behavior. He also did shadowboxing in a quiet corner, which helped him to calm down.

Restitution sessions: In the final section, attributional processing is repeatedly improved in role-plays addressing actions of daily life (e.g., "while sitting in a restaurant, someone at the next table is looking at me"). Patients should habituate to use less stressful attributions by practicing them in various situations of individual relevance in the group. Again, we use written short stories as stimuli or individual experiences of daily living described by group members. In parallel, patients are taught to repeatedly improve individualized stress reduction techniques that they have designed. This therapy sequence is later expanded to the real-world context through homework assignments.

TROUBLESHOOTING

Based on our experience with both IPT and INT, we think that one of the main problems in conducting such a group therapy occurs at the beginning, say, during the first five sessions: When group cohesion is low, it can be difficult to motivate patients to participate on a regular basis in the group sessions. Therefore, therapists should be well trained in cognitive and behavioral intervention techniques and therapy planning. They should also have some experience in group therapy and especially in handling group processes. Generally, the group should be well structured in the beginning by the main therapist supported by the co-therapist. In other words, the main therapist should be clearly defined as the leader of the group.

In the beginning, as well as in the following sections of INT, an ongoing difficulty is activating and motivating the participants. Against the background of therapists supporting group processes, INT always focuses closely on patients' resources, instead of deficits alone. Additionally, patients are allowed to take a time-out when an exercise seems to be too difficult or when they are not in the mood to participate actively. In this context, patients also have the option to choose between different exercises of various levels of difficulty. Here, it should be mentioned that a substantial minority of patients struggle with illiteracy or motor difficulties that hinder writing. Additionally, from our experience with IPT and INT groups, some patients may have problems reading and writing due to cognitive deficits or emotional strain. In this case, the co-therapist supports such a patient in writing down comments at the beginning of the therapy. After group cohesion has been established, other patients often help group mates with such deficits. Last, but not least, the daily-living experiences of each patient are strictly taken into consideration in the INT. All of these points should help to improve and maintain patients' intrinsic motivation during therapy, which prevents dropouts. In our groups, INT seems to be quite successful in attaining these goals since the dropout rate is always around 10%, and the session participation rate is more than 80%.

PATIENT SELECTION CONSIDERATIONS

INT was originally designed for stabilized outpatients. The criteria for optimal INT treatment differ in some points from its predecessor, IPT, as well as from

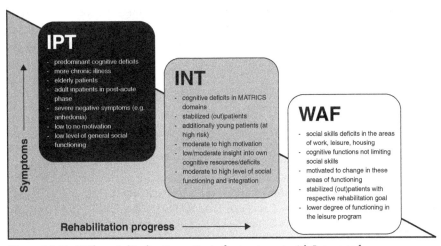

IPT
- predominant cognitive deficits
- more chronic illness
- elderly patients
- adult inpatients in post-acute phase
- severe negative symptoms (e.g. anhedonia)
- low to no motivation
- low level of general social functioning

INT
- cognitive deficits in MATRICS domains
- stabilized (out)patients
- additionally young patients (at high risk)
- moderate to high motivation
- low/moderate insight into own cognitive resources/deficits
- moderate to high level of social functioning and integration

WAF
- social skills deficits in the areas of work, leisure, housing
- cognitive functions not limiting social skills
- motivated to change in these areas of functioning
- stabilized (out)patients with respective rehabilitation goal
- lower degree of functioning in the leisure program

Symptoms

Rehabilitation progress ⟶

Figure 13.11 Differential indication criteria for treatment with Integrated Neurocognitive Therapy in comparison with Integrated Psychological Therapy (IPT) and WAF.

IPT's other sequel, WAF (Figure 13.11). Clinical experience implementing INT in various outpatient settings during an extensive international evaluation study clearly has demonstrated the benefit of INT to participants with low to moderate therapy motivation, insight into own resources and deficits in cognitive functioning, and moderate social integration and functioning. Additionally, INT could be an appropriate intervention for individuals in a prodromal phase of illness at a high-risk stage. On the other hand, the literature suggests that IPT may be more appropriate for more chronic patients with severe negative symptoms, as well as for elderly patients and patients in a more post-acute phase in inpatient settings. The social part of IPT and the WAF programs are both designed for patients first rehabilitated in cognitive functioning. In these programs, cognitive deficits should not limit social intervention. In contrast to IPT, patients participating in WAF procedures should be well stabilized. WAF is indicated when patients show unmet needs in work, residential, or leisure areas of daily living. Several studies indicate that patients benefit from IPT, INT and WAF independently of their age. Implementing INT showed that it is appropriate for young patients in their first episode of psychosis, due, in part, to the various therapy materials, including PC exercises. For this reason, we are currently modifying INT for use with patients at high risk for developing a psychosis. We have also found that middle-aged to older patients are often very motivated to work on a computer for the first time in their lives.

NOTE

INT includes various therapy materials: case vignettes, information sheets, worksheets, stimulus pictures, standardized written cards for group exercises, and a computer program for restitution sessions. Currently (Spring 2011), we only have

an unpublished research manual (Roder & Mueller, 2006). In the beginning of
2012, a German manual will be available from Springer Publishers, Heidelberg,
which will be immediately translated into English, French, and Spanish. In the
meantime, the research manual and materials can be ordered from the authors.

REFERENCES

Green, M. F., & Nuechterlein, K. H. (1999). Should schizophrenia be treated as a neuro-cognitive disorder? *Schizophrenia Bulletin, 25*, 309–319.

Green, M. F., & Nuechterlein, K. H. (2004). The MATRICS initiative: Developing a consensus cognitive battery for clinical trials. *Schizophrenia Research, 72*, 1–3.

Green, M. F., Olivier, B., Crawley, J. N., Penn, D. L., & Silverstein, S. (2005). Social cognition in schizophrenia: Recommendations from the Measurement and Treatment Research to Improve Cognition in Schizophrenia New Approaches Conference. *Schizophrenia Research, 31*, 882–887.

Mueller, D. R., & Roder, V. (2005). Social skills training in recreational rehabilitation of schizophrenia patients. *American Journal of Recreational Therapy, 4*(3), 11–19.

Mueller, D. R., & Roder, V. (2008). Empirical evidence for group therapy addressing social perception in schizophrenia. In J. B. Teiford (Ed.), *Social perception: 21st century issues and challenges* (pp. 51–80). New York: Nova Science Publishers.

Nuechterlein, K. H., Barch, D. M., Gold, J. M., Goldberg, T. E., Green, M. F., & Heaton, T. E. (2004). Identification of separable cognitive factors in schizophrenia. *Schizophrenia Research, 72*, 29–39.

Roder, V., Brenner, H. D., & Kienzle, N. (2008a). *Integriertes Psychologisches Therapieprogramm bei schizophren Erkrankten IPT*. Weinheim: Beltz.

Roder, V., Brenner, H. D., Mueller, D., Laechler, M., Zorn, P., Reisch, T., et al. (2002). Development of specific social skills training programmes for schizophrenia patients: Results of a multicentre study. *Acta Psychiatrica Scandinavica, 105*, 363–371.

Roder, V., & Mueller, D. (2006). *Integrated Neurocognitive Therapy (INT) for schizophrenia patients*. Unpublished manual. Bern, CH: University Psychiatric Hospital.

Roder, V., Mueller, D. R., Mueser, K. T., & Brenner, H. D. (2006). Integrated Psychological Therapy (IPT) for schizophrenia: Is it effective? *Schizophrenia Bulletin, 32*(Suppl. 1), 81–93.

Roder, V., Mueller, D. R., & Schmidt, S. J. (2011). Effectiveness of the Integrated Psychological Therapy (IPT) for schizophrenia patients: A research up-date. *Schizophrenia Bulletin, 37*, 71–79.

Roder, V., Mueller, D. R., Spaulding, W., & Brenner, H. D. (2010). *Integrated Psychological Therapy (IPT) for schizophrenia patients* (2nd ed.). Goettingen/Cambridge, MA: Hogrefe.

Roder, V., Zorn, P., Pfammatter, M., Andres, K., Brenner, H. D., & Mueller, D. R. (2008b). *Praxishandbuch zur verhaltenstherapeutischen Behandlung schizophren Erkrankter, 2. Aktualisierte Auflage*. Bern, CH: Huber.

Roder, V., Mueller, D. R., & Zorn, P. (2006b). Therapieverfahren zu sozialen Fertigkeiten bei schizophren Erkrankten in der Arbeitsrehabilitation. Vorteile des Aufbaus arbeitsspezifischer gegenüber unspezifischer sozialer Fertigkeiten. *Zeitschrift für Klinische Psychologie, Psychiatrie und Psychotherapie, 35*, 256–266.

14

Cognitive Enhancement Therapy

SHAUN M. EACK ■

Social cognition is pervasively and markedly impaired in individuals with schizophrenia (Green et al., 2008; Penn et al., 1997), and a growing body of evidence indicates that these impairments are significant contributors to functional disability in the disorder (Couture, Penn, & Roberts, 2006). Unfortunately, pharmacotherapeutic interventions designed to enhance cognition, social or nonsocial, have had a limited impact on these deficits (Keefe et al., 2007; Sergi et al., 2007a). However, cognitive rehabilitation approaches that utilize computerized and/or group-based training methods have emerged as effective approaches for enhancing cognition in schizophrenia (Horan et al., 2009; McGurk, Twamley, Sitzer, McHugo, & Mueser, 2007). Cognitive Enhancement Therapy (CET; Hogarty & Greenwald, 2006) is a comprehensive approach to the remediation of social and nonsocial cognitive impairments in schizophrenia, which has demonstrated considerable efficacy in clinical trials with this population (Eack et al., 2009; Hogarty et al., 2004).

CET is an integrated, small-group intervention designed to enhance the neurocognitive and social-cognitive impairments that limit functional recovery from schizophrenia. The treatment integrates 60 hours of computer-based neurocognitive training in attention, memory, and problem solving, with 45 structured social-cognitive group sessions designed to improve perspective taking, gistfulness, social context appraisal, and other core social-cognitive processes needed to succeed in adult life. Although the enhancement of social cognition is a primary focus of CET, targeting impairments in neurocognition is seen as necessary to support the attention, memory, and executive functions that provide a foundation for social information processing. It is through the unique integration of these two methods of intervention that CET has conferred significant benefits for patients with schizophrenia to improve cognition and functional outcome, and even protect against brain loss in this population (Eack et al., 2009; Eack et al., 2010b; Hogarty et al., 2004). This chapter provides an overview of CET, its theoretical foundations, targets, and treatment methods for patients with schizophrenia. A complete and detailed description of CET is available in *Cognitive Enhancement Therapy: The Training Manual* (Hogarty & Greenwald, 2006).

THEORETICAL FOUNDATIONS

CET is based upon a neurodevelopmental theory of cognitive development, which draws from disciplines ranging from neuroscience to sociology, and lays the foundation for the principles of treatment employed in the approach (Hogarty & Flesher, 1999a). This theoretical framework begins with recognition of the developmental nature of the brain and cognition (Gogtay et al., 2004), and increasing evidence characterizing schizophrenia as a disorder of neurodevelopment (Lewis & Levitt, 2002; Weinberger, 1987). The cognitive impairments experienced by people with schizophrenia do not begin at the onset of psychosis; rather, their origins are clearly evident years before the onset of the clinical syndrome (Eack et al., 2010c; Keshavan, Diwadkar, Montrose, Rajarethinam, & Sweeney, 2005). Studies have implicated prenatal (Kunugi, Nanko, & Murray, 2001), perinatal (Seidman et al., 2000), and postnatal (Prasad et al., 2011) insults in the development of schizophrenia, all suggesting a neurodevelopmental pathogenesis. The onset of schizophrenia typically occurs during a key maturational period for the development of social cognition, as individuals are learning to transition to adulthood and assume adult social roles. The timing of illness onset at this period has a significant neurodevelopmental impact and places schizophrenia patients at a profound disadvantage compared to their nonaffected peers. Indeed, when comparing the neurocognitive abilities of adult patients with schizophrenia to preadolescent children, striking similarities exist. Slowness of processing, inattentiveness, and poor cognitive flexibility are the norm in preadolescent children (Lezack, 1983). In addition, individuals at this age routinely exhibit egocentric behavior that is incongruent with situational norms and indicative of an underdeveloped capacity for perspective taking, foresight, and social context appraisal (Selman & Schultz, 1990). These characteristics of early cognitive development are hallmark signs of adults with schizophrenia, and, when combined with evidence on the neurodevelopmental nature of the condition, increasingly suggest that patients with schizophrenia suffer from a developmental delay in higher order cognitive processes, particularly social cognition.

By conceptualizing the cognitive impairments experienced by patients with schizophrenia in a neurodevelopmental context, Hogarty and colleagues then created CET as a method to "jump start" the developmental delay in cognitive functioning in schizophrenia. Methods for addressing this delay and enhancing cognition were based upon the emerging literature of brain plasticity (Karni et al., 1995) and the classic literature on social development (Selman & Schultz, 1990). Studies have increasingly documented the remarkable capacity of the brain to respond to enriched environmental experiences and reorganize itself for functional specialization and to compensate for injuries. The repetitive and strategic practice of motor tasks were shown to result in changes in the motor cortex and improved motor function in those who had experienced a stroke (Johansson, 2000). These principles were also successfully used to remediate other cognitive problems, such as attention deficits in patients with a traumatic brain injury (Ben-Yishay, Piasetsky, & Rattok, 1985). In CET, schizophrenia is viewed as a brain disorder, and the emerging evidence on brain plasticity points to the possibility of altering brain function through the practice of tasks designed to challenge the very cognitive processes that are impaired in the disorder. CET capitalizes on the growing evidence supporting the brain's capacity for plasticity and its ability to benefit from enriched environmental experiences, and provides a comprehensive approach employing innovative experiential methods to improve social and nonsocial cognitive functioning for schizophrenia patients.

Although studies on brain plasticity helped provide a meaningful organization of how cognition might be improved in schizophrenia, models and theories of information processing provided a meaningful organization to these methods. Contemporary information processing models structure cognitive processes in a hierarchical fashion and outline their many interdependencies (Simon, 1979). For example, the ability to hold a piece of information in working memory is highly dependent upon intact attentional abilities. Higher order social-cognitive processes are also dependent upon intact basic information processes. Individuals are unlikely to ever succeed in the interpretation and recognition of social cues if they cannot attend to them in the first place. Social-cognitive abilities also necessitate a rapid, gistful, and parallel processing of information that is in contrast with the slow, serial, and concrete processing style of many patients with schizophrenia. Evidence of the interdependent nature of cognitive processes, as well as the interrelations between cognitive impairments in schizophrenia (Eack et al., 2010a; Sergi et al., 2007b), clearly establishes the need for an integrated approach to improving cognition in the disorder, one that focuses on both neurocognitive and social-cognitive functioning. This evidence also indicates that some remediation of basic deficits in attention and processing speed are likely to be necessary for individuals to benefit from social-cognitive training. As such, CET begins with training in attention and processing speed for several months before individuals engage in the social-cognitive group curriculum.

Finally, the methods used to enhance social cognition in CET have relied on well-established theories of social development, particularly the sociological principles of secondary socialization (Parsons & Bales, 1956). Individuals develop an understanding of the social world in a variety of ways that usually involves a nonlinear trajectory. In early childhood, primary socialization is the mainstay for gaining social knowledge and consists of direct instruction about concrete rules of behavior by others, often parents or caregivers, such as "don't talk with your mouth full" and "say please and thank you" (Hogarty & Flesher, 1999a). However, as individuals enter into the adult social world, strict rules for behavior become less commonplace and primary socialization becomes insufficient for successful interpersonal interactions. In fact, a hallmark of adult social cognition is the ability to be cognitively flexible and recognize that the rules and norms that govern one social situation may not apply to others. Frequently, individuals find themselves needing to spontaneously appraise the informal rules that govern many social contexts. Information about these informal rules and norms for behavior are gained through accumulating secondary socialization experiences, or those experiences in which an individual is able to observe the situational context;

identify the perspectives, intentions, and emotional tone of others; and abstract the informal social rules that govern these situations. Unlike primary socialization, secondary socialization does not involve direct instruction of specific rules, but relies on individuals using a variety of social-cognitive abilities (e.g., perspective taking, social context appraisal) to learn how to behave.

The observation that much of adult social life is guided by informal rules of behavior obtained through secondary socialization experiences led Hogarty and colleagues to posit that the provision of such experiences within a therapeutic context could be of substantial value for enhancing social cognition in schizophrenia. As a result, CET makes use of a small-group context to facilitate the process of secondary socialization in schizophrenia. In the social-cognitive groups, individuals must not only learn the formal rules and norms of behavior that govern the group, but also the informal rules that characterize their interactions with their peers and CET coaches. Teamwork during in-group exercises, the presentation of homework, and the expression of feedback to peers are all based on formal and informal rules of conduct that must be extracted by observing others and taking their perspectives, appraising the group context, and relying on previous social knowledge from related experiences. Through the integration of these enriched secondary socialization experiences, along with the computer-based training in neurocognition, CET is able to facilitate improved social cognition among its recipients.

TREATMENT GOALS AND TARGETS

CET addresses the social and nonsocial cognitive impairments that limit functional outcome in schizophrenia. Cognitive impairments are viewed as rate-limiting factors to functional recovery in the disorder, and their amelioration is essential to supporting the personal goals of individuals with schizophrenia and improving their quality of life. This overall goal of enhancing cognition in CET is divided into the following two major subgoals during treatment: (1) fostering higher order thinking and (2) the development of social wisdom. The goal of facilitating higher order thinking among recipients is reflective of the neurodevelopmental theory guiding CET, which views cognitive impairment in schizophrenia as a developmental delay. The first goal of CET is then to support the transition to an adult cognitive style. The higher order thinking that characterizes adult cognition is fluid, abstract, and gistful, as opposed to concrete. Adult thinking is also active and flexible, and does not rely on rigid rules for behavior. Further, adults respond spontaneously to unrehearsed social situations and take the initiative to learn about their social environment in order to accomplish their goals. One of the primary goals of CET is to facilitate a mental shift to these characteristics of adult cognition through the provision of targeted therapeutic experiences and structured cognitive activities designed to facilitate higher order thinking.

The second goal of CET is to help individuals with schizophrenia develop social wisdom through the provision of enriched secondary socialization experiences.

CET focuses on helping individuals learn how to abstract the rules and norms for behavior in unrehearsed social exchanges, appraise the social context to identify appropriate behavior, take the perspective of others to assess their feelings and intentions, and assess the effectiveness of likely responses. CET fosters the development of foresightfulness to evaluate potential options for discourse/behavior and their likely consequences, and then to choose a course of action accordingly. These social-cognitive abilities become the foundation that CET uses to help individuals become more interpersonally wise. In addition, individuals develop social knowledge in CET by coming to appreciate the importance of social and emotional reciprocity in interactions. Many patients are accustomed to being the one who is cared for, and they rarely recognize the critical role of providing support and empathy to others in building and maintaining relationships. Finally, through this process of becoming more knowledgeable about the adult social context, CET aims to demystify the socialization process and increase social comfort among participants.

The therapeutic targets of CET address its goals of fostering higher order thinking and developing social wisdom. Clearly, impaired cognition is the primary target of CET. Unfortunately, the heterogeneity of schizophrenia results in many types of cognitive impairments, which must be taken into account to personalize the approach to the unique strengths and difficulties of each individual being treated. To parse the heterogeneity of cognitive impairment in schizophrenia and provide a personally meaningful framework for treatment targets, CET views impaired cognition as belonging to three dysfunctional cognitive styles of thinking (Hogarty & Flesher, 1999b). These include unmotivated, disorganized, and inflexible cognitive styles. Each style has its own behavioral characteristics that are meaningful and recognizable to patients.

An *unmotivated cognitive style* is characterized by difficulties with motivation and impoverished thinking and speech. For individuals with this cognitive style, CET aims to help them generate ideas, become more motivated, use elaborated speech, and think actively in social situations. Individuals with a *disorganized style* of thinking have difficulty organizing their ideas and often experience emotional dysregulation or "flooding." The focus for individuals with a disorganized style in CET is to help them organize their ideas by abstracting the main point or "gist" out of social situations and discarding irrelevant details, as well as helping individuals learn and practice the use of autoprotective strategies to regulate their emotions. The third cognitive style, *inflexible thinking*, is characterized by difficulty considering alternative points of view and explanations, and following rigid routines and rules for behavior. In CET, individuals with an inflexible style of thinking learn how to identify alternative solutions to problems, tolerate ambiguity, cope with the arousal associated with modifying routines, and become more cognitively flexible. These cognitive styles exist along a continuum of severity. Individuals may have characteristics of multiple cognitive styles, although one style is usually predominant. The identification of a person's dysfunctional cognitive style provides a personally meaningful set of treatment targets that individuals can address throughout CET.

PATIENT POPULATION

CET was developed for individuals diagnosed with schizophrenia or schizoaf-fective disorder, who are in the recovery phase of their condition. Schizophrenia is a phasic disorder characterized by prodromal, acute, and recovery phases (McGlashan & Johannessen, 1996). When individuals are acutely psychotic, the need for hospitalization and pharmacotherapeutic and psychosocial approaches to help stabilize positive symptoms is paramount, and CET would likely be of little benefit for such individuals at that time. However, the majority of patients with schizophrenia recover from the positive symptoms psychosis with adequate pharmacologic and psychosocial treatment, and most schizophrenia patients are able to enter the recovery phase of the disorder. CET was developed specifically for this population, as Hogarty and colleagues had previously developed several highly effective psychosocial approaches to be used in conjunction with antip-sychotic medication for individuals in the earlier, more acute phases of schizo-phrenia (Hogarty et al., 1974, 1986; Hogarty, 2002), and they sought to create in CET a recovery-phase intervention that would directly target the social and non-social deficits that kept patients from achieving improved functioning and a bet-ter quality of life. It is important to note that the recovery phase of illness is not synonymous with a complete absence of positive symptoms, but rather reflects that these symptoms have been stabilized and are reasonably well-controlled. Individuals who still experience frequent psychotic exacerbations leading to hos-pitalization or who are not adherent to medication are in need of treatment more specific to the acute phase of schizophrenia, such as Personal Therapy (Hogarty, 2002).

In addition, CET was developed for patients with schizophrenia who do not have a comorbid intellectual disability, which is operationalized as an IQ of 80 or below. Early trials of CET included some individuals with schizophrenia who had borderline intellectual functioning, and it was observed that such individuals had greater difficulty in grasping the concepts of the intervention, particularly the social-cognitive group curriculum, and were less likely to benefit from the treat-ment (Hogarty et al., 2004). Further, CET was not developed for patients with active substance use problems, due to the negative impact of substances on cogni-tion and brain function. Importantly, it must be established that a potential recipi-ent of CET experiences significant cognitive and social disability, and since the majority of schizophrenia patients experience disability in these two areas, CET is indicated for many patients. It is also important to note that CET has shown efficacy in patients with chronic (Hogarty et al., 2004) and early-course (Eack et al., 2009) schizophrenia, indicating its broad applicability across the course of the illness.

Finally, since the development of CET, two new advances have begun to expand the population of individuals for whom CET could be effective and available. The first initiative targets persons with schizophrenia and substance use problems, the most frequent of which are cannabis and alcohol (Volkow, 2009). Recognizing the frequency and impact of substance use on people with schizophrenia, Eack and colleagues have begun to integrate and expand the cognitive and social-cognitive methods employed in CET with the affect regulation strategies of Personal Therapy (Hogarty, 2002) to address cognitive impairment, affect dysregulation, and functional problems in patients with schizophrenia who misuse substances. The second CET initiative concerns individuals with autism spectrum disorders. Recently, Eack, Greenwald, Hogarty, and Minshew have begun adapting CET for verbal adults with autism spectrum disorders, who also experience significant impairments in neurocognitive and social-cognitive functioning (Baron-Cohen, Leslie, & Frith, 1985; Minshew & Goldstein, 1998). Although these developments are still in progress and not currently available outside of our research setting, evidence of the potential benefits of CET for substance misusing schizophrenia patients and adults with autism spectrum disorders is eagerly awaited.

INTERVENTION METHODS

Initial Assessment

The process of CET begins with a collaborative assessment between the patient and treating coach to identify strengths and areas in need of improvement. As with all effective interventions, the treatment process cannot begin without a careful assessment of the presenting problems and goals for the patient. A careful assessment of the patient helps to establish both the need and readiness for CET. In addition, since CET is primarily a small-group–based intervention, assessment becomes essential not only for directing individual treatment, but also for considering the composition of the neurocognitive and social-cognitive groups.

Assessment in CET begins with a review of the patient's history and the characteristics that indicate eligibility for the program, which usually includes a thorough psychiatric diagnostic assessment, an assessment of general intellectual ability (by an IQ test), and some inquiry into basic resources and housing stability. After this initial review, a semi-structured interview is conducted to provide a formal assessment of patient's cognitive and social difficulties. This interview is known as the Cognitive Styles and Social Cognition Eligibility Interview, and is published in the CET training manual (Hogarty & Greenwald, 2006). During the interview, patients are asked a series of questions about problems they may experience in thinking, socialization, role adjustment, and goal attainment. Questions are open-ended and provide information on the three cognitive styles (impoverished, disorganized, and inflexible) that are the targets of CET. In addition, questions regarding social-cognitive and functional difficulties are also asked to assess problems in vocational and social functioning, as well as the patient's adjustment to his to her disability. It is often helpful to videotape this interview so that it can be reviewed by other members of the CET treatment team, who may identify additional problems and areas of difficulty that the patient is experiencing. At a minimum, the finalization of clinical ratings on this assessment should be reviewed and discussed with the larger clinical team, as this assessment becomes important to the treatment planning process necessitating as accurate an assessment as possible.

After a patient has been admitted to the program, it is customary for them to be assigned a CET coach, who reviews the overall results of the Cognitive Styles and Social Cognition Eligibility Interview with them, as well as any neuropsychological testing results that were completed. This initiates a productive dialog with the patient about the impact of cognitive impairment on his or her life, and how the treatment of such impairments can support the achievement of broader life goals. In addition to the eligibility interview, participants also undergo a brief (5-minute) test of simple reaction time developed as part of one of the CET software packages (Ben-Yishay et al., 1985). This assessment provides a gauge of pretreatment attention and processing speed ability, which is important for constructing neurocognitive training pairs, as the first neurocognitive training module in CET is an attention and processing speed module. The pairing of individuals who have faster processing speeds (200–250 ms) with those who have slower processing speeds (350–450 ms) could be potentially demoralizing to the slower participant and frustrating to the faster participant, who would most likely be able to move at a faster pace. Since attention and processing speed are the foundations for many more complex cognitive abilities, the matching of individuals in reaction time is often helpful in subsequent memory and problem-solving exercises that occur during the later stages of CET. Consideration of other aspects, such as age and common interests, is also useful when pairing participants for computer work.

Finally, it is important to mention that collecting some assessment of outcome data is helpful during the CET program. For agencies with access to neuropsychological testing services, repeated testing using standardized neuropsychological tests such as the Wechsler Memory Scale (Wechsler, 1987), the Wisconsin Card Sorting Test (Heaton, Chelune, Talley, Kay, & Curtiss, 1993), the California Verbal Learning Test (Delis, Kramer, Kaplan, & Ober, 1987), and Trials B (Reitan & Waltson, 1985) at annual or 9-month intervals has been helpful for assessing treatment progress. Other agencies that do not have resources or access to neuropsychologists can assess progress by repeating the initial reaction time assessment, as well as using two CET clinician rating measures (Cognitive Styles Inventory and Social Cognition Profile) at initial assessment and at annual or 9-month intervals. These assessments have been shown to be sensitive to CET treatment effects in previous research studies (Eack et al., 2009; Hogarty et al., 2004). In this age of evidence-based practice, the systematic collection of outcome data is imperative for program evaluation and in assessing the gains and future needs of individual patients.

Neurocognitive Training

The computer-based neurocognitive training is the first systematic CET experience that patients encounter. This consists of a comprehensive training program that employs exercises in attention, memory, and problem solving designed to

Table 14.1 OVERVIEW OF COGNITIVE ENHANCEMENT THERAPY

Component/Timeline[a]	Description
NEUROCOGNITIVE TRAINING	
Attention Training (months 0–4)	Computer-based exercises designed to improve processing speed, the ability to maintain a cognitive set, and sustained attention
Memory Training (months 5–11)	Computer-based exercises designed to improve working memory, strategic encoding of information, and use of compensatory memory aids
Problem-Solving Training (months 12–18)	Computer-based exercises designed to improve planning, cognitive flexibility, and reasoning and logic
SOCIAL-COGNITIVE GROUP CURRICULUM	
Basic Concepts (months 4–8)	Focuses on understanding and coping with schizophrenia, motivation, using gistful thinking, improving memory, and cognitive flexibility
Social Cognition (months 9–14)	Focuses on acting wisely in social situations, social context appraisal, perspective-taking, reading nonverbal cues, and other important aspects of social cognition
CET Applications (months 15–18)	Focuses on generalizing CET to new situations, overcoming obstacles to using CET, and applying CET to respond to common social dilemmas, build social relationships, initiate meaningful activities

CET, Cognitive Enhancement Therapy
[a]Timelines are approximate and intended to provide an illustration of the timing of treatment components delivered during CET.

address the neurocognitive impairments experienced by patients with schizophrenia. Neurocognitive training in CET makes use of a "bottom-up" process, in which problems in attention and processing speed are targeted first using the Orientation Remediation Module (Ben-Yishay et al., 1985), followed by impairments in memory, and ultimately difficulties in reasoning, planning, and problem solving using software developed by Bracy (1994) (see Table 14.1). Unlike most neurocognitive training programs in which patients participate in neurocognitive training as a solitary activity, patient pairs are formed for neurocognitive training in CET. The pairing of patients has numerous benefits, including promoting treatment engagement; providing an early opportunity for socialization and the practicing of basic social-cognitive abilities, such as giving support; and making the computer training process more enjoyable for the participants. In addition, unlike other programs, neurocognitive training in CET is not a "hands-off" activity, but is actively facilitated by a therapist/coach who guides participants through the exercises and challenges them to think strategically about their performance.

A coach facilitates only one neurocognitive session at a time in a private office with a single pair of participants. All neurocognitive training sessions are held for approximately 1 hour per week, and proceed in this fashion for a total of 60 hours over the course of treatment.

An example neurocognitive training exercise is the Attention Reaction Conditioner in the Orientation Remediation Module suite, which is designed to improve sustained attention and processing speed (Ben-Yishay et al., 1985). In this exercise, participants view a screen that contains a critical stimulus light in the center and nine feedback lights that form a pyramid across the screen (see Figure 14.1). The task for participants is to press the space bar as soon as the center light appears. Participants receive a preparatory auditory cue (a "warning" tone) to let them know the task is beginning, and then, 5 seconds later, the critical stimulus or target light illuminates. Based on their performance (speed), feedback lights will then illuminate, telling participants whether or not they responded quickly enough. If participants do not respond within a given window (e.g., 300 ms) only a portion of the feedback lights will appear, with the number illuminated depending on how far outside the stimulus window participants responded. The faster participants respond, the more feedback lights will appear, and all nine feedback lights will illuminate if the participant responds within the stimulus window.

To aid participants in the exercise, auditory cues are given before the target light presents. At the beginning of attention training with this exercise, participants are given five auditory cues (one for each second) before the target appears. Gradually, these cues are faded, so that participants must begin to internalize the timing of when the target will appear. This greatly increases the difficulty of the task and promotes sustained attention. As participants progress further, the stimulus window is also reduced (e.g., from 300 ms to 170 ms), requiring them to not only sustain their attention for longer periods of time without cues, but to respond faster to the presentation of the target stimulus. In this fashion, the Attention Reaction Conditioner becomes a highly effective method for enhancing

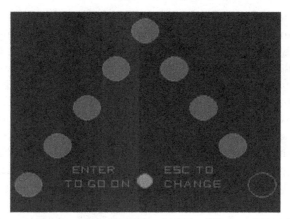

Figure 14.1 Example neurocognitive training exercise used in cognitive enhancement therapy: attention reaction conditioner. (Reprinted from the Orientation Remediation Module, with permission from Yehuda Ben-Yishay, Ph.D.)

processing speed and sustained attention. It is important to note that throughout the neurocognitive training (attention, memory, and problem solving) participants are encouraged to generate their own personal strategies for succeeding at the computer exercises. The role of the coach is to help facilitate this process, not to provide the strategy for the participant. Indeed, the process of developing strategies for solving the exercises is just as important as the particular strategy used in CET. The CET coach facilitates this process by encouraging self-reflection, suggesting consultation with the participant's computer partner, and the use of Socratic questioning to help individuals generate their own strategies.

Social-Cognitive Training

OVERVIEW
The enhancement of social cognition lies at the heart of CET. Neurocognitive training is designed to provide the requisite cognitive abilities needed to facilitate improved social cognition, but neurocognitive training alone does not provide the necessary strategies to address the social-cognitive deficits experienced by patients with schizophrenia. Targeted strategies for enhancing social cognition specifically are needed, and in CET this accomplished through the social-cognitive group experience. After approximately 3–6 months of attention training, three or four participant pairs join to form a social-cognitive group. A group-based approach to social-cognitive training, as opposed to individual or computer-based training, was adopted in CET because of the social nature of groups and their power for facilitating secondary socialization experiences. Much of the "social" in social cognition would be lost from an individual or computer-based experience, whereas a group setting affords many opportunities to learn and practice social-cognitive abilities in a more complex social setting. In addition, although studies have identified individual deficits in social cognition in schizophrenia (e.g., emotion perception, perspective taking), social-cognitive abilities are rarely performed in isolation in the real world, and the application of these abilities in a social setting often necessitates the use multiple aspects of social cognition in an integrated fashion that more closely resembles daily social interactions.

GROUP CONTENT
There are a total of 45 structured social-cognitive group sessions in CET, which are designed to facilitate key aspects of social cognition, including perspective taking, social context appraisal, foresightfulness, and emotion management. Social-cognitive groups integrate key psychoeducational content on social cognition with experiential learning opportunities through various in-group cognitive exercises, coaching, and homework assignments. The social-cognitive group curriculum is divided into three interrelated modules (see Table 14.1). The first module (Basic Concepts) focuses on schizophrenia and its management and introduces foundational concepts that are critical to subsequent sessions. Areas covered range from emotion regulation and stress management through the identification

of early distress cues and implementation of autoprotective coping strategies (e.g., diaphragmatic breathing) to increasing cognitive flexibility, enhancing motivation, and obtaining the main point or "gist" in communications.

The second module (Social Cognition) focuses on key social-cognitive abilities (e.g., perspective taking, social context appraisal, reading nonverbal cues, using elaborated speech, and giving support) and encourages participants to practice using these abilities in their everyday life through related and structured homework assignments. Social-cognitive enhancement in CET centers around improving the ability of participants to take the perspective of others in unrehearsed social situations. As such, perspective taking becomes the unifying theme around which other social-cognitive concepts and abilities are learned. For example, social context appraisal refers to the ability to spontaneously extract the rules and norms of behavior in a given social situation, which requires effortful observation and understanding the perspectives of all participants involved in the interaction. Reading nonverbal cues is another essential social-cognitive ability emphasized in CET. As participants learn to understand the perspectives of others, they are coached to observe others' feelings and behaviors, which are often most clearly stated through nonverbal behaviors such as facial expressions, posture, and tone of voice. Elaborated speech, which provides a shared context and allows others to understand the participant's own perspective, is also a core social-cognitive strategy learned in the CET group. Many of these concepts are strengthened when participants learn the social-cognitive strategies of giving emotional support, including reading the nonverbal cues of the person in need of support, taking their perspective and "emotional temperature," and conveying empathy. Experiential learning exercises are practiced to enhance these and other social-cognitive abilities learned throughout the second module, along with psychoeducation on their use and importance.

Finally, the third module of the social-cognitive group curriculum (CET Applications) focuses on the generalization and application of CET concepts and social-cognitive abilities in daily life, and how to use the strategies and abilities learned in CET to enhance the quality of one's life (e.g., expanding social networks, initiating new vocational or educational activities, deepening existing relationships). Obstacles to implementing CET strategies are also identified and addressed.

Group Structure

Each social-cognitive group session follows a very specific agenda that was designed to keep the group predictable and productive. Although the group sessions are highly structured, there remains ample opportunity for spontaneity and creativity within this format, while at the same time accomplishing the tasks of the particular group session. A typical social-cognitive group session includes several core components. First, one of the CET coaches provides a "Welcome Back" to participants and reviews the agenda for the session. Next, a group member volunteers to be the chairperson for the previous week's homework assignment. The chairperson role is one of the many opportunities for active participation in the group, as CET requires a great deal of active thinking and participation from group members, as opposed to a passive therapy group that only provides didactic instruction and problem solving for patients. The chairperson is in charge of calling on his or her peers to present their homework, as are the coaches who ask questions about the particular homework that is presented. The chairperson role provides many opportunities to integrate and utilize concepts that participants are learning in CET, such as motivation (e.g., volunteering to chair), strengthening working memory (e.g., keeping an online representation of the role of the chair and who has yet to present), and cognitive flexibility (e.g., deciding how to handle situations in which multiple participants volunteer to present their homework at the same time). Elaboration and a deeper understanding of the concepts involved in the homework assignment are encouraged by the coaches, who always ask follow-up questions of each presenting participant and use Socratic questioning to increase his or her understanding of the concepts. It is particularly rewarding as a CET coach to observe the growth in active thinking, abstraction, expressive language, and social understanding that participants exhibit during their homework presentations as they progress throughout the program. Once all participants, including the chair, have presented their homework assignment, the homework presentation component of the session is concluded.

After the homework presentation, selected participants engage in a cognitive exercise designed to provide direct experiential learning opportunities for enhancing social cognition. There are a total of nine thematic in-group exercises, each of which challenges participants to integrate and utilize the social-cognitive abilities that are being learned in the group. Variations of the nine thematic exercises are repeated across a number of group sessions, so that all participants will have the opportunity to perform each exercise at least once. Exercises are center stage, and consist of designated group members moving to the front of the group to perform the activity. Participants are given a brief introduction to the exercise by one of the coaches, and then encouraged to "think on their feet" to solve the given problem in these minimally rehearsed and novel interpersonal situations. Every exercise requires, at a minimum, the use of perspective taking for its successful completion. One example of an exercise that occurs during the second module of the group is known as "Condensed Messages." In this exercise, two participants are given the background of a social problem that ultimately involves someone who needs to send a message to persuade another person to act in a specific way. For example, an individual traveling overseas for an important business deal becomes sick with the flu and needs his spouse to travel immediately to his location to close the deal for him. Participants are given relevant information about the social context (e.g., that the husband and wife have an excellent relationship, and that the wife can take a leave from her job at a moment's notice), and are asked to construct a message that gets the recipient to act to solve the problem. A key challenge of this exercise is that the message must be brief (e.g., the husband can only send a 10-word telegram), but at the same time meaningful enough to encourage appropriate action.

The Condensed Message exercise requires the simultaneous use of many social-cognitive abilities. Participants must take the perspective of the sender to identify what action he would like the recipient to take (e.g., "come help close the business deal immediately"), as well as the perspective of the recipient to decipher what she must hear in order to act appropriately (e.g., that the husband needs immediate in-person help with the deal). The two participants must also appraise the social context and consider this information when formulating their message. For example, sending a message only indicating that the husband was sick and the wife needed to come quickly could lead her to believe he is seriously ill and prompt distress and perhaps a different course of action than the desired one. Participants must work together to determine the main gist of the message they would like to send, within the allotted number of words that are permitted. Throughout this and all other exercises in the social-cognitive group, participants must also be aware of their own emotions and anxieties about performing the exercise in front of the group, and work to manage these emotions to successfully complete the task. In this manner, the cognitive exercises become a primary vehicle for practicing and promoting the use of various social-cognitive abilities and other concepts learned throughout CET.

During the final module of the social-cognitive group curriculum, in-group cognitive exercises become particularly focused on facilitating the use of CET concepts and strategies in everyday life, which is a theme that is repeated throughout the CET program. One example of a cognitive exercise in this module is "Using CET to Help a Friend." In this exercise, participants are presented with a scenario (adapted from real-life situations encountered by previous patients) of a friend who is having difficulty in a social situation and is asking for help on what he or she might do to address the problem. For example, in one exercise, a friend who has been doing well and is hoping to move out of the family home to his own apartment comes to the participant asking for advice when his family is discouraging his move. The friend feels hurt, as though his family is being negative and does not trust him. He would like to become more independent, but at the same time wants to keep the peace at home. Participants complete this exercise in pairs, with one of the participants presenting the problem and the other trying to help using CET strategies, such as perspective taking (e.g., of the friend with the problem and family members who have a valid concern), giving a motivational account (e.g., helping the friend develop a convincing explanation of why he feels ready to move that acknowledges the perspective of the family), active listening (e.g., not rushing to give advice and displaying empathic concern), cognitive flexibility (e.g., that multiple perspectives are present in the scenario, and they must all be considered), and providing support (e.g., to the friend and the family). All participants eventually complete an exercise in which they have assumed both roles. The goal of this exercise is to facilitate the generalization of key CET "gists" and the use of independent, unrehearsed problem solving in common social dilemmas. Taken together, this exercise facilitates the review and consolidation of social-cognitive abilities learned throughout CET and promotes the generalization of these abilities to common social dilemmas.

While the selected participants complete the cognitive exercises, the remaining group members are tasked with organizing feedback to their peers about their performance using structured feedback sheets. This requires engagement and sustained attention for those not completing the exercise, and facilitates the use of social-cognitive abilities required in delivering feedback in a supportive and tactful manner. After each participant provides feedback, the coaches in the group provide their feedback on the strengths they observed during the exercise, as well as on any areas that could be improved. As with any therapeutic message, feedback from the coaches (and peers) is largely positive and always supportive. Any critical feedback that is provided is accompanied by a clear and genuine identification of the strengths of the participant's performance and offered in the spirit of helping the individual to continue to develop social wisdom and interpersonal effectiveness.

After the completion of the cognitive exercise and feedback has been provided, a coach delivers a brief (10- to 15-minute) psychoeducational lecture on a new topic in social cognition. Topics for these lectures were gleaned from the larger developmental literature on the social-cognitive abilities needed for interpersonal success (e.g., Baldwin, 1992; Selman & Schultz, 1990). Careful attention is paid by the coach to deliver the lecture in an engaging manner and to direct the focus of the lecture to real-world considerations that are of importance to participants (e.g., why perspective-taking is important for improving relationships with family members or succeeding at a job interview). When the lecture is completed, the coach asks for any clarifying questions (which is also done frequently throughout the lecture), then assigns a homework assignment for the following week based on the lecture content. Homework is intended to facilitate the application of CET concepts to everyday life outside of the therapeutic context. A typical homework assignment asks participants to think about the social-cognitive concept under consideration and how it applies to their personal lives. For example, when learning about perspective taking, individuals are asked to think of a person whose perspective is particularly important to understand, and then discuss how they would arrive at an understanding of that person's perspective given what they learned in the group. Finally, the time and date for the following group session is announced, and the group is adjourned. Each group session lasts 1.5 hours, and, given the amount of information covered in the social-cognitive groups, time management is essential.

RECOVERY PLANS

As with any effective treatment, patients arrive at CET with a unique set of personal goals and difficulties, and an effective treatment must incorporate these personal considerations to tailor intervention strategies to the different circumstances of the patient. In CET, treatment is individualized through the development of recovery plans, which target a participant's goal, the problem he or she is encountering that stands in the way of achieving the goal, and the CET strategies that he or she can use to work toward overcoming the problem and improving his or her life. With the help of the coach, participants develop recovery plans

Table 14.2 EXAMPLE COGNITIVE ENHANCEMENT THERAPY RECOVERY PLAN

EXAMPLE 1	
Goal:	To improve my motivation
Problem:	Difficulty convincing myself to remember and do things
Strategies:	1. Volunteer to be chairperson in the CET group and be an active participant in the CET computer sessions
	2. Create a list or calendar of tasks to be completed and review daily
	3. Break tasks down into smaller steps (focus on one step at a time)
	4. Be foresightful and think about the consequences of not completing tasks
	5. Use an internal yardstick to regularly review my progress
	6. Reward myself for completing tasks
EXAMPLE 2	
Goal:	To better understand how to act and what to say in social situations
Problem:	Difficulty with social context appraisal
Strategies:	1. Ask questions about what is appropriate
	2. Observe and listen to others for cues
	3. Take the perspective of others
	4. Think about how what I say might affect others, and adjust my behavior accordingly
	5. Practice giving tactful feedback in CET group

that are specific to each individual and obtainable in the time frame of CET. If long-term goals that are beyond the scope of CET are identified, the coach helps participants break these into a series of short-term goals that can be addressed in CET. Example recovery plans are provided in Table 14.2. The recovery plans are written on large poster boards and displayed during the social-cognitive group sessions, to help apply the content of the group to the personal goals of each of the members. Initial recovery plans are created at the beginning of the social-cognitive groups. Midway through the CET program, participants are asked to review the progress they have made on their initial recovery plan, and then a new recovery plan is formulated that incorporates their increased understanding of their social-cognitive difficulties in light of what they have learned thus far during the group. Final recovery plans are developed near the completion of the group, and serve to provide guidance and direction to participants as they graduate from CET and move toward an independent application of what they have learned to their daily lives. When helping individuals develop their recovery plan, the coach integrates the comprehensive neurocognitive and social-cognitive training strategies of CET to provide a meaningful treatment experience to participants that is clear in its aim to help them achieve their own personal goals and enhance their quality of life.

Individual Therapy

The primary therapeutic components of CET are the neurocognitive computer training and social-cognitive group curriculum. All of these aspects of the intervention are conducted in groups, whether they be a pair (for neurocognitive training) or a small group (for social-cognitive training) of participants. Individual meetings between participants and CET coaches address personal issues in the participant's life, review initial assessments, assist with developing recovery plans, and provide individual coaching on some CET homework assignments and exercises. All participants who enter the CET program are assigned a primary coach, who meets with the participant individually and frequently leads exercises involving the participant in the social-cognitive group. The need for individual sessions varies among participants; however, in the beginning of treatment, it is essential that coaches meet with their participant weekly to begin building a strong therapeutic relationship.

Individual therapy sessions also provide the opportunity to reinforce key CET concepts that are learned throughout the group. For example, during the early stages of the social-cognitive group curriculum, participants may still have considerable ambivalence about the need for medications, which would be inappropriate to discuss at length during group sessions. The coach uses individual sessions with the participant to review his or her medication history, note patterns of emerging illness that are associated with medication nonadherence, and share information about the likelihood of psychotic relapse when medication is not used. As individuals learn autoprotective strategies for managing stress and arousal during the early group curriculum, the coach encourages participants to recognize their early cues of stress and to apply healthy autoprotective strategies promptly. As participants gain more understanding of social cognition, the coach is always mindful to reinforce such CET strategies as perspective taking, giving a motivational account, and social context appraisal when participants discuss their interpersonal and social activities or concerns. In this fashion, the individual sessions help to further tailor CET to the individual needs of the participant.

Finally, individual sessions are particularly helpful when issues arise that are not the focus of the neurocognitive training or social-cognitive curriculum. The emphasis of CET is on improving cognition, not discussing residual symptomatology, paranoid delusional systems, or difficulties obtaining needed resources. Of course, during the 18- to 24-month period of receiving CET, it is not uncommon for these issues to occur among individuals with schizophrenia, and the coach should actively address these issues in individual sessions. The recurrence of psychotic symptoms can happen even when individuals faithfully take medication as prescribed, and the CET coach may be the first to discuss these symptoms with the participant. Changes in entitlements, housing, and other resource issues also can lead to stress and very significant life problems. Individual sessions give the participant an opportunity to discuss these issues in a more private setting. Since the emphasis of CET is on the improvement of cognition, the CET coach usually does not attempt to address these problems themselves, but calls upon local psychiatric and other resources that specialize in treating the presenting problem.

IMPLEMENTATION

The implementation of evidence-based practices in community mental health settings is of paramount importance, and it remains an area in which providers, policymakers, and researchers have not traditionally excelled. CET contains several key elements that facilitate its implementation in the community mental health centers that provide the majority of care for patients with schizophrenia. A group-based approach is often more economically feasible than an approach that consists primarily of individual-based therapy. This enables a greater patient-to-session ratio, which maximizes the use of therapist time, while still providing substantial benefits to the patient. In addition, a comprehensive treatment and training manual has been developed for CET (Hogarty & Greenwald, 2006), which includes highly specific, session-by-session guidance on the implementation of CET. Further, the evidence of the benefits of CET from two National Institutes of Health (NIH)-supported clinical trials (Eack et al., 2009; Hogarty et al., 2004) has supported third-party reimbursement of the treatment, which is essential for sustained implementation.

Community agencies interested in implementing CET will need a few additional resources. The CET training manual and accompanying supplemental CD-ROM are essential for obtaining information on how to implement and use the approach in patients with schizophrenia, as well as in obtaining the treatment materials that are utilized in the neurocognitive and social-cognitive groups. In addition, the neurocognitive training software from Ben-Yishay (Orientation Remediation Module) and Bracy (PSSCogRehab) are required for the attention, memory, and problem-solving training that occurs in CET. Beyond these initial costs, most community agencies already have the necessary resources for implementing CET. An office with a single computer is needed for neurocognitive training, and a medium-sized conference or group room is needed for conducting the social-cognitive groups. The neurocognitive training software is designed to operate on almost any existing PC-compatible computer. A white board is needed in the group room for cognitive exercises and developing patients' recovery plans, and large poster boards are needed for displaying finalized versions of the initial and interim recovery plans during the group. A Velcro board or cork board is also needed for one of the group exercises. A black-and-white printer is necessary for printing agendas, treatment handouts, and computer scoring sheets for participants, and three-ring binders are used to help participants organize the treatment materials they receive.

Staffing considerations are very important in conducting CET. Effective CET coaches can come from many disciplines, as social workers, psychologists, nurses, and other mental health professionals have all been trained to successfully provide CET in previous research studies. An interdisciplinary team is preferred, if possible, to bring in the different background and training experiences that often create a rich and effective treatment team. Individual coaches should have, at a minimum, master's-level preparation in a mental health profession and several years of direct clinical experience with patients with schizophrenia. Beyond these basic qualifications, individuals must be interested in learning a new approach, open to different styles of treatment, and passionate about helping patients with schizophrenia. The active nature of the social-cognitive groups places significant demands on the coaches, and thus at least two coaches are necessary for conducting these groups. CET is an agency- or center-based intervention. It is unlikely that it would be feasible to implement CET in a private practice setting. Support from agency leadership to provide the time and resources necessary for staff to learn and provide CET is essential for effective implementation.

CONCLUSION

CET is a unique and comprehensive approach to the remediation of social and nonsocial cognitive impairments in schizophrenia. The intervention effectively integrates computer-based training in attention, memory, and problem solving, with a social-cognitive group curriculum designed to enhance perspective taking, social context appraisal, gistfulness, and other important aspects of social cognition. Clinical trials of CET in schizophrenia have consistently documented its benefits on cognition and functioning (Eack et al., 2009; Hogarty et al., 2004), with recent evidence indicating a neuroprotective benefit of CET for patients in the early course of the disorder (Eack et al., 2010b). The integration of neurocognitive and social-cognitive training is viewed as a helpful combination by patients, who consistently engage and succeed in the program. Patients appreciate that CET is personalized, targets areas that are problematic for them, and increases their strengths. The demonstrated efficacy of CET, its emphasis on personal recovery, and its acceptability to patients all make this cognitive rehabilitation approach a particularly effective adjunct to pharmacotherapy for enhancing quality of life and facilitating a greater functional recovery among the many patients who live with schizophrenia.

REFERENCES

Baldwin, M. W. (1992). Relational schemas and the processing of social information. *Psychological Bulletin, 112*(3), 461–484.

Baron-Cohen, S., Leslie, A. M., & Frith, U. (1985). Does the autistic child have a theory of mind? *Cognition, 21*(1), 37–46.

Ben-Yishay, Y., Piasetsky, E. B., & Rattok, J. (1985). A systematic method for ameliorating disorders in basic attention. In M. J. Meir, A. L. Benton, & L. Diller (Eds.), *Neuropsychological rehabilitation* (pp. 165–181). New York: Guilford Press.

Bracy, O. L. (1994). *PSSCogRehab* [computer software]. Indianapolis, IN: Psychological Software Services Inc.

Couture, S. M., Penn, D. L., & Roberts, D. L. (2006). The functional significance of social cognition in schizophrenia: A review. *Schizophrenia Bulletin, 32*(Suppl.1), S44–S63.

Delis, D. C., Kramer, J. H., Kaplan, E., & Ober, B. A. (1987). *California verbal learning test manual*. San Antonio, TX: Psychological Corp.

Eack, S. M., Dworakowski, D., Montrose, D. M., Miewald, J., Gur, R. E., Gur, R. C., et al. (2010c). Social cognition deficits among individuals at familial high risk for schizophrenia. *Schizophrenia Bulletin, 36*(6), 1081–1088.

Eack, S. M., Greeno, C. G., Pogue-Geile, M. F., Newhill, C. E., Hogarty, G. E., & Keshavan, M. S. (2010a). Assessing social-cognitive deficits in schizophrenia with the Mayer-Salovey-Caruso Emotional Intelligence Test. *Schizophrenia Bulletin, 36*(2), 370–380.

Eack, S. M., Greenwald, D. P., Hogarty, S. S., Cooley, S. J., DiBarry, A. L., Montrose, D. M., et al. (2009). Cognitive Enhancement Therapy for early-course schizophrenia: Effects of a two-year randomized controlled trial. *Psychiatric Services, 60*(11), 1468–1476.

Eack, S. M., Hogarty, G. E., Cho, R. Y., Prasad, K. M. R., Greenwald, D. P., Hogarty, S. S., et al. (2010b). Neuroprotective effects of Cognitive Enhancement Therapy against gray matter loss in early schizophrenia: Results from a two-year randomized controlled trial. *Archives of General Psychiatry, 67*(7), 674–682.

Gogtay, N., Giedd, J. N., Lusk, L., Hayashi, K. M., Greenstein, D., Vaituzis, A. C., et al. (2004). Dynamic mapping of human cortical development during childhood through early adulthood. *Proceedings of the National Academy of Sciences of the United States of America, 101*(21), 8174–8179.

Green, M. F., Penn, D. L., Bentall, R., Carpenter, W. T., Gaebel, W., Gur, R. C., Kring, A. M., Park, S., Silverstein, S. M., & Heinssen, R. (2008). Social cognition in schizophrenia: An NIMH Workshop on Definitions, Assessment, and Research Opportunities. *Schizophrenia Bulletin, 34*(6), 1211–1220.

Heaton, R. K., Chelune, G. J., Talley, J. L., Kay, G. G., & Curtiss, G. (1993). *Wisconsin card sorting test manual: Revised and expanded*. Odessa, FL: Psychological Assessment Resources Inc.

Hogarty, G. E. (2002). *Personal therapy for schizophrenia and related disorders: A guide to individualized treatment*. New York: Guilford.

Hogarty, G. E., Anderson, C. M., Reiss, D. J., Kornblith, S. J., Greenwald, D. P., Javna, C. D., et al. (1986). Family psychoeducation, social skills training, and maintenance chemotherapy in the aftercare treatment of schizophrenia: I. One-year effects of a controlled study on relapse and expressed emotion. *Archives of General Psychiatry, 43*(7), 633–642.

Hogarty, G. E., & Flesher, S. (1999a). Developmental theory for a cognitive enhancement therapy of schizophrenia. *Schizophrenia Bulletin, 25*(4), 677–692.

Hogarty, G. E., & Flesher, S. (1999b). Practice principles of cognitive enhancement therapy for schizophrenia. *Schizophrenia Bulletin, 25*(4), 693–708.

Hogarty, G. E., Flesher, S., Ulrich, R., Carter, M., Greenwald, D., Pogue-Geile, M., et al. (2004). Cognitive enhancement therapy for schizophrenia. Effects of a 2-year randomized trial on cognition and behavior. *Archives of General Psychiatry, 61*(9), 866–876.

Hogarty, G. E., Goldberg, S. C., Schooler, N. R., & the Collaborative Study Group. (1974). Drug and sociotherapy in the aftercare of schizophrenic patients: III. Adjustment of nonrelapsed patients. *Archives of General Psychiatry, 31*(5), 609–618.

Hogarty, G. E., & Greenwald, D. P. (2006). *Cognitive enhancement therapy: The training manual.* Pittsburgh, PA: University of Pittsburgh Medical Center. Available from www.CognitiveEnhancementTherapy.com.

Horan, W. P., Kern, R. S., Shokat-Fadai, K., Sergi, M. J., Wynn, J. K., & Green, M. F. (2009). Social cognitive skills training in schizophrenia: an initial efficacy study of stabilized outpatients. *Schizophrenia Research, 107*(1), 47–54.

Johansson, B. B. (2000). Brain plasticity and stroke rehabilitation: The Willis lecture. *Stroke, 31*(1), 223–230.

Karni, A., Meyer, G., Jezzard, P., Adams, M. M., Turner, R., & Ungerleider, L. G. (1995). Functional MRI evidence for adult motor cortex plasticity during motor skill learning. *Nature, 377*(6545), 155–158.

Keefe, R. S. E., Bilder, R. M., Davis, S. M., Harvey, P. D., Palmer, B. W., Gold, J. M., et al. (2007). Neurocognitive effects of antipsychotic medications in patients with chronic schizophrenia in the CATIE trial. *Archives of General Psychiatry, 64*(6), 633–647.

Keshavan, M. S., Diwadkar, V. A., Montrose, D. M., Rajarethinam, R., & Sweeney, J. A. (2005). Premorbid indicators and risk for schizophrenia: A selective review and update. *Schizophrenia Research, 79*(1), 45–57.

Kunugi, H., Nanko, S., & Murray, R. M. (2001). Obstetric complications and schizophrenia: Prenatal underdevelopment and subsequent neurodevelopmental impairment. *British Journal of Psychiatry, 178*(40), S25–S29.

Lewis, D. A., & Levitt, P. (2002). Schizophrenia as a disorder of neurodevelopment. *Annual Review of Neuroscience, 25*, 409–432.

Lezack, M. D. (1983). *Neuropsychological assessment.* New York: Oxford University Press.

McGlashan, T. H., & Johannessen, J. O. (1996). Early detection and intervention with schizophrenia: rationale. *Schizophrenia Bulletin, 22*(2), 201–222.

McGurk, S. R., Twamley, E. W., Sitzer, D. I., McHugo, G. J., & Mueser, K. T. (2007). A meta-analysis of cognitive remediation in schizophrenia. *American Journal of Psychiatry, 164*(12), 1791–1802.

Minshew, N. J., & Goldstein, G. (1998). Autism as a disorder of complex information processing. *Mental Retardation and Developmental Disabilities Research Reviews, 4*(2), 129–136.

Parsons, T., & Bales, R. (1956). *Family, socialization and interaction process.* London: Routledge and Kegan Paul.

Penn, D. L., Corrigan, P. W., Bentall, R. P., Racenstein, J., & Newman, L. (1997). Social cognition in schizophrenia. *Psychological Bulletin, 121*(1), 114–132.

Prasad, K. M. R., Eack, S. M., Goradia, D., Pancholi, K. M., Keshavan, M. S., Yolken, R. H., et al. (2011). Progressive grey matter loss and changes in cognitive functions associated with exposure to HSV1 in schizophrenia: A longitudinal study. *American Journal of Psychiatry, 168*(8), 822–830.

Reitan, R. M., & Waltson, D. (1985). *The Halstead-Reitan Neuropsychological Test Battery.* Tucson, AZ: Neuropsychology Press.

Seidman, L. J., Buka, S. L., Goldstein, J. M., Horton, N. J., Rieder, R. O., & Tsuang, M. T. (2000). The relationship of prenatal and perinatal complications to cognitive functioning at age 7 in the New England Cohorts of the National Collaborative Perinatal Project. *Schizophrenia bulletin, 26*(2), 309–321.

Selman, R. L., & Schultz, L. H. (1990). *Making a friend in youth.* Chicago, IL: University of Chicago Press.

Sergi, M. J., Green, M. F., Widmark, C., Reist, C., Erhart, S., Braff, D. L., et al. (2007a). Cognition and neurocognition: Effects of Risperidone, Olanzapine, and Haloperidol. *American Journal of Psychiatry, 164*(10), 1585–1592.

Sergi, M. J., Rassovsky, Y., Widmark, C., Reist, C., Erhart, S., Braff, D. L., et al. (2007b). Social cognition in schizophrenia: Relationships with neurocognition and negative symptoms. *Schizophrenia Research, 90*(1–3), 316–324.

Simon, H. A. (1979). Information processing models of cognition. *Annual Review of Psychology, 30*(1), 363–396.

Volkow, N. D. (2009). Substance use disorders in schizophrenia—Clinical implications of comorbidity. *Schizophrenia Bulletin, 35*(3), 469–472.

Wechsler, D. (1987). *Manual for the Wechsler Memory Scale-Revised.* San Antonio, TX: Psychological Corp.

Weinberger, D. R. (1987). Implications of normal brain development for the pathogenesis of schizophrenia. *Archives of General Psychiatry, 44*(7), 660–669.

APPENDIX

RESOURCES AND MATERIALS ON COGNITIVE ENHANCEMENT THERAPY

Treatment Resources

Hogarty, G. E. &Greenwald, D. P. (2006). Cognitive Enhancement Therapy: The Training Manual. Available through www.CognitiveEnhancementTherapy.com
Ben-Yishay, Y. Orientation Remediation Module. Available through Yehuda Ben-Yishay, Ph.D. (212) 263-7156/(212) 263-6028, Yehuda.Ben-Yishay@ msnyuhealth.org or David J. Biderman, Ph.D. (212) 263-0309, David.Biderman@ nyumc.org.
Bracy, O. L. (1994). PSSCogRehab. Available through Psychological Software Service, www.neuroscience.cnter.com/pss/psscr.html

Research on Cognitive Enhancement Therapy

Eack, S. M. ,Greenwald, D. P., Hogarty, S. S.,Cooley, S. J., DiBarry, A. L., Montrose, D. M., & Keshavan, M. S. (2009). Cognitive Enhancement Therapy for early-course schizophrenia: Effects of a two-year randomized controlled trial. *Psychiatric Services, 60*(11), 1468–1476.

Eack, S. M. ,Greenwald, D. P. ,Hogarty, S. S., &Keshavan, M. S. (2010). One-year durability of the effects of Cognitive Enhancement Therapy on functional outcome in early schizophrenia. *Schizophrenia Research, 120*(1), 210–216.

Eack, S. M., Hogarty, G. E., Cho, R. Y., Prasad, K. M. R., Greenwald, D. P., Hogarty, S. S., & Keshavan, M. S. (2010). Neuroprotective effects of Cognitive Enhancement Therapy against gray matter loss in early schizophrenia: Results from a two-year randomized controlled trial. *Archives of General Psychiatry, 67*(7), 674–682.

Hogarty, G. E., Flesher, S., Ulrich, R., Carter, M., Greenwald, D., Pogue-Geile, M., et al. (2004). Cognitive enhancement therapy for schizophrenia. Effects of a 2-year random-ized trial on cognition and behavior. *Archives of General Psychiatry, 61*(9), 866–876.

Hogarty, G. E., Greenwald, D. P., & Eack, S. M. (2006). Durability and mechanism of effects of Cognitive Enhancement Therapy. *Psychiatric Services, 57*(12), 1751–1757.

15

Metacognitive Training in Schizophrenia

Theoretical Rationale and Administration

STEFFEN MORITZ, RUTH VECKENSTEDT, FRANCESCA BOHN,
ULF KÖTHER, AND TODD S. WOODWARD ■

Despite their widespread usage, neuroleptic agents do not provide lasting and comprehensive treatment success in many patients with schizophrenia. One-third of all patients are neuroleptic-resistant (Elkis, 2007; Lindenmayer, 2000), and the mean effect size of neuroleptics above placebo is only in the medium range (Leucht, Arbter, Engel, Kissling, & Davis, 2009). Even for those who benefit from neuroleptic administration, treatment can often come at a considerable cost in view of side effects, particularly neurological symptoms under first-generation neuroleptic agents, and metabolic symptoms, such as weight gain and diabetes under some second-generation agents (Haddad & Sharma, 2007; Rummel-Kluge et al., 2010). In addition to side effects, poor therapeutic alliance, lack of insight (Bora, Sehitoglu, Aslier, Atabay, & Veznedaroglu, 2007; Buchy, Malla, Joober, & Lepage, 2009), and memory problems (Moritz et al., 2009) are reasons why up to three-quarters of patients withdraw medication after hospital discharge (Byerly, Nakonezny, & Lescouflair, 2007; Lieberman et al., 2005).

The complacency that followed the introduction of atypical neuroleptics has led to a sober reassessment of the benefits and risks of neuroleptic treatment. The initial enthusiasm about the benefits of atypical drugs has markedly diminished in recent years (Davis, Chen, & Glick, 2003; Lehrer, 2010). In addition, the role of psychotherapy is being reconsidered, and psychological models and treatment approaches now face less skepticism. An extensive line of research has put forward evidence for contributions of neuropsychological deficits (Schretlen et al., 2007) and, more recently, cognitive biases (Bell, Halligan, & Ellis, 2006; Freeman, 2007) in the pathogenesis of psychosis. Results from basic research are increasingly translated into treatment programs (Roder & Medalia, 2010). So far, the most effective psychological treatment of psychosis appears to be cognitive-behavioral therapy (CBT), which exerts a small to medium effect size as an add-on treatment to neuroleptics (Wykes, Steel, Everitt, & Tarrier, 2008), although—as in other psychological disorders—dissemination is scarce (Shafran et al., 2009).

Psychopharmacology and psychotherapy should be seen as complementary rather than as rivals or counterexclusive interventions. For example, psychopharmacology is often a prerequisite for psychotherapy in order to mute agitation, formal thought disorder, and hostility, which may undermine or even preclude a therapeutic relationship. Psychotherapy, in turn, improves the person's understanding of his or her symptoms and thereby often ameliorates medication adherence. Tentative evidence suggests that the routes of action are very different (Birchwood & Trower, 2006; Moritz et al., 2009); neuroleptics provide some detachment and emotional numbing but do not alter belief conviction (Mizrah et al., 2006), whereas psychotherapy can enhance illness insight and decreases stress.

METACOGNITIVE TRAINING FOR SCHIZOPHRENIA: OVERVIEW

Metacognitive training (MCT; from *metacognition*, "thinking about one's thinking") is a novel approach founded in the tradition of psychoeducation, cognitive remediation, social cognition training and CBT. It is now in its fourth edition, and has been translated into 29 languages. MCT targets cognitive biases putatively involved in delusion formation, for which patients often lack adequate awareness (see next section). Another explicit aim of MCT is to foster improved social cognition and theory of mind (ToM; for an overview see Moritz, Vitzthum, Randjbar, Veckenstedt, & Woodward, 2010; Moritz & Woodward, 2007b). The training is highly structured, as we endeavored to keep preparation time short and thus facilitate its dissemination. Depending on the group's level of understanding, the text should be read or paraphrased. A friendly and humorous atmosphere should be created, and the exercises should be delivered in an entertaining, interactive, and playful fashion. The present program can be downloaded free of charge via the following link: www.uke.de/mkt. Table 15.1 summarizes the eight modules of the MCT along with target domains and learning aims.

The main objective of the MCT program is to raise the patient's awareness of cognitive biases (e.g., jumping to conclusions) and to prompt him or her to critically reflect on, complement, and alter his or her current repertoire of problem-solving and thinking skills. Longitudinal studies (Klosterkötter, 1992) assert that psychosis is not a sudden and inevitable event but is often preceded by a gradual change in the evaluation of one's cognitions and (social) environment over several weeks. The route into psychotic breakdown is thus not necessarily a one-way street, but is a potentially reversible process. Empowering metacognitive competency by raising awareness for cognitive biases may then act prophylactically against psychotic breakdown.

The training is delivered by a health care professional in a group of 3–10 schizophrenia spectrum patients. Although trainers should preferably be psychologists

Table 15.1 SUMMARY OF EACH METACOGNITIVE TRAINING MODULE (GROUP SESSIONS)

Module	Target domain	Description of core exercises and learning aims
(1) Attribution: blaming and taking credit	Monocausal inferences	Different causes of positive and negative events should be contemplated. Participants are taught to consider various causes instead of converging on monocausal explanations. For example, "a friend was talking behind your back"; dominant interpretation: "friend is not trustworthy" (blaming others); alternatives: "I have done something bad" (blaming self), "she is preparing a surprise party for my birthday" (circumstances). The negative consequences of a self-serving attribution are repeatedly highlighted.
(2) Jumping to conclusions I	Jumping to conclusions/ liberal acceptance	Motifs contributing to hasty decision making are discussed and disadvantages of jumping to conclusions are highlighted. Fragmented pictures are shown that eventually display objects. Premature decisions often lead to errors, emphasizing the benefits of cautious data gathering.
		In the second part, ambiguous pictures are displayed. Here, a quick survey leads to the omission of details, demonstrating that first impressions, in many cases, only reveal half the truth.
(3) Changing beliefs	Bias against disconfirmatory evidence	Cartoon sequences are shown in reverse order, which increasingly disambiguate a complex scenario. After each (new) picture, participants are asked to (re-)rate the plausibility of four interpretations. On some pictures, participants are "led up the garden path." Thus, participants learn to withhold strong judgments until sufficient evidence has been collected, and they are encouraged to maintain an open attitude toward counterarguments and alternative views.
(4) To empathize I	Theory of mind first order	Facial expression and other cues are discussed for their relevance to social reasoning. Then, pictures of human faces are presented in the exercises. The group should guess what emotions the depicted character(s) may feel. The correct solution often violates the first intuition, demonstrating that reliance on facial expression alone can be misleading and that response confidence needs to be attenuated when the available evidence is insufficient.
		In the second part, cartoon strips are shown that either must be completed or brought into the correct order. Participants are shown that social inferences should involve multiple pieces of evidence.

(5) Memory	Over-confidence in errors	Factors that foster or impair memory acquisition are discussed first, and examples for common false memories are presented. Then, prototypical scenes (e.g., beach) are displayed with two typical elements each removed (e.g., towel, ball). Owing to logical inference, gist-based recollection, and liberal acceptance, many patients falsely recognize these lure items in a later recognition trial with high confidence. The constructive rather than passive nature of memory is thus brought to the participants' attention. Participants are taught to differentiate between false and correct memories by means of the vividness heuristic.
(6) To empathize II	Theory of mind second order/need for closure	Different aspects guiding theory of mind (e.g., language) are discussed with respect to both their heuristic value and fallibility for social decision making. Then, cartoon sequences are presented, and the perspective of one of the protagonists must be taken, which involves discounting knowledge available to the observer but not available to the protagonist. For the majority of sequences, no definitive solutions can be inferred, which is unsatisfactory for patients with an enhanced need for closure.
(7) Jumping to conclusions II	Jumping to conclusions/ liberal acceptance	As in module 2, the disadvantages of quick decision making are emphasized with multiple examples. In the exercises, paintings are displayed for which the correct title must be deduced from four response options. On superficial inspection, many pictures tempt false responses.
(8) Mood and self-esteem	Mood and self-esteem	First, depressive symptoms, causes for depression, and treatment options are discussed. Then, typical depressive cognitive patterns are presented (e.g., overgeneralization, selective abstraction), and the group is asked to come up with more constructive and positive ones. At the end, some strategies are conveyed to help patients transform negative self-schemata and elevate their mood.

or psychiatrists who have experience with schizophrenia spectrum disorder patients, psychiatric nurses, social workers, and occupational therapists may also be eligible. For example, our groups in Hamburg are run by psychology students receiving extensive training and supervision.

The MCT comprises eight modules that consist of a series of PDF-converted slide shows that should be displayed via a video projector onto a white wall or screen. For several languages, two parallel cycles are now available that allow participants to undergo two sessions for each target domain, with new examples. Each session should not last longer than 60 minutes, as many patients have a poor attention span. As each module contains more exercises than can be accomplished in this timeframe, the trainer can choose among the extensive material and should skip ahead to the learning aims when the allotted 45–60 minutes is nearing completion. Trainers may well deviate from the slides, or blend the MCT with alternative therapeutic techniques. For example, the vignettes in module 1 which deal with attributional style (e.g., you failed an exam) can be used to stage role-play, as in social competence training. An administration mode of two sessions per week is advantageous (at one module per session, a full cycle can be completed in 4 weeks) to ensure that participants undergo as many sessions as possible. The group is open; that is, participants may enter at any module (each module deals with a separate bias and the contents are independent), so that there is no fixed group. This procedure has some advantages over fixed groups, as open groups do not as easily "dry out."

Each module follows a certain sequence: (1) an introduction demonstrating how cognitive biases and social misinterpretations/misunderstandings impact our everyday lives (the "normalizing" phase); (2) relationship of extreme forms of the respective bias/problem with mental illness in general and psychosis in particular (the slide entitled "Why are we doing this?"); (3) exercises highlighting the dysfunctionality of the respective bias/problems (corrective experiences); (4) summary of learning aims; and (5) case example(s) emphasizing the relationship between cognitive biases and psychosis. During the training, videos may be shown that can be downloaded at Google/video (search with the key term "metacognitive training") or are available at the bottom of our webpage at www.uke.de/mkt. Finally, leaflets with homework are handed out.

After his or her first session, each participant should receive a yellow card and a red card (again, templates can be downloaded from the MCT website). The yellow card raises three fundamental questions that a patient should consider when feeling offended, persecuted, or insulted:

1. What is the evidence?
2. Are there alternative views?
3. Even if it's like that...am I overreacting?

These questions are intended to prompt participants to master critical situations and to avoid hasty and consequential decisions. On the red card, the patient is encouraged to write down names and telephone numbers of persons and/or institutions that may help in case of crisis or breakdown.

The exercises demonstrate how cognitive biases—which are almost normal, benign, and sometimes even functional when presenting in a subtle degree (decisiveness as the bright side of jumping to conclusions; perseverance as the bright side of incorrigibility; self-certainty as the bright side of overconfidence in errors)—as well as problems with social cognition can escalate into troublesome situations. It is assumed that these biases may separately or in combination culminate in the formation of beliefs that may eventually become delusions (Bentall et al., 2009; Moritz, Veckenstedt, Hottenrott et al., 2010). In the next section, empirical evidence for the presence of problematic thinking styles in schizophrenia is summarized. We also subsequently explain how these are dealt with in the different modules of the MCT (for a summary, see Table 15.1). The following biases and problems are at the core of the MCT: attributional style (module 1), jumping to conclusions (JTC; modules 2 and 7), bias against disconfirmatory evidence (BADE; module 3), social cognition/ToM (modules 4 and 6), overconfidence in memory errors (module 5), and depressive cognitive patterns and low self-esteem (module 8). In the closing section, several recommendations for administration are provided.

COGNITIVE BIASES IN SCHIZOPHRENIA

A psychological or cognitive understanding of delusion formation has long been obstructed by claims that delusions are not amenable to understanding. Beginning in the 1980s, however, cognitive research has questioned strong formulations of this account. Several meaningful cognitive mechanisms have been implicated in the pathogenesis of fixed false beliefs (i.e., delusions). These will be described in the following sections, which will first present the theory and empirical evidence and then show how they are dealt with in the MCT.

Attributional Style: Theory

As dynamic theorists like Adler (1914/1929) had already reasoned at the beginning of the last century, patients with schizophrenia show deviances in attributional style, specifically a tendency to blame others for own failure (*scapegoating*). In contrast, healthy people are more likely to attribute blame to circumstances and are less prone to monocausal inferences than are patients (Randjbar, Veckenstedt, Vitzthum, Hottenrott, & Moritz, 2011). Deviances of attributional style in schizophrenia are virtually undisputed, but the exact signature is not consensually determined. Early research (Bentall, 1994) found a self-serving bias (attribution of success to oneself, attribution of failure to others or circumstances), whereas a common denominator of more recent research, which often used the Internal, Personal and Situational Attributions Questionnaire (IPSAQ; Kinderman &

Bentall, 1997) was the personalization of blame to others (Kinderman & Bentall, 1997). Our group (Moritz, Woodward, Burlon, Braus, & Andresen, 2007) and Lincoln et al. (2010) found a general externalization style indicating a form of helplessness and loss of control: Patients deem others responsible for good and bad things in their lives more than do healthy subjects.

Problems with attributional style have been linked with self-uncertainty and a deep-rooted low self-esteem (Bentall, Corcoran, Howard, Blackwood, & Kinderman, 2001) that is addressed in module 8 of the MCT.

Dealing with Attributional Style in the MCT (Modules 1 and 8)

In module 1 (Attribution: Blaming and Taking Credit), participants are first familiarized with the concept of attribution. It is made clear that three major sources may determine or influence an outcome: oneself, other persons, and/or circumstances. These influences usually act in combination rather than alone, and participants should thus resist the tendency to rely on only one explanation. The social consequences of different attributional styles are highlighted (e.g., blaming others for failure may lead to interpersonal tensions). The following exercises are inspired by the IPSAQ, which confronts the subject with complex social events for which situational as well as personal factors have to be taken into account (for an example, see Figure 15.1). Different possible explanations should be considered (e.g., "A friend says you do not look good"; possible explanations may be that you have been ill, harsh neon light, an insult, true concern). Group members are made aware that monocausal inferences are unlikely, and that it can be helpful to generate alternative explanations.

A policeman stops your car.

What caused the policeman to stop your car?

What is the main reason for this event?

Yourself?

Another person or other people?

Circumstances or chance?

Figure 15.1 In module 1 (attributional style), group members must discuss possible reasons for the occurrence of complex scenarios. Here: routine control (possible), driving at too high speed (possible), policeman is in bad mood and stops people driving non-U.S. car brands (unlikely). Monocausal inferences should be avoided. (Permission to reproduce photo granted under a creative commons license.)

Jumping to Conclusions and Need for Closure: Theory

Garety and coworkers were among the first (e.g., Garety, Hemsley, & Wessely, 1991; Huq, Garety, & Hemsley, 1988) to systematically investigate information acquisition preferences in schizophrenia. Following their seminal work, an extensive literature has asserted that patients with schizophrenia are hasty in their decision making (for a review, see Fine, Gardner, Craigie, & Gold, 2007). This line of research has been mainly conducted with the beads task, and a variant of the task is illustrated in Figure 15.2. Usually, 40%–70% of the patients show jumping to conclusions (JTC) in this task. In recent studies, we found that patients do not only collect less information but also weigh information inadequately (Glöckner & Moritz, 2009). Jumping to conclusions is intuitive and almost a literal description of schizophrenia delusions, which often rely on scarce pseudo-"evidence" (e.g., a sudden police siren and an unfriendly remark by a waitress are taken as solid evidence that the village is populated by "evil rednecks" who will hunt the patient down at night), but according to several studies, JTC, is also measurable in nondelusional scenarios.

Jumping to conclusions is thought to play an important role in the formation and maintenance of the disorder and is unlikely to represent a mere epiphenomenon of delusions. This is supported by the fact that it occurs in psychosis-prone but nonclinical participants (Freeman, Pugh, & Garety, 2008; Van Dael et al., 2006) and can be detected using delusion-neutral material, such as the beads task.

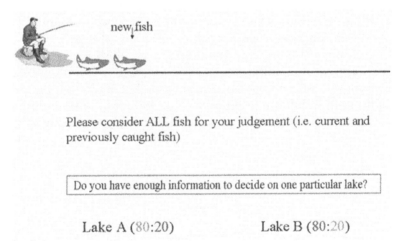

Figure 15.2 Example of the so-called Fish task, a variant of the "Beads task" (Moritz, Veckenstedt, Hottenrott et al., 2010; Speechley, Whitman, & Woodward, 2010; Woodward, Munz, Leclerc, & Lecomte, 2009). Subjects are asked to deduce from which of two lakes a fisherman is catching fish. A decision after only one (or sometimes two) fish is considered evidence for jumping to conclusions. Approximately 40%–70% of schizophrenia patients arrive at a decision after only one fish (or bead), whereas most controls wait for several fish or beads until they decide. Figure created for MCT Working Group.

Although poor motivation and memory have been ruled out as contributors to JTC, some authors implicate low intelligence as a moderator (Lincoln, Ziegler, Mehl, & Rief, 2010). Other research findings suggest that JTC is a special case of liberal acceptance (Moritz & Woodward, 2004; Moritz, Woodward, & Hausmann, 2006; Moritz, Woodward, & Lambert, 2007) or hypersalience of evidence-hypothesis matches (Speechley, Whitman, & Woodward, 2010; Balzan et al., 2012). Interestingly, recent evidence suggests that patients are largely unaware of their hastiness and often view themselves as rather hesitant and indecisive (Freeman et al., 2006; Moritz, Kuepper, Veckenstedt, Randjbar, & Hottenrott, unpublished manuscript).

Dealing with Jumping to Conclusions in the MCT (Modules 2 and 7)

After discussing the advantages (e.g., saving time and cognitive effort) and disadvantages of JTC (e.g., risk to make false decisions) at the start of both module 2 and 7, participants are introduced to drastic historical errors induced by JTC. Then, "urban legends" are discussed (e.g., that the Ku Klux Klan owns Marlboro). Arguments for and especially against these beliefs are displayed, exchanged, and evaluated for their plausibility among group members.[1]

The exercises from the first task set of module 2 are picture fragments that eventually display common objects (e.g., a pig; see Figure 15.3). At each stage, the plausibility of either self-generated or prespecified response alternatives should be rated. Participants are encouraged to make a decision once they feel entirely sure, and all the material was created in such a way that premature decisions lead to errors, thus providing corrective experiences ("seeing is believing").

An edited example of the second task set is shown in Figure 15.4. Here, complex pictures are shown, which, depending on the observer's perspective, contain two different objects/scenes. Group members are asked to give their first impression of the picture, and then to change their perspective in order to generate an alternative solution. Thus, participants are trained to avoid succumbing to first

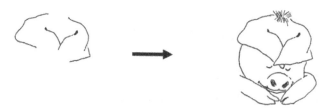

excluded, improbable, possible, probable, DECISION   excluded, improbable, possible, probable, DECISION

Figure 15.3 Brain, back of a man… or pig? In module 2 (jumping to conclusions I), participants are shown a fragmented object that is displayed with increasing details (for display purposes only, two out of the eight stages are shown). Hasty decisions often lead to wrong judgments, thus demonstrating the dysfunctionality of jumping to conclusions. Figure created for MCT Working Group.

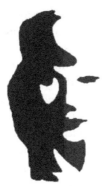

Figure 15.4 In task set 2 of module 2 (jumping to conclusions I), picture puzzles with two different objects or scenes are presented (e.g., saxophone player vs. woman's face). The learning aim is to point out that hasty decisions often reveal only half the truth.

impressions, which may turn out to be incorrect (first task set) or reveal only half truths (second task set). These perhaps abstract examples are substantiated by case stories and videos (see bottom of www.uke.de/mkt or enter "metacognitive training" as a keyword when searching in http://video.google.de).

In the exercises of module 7 (jumping to conclusions II), participants have to deduce the correct title for classical paintings (see Figure 15.5). Many of them contain cues for the correct solution that may be easily missed upon superficial inspection. Here, participants should be shown that a thorough search is perhaps more time-consuming but ensures a more reliable judgment.

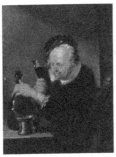

a. The monk
b. The drunkard
c. The reading chemist
d. The bookworm

Figure 15.5 In module 7 (jumping to conclusions II), participants are shown paintings. The pros and cons of potential titles are discussed. Then, the correct title (here, c) is revealed. Premature decisions often prompt false decisions (in this example, especially response option b). Closer inspection often reveals several hints that speak for the correct solution (here, book, devices on the table) and at the same time speak against alternative titles. (Figure created by Johann Peter von Langer.)

Bias Against Disconfirmatory Evidence (BADE): Theory

Incorrigibility is a hallmark criterion feature of delusions. The strong inflexibility seen during delusions (e.g., dismissing arguments proposed by relatives about why the CIA is, in fact, not interested in the patient) extends to nondelusional contents. For this line of research, the bias against disconfirmatory evidence (BADE) paradigm has been employed (Veckenstedt et al., 2001; Woodward, Buchy, Moritz, & Liotti, 2007; Woodward, Moritz, & Chen, 2006; Woodward, Moritz, Cuttler, & Whitman, 2006; Woodward, Moritz, Menon, & Klinge, 2008). In a standard BADE item, the subject is confronted with increasing pieces of information (sequences of three sentences or pictures). The first and sometimes also the second sentence or picture lures the subject into false assumptions that are eventually disconfirmed by subsequent information. In order to obscure the rationale of the test, control trials are presented in which the first sentence correctly suggests the solution. Patients with schizophrenia typically are more easily "led up the garden path" for BADE items than are healthy and even psychiatric controls. Patients with schizophrenia are less able to disengage from initially plausible interpretations, which, over the course of three trials, become more and more implausible. This effect was demonstrated in both first-episode (Woodward, Moritz, & Chen, 2006) and predominantly chronic patients (Moritz & Woodward, 2006), as well as in healthy participants scoring high on delusional ideation (Buchy, Woodward, & Liotti, 2007). In some studies, this bias was more pronounced in currently deluded patients (Woodward, Moritz, & Chen, 2006; Woodward, Moritz, Cuttler et al., 2006), but it is as yet unclear under which conditions a BADE is a state or trait marker of the illness.

Dealing with Bias Against Disconfirmatory Evidence in Schizophrenia in the MCT (Module 3)

At the beginning of module 3, participants are encouraged to discuss the advantages and disadvantages of inflexibility. For example, hard-headedness is a common human feature and, in a mild form, can also be functional (e.g., to overcome obstacles when pursuing one's goals). Then, historical examples and case samples are conveyed showing how incorrigibility has led to big problems, to the point of disastrous events or delusions (case examples). Following this, an example of the so-called confirmation bias is presented: three (different) types of flowers are displayed (parallel version: fruits). Subjects are asked to deduce the corresponding higher level category by proposing items that may also fit that category (superordinate categories: living beings; parallel version: food). The presented objects mislead many persons to believe the to-be-identified superordinate category is *flowers*. Therefore, most people generate objects that *only* fit this category, instead of contemplating alternative hypotheses. The confirmation bias reflects the human tendency to ignore information that does not match a person's attitudes or expectations.

The subsequent exercises consist of a series of three pictures shown in reverse order. Some of these were employed in the studies mentioned above. The sequences of pictures gradually disambiguate a complex plot (see Figure 15.6). For each picture, participants are asked to discuss the plausibility of four

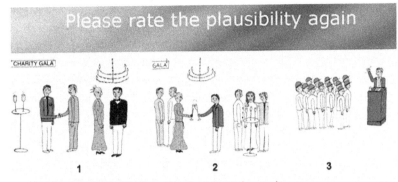

Please rate the plausibility again

1) The politician helps disadvantaged people.

2) The politician encourages the workers to work harder.

3) The preacher is proclaiming the end of the world.

4) The boss announces that there is no money to increase salaries, although he lives in luxury.

Figure 15.6 Preach water, drink wine? Module 3 teaches that things are often different than they appear at first sight. Three pictures are shown successively along with four response alternatives (first, picture 3 only; then, pictures 3 and 2 together; subsequently, all pictures together; the correct solution is highlighted at the end). Information in the first picture (marked with the number 3) misleads to false responses (especially response options 2 or 4). However, the subsequent pictures make clear that option 1 is the most plausible alternative, thereby demonstrating the dysfunctionality of inflexibility. (Figure created by Benny-Kristin Fischer for MCT Working Group.)

different interpretations. After each picture, they should state if their opinions have changed. The correct interpretation is highlighted at the end of each trial. For the BADE trails, which represent the majority of items, one of the four interpretations appears improbable upon the presentation of the first picture, but eventually is true. Two of the other interpretations seem plausible upon the presentation of the first (and sometimes even second) picture, but are eventually incorrect (lure interpretations). Participants should learn to search for more information before making definite judgments, and to stay open-minded and correct themselves if disconfirmatory evidence is encountered.

Social Cognition: Theory

Perhaps beginning with the pioneer work of Frith and coworkers (Frith, 1994; Frith & Corcoran, 1996), cognitive research on schizophrenia has increasingly embraced the social cognitive domain, which is often subsumed under the umbrella term "theory of mind." Theory of mind encompasses a wide range of aspects, including knowledge about "unwritten social rules," social competence, emotion recognition, and social reasoning. (For a more in-depth overview on ToM, see Abu-Akel & Shamay-Tsoory [2013], Chapter 8, this volume.) Although perhaps not specific to patients with schizophrenia (e.g., Kerr, Dunbar, & Bentall, 2003; Uekermann et al., 2008), deficits in social cognition are frequently observed in psychosis (Brüne, 2005), and interpersonal conflicts deriving from social cognitive impairments are likely to fuel psychotic symptoms (Moritz, Veckenstedt, Hottenrott et al., 2010). In recent years, programs have been developed, for example, Social Cognition and Interaction Training (SCIT; see Combs, Torres, & Basso [2013], Chapter 16, this volume), that target this important aspect. As with other cognitive deficits and biases, patients are mostly not adequately aware that their behavior is inappropriate or maybe even appear impolite at times. Reviews and meta-analyses assert substantial deficits for ToM in schizophrenia. The symptom correlates are equivocal, however (Brüne, 2005). Although some studies found correlations with positive symptoms (Mehl et al., 2010), the preponderance of the evidence suggests that ToM deficits are tied to disorganized patients (Sprong, Schothorst, Vos, Hox, & van Engeland, 2007) or negative symptoms (Brune, 2005; Woodward et al., 2009). The question of whether ToM is a state or trait has not yet been resolved, but there is evidence that ToM deficits are also present in remission (Bora, Yucel, & Pantelis, 2009).

Dealing with Social Cognition in the MCT (Modules 4 and 6)

Module 4 is primarily devoted to first-order ToM and emotion recognition, whereas module 6 primarily deals with second-order ToM, need for closure,

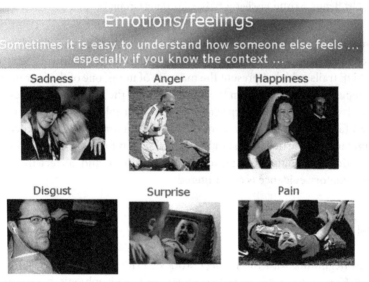

Figure 15.7 Example from module 4 (To empathize...I). Participants are asked to deduce emotional states. As these pictures provide rich contextual information, participants often arrive at correct conclusions. However, subsequent pictures (see Figure 15.8) in module 4 only show faces without context, which often mislead to wrong inferences. Participants are encouraged to attenuate their level of conviction in case information is incomplete. Permission to reproduce photos granted under a creative commons license.

and complex social reasoning. First-order ToM may involve guessing a person's intentions (e.g., based on their facial expressions), and second-order ToM may involve determining another person's guess about a third person's intentions (e.g., based on the situation). In module 4, participants are first familiarized with different cues for social cognition (e.g., appearance, language) and their validity. It is made clear that each social cue alone is fallible (e.g., face: happiness is not always expressed with a smile; anxiety and surprise often have a similar facial signature) and that social cognition is best when a range of different cues is used in combination. Participants are then asked to identify basic human emotions and assign them to facial expressions (see Figure 15.7). This task set is easily solved by most participants as context information is provided (e.g., a smiling woman in a wedding dress). However, subsequent items do not contain contextual information, thereby commonly prompting misinterpretations (see Figure 15.8). The manual advises the trainer not only to ask for the most likely response option, but also to rate the patient's degree of confidence. Participants are asked to withhold strong judgments in order to prevent overconfidence in errors. Other tasks of module 4 have been adopted from Sarfati and Hardy-Baylé (1999), depicting a sequence of black-and-white pictures that have to be logically terminated with one out of three response options (these exercises are not recommended anymore). Module 4 conveys the message that although facial expressions are very important for identifying the feelings of a person, they can also lead to false assumptions.

In module 6, comic sequences are presented. Participants are required to take the perspective of one of the protagonists and to deduce what the character may think about another person or a certain event (see Figure 15.9). As mentioned before, this task taps into second-order ToM constructs: The subject has to deduce what a second person is thinking about a third person. In other words, the subject has to socially think outside the box.

In the style of the BADE exercises in module 3 (see above), most slides are presented in reverse temporal order: The picture showing the final action or situation is presented first. Each novel picture reveals more about the storyline, and explanations that initially seem plausible eventually prove wrong and have to be corrected. For the majority of items, several interpretations remain possible

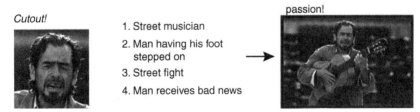

Figure 15.8 This item is taken from the second task set of module 4 and shows that facial information can mislead to false responses. Only a few people assume the correct response (*right image*) from the picture (*left*) shown first. Participants are taught to withhold strong judgments and collect additional information in ambiguous and unclear situations. Permission to reproduce photos granted under a creative commons license.

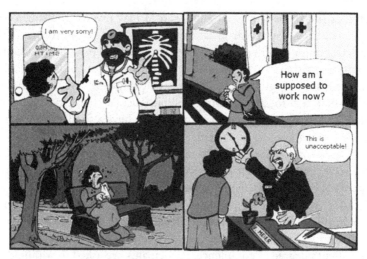

Is the boss cold-hearted? Do we need additional
information to decide?

Figure 15.9 Cold-hearted boss? The example is taken from module 6 (To empathize . . . II). The pictures are viewed one after the other (the lower right picture is
presented first). In this example, participants sometimes do not understand that the
viewer has more information than the boss. Whereas the boss' reaction may seem
adequate initially (the woman is obviously late), the other pictures cast some doubt on
this. The woman has apparently received a bad message from her doctor and is visibly
devastated in the two pictures before. Likely manifestations of crying (especially red
eyes, bad make-up) may be visible to the boss, who might therefore have reacted more
compassionately even if he was unaware of the doctor's message. Figure created by
Marina Ruiz-Villarreal for MCT Working Group.

until the end, which is unsatisfactory for patients with an enhanced need for
closure (i.e., intolerance for ambiguity). For such items, participants should
propose what additional information is needed to make a reliable judgment.
Nevertheless, it should be discussed which interpretation is best supported by
the available evidence.

Metamemory Problems in Schizophrenia: Theory

Memory problems are ubiquitous in most psychiatric disorders, but are especially pronounced in patients with schizophrenia (Aleman, Hijman, de Haan, &
Kahn, 1999; Heinrichs & Zakzanis, 1998). Memory dysfunctions impact negatively on functional (Green, Kern, & Heaton, 2004) and symptomatic outcome
(Moritz et al., 2000) in the disorder. Unlike in the amnestic syndrome, memory
deficits in schizophrenia reflect problems with encoding and learning information rather than rapid forgetting (Moritz, Heeren, Andresen, & Krausz, 2001).
Patients are not usually aware of their memory problems. In fact, our group

found a zero-correlation between subjective and objective memory impairments (Moritz, Ferahli, & Naber, 2004).

A new line of literature has turned to *metamemory*, which is concerned with the subjective appraisal of one's memory performance, particularly response confidence (Moritz & Woodward, 2006) and memory vividness rather than memory accuracy. As shown by Danion and others (2005), the recollections in schizophrenia patients are often vague and lack detail. Further, our group has repeatedly demonstrated that patients with schizophrenia are overconfident in memory errors, while at the same time being underconfident in correct responses (for a review, see Moritz & Woodward, 2006). This response pattern has now been independently replicated (Bhatt, Laws, & McKenna, 2010; Doré, Caza, Gingras, & Rouleau, 2007; Peters et al., 2007). Some of the more recent studies have been conducted with items from the Deese-Roediger-McDermott (DRM) paradigm, which readily elicits false memories (see below for an example). Although in most investigations patients with schizophrenia did not differ from controls in *accuracy* on the DRM paradigm (e.g., Huron & Danion, 2002), their conviction for error responses was disproportionately increased (Moritz, Woodward, & Rodriguez-Raecke, 2006). Importantly, overconfidence in errors has been found with nondelusional material and likely represents a risk factor and not a consequence of paranoid symptoms. We have put forward that this twofold response pattern mirrors liberal acceptance for response alternatives and JTC, respectively (Moritz, Woodward, Jelinek, & Klinge, 2008; Moritz, Woodward, & Lambert, 2007): Premature termination of cognitive search processes and liberal decision criteria may result in a neglect of essential cues that might have indicated the fallibility of an incorrect response option, thereby promoting overconfidence in errors. In contrast, controls adopt more careful and deliberate strategies, expressed as a reluctance to fully endorse a response option when the available evidence is ambiguous. Along the same lines, we assume that healthy control participants exhibit greater confidence in correct responses relative to patients, as the detection of multiple supportive cues raises response confidence. A recent study identified a general pattern of overconfidence in schizophrenia patients, which, however, was more pronounced for errors (Kircher, Koch, Stottmeister, & Durst, 2007).

Dealing with Metamemory Problems in the MCT (Module 5)

Module 5 first introduces mnemonic strategies to help the patient recall information, and it provides examples for the fallibility of human memory (e.g., in contrast to popular belief, the line "Play it again, Sam" was never uttered in the movie Casablanca): Healthy subjects also forget, mix up, embellish, or recall memory information falsely. In the main part of the module, complex visual scenes are displayed. Many of the stimuli have been utilized in prior basic research studies on the false memory paradigm (Miller & Gazzaniga, 1998; Roediger & McDermott, 1995). This material prompts a high frequency of false memories, even in 50%–80% of healthy subjects, as core items that you would expect in the picture are in

Classroom

- ➤ backpack
- ➤ teacher
- ➤ map
- ➤ books
- ➤ benches
- ➤ teacher´s chair
- ➤ blackboard
- ➤ teacher´s bag

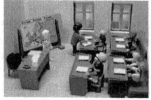

© geobra Brandstätter

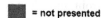 = not presented

Figure 15.10 Module 5 shows complex and rather prototypal scenes. These pictures elicit false memories in most subjects, as strongly suggested items are not displayed (here, blackboard or backpacks are expected from the context but, in fact, are not shown). Exercises teach participants to base their judgments on perceptual recollections rather than gist or on logical inferences. When the recollection is vague, confidence should be attenuated.

fact removed. Group members are instructed to study the pictures carefully (see Figure 15.10) and to memorize each item as vividly as possible. Each scene is followed by a recognition task asking participants to decide whether an item was displayed or not. Subjects are also asked about their response confidence, and the trainer should later ask for perceptual details and for participants to adopt "vividness heuristics" (i.e., the recollection of perceptual details is a good proxy that an object has indeed been shown, whereas "pale" recollections often indicate false memories. Here, response confidence should be attenuated). It is made clear to participants that our memory can play tricks on us, as it is constructive and does not work passively like, for example, a video recorder. Participants should learn to doubt their memories and collect additional information if a vivid recollection is not available.

Mood and Self-Esteem in Schizophrenia

It is now well-established that approximately 50% (Buckley, Miller, Lehrer, & Castle, 2009) of the schizophrenia population (in contrast to accounts by, for example, Kraepelin) share affective disturbances. Other studies estimate that two (Moritz, Veckenstedt, Randjbar et al., 2010) to three (Freeman et al., 1998) out of four patients have low self-esteem, which may be one reason (among others) for the high suicide rate in schizophrenia, which is in the range of 5%–15% (for overviews, see Preston & Hansen, 2005; Siris, 2001).

Dealing with Low Mood and Self-Esteem in the MCT (Module 8)

In view of the high prevalence of depression and low self-esteem in schizophrenia, module 8 specifically targets depressive cognitive schemata (overgeneralization and selective abstraction), unhelpful coping strategies (especially rumination, thought suppression), underlying depression, and low self-esteem (see Figure 15.11). The trainer provides more realistic and helpful strategies and encourages participants to use detached mindfulness (this technique plays a prominent role in the treatment program devised by Fisher and Wells [2009]) instead of thought suppression and rumination for dealing with negative thoughts. Finally, some simple techniques derived from CBT of depression are provided that, if used regularly, help to alter low self-esteem and raise depressed mood (e.g., writing down positive events during the day, engaging in social activities).

INTRODUCING THE PROGRAM TO PARTICIPANTS

As mentioned earlier, the MCT is designed as an open group therapy program, so participants enter at any module within a cycle. New participants are first welcomed by all members and informed about the goal of the program—preferably by participants who have already attended some sessions. Most participants will not know what metacognition signifies, which can be explained as follows: "*Meta* is Greek for about and *cognition* refers to higher mental processes, such as attention

Tips to improve depressed mood/low self-esteem	6. Suppression of negative thoughts Does it work? No!
➤ Try to remember situations, in which you felt really good—try to remember these with all your senses (visual, feeling, smelling...), perhaps with the help of a photo album.	
➤ Do things you really enjoy – ideally with others (e.g. movies, go to a cafe).	Most of you had probably thought of an elephant and/or of something which has to do with an elephant (e.g. zoo, safari, Africa etc.)
➤ Workout (at least 20 minutes) – but no struggling – if possible stamina training, for example, a long walk or jogging.	This effect grows even stronger if one tries to deliberately suppress upsetting thoughts ("I am a loser" etc.). Those thoughts can then become so strong that they seem strange or out of one's control!
➤ Listen to your favourite music.	

Figure 15.11 In module 8 (mood and self-esteem), participants are taught how to replace negative appraisals with more positive and constructive ones. At the end of the module, some recommendations are provided on how to raise one's mood (part 1 of this exercise is shown on the left). In addition, alternatives for dysfunctional coping strategies (e.g., thought suppression, see right side) are conveyed (e.g., detached mindfulness for worries).

and problem solving. In brief, *metacognition* is thinking about our thinking. The aim of the program is to learn more about human cognition, and how we can observe and change it to optimize our problem-solving abilities. At the heart of the program are several thinking styles that may contribute to the formation of odd ideas and psychotic symptoms."

Inclusion Criteria, Problematic Situations, and Individualized Treatment

Inclusion criteria for the MCT group are very liberal. As a rule of thumb, all schizophrenia spectrum patients can participate who are able to attend and follow other group programs as well (e.g., occupational therapy). In our view, important inclusion criteria are past or current delusional ideas or hallucinations. Patients with primary diagnoses other than schizophrenia, depression with psychotic features, and bipolar disorder with beliefs of grandiosity may also be included.

According to our experience and that of our collaborators, groups may comprise first-episode and chronic patients, in- and outpatients, and male and female patients at the same time. Patients with a short attention span or inappropriate/eccentric behavior, aggression/hostility, and severe formal thought disorder should not take part until symptoms have at least declined somewhat. Although we have successfully run groups with patients diagnosed with oligophrenia, here, a stronger focus on the main exercises and frequent repetition is advisable.

Good feasibility and treatment fidelity are now well-established in both in- and outpatients samples (Favrod et al., 2009; Favrod, Maire, Bardy, Pernier, & Bonsack, 2011; Gaweda, Moritz, & Kokoszka, 2009; Moritz & Woodward, 2007a). Nevertheless, problematic situations can occur. Here, general treatment guidelines apply. For example, if a group member displays severe psychotic symptoms during sessions, these should neither be supported nor openly challenged. However, if patients are already distanced a bit from their symptoms, such experiences may be picked up with MCT exercises containing delusional themes (e.g., module 1, scenario "A friend is talking behind your back"; module 6, scenario in which two men appear to talk about a third man). At the start and at the end of each module, we also raise the questions "Why are we doing this?" and "What does this have to do with psychosis?" These slides translate knowledge from basic research to patients and provide an opportunity for further reflections on personal experiences of psychosis; participants are encouraged to talk in a nonjudgmental climate about their past and present psychotic experiences. However, an in-depth analysis and exchange about individual delusional ideas is best addressed in the framework of face-to-face sessions, as in CBT. An alternative is individualized Metacognitive Therapy (MCT+), which is available in a German-language version and as a beta version in English and Dutch at www.uke.de/mct_plus. The MCT+ is more focused on individual symptoms and combines elements of CBT (dispute of fixed beliefs by means of Socratic dialogue, response prevention, establishment of an illness model) with core features of the MCT. As in the group training, a "back-door approach" is adopted: Instead of challenging symptoms and delusional appraisals directly, which may undermine the therapeutic alliance, cognitive biases are addressed first before the therapy continues to challenge individual biases and delusions.

Metacognitive Training: Feasibility, Subjective Feedback, & Efficacy

As described in further detail in Chapter 12 (Fizdon, 2013, this volume), various studies have now asserted the feasibility of the MCT in German (Moritz, Vitzthum et al., 2010; Moritz & Woodward, 2007b) and other languages (Favrod et al., 2009; Gaweda et al., 2009). Participants consider the training to be both entertaining and (subjectively) effective. Attendance rates are usually high. Moreover, studies from our group, as well as from other researchers, have shown a positive impact on symptoms (Aghotor, Pfueller, Moritz, Weisbrod, & Roesch-Ely, 2010; Kumar et al., 2010; Moritz, Veckenstedt et al., in press; Moritz, Veckenstedt, Randjbar, Vitzthum, & Woodward, in press; Ross, Freeman, Dunn, & Garety, 2011), cognitive biases (Aghotor et al., 2010; Moritz, Kerstan et al., in press; Moritz, Veckenstedt et al., in press; Ross et al., 2009), and quality of life (Briki et al., 2008; Moritz, Kerstan et al., in press). Still, follow-up analyses are needed to provide insight into the stability of the effects.

CONCLUSION

Over the last two decades, increasing support has been gathered for both psychological theories and interventions of schizophrenia. MCT is one manifestation of this new trend. Cognitive biases and social cognitive impairments are likely involved in the formation and maintenance of the disorder and thus represent important treatment targets. The goal of the MCT is to sharpen patients' (metacognitive) awareness of these biases and impairments and to carry over the learning aims into their daily life. Although there is increasing support for the efficacy of the MCT as a stand-alone program, we advise clinicians to complement MCT with personal therapy, for example CBT or MCT+ (Moritz, Veckenstedt, Randjbar, & Vitzthum, 2010; Moritz, Veckenstedt et al., in press). Against the background of high rates of relapse and only modest symptom decline under antipsychotic medication alone, we hope that (adjunct) cognitive interventions someday will be the norm rather than the exception in treatment.

ACKNOWLEDGMENTS

The authors would like to thank Katharina Struck for helpful comments on an earlier version of the manuscript.

NOTE

1. Clearly, all discussed urban legends are falsifiable and serve to illustrate, via a minia-
ture model of delusions, how JTC and other biases (e.g., selective attention to certain
information) promote delusional beliefs.

REFERENCES

Abu-Akel, A., & Shamay-Tsoory, S. G. (2013). Characteristics of theory of mind impairments in schizophrenia. In D. L. Roberts & D. L. Penn (Eds.), *Social cognition in schizophrenia: From evidence to treatment* (Chapter 8). New York: Oxford University Press.
Adler, A. (1914/1929). Melancholia and paranoia. In A. Adler (Ed.), *The practice and theory
of individual psychology*. London: Routledge & Kegan Paul Ltd.
Aghotor, J., Pfueller, U., Moritz, S., Weisbrod, M., & Roesch-Ely, D. (2010). Metacognitive
training for patients with schizophrenia (MCT): Feasibility and preliminary evidence
for its efficacy. *Journal of Behavior Therapy and Experimental Psychiatry, 41,* 207–211.
Aleman, A., Hijman, R., de Haan, E. H., & Kahn, R. S. (1999). Memory impairment in
schizophrenia: A meta-analysis. *American Journal of Psychiatry, 156,* 1358–1366.
Balzan, R., Delfabbro, P., Galletly, C., & Woodward, T. S. (2012). Reasoning heuristics
across the psychosis continuum: The contribution of hypersalient evidence-hypothesis
matches. *Cognitive Neuropsychiatry.* doi:10.1080/13546805.2012.663901
Bell, V., Halligan, P. W., & Ellis, H. D. (2006). Explaining delusions: A cognitive perspective.
Trends in Cognitive Sciences, 10, 219–226.
Bentall, R. P. (1994). Cognitive biases and abnormal beliefs: Towards a model of persecu-
tory delusions. In A. S. David & J. C. Cutting (Eds.), *The neuropsychology of schizophre-
nia* (pp. 337–360). Mahwah, NJ: Lawrence Erlbaum Associates.
Bentall, R. P., Corcoran, R., Howard, R., Blackwood, N., & Kinderman, P. (2001).
Persecutory delusions: a review and theoretical integration. *Clinical Psychology Review,
21,* 1143–1192.
Bentall, R. P., Rowse, G., Shryane, N., Kinderman, P., Howard, R., & Blackwood, N. (2009).
The cognitive and affective structure of paranoid delusions: A transdiagnostic investi-
gation of patients with schizophrenia spectrum disorders and depression. *Archives of
General Psychiatry, 66,* 236–247.
Bhatt, R., Laws, K. R., & McKenna, P. J. (2010). False memory in schizophrenia patients
with and without delusions. *Psychiatry Research, 178,* 260–265.
Birchwood, M., & Trower, P. (2006). The future of cognitive-behavioural therapy for psy-
chosis: Not a quasi-neuroleptic. *British Journal of Psychiatry, 188,* 107–108.
Bora, E., Sehitoglu, G., Aslier, M., Atabay, I., & Veznedaroglu, B. (2007). Theory of mind
and unawareness of illness in schizophrenia: Is poor insight a mentalizing deficit?
European archives of psychiatry and Clinical Neuroscience, 257, 104–111.
Bora, E., Yucel, M., & Pantelis, C. (2009). Theory of mind impairment in schizophrenia:
Meta-analysis. *Schizophrenia Research, 109,* 1–9.
Briki, M., Pahin, A., Trossat, V., Hummel, M. -P., Haffen, E., & Vandel, P. (2008). *Evaluation
of a metacognitive training in a schizophrenic outpatient's group: Social skills and mood.*
Paper presented at the European College of Neuropsychopharmacology, Barcelona.
Brüne, M. (2005). "Theory of mind" in schizophrenia: A review of the literature.
Schizophrenia Bulletin, 31, 21–42.

Brune, M. (2005). Emotion recognition, 'theory of mind', and social behavior in schizophrenia. *Psychiatry Research, 133*, 135–147.

Buchy, L., Malla, A., Joober, R., & Lepage, M. (2009). Delusions are associated with low self-reflectiveness in first-episode psychosis. *Schizophrenia Research, 112*, 187–191.

Buchy, L., Woodward, T. S., & Liotti, M. (2007). A cognitive bias against disconfirmatory evidence (BADE) is associated with schizotypy. *Schizophrenia Research, 90*, 334–337.

Buckley, P. F., Miller, B. J., Lehrer, D. S., & Castle, D. J. (2009). Psychiatric comorbidities and schizophrenia. *Schizophrenia Bulletin, 35*, 383–402.

Byerly, M. J., Nakonezny, P. A., & Lescouflair, E. (2007). Antipsychotic medication adherence in schizophrenia. *Psychiatric Clinics of North America, 30*, 437–452.

Combs, D. R., Torres, J., & Basso, M. R. (2013). Social cognition and interaction training. In D. L. Roberts & D. L. Penn (Eds.), *Social cognition in schizophrenia: From evidence to treatment* (Chapter 16). New York: Oxford University Press.

Danion, J. M., Cuervo, C., Piolino, P., Huron, C., Riutort, M., & Peretti, C. S. (2005). Conscious recollection in autobiographical memory: An investigation in schizophrenia. *Consciousness and Cognition, 14*, 535–547.

Davis, J. M., Chen, N., & Glick, I. D. (2003). A meta-analysis of the efficacy of second-generation antipsychotics. *Archives of General Psychiatry, 60*, 553–564.

Doré, M. C., Caza, N., Gingras, N., & Rouleau, N. (2007). Deficient relational binding processes in adolescents with psychosis: Evidence from impaired memory for source and temporal context. *Cognitive Neuropsychiatry, 12*, 511–536.

Elkis, H. (2007). Treatment-resistant schizophrenia. *Psychiatric Clinics of North America, 30*, 511–533.

Favrod, J., Bardy- Linder, S., Pernier, S., Mouron, D., Schwyn, C., & Bonsack, C. (2009). Entraînement des habiletés métacognitives avec des personnes atteintes de schizophrénie. In J. Cottraux (Ed.), *TCC et neurosciences* (pp. 103–114). Issy-les-Moulineaux: Elsevier Masson SAS.

Favrod, J., Maire, A., Bardy, S., Pernier, S., & Bonsack, C. (2011). Improving insight into delusions: A pilot study of metacognitive training for patients with schizophrenia. *Journal of Advanced Nursing, 67*(2), 401–407.

Fine, C., Gardner, M., Craigie, J., & Gold, I. (2007). Hopping, skipping or jumping to conclusions? Clarifying the role of the JTC bias in delusions. *Cognitive Neuropsychiatry, 12*, 46–77.

Fisher, P., & Wells, A. (2009). *Metacognitive therapy*. Hove, UK: Routledge.

Fiszdon, Joanna M. (2013). introduction to social cognitive treatment approaches for schizophrenia. In D. L. Roberts & D. L. Penn (Eds.), *Social cognition in schizophrenia: From evidence to treatment* (Chapter 12). New York: Oxford University Press.

Freeman, D. (2007). Suspicious minds: the psychology of persecutory delusions. *Clinical Psychology Review, 27*, 425–457.

Freeman, D., Garety, P., Fowler, D., Kuipers, E., Dunn, G., & Bebbington, P. (1998). The London-East Anglia randomized controlled trial of cognitive-behaviour therapy for psychosis. IV: Self-esteem and persecutory delusions. *British Journal of Clinical Psychology, 37*, 415–430.

Freeman, D., Garety, P., Kuipers, E., Colbert, S., Jolley, S., & Fowler, D. (2006). Delusions and decision-making style: Use of the Need for Closure Scale. *Behaviour Research and Therapy, 44*, 1147–1158.

Freeman, D., Pugh, K., & Garety, P. (2008). Jumping to conclusions and paranoid ideation in the general population. *Schizophrenia Research, 102*, 254–260.

Frith, C. D. (1994). Theory of mind in schizophrenia. In A. S. David & H. J. Cutting (Eds.), *The neuropsychology of schizophrenia* (pp. 147–161). Mahwah, NJ: Lawrence Erlbaum Associates.

Frith, C. D., & Corcoran, R. (1996). Exploring 'theory of mind' in people with schizophrenia. *Psychological Medicine, 26*, 521–530.

Garety, P. A., Hemsley, D. R., & Wessely, S. (1991). Reasoning in deluded schizophrenic and paranoid patients. Biases in performance on a probabilistic inference task. *Journal of Nervous and Mental Disease, 179*, 194–201.

Gaweda, Ł., Moritz, S., & Kokoszka, A. (2009). [The metacognitive training for schizophrenia patients: description of method and experiences from clinical practice]. *Psychiatria Polska, 43*, 683–692.

Glöckner, A., & Moritz, S. (2009). A fine-grained analysis of the jumping to conclusions bias in schizophrenia: Data-gathering, response confidence, and information integration. *Judgment and Decision Making, 4*, 587–600.

Green, M. F., Kern, R. S., & Heaton, R. K. (2004). Longitudinal studies of cognition and functional outcome in schizophrenia: Implications for MATRICS. *Schizophrenia Research, 72*, 41–51.

Haddad, P. M., & Sharma, S. G. (2007). Adverse effects of atypical antipsychotics: Differential risk and clinical implications. *CNS Drugs, 21*, 911–936.

Heinrichs, R. W., & Zakzanis, K. K. (1998). Neurocognitive deficit in schizophrenia: A quantitative review of the evidence. *Neuropsychology, 12*, 426–445.

Huq, S. F., Garety, P. A., & Hemsley, D. R. (1988). Probabilistic judgements in deluded and non-deluded subjects. *Quarterly Journal of Experimental Psychology, 40A*, 801–812.

Huron, C., & Danion, J. M. (2002). Impairment of constructive memory in schizophrenia. *International Clinical Psychopharmacology, 17*, 127–133.

Kerr, N., Dunbar, R. I., & Bentall, R. P. (2003). Theory of mind deficits in bipolar affective disorder. *Journal of Affective Disorders, 73*, 253–259.

Kinderman, P., & Bentall, R. P. (1997). Causal attributions in paranoia and depression: Internal, personal, and situational attributions for negative events. *Journal of Abnormal Psychology, 106*, 341–345.

Kircher, T. T., Koch, K., Stottmeister, F., & Durst, V. (2007). Metacognition and reflexivity in patients with schizophrenia. *Psychopathology, 40*, 254–260.

Klosterkötter, J. (1992). The meaning of basic symptoms for the genesis of the schizophrenic nuclear syndrome. *Japanese Journal of Psychiatry & Neurology, 46*, 609–630.

Kumar, D., Zia, U. I., Haq, M., Dubey, I., Dotiwala, K., Siddiqui, S. V., et al. (2010). Effect of meta-cognitive training in the reduction of positive symptoms in schizophrenia. *European Journal of Psychotherapy & Counselling, 12*, 149–158.

Lehrer, J. (2010). The truth wears off: Is there something wrong with the scientific method? *The New Yorker*, 1–7. Retrieved from http://www.newyorker.com/reporting/2010/12/13/101213fa_fact_lehrer

Leucht, S., Arbter, D., Engel, R. R., Kissling, W., & Davis, J. M. (2009). How effective are second-generation antipsychotic drugs? A meta-analysis of placebo-controlled trials. *Molecular Psychiatry, 14*, 429–447.

Lieberman, J. A., Stroup, T. S., McEvoy, J. P., Swartz, M. S., Rosenheck, R. A., & Perkins, D. O. (2005). Effectiveness of antipsychotic drugs in patients with chronic schizophrenia. *New England Journal of Medicine, 353*, 1209–1223.

Lincoln, T., Mehl, S., Exner, C., Lindenmeyer, J., & Rief, W. (2010). Attributional style and persecutory delusions. Evidence for an event independent and state specific external-personal attribution bias for social situations. *Cognitive Therapy and Research*, *34*, 297–302.

Lincoln, T. M., Ziegler, M., Mehl, S., & Rief, W. (2010). The jumping to conclusions bias in delusions: specificity and changeability. *Journal of Abnormal Psychology*, *119*, 40–49.

Lindenmayer, J. P. (2000). Treatment refractory schizophrenia. *Psychiatric Quarterly*, *71*, 373–384.

Mehl, S., Rief, W., Lullmann, E., Ziegler, M., Kesting, M. L., & Lincoln, T. M. (2010). Are theory of mind deficits in understanding intentions of others associated with persecutory delusions? *Journal of Nervous and Mental Disease*, *198*, 516–519.

Miller, M. B., & Gazzaniga, M. S. (1998). Creating false memories for visual scenes. *Neuropsychologia*, *36*, 513–520.

Mizrahi, R., Kiang, M., Mamo, D. C., Arenovich, T., Bagby, R. M., & Zipursky, R. B. (2006). The selective effect of antipsychotics on the different dimensions of the experience of psychosis in schizophrenia spectrum disorders. *Schizophrenia Research*, *88*, 111–118.

Moritz, S., Ferahli, S., & Naber, D. (2004). Memory and attention performance in psychiatric patients: Lack of correspondence between clinician-rated and patient-rated functioning with neuropsychological test results. *Journal of the International Neuropsychological Society*, *10*, 623–633.

Moritz, S., Heeren, D., Andresen, B., & Krausz, M. (2001). An analysis of the specificity and the syndromal correlates of verbal memory impairments in schizophrenia. *Psychiatry Research*, *101*, 23–31.

Moritz, S., Kerstan, A., Veckenstedt, R., Randjbar, S., Vitzthum, F., Schmidt, C., Heise, M., & Woodward, T. S. (2011). Further evidence for the efficacy of a metacognitive group training in schizophrenia. *Behaviour Research and Therapy*, *49*, 151–157.

Moritz, S., Krausz, M., Gottwalz, E., Lambert, M., Perro, C., Ganzer, S. (2000). Cognitive dysfunction at baseline predicts symptomatic 1-year outcome in first-episode schizophrenics. *Psychopathology*, *33*, 48–51.

Moritz, S., Kuepper, R., Veckenstedt, R., Randjbar, S., & Hottenrott, B. (unpublished manuscript). *Lack of awareness for the "jumping to conclusions" bias in schizophrenia.*

Moritz, S., Peters, M. J. V., Karow, A., Deljkovic, A., Tonn, P., & Naber, D. (2009). Cure or curse? Ambivalent attitudes towards neuroleptic medication in schizophrenia and non-schizophrenia patients. *Mental Illness*, *1*, 4–9.

Moritz, S., Veckenstedt, R., Hottenrott, B., Woodward, T. S., Randjbar, S., & Lincoln, T. M. (2010). Different sides of the same coin? Intercorrelations of cognitive biases in schizophrenia. *Cognitive Neuropsychiatry*, *15*, 406–421.

Moritz, S., Veckenstedt, R., Randjbar, S., & Vitzthum, F. (2010). *MKT+: Individualisiertes metakognitives Therapieprogramm für Menschen mit Psychose [MCT+: Individualized metacognitive therapy program for people with psychosis]*. Heidelberg, GR: Springer.

Moritz, S., Veckenstedt, R., Randjbar, S., Vitzthum, F., Karow, A., & Lincoln, T. M. (2010). Course and determinants of self-esteem in people diagnosed with schizophrenia during psychiatric treatment. *Psychosis*, *2*, 1752–2439.

Moritz, S., Veckenstedt, R., Randjbar, S., Vitzthum, F., & Woodward, T. S. (2011). Antipsychotic treatment beyond antipsychotics: Metacognitive intervention for schizophrenia patients improves delusional symptoms. *Psychological Medicine*, *41*(9), 1823–1832.

Moritz, S., Vitzthum, F., Randjbar, S., Veckenstedt, R., & Woodward, T. S. (2010). Detecting and defusing cognitive traps: Metacognitive intervention in schizophrenia. *Current Opinion in Psychiatry*, *23*, 561–569.

Moritz, S., & Woodward, T. S. (2004). Plausibility judgment in schizophrenic patients: Evidence for a liberal acceptance bias. *German Journal of Psychiatry, 7,* 66–74.

Moritz, S., & Woodward, T. S. (2006). A generalized bias against disconfirmatory evidence in schizophrenia. *Psychiatry Research, 142,* 157–165.

Moritz, S., & Woodward, T. S. (2006). Metacognitive control over false memories: A key determinant of delusional thinking. *Current Psychiatry Reports, 8,* 184–190.

Moritz, S., & Woodward, T. S. (2007a). Metacognitive training for schizophrenia patients (MCT): A pilot study on feasibility, treatment adherence, and subjective efficacy. *German Journal of Psychiatry, 10,* 69–78.

Moritz, S., & Woodward, T. S. (2007b). Metacognitive training in schizophrenia: From basic research to knowledge translation and intervention. *Current Opinion in Psychiatry, 20,* 619–625.

Moritz, S., Woodward, T. S., Burlon, M., Braus, D. F., & Andresen, B. (2007). Attributional style in schizophrenia: Evidence for a decreased sense of self-causation in currently paranoid patients. *Cognitive Therapy and Research, 31,* 371–383.

Moritz, S., Woodward, T. S., & Hausmann, D. (2006). Incautious reasoning as a pathogenetic factor for the development of psychotic symptoms in schizophrenia. *Schizophrenia Bulletin, 32,* 327–331.

Moritz, S., Woodward, T. S., Jelinek, L., & Klinge, R. (2008). Memory and metamemory in schizophrenia: A liberal acceptance account of psychosis. *Psychological Medicine, 38,* 825–832.

Moritz, S., Woodward, T. S., & Lambert, M. (2007). Under what circumstances do patients with schizophrenia jump to conclusions? A liberal acceptance account. *British Journal of Clinical Psychology, 46,* 127–137.

Moritz, S., Woodward, T. S., & Rodriguez-Raecke, R. (2006). Patients with schizophrenia do not produce more false memories than controls but are more confident in them. *Psychological Medicine, 36,* 659–667.

Peters, M. J., Cima, M. J., Smeets, T., de Vos, M., Jelicic, M., & Merckelbach, H. (2007). Did I say that word or did you? Executive dysfunctions in schizophrenic patients affect memory efficiency, but not source attributions. *Cognitive Neuropsychiatry, 12,* 391–411.

Preston, E., & Hansen, L. (2005). A systematic review of suicide rating scales in schizophrenia. *Crisis, 26,* 170–180.

Randjbar, S., Veckenstedt, R., Vitzthum, F., Hottenrott, B., & Moritz, S. (2011). Attributional biases in paranoid schizophrenia: Further evidence for a decreased sense of self-causation in paranoia. *Psychosis: Psychological, Social and Integrative Approaches, 3,* 74–85.

Roder, V., & Medalia, A. (2010). *Neurocognition and social cognition in schizophrenic patients. Basic concepts and treatment.* Basel, CH: Karger.

Roediger, H. L., & McDermott, K. B. (1995). Creating false memories: Remembering words not presented in lists. *Journal of Experimental Psychology: Learning, Memory, and Cognition, 21,* 803–814.

Ross, K., Freeman, D., Dunn, G., & Garety, P. (2011). A randomized experimental investigation of reasoning training for people with delusions. *Schizophrenia Bulletin, 37*(2), 324–333.

Rummel-Kluge, C., Komossa, K., Schwarz, S., Hunger, H., Schmid, F., & Lobos, C. A. (2010). Head-to-head comparisons of metabolic side effects of second generation antipsychotics in the treatment of schizophrenia: A systematic review and meta-analysis. *Schizophrenia Research, 123,* 225–233.

Sarfati, Y., & Hardy-Baylé, M. C. (1999). How do people with schizophrenia explain the behaviour of others? A study of theory of mind and its relationship to thought and speech disorganization in schizophrenia. *Psychological Medicine, 29*, 613–620.

Schretlen, D. J., Cascella, N. G., Meyer, S. M., Kingery, L. R., Testa, S. M., & Munro, C. A. (2007). Neuropsychological functioning in bipolar disorder and schizophrenia. *Biological Psychiatry, 62*, 179–186.

Shafran, R., Clark, D. M., Fairburn, C. G., Arntz, A., Barlow, D. H., & Ehlers, A. (2009). Mind the gap: Improving the dissemination of CBT. *Behaviour Research and Therapy, 47*, 902–909.

Siris, S. G. (2001). Suicide and schizophrenia. *Journal of Psychopharmacology, 15*, 127–135.

Speechley, W. J., Whitman, J. C., & Woodward, T. S. (2010). The contribution of hypersalience to the "jumping to conclusions" bias associated with delusions in schizophrenia. *Journal of Psychiatry and Neuroscience, 35*, 7–17.

Sprong, M., Schothorst, P., Vos, E., Hox, J., & van Engeland, H. (2007). Theory of mind in schizophrenia: meta-analysis. *British Journal of Psychiatry, 191*, 5–13.

Uekermann, J., Channon, S., Lehmkämper, C., Abdel-Hamid, M., Vollmoeller, W., & Daum, I. (2008). Executive function, mentalizing and humor in major depression. *Journal of the International Neuropsychological Society, 14*, 55–62.

Van Dael, F., Versmissen, D., Janssen, I., Myin-Germeys, I., van Os, J., & Krabbendam, L. (2006). Data gathering: Biased in psychosis? *Schizophrenia Bulletin, 32*, 341–351.

Veckenstedt, R., Randjbar, S., Vitzthum, F., Hottenrott, B., Woodward, T. S., & Moritz, S. (2011). Incorrigibility, jumping to conclusions, and decision threshold in schizophrenia. *Cognitive Neuropsychiatry, 16*, 174–192.

Woodward, T. S., Buchy, L., Moritz, S., & Liotti, M. (2007). A bias against disconfirmatory evidence is associated with delusion proneness in a nonclinical sample. *Schizophrenia Bulletin, 33*, 1023–1028.

Woodward, T. S., Mizrahi, R., Menon, M., & Christensen, B. K. (2009). Correspondences between theory of mind, jumping to conclusions, neuropsychological measures and the symptoms of schizophrenia. *Psychiatry Research, 170*, 119–123.

Woodward, T. S., Moritz, S., & Chen, E. Y. (2006). The contribution of a cognitive bias against disconfirmatory evidence (BADE) to delusions: A study in an Asian sample with first episode schizophrenia spectrum disorders. *Schizophrenia Research, 83*, 297–298.

Woodward, T. S., Moritz, S., Cuttler, C., & Whitman, J. C. (2006). The contribution of a cognitive bias against disconfirmatory evidence (BADE) to delusions in schizophrenia. *Journal of Clinical and Experimental Neuropsychology, 28*, 605–617.

Woodward, T. S., Moritz, S., Menon, M., & Klinge, R. (2008). Belief inflexibility in schizophrenia. *Cognitive Neuropsychiatry, 13*, 267–277.

Woodward, T. S., Munz, M., Leclerc, C., & Lecomte, T. (2009). Change in delusions is associated with change in "jumping to conclusions." *Psychiatry Research, 170*, 124–127.

Wykes, T., Steel, C., Everitt, B., & Tarrier, N. (2008). Cognitive behavior therapy for schizophrenia: Effect sizes, clinical models, and methodological rigor. *Schizophrenia Bulletin, 34*, 523–537.

16

Social Cognition and Interaction Training

DENNIS R. COMBS, JOHANNA TORRES, AND
MICHAEL R. BASSO ■

Social Cognition and Interaction Training (SCIT) is a comprehensive, stand-alone manual-based group intervention that targets the three core social cognitive deficits in schizophrenia: emotion perception, theory of mind (ToM), and attributional style (Roberts, Penn, & Combs, 2009). By targeting these deficits in social cognition, it is believed that social and community functioning will ultimately improve (Combs et al., 2007; Wölwer, Combs, Frommann, & Penn, 2010). SCIT is comprised of three distinct phases, lasts 20–24 weeks, and is built around a weekly 1-hour group therapy session. SCIT has shown improvements in both inpatients and outpatients with schizophrenia (Combs et al., 2007; Penn et al., 2005; Roberts et al., 2009), and these gains persist at 6-month follow-up (Combs et al., 2009). SCIT has the potential to become an evidence-based treatment for schizophrenia (Penn, Roberts, Combs, & Sterne, 2007). SCIT involves the use of didactic instruction, videotape and computerized learning tools, and role-play methods to improve social cognition. SCIT involves weekly homework assignments and uses optional phone-in contacts and practice partners to consolidate gains made in the sessions. The theoretical underpinnings of SCIT will now be discussed.

THEORETICAL ORIENTATION

Deficits in social cognition have been shown to be closely related to poor social and community functioning (Penn, Addington, & Pinkham, 2006). SCIT is based on empirically derived social cognitive models of schizophrenia, particularly as they apply to paranoid processes (Combs & Penn, 2008). SCIT emphasizes several key social cognitive domains that appear to interact in hindering effective social behavior in schizophrenia. First, a need for closure (i.e., intolerance of ambiguity) is associated with the tendency to truncate searches for explanatory evidence and jump to hasty conclusions in many social situations. Second, externalizing and personalizing attributional biases are used in explaining negative events. When many individuals with schizophrenia experience negative events, they are vulnerable to hastily blaming factors outside of themselves and blaming other people, as opposed to blaming situations. This is especially true for persons with paranoia (Combs & Penn, 2008). Third, ToM is the ability to simulate in one's own mind the mental states of people other than oneself. This includes the ability to infer the intentions, perspectives, desires, and emotions of other people (i.e. "to put oneself in another's shoes"). It also includes the ability to imagine oneself in a different situation from the here-and-now, and to evaluate one's current thoughts and emotions nonsubjectively, as if looking at oneself from the outside. It has been widely demonstrated that persons with schizophrenia have deficits in ToM, and these deficits are linked to social functioning (Brune, 2005). This latter aspect of ToM overlaps with the concept of *metacognition*. Fourth, emotion perception abnormalities include difficulties identifying facially expressed emotions. Abnormalities in emotion perception are thought to exacerbate the above constellation of difficulties as they apply to interpersonal functioning.

Conceptually, SCIT is structured hierarchically, such that training on recognizing emotions is presented first in phase 1. It is believed that obtaining accurate information on emotional expressions provides important "data" that can be used to "figure out" situations (how people are feeling, in order to make better decisions), which is the focus of phase 2. Phase 3 focuses on problems in the participant's real life, and participants can use data to figure these situations out. SCIT achieves change by correcting the inherent social cognitive deficits and biases found in schizophrenia and makes adaptive processes more automatic in nature.

OVERVIEW OF SCIT

SCIT is designed to meet at least once per week for 45–60 minutes, for 20–24 sessions. This manual is structured around a 20-session treatment phase. However, facilitators may elect to add up to four "catch-up" sessions within the treatment if they decide that it would be useful to spend more than the allotted time working through specific content areas.

SCIT is divided into three distinct treatment phases, as shown in Table 16.1.

Table 16.1 SOCIAL COGNITION AND INTERACTION TRAINING (SCIT) PHASES

Sessions	Phase	Content
1 to 7	I—Introduction and Emotions	Introduce SCIT and social cognition, establish group alliance, review the role of emotions in social situations, develop emotion recognition skills
8 to 15	II—Figuring Out Situations	Address jumping to conclusions, attributional biases, tolerating ambiguity, distinguishing facts from guesses, and gathering data to make better guesses
16 to 20	III—Integration: Checking It Out	Skill consolidation and generalization to everyday problems

Phase I: Introduction and Emotions

The initial two sessions are spent building group alliance and introducing participants to the SCIT group and the concept of social cognition. After this introduction, the remainder of phase I is spent defining basic emotions, discussing the relationship between emotions and social situations, and identifying facial expressions of emotion. The goals of phase I are to:

1. Begin building group alliance.
2. Introduce SCIT and the concept of social cognition.
3. Share personal experiences of emotion and link them to social contexts.
4. Define seven basic emotions.
5. Flexibly distinguish between different facial expressions of emotion and improve attention to crucial areas of the face needed for emotion perception.
6. Conceptualize paranoia as an emotion.

Phase II: Figuring Out Situations

Phase II presents social cognitive strategies to avoid the pitfalls associated with "jumping to conclusions" (JTC) in social situations. These strategies include generating multiple attributions for negative events, perspective taking, distinguishing social facts from social guesses, tolerating ambiguity in social situations, and utilizing new information to improve interpretation of social situations. The goals of phase II are to:

1. Learn to recognize "jumping to conclusions."
2. Learn the difference between internal/personal, external/personal, and external/situational attributions.
3. Learn to generate causal attributions from these three perspectives.
4. Appreciate the difficulty of interpreting ambiguous situations.
5. Recognize the difference between social facts and guesses.
6. Practice gathering evidence instead of JTC.
7. Learn to judge the likelihood that a conclusion is right.

Phase III: Checking It Out

This final phase of SCIT is a consolidation of skills learned up to this point and an application of these skills to participants' own lives. This is achieved by learning, rehearsing, and applying a step-by-step problem-solving algorithm called the "checking it out" process. Participants are encouraged to bring in problematic situations from their daily lives. The group then analyzes the situations and develops behavioral strategies for "checking out" problems with other people based on SCIT skills. The goals of phase III are to:

1. Collaboratively assess the facts surrounding social events in different members' lives that cause them distress.
2. Recognize that sometimes it is not possible to understand a situation without gathering more information.
3. Appreciate that "checking out" guesses with another person can prevent you from jumping to conclusions that make you feel bad.
4. Identify appropriate questions to check out guesses in specific social situations.
5. Role-play "checking it out" in response to events in members' lives.

DESCRIPTION OF INDIVIDUAL SCIT SESSIONS

Check-In

Each SCIT session begins with a 10-minute group check-in, during which members are asked how they are feeling (participants are asked "are you feeling mostly good, mostly bad, or neutral?"). This check-in procedure occurs in all SCIT sessions. The check-in sets the tone early on that members are expected to share their feelings openly in the group and also provides examples for SCIT leaders to draw upon if needed. A secondary goal is to promote awareness of emotional reactions in social situations (to help address possible alexithymia) and the effect that emotions can have on social judgments and behavior. After check-in, the leaders review the previous week's homework and then begin the material for the current session.

Phase 1: Emotion Training

SESSIONS 1 AND 2: INTRODUCTION
These initial sessions orient participants to the general goals of the SCIT intervention and provide a shared model of thinking that will be emphasized throughout the intervention. The group leaders introduce themselves and the goals of SCIT. Participants are informed that the group will help them enhance their social lives by avoiding misunderstandings with others. The group sessions will consist of a number of different activities, such as watching and discussing videos, doing puzzles and games, and having conversations about participants' lives and problems. Participants then introduce themselves and, if possible, state goals for themselves. Then the leaders collaboratively discuss the group rules, attendance, homework, and the role of practice partners to lay the foundation for a successful group. After the basic information about SCIT is presented, the session then shifts to the first main point, which is illustrated by use of the SCIT triangle. The SCIT triangle (Figure 16.1) depicts the causal connections among emotions, thoughts, and actions. An example serves to illustrate the relationships to the participants.

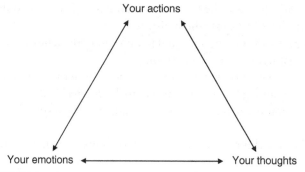

Figure 16.1 SCIT triangle.

So, let me give you an example of how this triangle works. Yesterday, I was in a bad mood for some reason. A friend of mine called me on the phone and asked if I wanted to go see a certain movie with him. I said no and told him that it sounded like a stupid movie. Afterward, I felt bad because I realized that my bad mood made me treat my friend badly. It also made me think that it was a dumb idea to go see that movie.

Every time we talk to somebody, all three of these things are happening— emotions, thoughts, and actions— and they're all affecting each other.

Following the above example from the group leader, a video vignette is shown and the members discuss how emotions, thoughts, and behaviors are interrelated. Then, group members are asked to apply the SCIT triangle to their own lives in a group discussion. Members are asked to write down two things they would like to improve about their own lives as homework.

SESSION 3: EMOTIONS AND SOCIAL SITUATIONS

This session continues the psychoeducational lesson from the previous sessions, with an emphasis on the causal links between emotions and social situations. Participants are primed to conceptualize emotions as factors that can affect one's perception of a situation. They are challenged to employ a metacognitive perspective in thinking about how emotions in their own lives may affect their behavior. The group leader provides an example to discuss how our feelings affect thoughts and behaviors. This exercise explicitly counteracts the temptation to use "affect as information" in interpreting social situations, by contrasting emotional and cognitive influences. Many persons feel unhappy and then use this emotion to create paranoid beliefs about the situation. At the end of the session, the use of facial mimicry is introduced as a tool for understanding others' emotional states. A structured activity called "How Would You Feel in Their Shoes" is completed in session. Participants read a short vignette such as "Carrie just heard that her pet dog was just hit by a car" and are asked to decide which emotion Carrie might be feeling and to mimic that emotion as well. The use of facial cues can provide important data to help recognize emotions and later in SCIT help participants understand the role of social context.

SESSION 4: DEFINING EMOTIONS

This session develops basic conceptual knowledge about seven basic emotions (happy, anger, sadness, surprise, fear, shame, and disgust). The session is devoted to describing how these emotions are expressed on the faces of others and to developing a shared definition of different emotional expressions. These facial "cues" are then placed on an "Emotion Poster," which is used for the remainder of SCIT. Consistent with the SCIT triangle, to initiate the discussion, a situation is presented that then evokes an emotion. For example, "We hear a loud bang. What emotion would be present?" Time is also spent discussing paranoia as an emotion, as many participants have paranoid beliefs about others. For homework, participants complete an exercise called "Emotions in My Life," in which they write down the meaning of each emotional state.

SESSION 5: GUESSING PEOPLE'S EMOTIONS

Following the creation of the Emotion Poster, session 5 provides more practice in emotion recognition. Participants view a PowerPoint slide show presentation that contains different facial depictions of the seven basic emotional states. Participants are asked to look at each image and make a "guess" about the emotion being presented. Facial "cues" are used to provide the data that informs their guess, and participants can refer to the emotion poster for assistance. It is important to note that participant answers are viewed as guesses since we cannot be 100% confident which emotion someone is feeling. After a guess, participants then rate on a scale of 0%–100% how confident they are with their guess. If participants are not sure of the emotional expression, they can mimic the emotional expression to receive facial feedback.

An optional exercise comes from research on attention shaping as a means to improve emotion recognition (Combs et al., 2006, 2008, 2011). The center of the face contains a wealth of important information, and persons with schizophrenia often look at nonrelevant areas of the face when recognizing emotions. By focusing attention on the eyes, nose, and mouth areas, emotion perception can improve. Thus, visual attention is shaped or directed toward these areas. Attention is directed by using a visual prompt that focuses the participants on the right areas to view. A PowerPoint demonstration of how attention shaping works can be shown that contains five practice and 12 training faces in which an attentional prompt directs attention to the center of the face. As evident, session 5 contains a wealth of material, and participants find this session especially challenging yet informative.

SESSION 6: UPDATING EMOTION GUESSES

During session 6, participants continue to practice identifying emotional expressions. In this session, they are asked to make guesses about emotional expressions that change or "morph" over time. Since most emotional expressions can rapidly change, it is beneficial to see how facial expressions change from a neutral to a strongly expressive emotion. An example of several emotion morph slides is presented in Figure 16.2 to illustrate this activity.

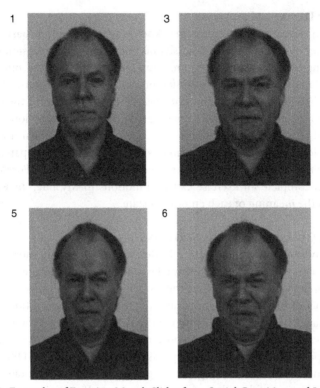

Figure 16.2 Examples of Emotion Morph Slides from Social Cognition and Interaction Training (SCIT) session 6. Participants are asked to identify each emotion and rate how confident they are in their guess on a scale of 0%–100%. Expressions increase in saliency from neutral to very intense. (Picture provided courtesy of Christian Kohler.)

Participants view a series of six images that increase in saliency, and, at each step, they make a "guess" about which emotion is present and how confident they are in their guess. As emotions become more intense, the facial cues become more evident to participants. Five different slide shows can be used for training purposes to provide ample practice. In addition to reinforcing the techniques from the previous session, this exercise is designed to improve social cognitive flexibility and to decrease rigid responding. Such responding may be due to neurologically based perseveration, especially among participants with pronounced negative symptoms. However, according to the SCIT model, inflexible, repetitive responding may also be due to psychological factors, such as a high need for closure. This is especially true among participants who are emotionally aroused by the social context and the evaluative implications of the exercise.

SESSION 7: SUSPICIOUS FEELINGS
Paranoia is especially common in SCIT participants and engenders a wide range of emotions such as anger, fear, or even sadness. Session 7 focuses specifically on paranoia and suspiciousness as an emotion. For participants to benefit from SCIT, they must be able to identify fluctuations in emotional states, including

paranoia, that influence how they interpret situations and behave. This session is aimed at normalizing the experience of paranoia by framing it as an emotion that is continuous with more normative experiences, such as wariness and suspicion. Participants collaboratively come up with different reasons for paranoia, and answers are grouped into three categories: (1) Characteristics of others (past lying behaviors, ambiguous behaviors), (2) situational factors (being in a dangerous situation), and (3) internal factors (anxiety, drug use, lack of sleep). The point is that paranoia has a number of causes and may not reflect the actual or true belief of the other person.

Paranoia as applied to social situations can be justified, inappropriate, or ambiguous. Three video vignettes are used to discuss each type of paranoia, and participants discuss the vignettes. Two homework assignments are used to consolidate gains, and these involve an introspection of times in their lives when participants were mistrustful of others and situations in their lives that were ambiguous in terms of others' intentions.

Phase 2: Figuring Out Situations

SESSION 8: JUMPING TO CONCLUSIONS

As phase 2 begins, the focus of SCIT shifts to teaching strategies and skills to figure out social situations. The initial session focuses on identifying and defining the JTC bias. The JTC bias involves making hasty decisions using very little data. Persons with delusions and paranoia often rush the decision-making process and do not seek out other pieces of information that might lead to a different and, more likely, accurate conclusion. Participants take the role of a "social detective," and it is emphasized that detectives examine all sources of data before making a decision. Detectives often work slowly, and participants should too in social situations. The JTC bias is normalized as a common human error that is more likely to occur in situations that are ambiguous in nature (e.g., where intention is not clear). The JTC bias often leads to negative judgments about people and, more specifically, paranoid beliefs. Using the SCIT triangle (Figure 16.1), paranoia is placed in the "Emotion" corner while JTC is placed in the "Thoughts" corner of the triangle. In other words, just as paranoia is a kind of emotion that can lead to social problems, JTC is a kind of thinking that can also lead to social problems. People who jump to conclusions often believe they are right but are often wrong, and this kind of thinking can create bad feelings in others. Through two video vignettes, participants begin to develop skills at recognizing this error in fictional characters, so that they may later identify it in their own lives. Homework consists of having the participants generate times in their lives when they engaged in JTC and the consequences of this type of decision making.

SESSIONS 9 AND 10: THINK UP OTHER GUESSES

Following a discussion of the JTC, participants are taught a strategy to possibly remediate this social cognitive bias that focuses on "thinking up other guesses as means to avoid jumping to conclusions." This approach is a modified form of "generating alternatives," a common cognitive-behavioral therapy (CBT) technique that is familiar to many clinicians. Generating alternatives is used primarily to decrease a client's conviction in a maladaptive belief or conclusion and to slow down the decision-making process. The SCIT approach is unique in two ways. First, individuals with cognitive limitations often have difficulty engaging in open-ended brainstorming. Therefore, we have deliberately constrained the brainstorming exercise so that participants must only think of three possible guesses and can use a simple heuristic in generating these guesses by adopting the perspective of three fictional characters (i.e., Blaming Bill, My-Fault Mary, and Easy Eddie; see below). The goal is to make this process less cognitively taxing and more automatic in nature. Second, we have linked this approach to research on attributional style among individuals with persecutory delusions. Thus, the three characters reflect the different types of attributional styles found in research studies. "Blaming Bill" exhibits the personalizing bias that involves blaming others for negative events (external-personal) and is often angry. Blaming Bill reflects the attributional style of most paranoid persons. "My-Fault Mary" blames herself for negative events (internal-personal) and gets depressed over her perceived failures. Finally, Easy Eddie blames the situation and tends to remain calm (external-situational). Participants are also asked to describe what types of emotional expressions and behaviors these three characters would exhibit. These questions about thoughts, emotions, and behaviors perfectly align with the SCIT triangle. Participants practice generating alternative explanations for a number of negative fictional events to reinforce this skill. An example of this activity is provided here:

Tasia said she would go to Betty's party. But on the night of the party, Tasia didn't come.

Questions:

What does Betty think?
How would Blaming Bill, My-Fault Mary, and Easy Eddie interpret the situation, and what emotions they would feel?

The responses are organized into a three-column table with the headings Facts, Guesses, and Feelings for each character.

Participants continue to practice with fictional scenarios and then provide examples from their own life. For these exercises, after the three alternatives are discussed, participants must decide which one they believe is most correct (based on the facts and evidence) and then rate how certain they are of the correct decision on a 10-point scale to make "gradients of certainty" judgments. This metacognitive process should increase the dissonance that participants experience when they jump to conclusions, and therefore it should increase the likelihood of their entertaining other guesses.

Table 16.2 THINKING UP OTHER GUESSES RESPONSES

Facts	Guesses	Feelings
Tasia said she would go to Betty's party. Tasia didn't go.	My-fault Mary: *"Tasia doesn't like me."*	Sad
	Blaming Bill: *"Tasia is a mean, inconsiderate person."*	Angry
	Easy Eddie: *"Tasia got caught in traffic."*	Fine

SESSIONS 11, 12, AND 13: SEPARATE FACTS FROM GUESSES

These sessions extend the work of sessions 9 and 10 by presenting another strategy for avoiding jumping to conclusions: separating facts from guesses. Individuals with psychotic disorders often make poor judgments, even when they possess sufficient information to make good judgments. Participants are taught the differences between objective facts and a guess. Objective facts are things that almost all people agree on (often what is visible or known), and guesses are things that we cannot know for certain, such as feelings, motivations, and thoughts. Guesses are usually inferences or attributions about why people do things or how they are feeling. By identifying and then using the facts, we can make better social guesses; however, guesses could also be wrong. The difference between facts and guesses is illustrated by using a series of SCIT pictures (eight total). Participants are shown a picture and are asked to come up with facts, guesses, and feelings. A script for this activity is provided below.

> This is like the game we did a few weeks ago where we listed facts and guesses. Only this time, we are going to look at pictures instead of having me read you situations. We are going to try to name as many facts as we can about the pictures. Think of yourself as a detective at the scene of a crime. We want to list everything that we know for sure, things that everybody will agree on. These are the facts. I'll write the facts on the board. Make sure you don't jump to conclusions about things that you aren't 100% sure about.
>
> After we list facts, we are going to list guesses—things that we think might be true about the people in the situation, but might not. I have a sheet of paper that tells me what the real facts are "behind the scenes" in the pictures, so that we can see how many of our guesses are right and how many are wrong.

A sample picture similar to one used in SCIT is illustrated in Figure 16.3.

Once participants are comfortable discussing pictures, several videos are used. Then, at the end of session 13, participants discuss this activity in their own lives. A series of homework assignments are used after each session to practice this activity with a practice partner. One particular homework assignment centers on inferring what a person wants for his or her birthday using known facts (e.g., what they like to do) to make a good guess. For example, "Lonnie is in school, but wishes he was a chef. Every day he has class from 8:30 to 3:30. After school, he

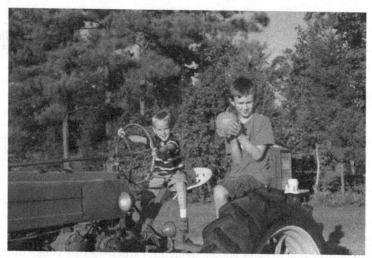

Figure 16.3 Example of a picture from *Facts Versus Guesses*. Participants are asked to identify the facts about the picture to make a guess about what the children are doing. (Picture provided courtesy of Dennis Combs.)

works at a convenience store. Sometimes he goes bowling because his friends like to bowl. But Lonnie doesn't like to bowl. What would be a good gift to get Lonnie, based on the information provided above?"

Sessions 14 and 15: Gather More Evidence

To reinforce all of the skills learned in phase II and continue to target the JTC bias, participants play the 20 Questions game, which emphasizes data gathering and making good guesses. This activity is designed to target participants' metacognitive abilities and tolerance of ambiguity in the context of a "hot" social cognitive situation—a competitive guessing game. By participating with others in a game in which points are won and lost, participants are at risk of performing poorly in front of their peers, and thus are at risk of increased social cognitive error. The rules of the game are presented, and the group leaders conduct the first several rounds. The leader thinks of an animal, a place, or a food. Participants can only ask "yes-or-no" type questions. Participants begin with 10 points and each yes/no question earns them an additional 1 point. After asking a question, each participant has the option of guessing what the correct answer is. If a player elects to guess the answer, he or she must decide how many points to bet on whether the guess is correct or incorrect. Players cannot bet more points than they have. After each round, players review their scores, discuss the strategies they used in the round, and state how it might be possible to improve their strategy for the next round. The focus is on players who jumped to conclusions by betting on a guess before enough information was available to make a good guess and/or by betting too many points on their guess, given how little information was available. An alternative version of the 20 Questions game is available using participant likes and dislikes. The use of points is optional for some groups.

Phase III

SESSIONS 16 TO 24: INTEGRATION (OR "CHECKING IT OUT")

The primary goals of phase III (integration) are to assess the certainty of facts and guesses surrounding events in participants' personal lives, recognize that it is sometimes necessary to obtain more information about social situations, and to teach effective social skills for checking out guesses. The essential purpose of the final phase is to put into practice what participants have learned in SCIT. Participants are taught a systematic method for making social decisions called "checking it out." The steps of the checking it out process are presented in Table 16.3.

Once the steps in the checking it out method are presented (usually in sessions 16 and 17), the rest of the sessions focus on applying these steps to problems in the participants' lives. For example, a participant arranges to go to a movie with a friend, and the friend does not show up. The participant is asked to make an attribution about why this occurred. The check it out process involves all of the tools learned in SCIT, such as separating facts from guesses, avoiding jumping to conclusions, and gathering good data, in order to make an informed guess about the situation. The participant can then choose to check out his or her guess by asking the person directly (or asking another person, write a letter or e-mail, or do nothing at all) to see if their guess was correct. Of course, the group discusses the

Table 16.3 HOW TO CHECK IT OUT

FOLLOW THESE STEPS TO CHECK OUT A SOCIAL SITUATION THAT LEFT YOU FEELING BAD OR CONFUSED
Tell the group about the situation.
On the board, make a FACTS column, a GUESSES column, a FEELINGS column, and an ACTION column.
List the key facts of the situation in the FACTS column.
List your guesses about what caused the problem in the GUESSES column.
Underline the one you believe most.
List the emotions that each guess would make you feel in the FEELINGS column.
Underline the one you feel most.
Get feedback from the group about what they think is the best guess based on the facts.
Work with the group to think of some actions you could take to make the bad feelings less.
Weigh the pros and cons of doing the different actions and decide which one is best.
Role-play the action with somebody in group.
Do the action that you decided on before next group.

Table 16.4 EXAMPLE FOR CHECKING IT OUT

Facts	Guesses	Feelings	Action
Called friend to go to a movie. He said he was busy, and would call me back.	(1) Bill doesn't like me **3 (how confident the person is in their guess on a scale of 1–10)**	(1) Sad	Call Bill again and check it out.
He never called me back. It's been 2 days.	(2) Bill forgot to call because he was busy **7**	(2) Maybe a little sad	Write him a letter.
Friend's name is Bill.	(3) Bill just didn't call because he isn't very thoughtful **5**	3) Angry	Ask someone who knows Bill if there is something bothering Bill.
	(4) Bill is angry at me **3**	4) Worried	Do nothing.

pros and cons of each proposed action before this is done in real life. For example, a person who is very angry may not be advised to confront the person about the event. Role-plays are often used at this point to practice the skills needed for an effective interaction. The participant is offered constructive feedback on his or her social skills and can practice as much as he or she desires with other people or practice partners. To assist with making a good decision, participants organize their thoughts into four columns: facts, guesses, feelings, and possible actions. Table 16.4 shows an illustrative example of such a chart.

TROUBLESHOOTING

Given that schizophrenia is a heterogeneous condition, SCIT was developed to be flexible in its methods and activities to accommodate the full range of symptoms and characteristics. Here, we review some of the issues that may affect group performance and the achievement of the learning objectives.

Symptom Heterogeneity

The activities in SCIT can be varied for persons with different symptom presentations, with special emphasis placed on working with persons with negative symptoms. Within the SCIT manual, a common symbol (yin-yang symbol) designates when symptoms may affect an activity. SCIT conceptualizes social cognitive dysfunction in the two broad syndromal subtypes of schizophrenia: type 1 (positive syndrome) and type 2 (negative syndrome). Behavioral techniques are more likely to be effective for participants with predominant negative syndrome features (type 2), whereas a combination of cognitive and behavioral techniques is recommended for participants with predominant positive syndrome features (type 1). More in-session activities are used with negative-symptom persons due to poor motivation for homework compliance after the session. Also, persons with negative symptoms require more attention from the group leaders to keep them engaged. At the beginning of SCIT, a special emphasis is placed on cultivating client motivation, engagement, and "buy in" throughout the course of treatment. Participants develop personal goals for how SCIT can improve their lives and are then reminded of these goals often. SCIT activities are designed to be fun and engaging, to make the groups more intrinsically motivating.

Homework

To reinforce gains, SCIT makes ample use of homework assignments following each session. However, we acknowledge that homework compliance tends to be low in this population, and pressuring participants to comply with homework may strain the therapeutic alliance. On the other hand, empirical research indicates that homework assignment and adherence has a modest impact on treatment outcome (Kazantzis, Deane, & Ronan, 2000). Additionally, a core assumption of SCIT is that most skill practice will take place outside of therapy sessions through participants using SCIT strategies in their day-to-day lives.

To balance these issues, SCIT takes a moderate approach to homework. SCIT facilitators should provide homework activities, encourage client adherence, and spend time at the beginning of each session reviewing homework. After all, if a group leader assigns homework but does not review it in session, the participants learn that it is not important. However, we suggest that facilitators honor a participant's decision if he or she decides not to do homework and refrain from requiring it or coercing him or her to complete it. Homework is given to the class at the end of each session. The directions for each assignment need to be clearly presented and discussed to troubleshoot any potential problems. Copies of the materials should always be handed out to improve compliance with the assignment as well.

Practice Partners

SCIT involves the optional use of "practice partners" to provide more practice in developing the skills taught in SCIT. A practice partner is a specific person from the participant's life outside of the group who has agreed to help him or her practice SCIT skills. This can include a family member, friend, individual therapist, case manager, or acquaintance. As with homework, the use of practice partners provides an increased opportunity for the consolidation of concepts, as well as for skill application and integration through social interaction. Depending on the population, it may not be feasible for all or some group members to identify an appropriate practice partner. Therefore, group leaders should use their judgment in deciding if it is appropriate to introduce this aspect of homework assignments. With consent, the group leaders should contact the practice partners and explain the goals and structure of SCIT. The practice partner must be aware of his or her weekly involvement. Ask the participant to identify another practice partner if it seems that the initially identified practice partner is not interested or does not have the time to be involved. At the end of the weekly session, the SCIT leaders either mail or e-mail the SCIT homework to the practice partner. The SCIT manual contains weekly activities for practice partners that mirror the content taught in the SCIT session. The activities instruct the practice partner on how to engage the client and provide an outline of topics to discuss. When required, the group leaders should call the practice partners weekly to update them on what happened in each SCIT group and check in with them about the homework.

PARTICIPANT SELECTION AND PRACTICAL ISSUES

SCIT is appropriate for individuals who are at least 18 years of age, suffering from a psychotic illness, and who have interpersonal difficulties as a result of their illness. SCIT is designed for individuals in both inpatient and outpatient treatment centers, and works well for both positive and negative symptoms (Roberts & Penn, 2009). SCIT is particularly appropriate for individuals with symptoms of suspiciousness and paranoia. SCIT is less useful for individuals with profound cognitive impairments (i.e., IQ below 70), profound depression, or for individuals with serious substance abuse or dependence problems.

We recommend including five to eight participants and two leaders in each SCIT group, although groups of 10–12 have been conducted. Having at least five participants will bring a variety of perspectives to the group and ensure that individual participants will not feel too much pressure to perform. Although the group can be run with one facilitator, with two facilitators, one can lead the group while the other keeps participants on task, hands out materials, and writes on the flipchart or board. SCIT can be administered by mental health professionals, such as psychologists, psychiatrists, social workers, and nurses with experience working with individuals with schizophrenia, who possess training in SCIT.

The following materials are needed to implement SCIT:

- A blackboard and chalk, dry-erase board, or flipchart and markers
- Poster (or flipchart) paper that can be posted on the classroom wall
- A television and DVD player
- SCIT manual
- The SCIT video vignettes DVD
- The SCIT photograph set
- A computer and an LCD projector

- The *Guessing People's Emotions* PowerPoint slide show
- The *Attention Shaping Emotions* PowerPoint slide show
- The *5 Emotion Morphs* PowerPoint slide shows
- The *Facts Versus Guesses* PowerPoint slide show

CONCLUSION

SCIT is a group intervention for schizophrenia. The training addresses many of the central social cognitive abnormalities found in schizophrenia. SCIT targets deficits in emotion perception, ToM, and attributional style, as well as the tendency to jump to conclusions. SCIT attempts to remediate these deficits by using a combination of didactic instruction and repeated practice. Participants hone their skills on practice vignettes, videos, and, finally, their real lives. The empirical evidence on SCIT has been promising, and SCIT fills the gap that many cognitive remediation interventions do not. In the end, SCIT may lead to changes in the person's quality of life and social and community functioning.

REFERENCES

Brune, M. (2005). Emotion recognition, 'theory of mind,' and social behavior in schizophrenia. *Psychiatry Research, 133*, 135–147.

Combs, D. R., Adams, S. D., Penn, D. L., Roberts, D., Tiegreen, J., & Stem, P. (2007). Social Cognition and Interaction Training (SCIT) for inpatients with schizophrenia spectrum disorders: Preliminary findings. *Schizophrenia Research, 91*, 112–116.

Combs, D. R., Chapman, D. C., Waguspack, J., Basso, M. R., & Penn, D. L. (2011). Attention shaping as a means to improve emotion perception deficits in outpatients with schizophrenia and impaired controls. *Schizophrenia Research, 127*(1), 151–156.

Combs, D. R., & Penn, D. L. (2008). Social cognition in paranoia. In D. Freeman, R. Bentall, & P. Garety (Eds.), *Persecutory delusions: Assessment, theory and treatment* (pp. 175–204). New York: Oxford University Press.

Combs, D. R., Penn, D. L., Ledet, S., Tiegreen, J., Nelson, A., Basso, M. R., et al. (2009). Social Cognition and Interaction Training (SCIT) for schizophrenia: Six month follow-up results. *Schizophrenia Research, 112*, 196–197.

Combs, D. R., Tosheva, A., Penn, D. L., Basso, M. R., Wanner, J. L., & Laib, K. (2008). Attentional-shaping as a means to improve emotion perception deficits in schizophrenia. *Schizophrenia Research, 105*, 68–77.

Combs, D. R., Tosheva, A., Wanner, J., & Basso, M. R. (2006). Remediation of emotion perception deficits in schizophrenia: The use of attentional prompts. *Schizophrenia Research, 87*, 340–341.

Kazantzis, N., Deane, F. P., & Ronan, K. R. (2000). Homework assignments in cognitive and behavioral therapy: A meta-analysis. *Clinical Psychology: Science and Practice, 7*, 189–202.

Penn, D. L., Addington, J., & Pinkham, A. (2006). Social cognitive impairments. In J. A. Lieberman, T. S. Stroup, & D. O. Perkins (Eds.), *American psychiatric association textbook of schizophrenia* (pp. 261–274). Arlington, VA: American Psychiatric Publishing Press, Inc.

Penn, D. L., Roberts, D. L., Combs, D. R., & Sterne, A. (2007). The development of the social cognition and interaction training (SCIT) program for schizophrenia spectrum disorders. *Psychiatric Services, 58,* 449–451.

Penn, D. L., Roberts, D., Munt, E. D., Silverstein, E., Jones, N., & Sheitman, B. (2005). A pilot study of social cognition and interaction training (SCIT) for schizophrenia. *Schizophrenia Research, 80,* 357–359.

Roberts, D. L., & Penn, D. L. (2009). Social cognition and interaction training (SCIT) for outpatients with schizophrenia: A preliminary study. *Psychiatry Research, 166,* 141–147.

Roberts, D. L., Penn, D. L., & Combs, D. R. (2009). *Social cognition and interaction training manual.* Unpublished manuscript.

Wölwer, W., Combs, D. R., Frommann, N., & Penn, D. L. (2010). Treatment approaches with a special focus on social cognition: Overview and empirical results. In A. Medalia & V. Roder (Eds.), *Neurocognition and social cognition in schizophrenia patients: Basic concepts and treatment* (pp. 61–78). Basel, CH: Karger Publishers.

APPENDIX

SCIT training materials and requests for research use can be obtained from the following persons:

David L. Penn, Ph.D.
University of North Carolina at Chapel Hill
Dpenn@email.unc.edu

David L. Roberts, Ph.D.
University of Texas Health Science Center at San Antonio
RobertsD5@uthscsa.edu

Dennis R. Combs, Ph.D.
The University of Texas at Tyler
Dcombs@uttyler.edu

The Future of Social Cognition in Schizophrenia

Implications from the Normative Literature

DAVID L. ROBERTS AND AMY E. PINKHAM ■

The study of social cognition in schizophrenia is a young and rapidly changing field. As in most new fields, researchers have made rapid and important progress while also encountering a range of vexing obstacles. In particular, the study of social cognition in schizophrenia has yet to develop a solid conceptual foundation or a conventionally accepted set of basic measurement tools. To address these issues, an expert consensus panel convened by the National Institute of Mental Health (NIMH) advised that schizophrenia researchers look to the literature on normal social cognition for guidance (Green et al., 2008). The current volume was designed to facilitate this process. Part I of this volume is dedicated to reviewing the normative literature on social cognition, including its developmental emergence (Chapter 1), manifestation in healthy adults (Chapter 2), cross-cultural variation (Chapter 3), and neural bases (Chapter 4). In Chapter 5, Tudusciuc and Adolphs (2013) provide a roadmap for translating this normative literature into the study of dysfunctional social cognition.

Part II of this volume describes research on mechanisms of abnormal social cognition in schizophrenia and their link to social functioning impairment. In Chapter 6, Horan and colleagues (2013) review research that establishes the importance of social cognition as an independent focus of study in schizophrenia—showing that it is relatively dissociable from neurocognition and is strongly and independently associated with functional outcome. In Chapter 7, Kohler and colleagues (2013) review the descriptive literature on emotion processing in schizophrenia. They conclude that there is strong evidence of impairment in the recognition of emotions, but that the research on emotional expression and experience is limited by variability in measurement approach. Chapter 8 reviews the literature on theory of mind (ToM), which provides consistent support for the existence of ToM deficits in schizophrenia. As in the emotion processing literature, however, Abu-Akel and

Shamay-Tsoory (2013, Chapter 8, this volume) emphasize that the use of widely varying measurement approaches and incompatible theoretical assumptions are important rate limiting factors in this area of study.

A common theme in the research on emotion perception and ToM is the tendency to conceptualize abnormal performance as a type of deficiency in information processing capacity. Less influential than this capacity-oriented literature is the literature, influenced by social psychology, that examines the role of social cognitive bias in explaining abnormalities in schizophrenia. If, from the cognitive perspective, *deficient capacity* refers to the inability to perform an information processing function, then *bias* refers to information-processing functions that produce *systematically distorted* output. This perspective is represented in Chapter 9, where Bentall and Udachina (2013) review research in which paranoid social cognition in schizophrenia is conceptualized as partly resulting from an exaggeration of normal social cognitive processes, including threat detection, need for cognitive closure, emotional arousal, and self-esteem maintenance. The possibility that social cognitive abnormality in schizophrenia may result from some combination of information-processing deficits and biases is also supported by the neuroimaging research reviewed by Pinkham (2013) in Chapter 11. For example, she reviews studies that have shown hypoactive amygdala function during emotion processing tasks, suggesting deficient function, along with other studies reporting *hyper*activity, which may lead to biased social inferences.

The chapters in Part II echo the conclusions of the expert consensus panel noted above. They highlight the need for a solid theoretical foundation that can guide the standardization of measurement instruments and provide a framework for integrating deficit- and bias-based research.

Our aim in this final chapter is to facilitate the application of the normative literature reviewed in Part I of this volume to address the issues with research on social cognition in schizophrenia, as reviewed in Parts II and III. First, we expand on a point made by Lundberg (2013) in Chapter 2—that social psychologists conceptualize social cognition in a markedly different way than do schizophrenia researchers, which has far-reaching implications for measurement, understanding of mechanisms, and treatment development. Second, and building on this first point, we describe the dual-process (DP) framework, a theoretical model that has taken hold in both social psychology (see Chapter 2) and social neuroscience (see Chapter 4) and which, we think, has particular promise as a guiding theoretical model for the study of social cognition in schizophrenia.

WHAT IS SOCIAL COGNITION?

We suspect that most schizophrenia researchers are like us in thinking of social cognition as the ability to infer the mental and emotional states of others, and that to the extent that our patients fail to do this accurately, it is due to their having either *capacity deficits* or *biases* (or both) in social cognition. When we turn to the social psychological literature, however, we see a very different perspective. Social psychologists do not appear to share the basic assumption that normal people have the capacity to infer others' mental and emotional states. And, although social psychologists do use concepts like *capacity* and *bias*, they have slightly different meanings—and starkly different implications for measurement and treatment development.

The Capacity to Infer Others' Mental and Emotional States

Social psychologists generally do not share the view that healthy people are endowed with the capacity to accurately infer others' mental and emotional states. Their perspective appears to have emerged from a confluence of empirical findings and theoretical principles. First, social psychologists have found that the social cognitive judgments of healthy adults exhibit only a mediocre level of accuracy (Ickes, 2003), and often, that accuracy does not appear to be the goal of judgment makers. Instead, normal adults' judgments often are influenced more by the subject's own goals and motives than by a desire to be correct (Fiske & Taylor, 2008; Kunda, 1990). Second, social neuroscience suggests that, not only are people often not motivated to be accurate, but even if we were, our brains aren't designed to achieve accuracy. Neural circuits that subserve social cognition appear to be involved in the processing of two types of information: socially relevant *external* features of others (such as facial configuration and biological motion), and socially relevant *inner* features of the self (such as emotional experience and metacognitive processes; see Chapter 4). Thus, rather than conferring access to others' inner states, our brains appear to be designed to draw on our own inner states when judging others'. This evidence from neuroscience is consistent with the long-held theoretical position of philosophers of mind that a brain-based capacity to perceive or otherwise gain objective knowledge of others' inner states is impossible (Dennett, 1987; Skinner, 1953; Wittgenstein, 1958). What is going on in others' heads is fundamentally intangible to us.

In sum, social psychologists tend toward the view that, whereas normal people are in the practice of drawing inferences about others' mental and emotional states, we are neither able to nor motivated to maximize *accuracy* in these inferences.

A Social Psychological View of Social Cognitive Capacity

What is the implication of this perspective for our understanding of social cognitive capacity? The concept of social cognitive capacity is foundational to our approach as schizophrenia researchers (i.e., poor performance on an emotion recognition task indicates an inability to judge the emotional expressions of others), but if even normal people cannot accurately infer others' mental and emotional states, then is capacity a bankrupt concept?

To our reading, the answer is no. Social psychologists do appear to be very interested in the role of capacity in social cognition, but in a different way than are schizophrenia researchers. Since its very early days, social psychology has been concerned with the distinctively human capacity to generate impressions about others' thoughts, feelings, beliefs, and motives. This is illustrated in Heider and Simmel's influential (1944) study of social attribution. Participants completed the social attribution task (SAT), which requires them to view and then describe "what happened" in a video of moving geometrical shapes. The authors found that normal subjects typically ascribed complex human motives and feelings to the shapes, and described a consistent storyline in which bullied small shapes escape from a tormenting larger shape. In the years since this study, the understanding of the human capacity to ascribe mental states has been refined, and its neural underpinnings are emerging through research in social neuroscience. This line of research supports the view that humans have the capacity to generate and manipulate mental and emotional state representations.

These two capacities have notable differences. The capacity to *generate* social cognitive representations comes easily and automatically to most adults. However, the capacity to *manipulate* these representations can be highly variable, even in high-functioning adults. Manipulating representations is a labor-intensive process mediated by prefrontal executive circuitry. Because this capacity is scarce, people use it judiciously, and frequently seek short-cuts to minimize the difficulty of social cognitive processing. These short cuts often take the form of *heuristics*, which are described below. The term "cognitive miser" is used in social psychology to describe this human tendency to resist effortful mental processing. In addition to being scarce, the capacity to manipulate representations also is vulnerable to being handicapped through situational factors such as cognitive load and emotional arousal. For example, in a classic study, described further below, Gilbert, Pelham, and Krull (1988) showed that forcing people to memorize a string of digits while making social cognitive judgments did not affect their ability to *generate* social cognitive attributions but diminished their capacity to strategically *manipulate* these attributions, which led to maladaptive judgments.

In sum, the social psychological literature appears to support a more circumscribed conceptualization of social cognitive capacity than does the schizophrenia literature. It includes the capacity to generate social cognitive representations, which is strong and stable in normal adults, and the capacity to manipulate these representations, which is variable and overlaps considerably with executive functioning. What is not included, however, is the identification of capacity with accuracy.

Social Cognitive Bias

In the schizophrenia literature, the concept of capacity has received more attention than the concept of bias. The opposite appears to be true in the social psychological literature. To our reading, social psychologists see the capacities to generate and manipulate representations as the parameters which constrain social cognition, whereas *biases* are the processes that drive social cognition. The most important type of bias process is called *heuristics*. Heuristics are guess-making strategies that enable people to efficiently make judgments about phenomena that are impossibly complex and inaccessible. Because nearly all social cognitive judgments involve evaluation of intangible phenomena (i.e., others' inner states), heuristics are a core social cognitive process. For example, Bob's emotional state is fundamentally intangible to you, but you still want to make a judgment about it. Using heuristics, you might take your own feeling, or your desire about Bob's feeling, to be a good enough guess about Bob's feeling ("Because I'd like to believe that Bob likes me, I'll take his smirk to mean that he is happy"). Heuristics are practically useful because they efficiently generate actionable social inferences that typically are in line with the subject's situational goals. However, heuristic social cognitive judgments are always biased due to the fact that they do not draw on the actual inner states of others (e.g., your judgment of Bob's feeling is biased by your own situational goal).

WHAT ARE THE IMPLICATIONS OF THIS PERSPECTIVE FOR SCHIZOPHRENIA RESEARCH?

The normative perspective described above has implications for both capacity-oriented and bias-oriented research in schizophrenia.

Implications for Capacity-Oriented Research

This perspective implies that efforts to quantify schizophrenia patients' social cognitive capacity in terms of the *accuracy* of their judgments may be off track. (After all, even healthy adults' judgments are as likely to be inaccurate as accurate.) Instead, it suggests that capacity should be quantified in terms of the ability to generate and manipulate social cognitive representations, irrespective of accuracy. Schizophrenia researchers interested in pursuing this implication could start by recalibrating how we score existing measures. For example, research shows that schizophrenia participants' responses on Heider and Simmel's SAT deviate from the norm (Bell, Fiszdon, Greig, & Wexler, 2010). The social psychological perspective would caution against interpreting deviation in story interpretation, in and of itself, as evidence of social cognitive deficit. Instead, it would recommend that the term "deficit" be used to describe only subjects who fail to generate mental state attributions at all.

Using this latter scoring approach, Klin (2000) found evidence of deficit among autistic participants on the SAT, who tended to attribute physical instead of intentional attributes to the shapes (e.g., "The triangle moved quickly toward the circle"). In contrast, our lab found that whereas people with schizophrenia did indeed generate abnormal story narratives (e.g., "The circle is me annoying my brother"), they did not exhibit evidence of deficiency. That is, they told unusual stories, but the stories included as many mental and emotional state attributions as those provided by healthy controls (Roberts, unpublished data). In contrast to our findings, Horan and colleagues (2009) used a task similar to the SAT and found evidence that people with schizophrenia do generate fewer and less elaborated mental and emotional state representations, suggesting a true deficit in this ability. Nevertheless, these conflicting results demonstrate the importance of the distinction between deficit (i.e., no representations) and accuracy (i.e., unusual representations) for understanding social cognitive abnormalities in schizophrenia, and they highlight the need for more research that will determine whether schizophrenia patients have true "deficits" in the ability to generate social cognitive representations.

Implications for Bias-Oriented Research

As noted above, in the schizophrenia literature, we generally view abnormal social cognitive judgments as resulting from deficient capacity, but a growing literature is examining the role that bias may contribute to poor social cognitive performance and is conceiving of bias as a mechanism of dysfunction. This view of bias differs from the social psychological perspective, in which bias is seen as a mechanism of normal functioning. That is, bias is not seen as an indicator of failed accuracy but rather of successful heuristic use. This perspective argues against research on bias in schizophrenia that focuses on why patients "got it wrong" and suggests that a more relativistic approach might be appropriate. Researchers may do well to ask questions like, "Why do some patients use heuristic strategies that lead to X bias, while non-ill subjects use heuristics that lead to Y bias?"

The potential value of this more relativistic perspective is illustrated in research using the *beads task*. The beads task is a measure of bias in probabilistic reasoning that requires subjects to judge from which of two jars a series of beads is drawn. The dependent variable is the number of successively presented beads the subject views before picking the jar. Patients with delusions exhibit a "jumping to conclusions" bias on this task, as indicated by the fact that they lock in their judgment after fewer beads than is optimal according to Bayesian logic. From a social psychological standpoint, however, it is notable that non-ill participants also exhibit a bias, but in the opposite, conservative direction. They wait to pick a jar until having viewed *more* beads than is probabilistically optimal (reviewed in Garety & Freeman, 1999). Thus, it is not the case that normal subjects make more accurate judgments, but rather that they use a different heuristic strategy in making their judgment. In holding with this, in Chapter 9 of the present volume, Bentall and Udachina (2013) conceptualize bias in schizophrenia as continuous with bias in non-ill individuals, and emphasize motivational factors that may contribute to patients' selection of judgment-making heuristics.

The Dual-Process Framework

Above, we described how social psychological research diverges from schizophrenia research in its conceptualization of social cognitive capacity and bias. In this section, we describe a theoretical model that is consistent with the social psychological perspective and that we believe holds promise for advancing research on social cognition in schizophrenia in the coming years. Already alluded to in several chapters in the present volume (Chapters 2, 4, and 11), the dual-process (DP) framework is parsimonious, empirically and methodologically robust, and coheres across behavioral and neural levels of analysis. Further, it suggests promising hypotheses regarding capacity- and bias-based mechanisms of social cognitive dysfunction in schizophrenia that have powerful implications for treatment development.

The DP framework holds that social cognitive judgments emerge from the interaction of *automatic* and *controlled* cognitive processing (Chaiken & Trope, 1999). Automatic processing is the primary mechanism for *generating* initial social cognitive representations, and plays a large role in heuristic *manipulation* of representations. It is fast and efficient, and takes place outside of the intention, awareness, and control of the subject. Automatic generation of social cognitive representations draws on early perception-based representations of others' facial features and bodily motion, mediated in part by fusiform gyrus and superior temporal sulcus, respectively. It also draws on well-rehearsed interpersonal scripts or stereotypes, and emotional experiences and representations of the subject's own bodily and physiological states, as mediated by subcortical structures such as the amygdala and insula (Lieberman, 2007).

The neural mechanisms by which automatic processes subserve heuristic manipulation and assignment of social cognitive representations are not well understood. One hypothesized mechanism that has gained empirical support in recent years is based in the mirror neuron system (Carr et al., 2003). It appears that when a subject observes another, the other's behavior is automatically represented in the subject's brain as if she were performing it herself. This spurs automatic generation of subjective inner state representations as proto-hypotheses regarding the other's possible inner states. It is as if the subject's brain is saying, "If I were in Bob's position, I would likely be thinking/feeling X. Therefore, I imagine that Bob is thinking/feeling X." As in the earlier example with Bob, this represents a heuristic process because it substitutes an unanswerable question (how Bob is thinking/feeling) with the answerable question (how the subject would be thinking/feeling if she were in Bob's place). Additionally, as with other heuristics, this is a highly efficient process, which occurs largely outside of the subject's awareness, intention, and control, thus furnishing an actionable impression of others' thoughts, intentions, and feelings without burdening conscious processing.

Automatic processing has the advantage of enabling rapid, holistic evaluation of social situations, providing people with gistful impressions to guide behavior in the real world of fast-paced social interaction. However, automatic processing has the disadvantage of being vulnerable to maladaptive biases because it is not influenced by conscious, reflective thought and is always based on partial, imperfect information.

In contrast to automatic processing, controlled social cognitive processing is slow, inefficient, and late to initiate after stimulus presentation. It takes place within the intention, awareness, and control of the subject, and includes self-monitoring, deliberative reasoning, and impulse inhibition. Overlapping considerably with executive functioning, controlled social cognition is mediated primarily by medial, lateral, and ventral prefrontal circuitry (Lieberman, 2007). Controlled processing supports the capacity to consciously manipulate social cognitive representations, conferring the advantage of enabling subjects to strategically evaluate, modify, and suppress automatic impressions that may be maladaptive or inconsistent with the subject's goals. However, controlled processing has the disadvantage of being inefficient and having severely restricted capacity.

The basic DP model of social cognition is illustrated in Figure 17.1. Automatic processing responds immediately to a social stimulus, quickly and unconsciously generating an actionable impression on the basis of whatever combination of percepts, emotion, cognitive schemas, and physiological inputs happen to be most salient at the time. After roughly 500 ms post stimulus onset, controlled processing *may or may not* be engaged to modify or suppress this initial impression, depending on multiple factors. Controlled processing is less likely to be engaged if the automatic impression is highly salient; if the subject is experiencing cognitive load, emotional arousal, or distraction; is cognitively impaired; is unaware that the initial impression may be maladaptive; or is not motivated to question the initial impression. Failure to actively engage controlled cognition results in passive endorsement of the automatic impression, and subsequent controlled processing will be biased toward its continued endorsement.

In the DP framework, social cognitive *capacities* comprise the automatic ability to generate mental and emotional state representations, and the controlled ability to manipulate these representations. *Biases* refer to systematic response tendencies that emerge out of the interaction of these capacities and automatic influences on judgment. The interaction of capacity and bias within the DP framework is illustrated in a study by Gilbert and colleagues (Gilbert et al., 1988) in which healthy participants were shown a film of a young woman behaving in an anxious manner and asked to judge the cause of her behavior. Subjects who were forced to answer the question while holding a string of numbers in memory judged her to be a constitutionally neurotic person, whereas subjects not under cognitive load judged her to be reacting to a situational stressor. The loaded group had

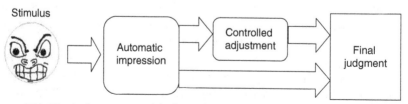

Figure 17.1 The dual-process model of social cognition.

controlled processing handicapped and thus were guided in their judgment by the *fundamental attribution error*, a normative heuristic in which people automatically assume that behavior is driven by intention and personality. The downside of this heuristic in this case is that it leads to an unfairly derogatory appraisal of the woman's character. In contrast, the nonloaded group deployed controlled processing to override this initial impression and make more prosocial situationalizing attributions for the woman's behavior (e.g., she just saw a scary movie). This study illustrates that when healthy adults evaluate others' inner states, their judgments often are guided by social goals rather than accuracy, but that their ability to use these goals to guide judgment may be moderated by the availability of controlled processing capacity, which, when unavailable, leaves judgments to be based on biased automatic impressions.

Applying the Dual-Process Framework to Social Cognition in Schizophrenia

To our thinking, the DP framework provides a strong basis for applying social psychological principles to the study of social cognition in schizophrenia. A plausible initial DP model is that social cognitive abnormality in schizophrenia results from two factors: (1) diminished controlled processing capacity and (2) excessively salient and aberrant automatic social cognitive impressions. There is broad support in the literature for the first factor, as schizophrenia is linked to diminished prefrontal functioning (Ragland, Yoon, Minzenberg, & Carter, 2007). There is also support for the second factor in the literature on dopamine-mediated aberrant salience experience (Kapur, 2003), including evidence that dysregulated neural signaling causes feelings of social threat, alien control, and other forms of aberrant intentionality (Roberts, Stutes, & Hoffman, in press). This two-factor model predicts the generation of highly salient but maladaptively biased automatic social cognitive impressions (e.g., the impression of being the object of hostility) in combination with a handicapped ability to evaluate, suppress, or modify these dysfunctional impressions. Other hypotheses may also be tested within the DP framework, such as those relating to reductions in the automatic capacity to generate social cognitive representations, as suggested by the Horan study above.

Researchers using the DP framework have developed a range of well-validated manipulation and measurement techniques. For example, automatic and controlled capacities can be dissociated through a range of experimental manipulations, including cognitive load (as described in the Gilbert study, above), speeded tasks, use of distraction, obfuscating the automatic source of an impression, and depletion of controlled resources (Bargh, 1994). From a data analytic standpoint, techniques such as signal detection (Green & Swets, 1966) and process dissociation (Payne & Stewart, 2007) have been developed that are capable of reliably dissociating capacity and bias parameters.

To be sure, application of DP techniques to schizophrenia research requires thoughtful and creative adaptation. Readers are referred to Martin and Penn's

(2002) study, an application of Gilbert et al.'s (1988) paradigm to schizophrenia, which shows both the potential value of the social psychological perspective and the difficulty of adapting it to schizophrenia.

Treatment Implications of the Dual-Process Framework

Part III of this volume addresses the research on social cognitive treatment in schizophrenia. Interventions such as Integrated Psychological Therapy (IPT)/Integrated Neurocognitive Therapy (INT) (Chapter 13) and Cognitive Enhancement Therapy (CET; Chapter 14) conceive of social cognition and neu-rocognition as closely related, and are designed to improve both in a synergistic manner. These represent the oldest and most intensive social cognitive interventions, and have amassed the most evidence of efficacy. More recently, interventions such as Metacognitive Therapy (MCT) and Social Cognition and Interaction Training (SCIT) have built off of evidence of the relative independence of social cognition, attempting to improve social functioning more efficiently by enhancing social cognition at the exclusion of neurocognition. Initial results from these new interventions are promising, but much more research is needed. Unfortunately, problems with measurement and theoretical integration are rate-limiting factors in the treatment literature, just as they are in the basic descriptive research.

In addition to its implications for research on the mechanisms of social cognitive abnormality, the DP framework has implications for treatment development in schizophrenia. Foremost, it suggests that the treatment goal of improving the accuracy of social cognitive judgments may be a red herring. Not only is accuracy not the typical goal or the outcome of normal social cognition, but completely accurate social cognitive judgment making is likely to be maladaptive. It is well established that adaptive social cognition is characterized by a range of biases (Haselton & Buss, 2003), including a self-serving bias for explaining positive events, a situationalizing bias for negative events, and a conservative bias for probabilistic judgments, among others (Fiske & Taylor, 2008). Further, given that the tendency to believe in mind reading is a common delusion in schizophrenia, it may be inadvisable for social cognition training to teach that it is possible to read others' minds and emotions. Instead of teaching patients how to "get it right" in social situations, the DP framework suggests that it may be preferable to design interventions that teach patients that it is impossible to know for sure what others might be thinking and feeling.

This goal would be in line with the broader trend in empirically supported psychological treatment development, which is moving away from an emphasis on correcting inaccurate thinking toward an emphasis on acceptance of uncertainty (Hayes, Villatte, Levin, & Hildebrandt, 2011). Initial applications of acceptance-based interventions in schizophrenia have been promising. For example, one preliminary study targeting psychotic symptoms found treatment-related decreases in the believability of symptoms and in symptom-related distress (Bach & Hayes, 2002). This finding was subsequently independently replicated

(Gaudiano & Herbert, 2006). One might hypothesize that an analogous social cognitive intervention would lead to patients having decreased confidence in their ability to infer others' mental and emotional states alongside decreased social anxiety and distress.

A second treatment implication of the DP model stems from the fact that controlled social cognitive capacity is a scarce resource, and that even healthy adults must often behave as "cognitive misers," relying more on automatic impressions than on controlled evaluation. From this perspective, interventions that teach patients to slow down and think carefully may not be likely to succeed (especially given the cognitive deficits associated with schizophrenia), and may be teaching a brand of social cognition that is itself abnormal and unlikely to be useful in dynamically evolving social situations. Instead, the DP framework suggests that social cognitive interventions of the future may do well to harness people's natural tendency toward quick, heuristic processing. For example, patients may benefit more from practice in manipulating social gestalts than from practice in gathering and evaluating pieces of social cognitive evidence.

The pitfalls of overemphasis on controlled processing are highlighted by emerging social psychological research on *cognitive fluency*, which refers to the experiences of ease or difficulty that accompany controlled cognition (Schwarz, 2004). This research has established that when people experience the act of thinking to be difficult, this experience in and of itself is interpreted by the subject as evidence *against* the product of the cognitive act. For example, the commonly used psychotherapeutic technique of *generating alternatives* requires patients to consciously think up alternative interpretations to compete with an existing dysfunctional belief or conclusion. If the patient generates a large number of alternatives, to the extent that the process of generating alternatives is experienced as difficult, the patient may essentially conclude, "It was so hard for me to imagine alternatives that my initial impression *must* be correct." This suggests the unsettling possibility that our widespread technique of teaching patients to use deliberate, strategic social cognition may not only be ineffective, but may actually be counterproductive!

In conclusion, we have shared two thoughts on how the social psychological literature may be used to advance research on social cognition in schizophrenia. First, the social psychological perspective suggests that our convention in schizophrenia research of operationalizing social cognitive capacity in terms of the *accuracy* of social cognitive judgments may be off base. As suggested by the recent expert consensus panel on social cognition in schizophrenia (Green et al., 2008), modifying our view of capacity to match the social psychological perspective may help us to address rate-limiting factors in our research. Second, a promising method for aligning our research with social psychological research is the DP framework. Attractive features include its basis in the normative research, parsimony, compatibility across behavioral and neural levels of analysis, established methods and research paradigms, ability to contextualize both capacity- and bias-based research, and its implications for social cognitive treatment development.

Social cognition has been a focus of research in the normative literature for over 80 years. We hope that this chapter, and this volume more broadly, will inspire schizophrenia researchers and clinicians to delve further into the rich normative literature in the years to come, so that we may speed progress in the understanding and treatment of social cognitive dysfunction in this illness.

REFERENCES

Abu-Akel, A., & Shamay-Tsoory, S. G. (2013). Characteristics of theory of mind impairments in schizophrenia. In D. L. Roberts & D. L. Penn (Eds.), *Social cognition in schizophrenia: From evidence to treatment* (Chapter 8). New York: Oxford University Press.

Bach, P., & Hayes, S. C. (2002). The use of acceptance and commitment therapy to prevent the rehospitalization of psychotic patients: A randomized controlled trial. *Journal of Consulting and Clinical Psychology, 70,* 1129–1139.

Bargh, J. A. (1994). The Four Horsemen of automaticity: Awareness, efficiency, intention, and control in social cognition. In R. S. Wyer, Jr., & T. K. Srull (Eds.), *Handbook of social cognition* (2nd ed., pp. 1–40). Hillsdale, NJ: Erlbaum.

Bell, M. D., Fiszdon, J. M., Greig, T. C., & Wexler, B. E. (2010). Social Attribution Test—Multiple Choice (SAT-MC) in schizophrenia: Comparison with community sample and relationship to neurocognitive, social cognitive and symptom measures. *Schizophrenia Research, 122,* 164–171.

Bentall, R. P., & Udachina, A. (2013). Social cognition and the dynamics of paranoid ideation. In D. L. Roberts & D. L. Penn (Eds.), *Social cognition in schizophrenia: From evidence to treatment* (Chapter 9). New York: Oxford University Press.

Carr, L., Iacoboni, M., Dubeau, M. -C., Mazziota, J., C., & Lenzi, G. L. (2003). Neural mechanisms of empathy in humans: A relay from neural systems for imitation to limbic areas. *Proceedings of the National Academy of Sciences, 100,* 5497–5502.

Chaiken, S., & Trope, Y. (1999). *Dual-process theories in social psychology.* New York: The Guilford Press.

Dennett, D. C. (1987). *The intentional stance.* Cambridge, MA: The MIT Press.

Fiske, S. T., & Taylor, S. E. (2008). *Social cognition: From brains to culture.* New York: McGraw-Hill.

Garety, P. A., & Freeman, D. (1999). Cognitive approaches to delusions: A critical review of theories and evidence. *British Journal of Clinical Psychology, 38,* 113–154.

Gaudiano, B. A., & Herbert, J. D. (2006). Acute treatment of inpatients with psychotic symptoms using Acceptance and Commitment Therapy: Pilot results. *Behaviour Research and Therapy, 44,* 415–437.

Gilbert D. T., Pelham B. W., & Krull D. S. (1988). On cognitive busyness: When person perceivers meet persons perceived. *Journal of Personality and Social Psychology, 54,* 733–740.

Green, M. F., Penn, D. L., Bentall, R., Carpenter, W. T., Gaebel, W., Gur, R. C., et al. (2008). Social cognition in schizophrenia: An NIMH workshop on definitions, assessment, and research opportunities. *Schizophrenia Bulletin, 34,* 1211–1220.

Green, D. M., & Swets J. A. (1966). *Signal detection theory and psychophysics.* New York: Wiley.

Hayes, S. C., Villatte, M., Levin, M., & Hildebrandt, M. (2011). Open, aware, and active: Contextual approaches as an emerging trend in the behavioral and cognitive therapies. *Annual Review of Clinical Psychology, 7*, 141–168.

Haselton, M. G., & Buss, D. M. (2003). Biases in social judgment: Design flaws or design features? In J. Forgas, K. Williams, & B. von Hippel (Eds.), *Responding to the social world: Implicit and explicit processes in social judgments and decisions* (pp. 23–43). Cambridge, UK: Cambridge University Press.

Heider, F., & Simmel, M. (1944). An experimental study of apparent behavior. *The American Journal of Psychology, 57*, 243–259.

Horan, W. P., Lee, J., & Green, M. F. (2013). Social cognition and functional outcome in schizophrenia. In D. L. Roberts & D. L. Penn (Eds.), *Social cognition in schizophrenia: From evidence to treatment* (Chapter 6). New York: Oxford University Press.

Horan, W. P., Nuechterlein, K. H., Wynn, J. K., Lee, J., Castelli, F., & Green, M. F. (2009). Disturbances in the spontaneous attribution of social meaning in schizophrenia. *Psychological Medicine, 39*, 635–643.

Ickes, W. (2003). *Everyday mindreading: Understanding what other people think and feel.* New York: Prometheus Books.

Kapur, S. (2003). Psychosis as a state of aberrant salience: A framework linking biology, phenomenology, and pharmacology in schizophrenia. *American Journal of Psychiatry, 160*, 13–23.

Klin, A. (2000). Attributing social meaning to ambiguous visual stimuli in higher-functioning autism and Asperger syndrome: The social attribution task. *Journal of Child Psychology and Psychiatry, 41*, 831–846.

Kohler, C. G., Hanson, E., & March, M. E. (2013). Emotion processing in schizophrenia. In D. L. Roberts & D. L. Penn (Eds.), *Social cognition in schizophrenia: From evidence to treatment* (Chapter 7). New York: Oxford University Press.

Kunda, Z. (1990). The case for motivated reasoning. *Psychological Bulletin, 108*, 480–498.

Lieberman, M. D. (2007). Social cognitive neuroscience: A review of core processes. *Annual Review of Psychology, 58*, 259–289.

Lundberg, K. (2013). Social cognition: Social psychological insights from normal adults. In D. L. Roberts & D. L. Penn (Eds.), *Social cognition in schizophrenia: From evidence to treatment* (Chapter 2). New York: Oxford University Press.

Martin, J. A., & Penn, D. L. (2002). Attributional style in schizophrenia: An investigation in outpatients with and without persecutory delusions. *Schizophrenia Bulletin, 28*, 131–141.

Payne, B. K., & Stewart, B. D. (2007). Automatic and controlled components of social cognition: A process dissociation approach. In J. A. Bargh (Ed.), *Social psychology and the unconscious: The automaticity of higher mental processes* (pp. 293–315). New York: Psychology Press.

Pinkham, A. E. (2013). The social cognitive neuroscience of schizophrenia. In D. L. Roberts & D. L. Penn (Eds.), *Social cognition in schizophrenia: From evidence to treatment* (Chapter 11). New York: Oxford University Press.

Ragland, J. D., Yoon, J., Minzenberg, M. J., & Carter, C. S. (2007). Neuroimaging of cognitive disability in schizophrenia: Search for a pathophysiological mechanism. *International Review of Psychiatry, 19*, 417–427.

Roberts, D. L., Stutes, D., & Hoffman, R. (in press). Alien intentionality in schizophrenia. In A. Mishara, M. Schwartz, P. Corlett, & P. Fletcher (Eds.), *Phenomenological neuropsychiatry: Bridging the clinic with clinical neuroscience.* New York: Springer.

Schwarz, N. (2004). When thinking feels difficult: Meta-cognitive experiences in judgment and decision making. *Medical Decision Making, 25*, 105–112.

Skinner, B. F. (1953). *Science and human behavior*. New York: Free Press.

Tudusciuc, O., & Adolphs, R. (2013). Social cognitive neuroscience: Clinical foundations. In D. L. Roberts & D. L. Penn (Eds.), *Social cognition in schizophrenia: From evidence to treatment* (Chapter 5). New York: Oxford University Press.

Wittgenstein, L. (1958). *The blue and brown books*. Oxford, UK: Blackwell.

INDEX

AAAS. *See* American Association for the Advancement of Science
abnormal beliefs, 215
Abu-Akel, A., 401–2
ACC. *See* anterior cingular cortex
acculturation, 73
across-task manipulations, 23
actions
  development and understanding of, 21
  goals and, 20
  intention and, 20
  ownership, 94–95
  units, 175
Addington, D., 163, 166
Addington, J., 163, 166, 248
Adler, A., 363
Adolphs, R., 2, 138, 401
adult cognition, 338
affect
  contextual modulation of, 110
  discrimination, 247
  facial affective flattening, 174–76
  as information, 388
  labeling, 109
  perception, 289–90
  valuation, 70
affective capacity, 71
affective traits, 184
affect recognition, 305. *See also* emotion perception and emotion recognition
  in clinical high risk of psychosis, 251
  in family high risk of psychosis, 254–55
  in first-episode psychosis, 247–48
  improvement of, 287
  malleability of, 287–88
agency, 94, 97
agenesis of corpus callosum, 140
aggression
  social understanding and, 33

ToM and, 33
agnosia, 135
AIHQ. *See* Ambiguous Intentions Hostility Questionnaire
allocentric coding system, 95
altruism, 76
Ambady, N., 51–52
Ambiguous Intentions Hostility Questionnaire (AIHQ), 252
ambivalence, 184
American Association for the Advancement of Science (AAAS), 124
amnestic syndrome, 372
amygdala, 5–6, 104, 106, 109, 136
  activation levels, 266
  calcification of, 125
  in emotion processing, 265
  lesions of, 126
  responsivity, 110
  in schizophrenia, 265–66
  in social cognition, 137–40
  in threat detection, 137
  trust and, 137
Andersen, S. M., 228
Anderson, C. M., 105
anger, 50, 105, 266
anhedonia, 181–84
animated shapes task, 207
anomalous perceptions, 228–29
anterior cingular cortex (ACC), 73, 132
  dorsal, 5, 272
  in emotional processing, 133
  rostral, 109
anterior insula, 95
  right, 79
antibiotics, 188
Anticevic, A., 265
anticipatory pleasure, 182–83
antipsychotic medications, 177, 221

anxiety, 182
  social, 185
apathy, 184
apparent mental causation, 58
application aspect of mentalizing, 199
APS. *See* attenuated positive symptoms
arousal, 187
Asch, S. E., 42
Asperger syndrome, 196, 205
ASQ. *See* Attributional Style Questionnaire
association, 57
Astington, J. W., 23
attention, 133
  in CET training, 343
  in INT Module A, 320–21
Attention Reaction Conditioner, 344
attenuated positive symptoms (APS), 246
attitude change, 43
attributions, 234. *See also* causal attri-
    butions; emotion attribution;
    fundamental attribution error;
    misattributions
  emotion, 201–2
  intention, 20–21
  in INT Module D, 330–32
  MCT and, 360
  in mentalizing, 198
  paranoia and, 229–31
  self-attribution, 95
  self-representations and, 226–27
  social cognition and, 330–32
  theory, 225
attributional style, 8, 152, 384
  in clinical high risk of psychosis, 252–53
  in first-episode psychosis, 249–50
  fMRI of, 271
  in MCT, 364
  in SCIT, 392
  in social cognitive neuroscience, 269–71
  theory of, 363–64
Attributional Style Questionnaire (ASQ),
    230, 249
attribution biases
  consensus in, 47
  consistency in, 47
  correspondent inference theory, 47
  covariation model, 47

distinctiveness in, 47
  formal social psychological models,
    47–48
  in schizophrenia research, 46–48
atypical neuroleptics, 358–59
auditory cues, 344
auditory deprivation, 84
autism, 97, 98, 196, 200
  connectivity in, 140
  in developing brain, 127–29
  WMS and, 130
autobiographical memory, 96
automatic processes, 6, 43, 57, 272, 407–8
Avenanti, A., 77
Awareness of Social Inference Test Part III,
    249, 253

BADE. *See* Bias Against Disconfirmatory
    Evidence
bad-me (BM) delusions, 218–19
Bailey. A. J., 98
Baillargeon, R., 28
Bandura, A., 121
Barch, D. M., 182
Bargh, J. A., 177
Baron-Cohen, S., 128
Barrowclough, C., 231
basal ganglia, 221
Bayesian analysis, 224
beads in a jar task, 224, 365, 406
Beck Depression Inventory, 231
behaviorism, 42–43, 121
belief. *See also* false-belief task
  abnormal, 215
  changing, 360
  desire and, 24
  incorrect, 23
  MCT and, 360
  understanding, 22, 24
Bell, M., 164, 294
Bentall, R. P., 222, 223, 225, 402, 406
Ben-Yishay, Y., 352
Ben-Zeev, D., 228
biases
  attribution, 46–48
  cognitive, 58, 363–75
  confirmation, 368

correspondence, 46
in DP models, 408
egocentric, 55
oriented research, 406
personalizing, 269
self-serving, 270–71
social cognitive, 404–5
Bias Against Disconfirmatory Evidence (BADE), 371
dealing with, 368–69
MCT and, 367–69
theory, 367–68
bilateral amygdala lesions, 126, 137
bilateral inferior frontal gyrus, 73–74
bipolar disorder, 216, 302
BIPS. *See* brief intermittent psychotic symptoms
Bleuler, E., 225
blood oxygen level-dependent (BOLD) signal, 137, 140
BM delusions. *See* bad-me delusions
Bobo doll experiments, 121
bodily expression, 75
BOLD. *See* blood oxygen level-dependent signal
Boone, S. E., 285
boss effect, 79
Bowen-Jones, K., 222
Bowler, D. M., 205
Bracy, O. L., 343, 352
brain. *See* human brain; social cognitive brain; *specific regions*
Brekke, J., 163
brief intermittent psychotic symptoms (BIPS), 246
Brittain, 165
broad-based treatments, 293–94
Brothers, L., 2
Brüne, M., 5, 201
bullying, 33, 219
Burbridge, J. A., 182

CAARMS. *See* Comprehensive Assessment of the At-Risk Mental State
Campbell, M. L. C., 218
capacity
affective, 71
cognitive, 71
in DP framework, 408
oriented research, 405–6
social cognitive brain and, 110–11
tendency and, 110–11
card-sorting exercise, 323
Carrington, S. J., 98
cartoon-based ToM tasks, 73
causal attributions, 41, 46, 57, 70
cross-cultural variation in, 75–77
dispositional, 56
focal objects in, 70
situational, 56
CBT. *See* cognitive-behavioral therapy
CET. *See* Cognitive Enhancement Therapy
Chadwick, P., 218
Chambers, J. R., 54
chameleon effect, 177
Chapman Anhedonia Scales, 182, 186
character intention task, 288
Chartrand, T. L., 177
Chawla, P., 51
check-in, SCIT, 387
checking it out phase, SCIT, 386, 395–96
Chiao, J. Y., 83
CHR. *See* clinical high risk
Christensen, B. K., 166
chronically accessible schemas, 52
chronic schizophrenia, 1–2, 247
Chung, Y. S., 252
Clément, F., 31
clinical high risk (CHR), 246
affect recognition in, 251
attributional style in, 252–53
multiple domains in, 253
social cognition in, 251–54
social knowledge in, 251–52
social perception in, 251–52
ToM in, 252
treatment approaches, 257
clinical psychology, 44
clinical vignettes, 1–2
closure, 365–66. *See also* need for closure
cognitive-behavioral therapy (CBT), 188, 302, 358–59, 392
cognitive biases, 58
in schizophrenia, 363–75

cognitive capacity, 71
cognitive change, 106
cognitive dissonance, 43
Cognitive Enhancement Therapy (CET),
    289
  Applications, 343
  Attention Reaction Conditioner, 344
  attention training, 343
  basic concepts, 343
  basis of, 335
  brain morphology changes from, 297
  CD-ROM, 352
  Condensed Messages, 347–48
  for early-course schizophrenia, 296
  effect durability, 295–96
  employment outcomes, 296
  evaluation of, 295–96
  fMRI and, 297
  follow-up from, 296–97
  friend-helping with, 348
  graduation from, 350–51
  group content, 345–46
  group structure, 346–49
  homework presentation, 347
  implementation, 352–53
  improvements from, 295
  individual therapy, 351–52
  initial assessment, 341–42
  intervention methods, 341–52
  memory training, 343
  methods used in, 337
  neurocognitive training, 342–45
  Orientation Remediation Module, 343
  overview of, 343
  patient population, 340–41
  problem solving training, 343
  recovery plans, 349–51
  research on, 294–97
  resources for, 352
  social cognitive training, 345–51
  social wisdom development in, 338–39
  theoretical foundations, 335–38
  training manual, 352
  treatment goals, 338–39
  treatment targets, 338–39
cognitive enhancers, 188
cognitive fluency, 411

cognitive miser, 411
cognitive processes, 337
  adult, 338
  disorganized, 339
  inflexible, 339
  unmotivated, 339
cognitive remediation therapy (CRT),
    289
cognitive revolution, 41, 121
cognitive therapy, 58
CogPack, 303, 316
collectivism, 83
Collip, D., 218
Coltheart, M., 234
Combs, D., 230, 394
community functioning, 159
comorbid symptoms, 231
  intellectual, 340
comparative psychology, 23
Comprehensive Assessment of the At-Risk
    Mental State (CAARMS), 245, 251
comprehensive treatments, 292–93
computer-room, INT, 316
conceptual self-knowledge, 97
Condensed Messages, 347–48
conditioned avoidance paradigm, 221
confirmation bias, 368
congruence, 48
congruous movements, 178
conscious will, 58–59
consensus, 47
consistency, 47
constructivism, 121
consummatory pleasure, 182–83
contexts
  in causal attribution, 70
  in perception, 70
  social, 78–79
  in visual perception, 70
contextual modulation, 108–10
  of affect, 110
controlled processes, 43, 57, 272, 407–8
  in schizophrenia, 44
control trials, 25
conversation, 26–27
Conway, M. A., 81
cooperation, 76

COPS. *See* Criteria of Psychosis-risk
    Syndromes
Corcoran, R., 222, 223, 233
Correll, J., 52
correspondence bias, 46
correspondent inference theory, 47
Corrigan, P. W., 163, 287
corrugator muscle, 176
corticospinal excitability (CSE), 74
Couture, S. M., 4, 156, 166
covariation model, 47
Criteria of Psychosis-risk Syndromes
    (COPS), 245–46
cross-cultural variation
    in bodily expression, 75
    in causal attributions, 75–77
    emotion in, 76
    in emotion processing, 50
    in empathy, 76–77
    gesture understanding in, 74
    human brain and, 84–85
    mental health implications, 85–86
    in mentalizing, 73–74
    in mental stage reasoning, 73–74
    paranoia and, 216
    perspective taking in, 71–72
    processes of, 84–85
    processing of others in, 71–77
    in self-face recognition, 78–80
    in self-processing, 77–84
    self-related memory in, 81–84
    in social cognition, 70
    in ToM, 73–74
CRT. *See* cognitive remediation therapy
CSE. *See* corticospinal excitability
Cui, X., 217
cultural neuroscience, 70
culture. *See also* cross-cultural variation;
    Eastern culture; Western culture
    human brain and, 70
Cutting, J., 3

dACC. *See* dorsal anterior cingulate cortex
Damasio, A., 124
Damasio, H., 124
Darwin, Charles, 50
David, N., 95

Davis, K. E., 47–48
deafness, 84, 228
deception, 98
    ToM and, 33
decision making, 41
Deese-Roediger-McDermott (DRM)
    paradigm, 373
defensiveness, 234
    paranoia and, 229–31
deficient capacity, 402
delusions, 94, 197, 207
    bad-me, 218–19
    defined, 215
    persecutory, 216
dementia, 216
depression, 139, 160, 182, 184, 216, 225
desires
    beliefs and, 24
    of others, 21
    predicting, 21
Determinants of Outcome of Severe
    Mental Disorders, 216
Dewey, M. E., 222
*Diagnostic and Statistical Manual of
    Mental Disorders* (DSM-IV), 151,
    215–16
didactic therapy components, 317–32
Dinnel, D. L., 86
disgust, 50
disorganized thinking, 339
dispositional causal attributions, 56
dissonant movements, 178
distancing, 108
distinctiveness, 47
distress, 50
dlPFC. *See* dorsolateral prefrontal cortex
DMPFC. *See* dorsal medial prefrontal
    cortex
domain-general accounts of ToM, 25
domain-specific accounts of ToM, 25
dominance, 75
dopamine, 221, 409
dorsal anterior cingulate cortex (dACC),
    5, 272
dorsal medial prefrontal cortex (DMPFC),
    73, 74, 96
dorsal prefrontal cortex, 5

dorsolateral prefrontal cortex (dlPFC), 73, 95

double bluff, 98

DP models. *See* dual-processing models

DRM paradigm. *See* Deese-Roediger-McDermott paradigm

DSM-IV. *See Diagnostic and Statistical Manual of Mental Disorders*

dualism, 120

dual-processing (DP) models, 56–57, 271–72, 407–9
  basic representation of, 408
  bias in, 408
  capacity in, 408
  for social cognition, 409–10
  treatment implications of, 410–12

Duchenne smile, 175

Earnst, K. S., 182

Eastern culture, 70
  boss effect in, 79
  self-concept in, 77
  self-face recognition in, 78
  self in, 72
  self-judgments in, 82–83
  VMPFC in, 82

ecological validity, 9–10

EEG. *See* electroencephalography

egocentric bias, 55

Ekman, Paul, 50, 180

elaborated speech, 346

elastin, 129

El-Deredy, W., 229

electroencephalography (EEG), 123, 270

electromyography (EMG), 176

Ellington, K., 228

embarrassment, 50, 86

EMFACS. *See* Emotion FACS

EMG. *See* electromyography

emotion
  attribution, 201–2
  cross-cultural variation in, 76
  defining, 101, 389
  guessing, 389
  identifying, 371
  inferring, 403
  intentional regulation of, 105–8

in paranoia, 225–33
  in SCIT, 386
  social cognitive brain and, 101–10
  social situations and, 388

emotional contagion, 177–78

emotional regulation
  incidental, 108–10
  intentional, 105–8
  in INT Module D, 330–32

emotional Stroop task, 109

emotional support, 346

Emotion and ToM Imitation Training (ETIT), 291

emotion experience, 181–88
  assessment of, 186–87
  interview, 186
  questionnaires, 186–87
  treatment approaches, 187–88

emotion expression. *See also* facial expression
  clinical course associations, 176–77
  in schizophrenia, 174–78
  social cognitive brain and, 104–5

Emotion FACS (EMFACS), 175

Emotion Morph Slides, 390

emotion perception, 156, 384. *See also* affect recognition and emotion recognition
  in INT Module A, 321–24

emotion processing, 152
  ACC in, 133
  amygdala in, 265
  biological basis for, 50
  congruence in, 48
  cross-cultural universality in, 50
  of emotion-congruent words, 49
  face identification and, 136–37
  feelings-as-information approach, 49
  misattributions in, 49
  in schizophrenia, 48–50
  in social cognition, 48–49
  in social cognitive neuroscience, 263–66
  social functioning perspective of, 50
  social judgments and, 49
  treatment, 178

emotion recognition. *See also* affect recognition and emotion perception

clinical course association, 180–81
  facial channel, 179
  measurement of, 180
  in schizophrenia, 179–81
  speech channel, 179–80
emotion training studies, 287–88
  introduction to, 387–88
  SCIT, 387–91
empathy, 97, 111, 202, 372
  cross-cultural variation in, 76–77
  MCT and, 360, 361
Enriched Supportive Therapy (EST), 295
Epley, N., 54
ERPs. See event-related potentials
EST. See Enriched Supportive Therapy
ETIT. See Emotion and ToM Imitation
    Training
event-related potentials (ERPs)
  in false-belief task, 25–26
  in self-face recognition, 80
evolutionary psychology, 121
executive function, 25
  in schizophrenia, 44
  in ToM, 25–26
experience
  perception and, 22–23
  sampling, 187, 218
experiential avoidance, 229–31
expertise, 32
The Expression of Emotions in Man and
    Animals (Darwin), 50
externally focused processes, 272
extraversion, 51
extreme male brain hypothesis, 128
eye fixation, 72
Eyes task, 8, 249
eye tracking studies, 222

face identification, 135. See also self-face
    recognition
  emotion processing and, 136–37
  proof-of-concept studies, 287
face perception, 3
  domain-specificity of, 134
  social cognitive brain and, 102–4
FACES. See Facial Expression Coding
    System

Facial Action Coding System (FACS), 175
facial affective flattening, 174–76
facial channel, 179
Facial Emotion Discrimination Task
    (FEDT), 9
Facial Emotion Identification Task (FEIT),
    9
facial expression, 50, 135. See also emotion
    expression
  identification, 101
Facial Expression Coding System (FACES),
    175
facial muscles, 175
facilitated communication, 59
FACS. See Facial Action Coding System
Facts Versus Guesses, 394
false-belief task, 23–24, 26, 55, 97,
    199–200, 201–2
  ERPs in, 25–26
  in ToM, 53
false consensus effect, 54
false-sign task, 26
family-assisted SCIT (F-SCIT), 300–301
family high risk of psychosis
  affect recognition in, 254–55
  social cognition in, 254–56
  social knowledge in, 255
  social perception in, 255
  ToM in, 255–56
Farah, M. J., 94
faux pas, 24, 98
  task, 202
fear, 50, 136, 266
FEDT. See Facial Emotion Discrimination
    Task
feelings-as-information approach, 49
FEIT. See Facial Emotion Identification
    Task
Fett, A. K., 156
figuring out situations phase (of SCIT),
    386
  evidence gathering, 394–95
  fact and guessing separation, 393–94
  JTC in, 391
  thinking up other guesses section,
    392–93
filter model, 323

first-episode psychosis
  affect recognition in, 247–48
  attributional style in, 249–50
  correlates, 250
  social cognition in, 246–50
  social knowledge in, 248
  social perception in, 248
  ToM in, 248–49
Fischer, Benny-Kristin, 369
fish task, 365
Fiske, S. T., 2, 42
fMRI. See functional magnetic resonance
    imaging
focal objects
  in causal attributions, 70
  in visual perception, 70
Frank, R., 124
Freeman, Daniel, 75, 218, 227–28, 229
Freud, Sigmund, 121
Friesen, W. V., 180
Frith, C., 197, 223, 369
frontal-central area (N2), 80
frontal-parietal network, 100
F-SCIT. See family-assisted SCIT
functional attainment, 156, 183
  longitudinal prediction of, 158
functional competence, 156
functional impairments, 151–52
functional magnetic resonance imaging
    (fMRI), 72, 74, 76, 123, 134, 177
  of attributional style, 271
  CET and, 297
  of reappraisal, 106–7
  of self-face recognition, 79
  of self-reference task, 81
  ToM and, 98–99
functional outcome
  assessment of, 154
  neurocognition and, 160, 314
  objective appraisal of, 155
  in schizophrenia, 153–56
  self-reports of, 154
  social cognition and, 4–5, 156–58, 160
  subjective appraisals of, 154
fundamental attribution error, 46, 409
fusiform face area, 102, 134–35
fusiform gyrus

lateral, 102, 263
left, 79
right, 79

Gage, Phineas, 123, 124, 125, 133
Galaburda, A. M., 124
Galinsky, A. D., 55
Gambini, O., 203
Gard, D. E., 164
Garety, P. A., 224
gazes
  following, 29
  learning and, 30
Gelman, S. A., 32
gender discrimination task, 73–74
genetic risk and deterioration (GRD), 246
gesture understanding
  in cross-cultural variation, 74
  mentalizing in, 74
  mirror neurons in, 74
Gilbert, D. T., 404, 408, 410
Gillihan, S. J., 94
Girard, T. A., 166
goal-directed behavior, 100
goals, actions and, 20
Goldin, P. R., 107
Gopnik, A., 21, 23
Grabowski, T., 124
Granholm, E., 228
gray matter
  density, 85
  volumes, 267
GRD. See genetic risk and deterioration
Green, M. F., 160, 163, 164
Gross, J. J., 105, 107
group intervention room, INT, 316
guilt, 50
Gur, R. C., 180, 266
Gur, R. E., 180, 266

H. M., 123
hallucinations, 197
Han, S., 76, 78–79, 80
Happé, F., 204
happiness, 50
Hare, T. A., 110
Harris, P. L., 31

Hatfield, E., 177
Hebb, Donald, 139
Heider, Fritz, 46, 404
Hemsley, D. R., 224
Herbener, E. S., 184, 248
heuristics, 404, 407
  vividness, 374
higher-order mentalizing, 98
hippocampus, 5
Hoekert, M., 180
Hogarty, G. E., 336
homework, SCIT, 397
Horan, W. P., 248
Horton, H. K., 164
Hovland, C. I., 42–43
How Would You Feel in Their Shoes activity (in SCIT), 388
human brain. See also social cognitive brain; specific regions
  autism and development of, 127–29
  CET and, 297
  connectivity, 139–40
  cross-cultural variation and, 84–85
  culture and, 70
  developing, 127–31
  plasticity of, 70, 84–85, 337
  in social cognition, 84
  social interactions and, 70
  Williams syndrome in developing, 129–31
humor, 98
Humphreys, L., 231
Huq, S. F., 224
hyperaffective mental states, 207
hypermentalizing, 205
hyper-theory-of-mind, 205

IAPS. See International Affective Picture System
IFG. See inferior frontal gyrus
imitation, 21
Implicit Association Test, 43
implicit processes, 43
incidental emotion regulation, 108–10
incoherence, 197
indirect speech tasks, 198
individualism, 77, 83

individual therapy
  in CET, 351–52
  in MCT, 376–77
inferior frontal gyrus (IFG), 79
  right, 96
inferior occipital gyrus, 79
inferior parietal cortex, 95
inferior parietal lobule (IPL), 100
inflexible thinking, 339
information source reliability, 30–31
insight, 203–4
Integrated Neurocognitive Therapy (INT), 289, 410
  computer-room, 316
  consecutive sessions, 318
  development of, 311
  didactic therapy components of, 317–32
  differential indication criteria for, 333
  efficacy of, 298
  feasibility of, 298
  goals of, 315
  group intervention room, 316
  implementation of, 315–16
  information sheets, 318
  infrastructure needs, 316
  intervention description, 315–32
  intrinsic motivation in, 315
  introduction sessions, 318
  Module A, 319–24
  Module B, 324–27
  Module C, 327–29
  Module D, 329–32
  modules of, 316–17
  neurocognition targeted in, 313
  patient selection, 332–33
  prototypical case vignettes, 318
  research on, 297–98
  schematic presentation of, 317
  sequential steps in, 315
  social cognition targeted in, 313
  theoretical basis for, 313–15
  therapy materials, 317–32
  therapy rationale for, 314–15
  treatment concept of, 313
  treatment targets of, 313
  troubleshooting, 332
  worksheets, 318

Integrated Psychological Therapy (IPT), 293, 410
  development of, 311
  efficacy of, 294, 305
  evolution of, 312
  exercises, 312
  as group therapy approach, 312
  lessons from, 312
  manual for, 311
  neurocognition targeted by, 312
  patient selection, 332–33
  social cognition targeted by, 312
  subprograms, 311
  troubleshooting, 332
intention
  actions and, 20
  attribution of, 20–21
intentional emotion regulation, 105–8
intention-inferencing tasks, 198
interdisciplinary cross fertilization, 44
Internal, Personal, and Situational Attributions Questionnaire (IPSAQ), 230, 249, 270, 363
internally focused processes, 272
International Affective Picture System (IAPS), 182
intrapsychic processes, 154
intrinsic motivation, 315
introspective-based information, 198, 204
IPL. See inferior parietal lobule
IPSAQ. See Internal, Personal, and Situational Attributions Questionnaire
IPT. See Integrated Psychological Therapy
irony, 98

Janssen, I., 220
jealousy, 207
Jiang, Z., 217
job performance, 51
Jones, E. E., 47–48
JTC. See jumping to conclusions
Judd, C. M., 52
jumping to conclusions (JTC), 233, 373
  dealing with, 366–67
  in MCT, 303, 360, 361, 365–67
  paranoia and, 224–25

  in SCIT, 391
  theory of, 365–66

Kabat, L. G., 228
Kaney, S., 222
Kanske, P., 107
Kay, D. D., 163
Kayser, N., 288
Kee, K. S., 163
Keleman, O., 256
Kelley, H. H., 47
Kern, R. S., 285
Kerr, S. L., 180
Kim, H., 217
Kitayama, S., 81
Klin, A., 405
knowledge
  acquisition of, 22
  perception and, 22
  self, 97, 99
  social, 248, 251–52, 255
  understanding, 22
Koenig, M. A., 31
Kohler, Christian, 390, 401
Kraepelin, E., 216
Krauss, R. M., 51
Kring, A. M., 182
Kruger, J., 55
Krull, D. S., 404
Kucharska-Pietura, K., 3
Kurtz, M. M., 162
Kushnir, T., 32

labeling
  affect, 109
  object, 30
Langdon, R., 201, 203, 207
language development, 26–27
laptops, 316
lateral fusiform gyrus, 102
  in schizophrenia, 263
lateral prefrontal cortex (LPFC), 272
lateral temporal cortex (LTC), 272
learning
  gaze and, 30
  source reliability and, 30–31
  verbal, 324–25

visual, 324–25
  word, 31
left fusiform gyrus, 79
left lateral cerebellar hemisphere, 270
left lateral orbitofrontal cortex, 270
left middle temporal gyrus, 270
left superior temporal sulcus, 72, 73
left temporal pole, 72
lesion method, 123–24
Li, D., 217
Liddle, P. F., 200
Lieberman, M. D., 97, 101, 111
lies, 33
Liew, S., 79, 87
life satisfaction, 49
lingual gyrus, 72
  right, 270
Liu, C. H., 25
Lohmann, H., 27
longitudinal MRI, 85
looking time, 24, 28
LPFC. *See* lateral prefrontal cortex
LTC. *See* lateral temporal cortex

Ma, Y., 78–79, 87
Macaque monkeys, 133, 135
magnetoencephalography (MEG), 123
Maher, B. A., 228
maintenance deficit, 183
Mancuso, F., 5
manipulation, 404
Markham, R., 76
Markus, H. R., 81
Martin, J. A., 409–10
Maryland Assessment of Social
    Competence (MASC), 154, 155
MATRICS. *See* Measurement and
    Treatment Research to Improve
    Cognition in Schizophrenia
Mayberg, H. S., 139
Mayer Salovey Caruso Emotional
    Intelligence Test (MSCEIT) 2.0, 7, 253
McCabe, R., 206
MCT. *See* Metacognitive Therapy
Measurement and Treatment Research to
    Improve Cognition in Schizophrenia
    (MATRICS), 5, 7, 152, 298, 313

medial prefrontal cortex (mPFC), 54, 99,
    132, 272
  gray matter volumes in, 267
  reduced activation in, 268
  in self-knowledge, 99
  task-related activation of, 268–69
  in ToM tasks, 267–68
MEG. *See* magnetoencephalography
Mehl, S., 207
Melo, S., 219
memory. *See also* metamemory problems
  autobiographical, 96
  CET training, 343
  MCT and, 361
  neurocognition and, 324–25
  self-related, 81–84
  working, 25, 159, 329–30
mental health, cross-cultural variation and,
    85–86
mentalizing, 53, 152, 196. *See also* theory
    of mind
  analysis levels, 198
  application aspect of, 199
  attributional aspect of, 198
  cross-cultural variation in, 73–74
  in gesture understanding, 74
  higher-order, 98
  mirror neurons and, 100–101
  others and, 97
  representational aspect, 198
mental stage reasoning, cross-cultural
    variation in, 73–74
mesial superior parietal cortex, 72
metacognition, 7, 376
metacognitive experiences, 57–58
Metacognitive Therapy (MCT), 289, 410
  aim of, 302–3
  attributional style in, 364
  attribution and, 360
  BADE and, 365–67
  belief-changing, 360
  closure, 365–66
  cognitive biases in schizophrenia,
    363–75
  efficacy, 303–4
  empathizing in, 360, 361
  evaluation of, 304

Metacognitive Therapy (*Cont.*)
  feasibility of, 303, 376, 377
  inclusion criteria, 376–77
  individualized treatment, 376–77
  introduction of, 375–77
  JTC in, 303, 360, 361, 365–67
  memory and, 361
  metamemory problems, 372–74
  Module 1, 360
  Module 2, 360
  Module 3, 360
  Module 4, 360
  Module 5, 361
  Module 6, 361
  Module 7, 361
  Module 8, 361
  mood and, 374–75
  overview of, 359–63
  problematic situations in, 376–77
  research on, 302–4
  safety of, 303
  self-esteem and, 361, 374–75
  session structure, 362
  social cognition and, 369–72
  ToM and, 369–72
  training, 377
  treatment fidelity, 376
metamemory problems
  MCT and, 372–74
  in schizophrenia, 372–73
metarepresentation, 94
METT. *See* Micro-Expressions Training
    Tool
Meyer, M. B., 162
Micro-Expressions Training Tool (METT),
    288
middle temporal gyrus, 270
mimicry
  nonconscious, 60
  nonverbal behavior and, 51
  rapid facial, 177
mind perception, 53
Mirowsky, J., 220
mirror neurons, 54
  defined, 100
  in gesture understanding, 74
  mentalizing and, 100–101

misattributions, 58, 203
  in emotion processing, 49
  schizophrenia and, 49
Mitchell, J. P., 99
modeling studies of social cognition,
    160–67
moderate paranoia, 220
Module A, INT, 320–24
  attention in, 320–21
  emotion processing in, 321–24
  information sheet in, 323
  neurocognitive part, 319–21
  processing speed in, 319–21
  social cognition in, 321–24
  vigilance in, 320–21
  worksheet, 322
Module B, INT, 324–27
  group exercises in, 326
  memory, 324–25
  neurocognitive part, 324–25
  social cognitive part, 325–27
  social perception in, 325–27
  ToM in, 325–27
  verbal learning, 324–25
  visual learning, 324–25
Module C, INT, 327–29
  information sheet, 328
  neurocognitive part, 327–28
  social schema in, 328–29
Module D, INT, 329–32
  attributions, 330–32
  group exercise in, 330
  neurocognitive part, 329–30
  working memory in, 329–30
monism, 120
mood, 374–75
Morelli, S. A., 111
Moritz, S., 7
Morrison, A. P., 218
Moskowitz, G. B., 55
mother, 82
motor resonance, 74
Moutoussis, M., 229
Movie for the Assessment of
    Social Cognition (MASC),
    206
mPFC. *See* medial prefrontal cortex

MSCEIT, *See* Mayer Salovey Caruso
    Emotional Intelligence Test
Murphy, D., 3

N2, 80
Nakayama, K., 78
National Basic Research Program of
    China, 87
National Institute of Mental Health
    (NIMH), 7, 152, 155, 298, 313, 401
  clinical trials, 352
National Natural Science Foundation of
    China, 87
Nature, 120
Ndetei, D. M., 216
Neale, J. M., 180
neocortex, 70
NET. *See* Neurocognitive Enhancement
    Therapy
Neuchterlein, K. H., 160, 164
neurocognition
  attention and, 319–20
  CET, training, 342–45
  functional outcome and, 160, 314
  in INT Module A, 319–21
  in INT Module B, 324–25
  in INT Module C, 327–28
  in INT Module D, 329–30
  INT targeting of, 313
  IPT targeting of, 312
  memory and, 324–25
  neural substrates, 5–6
  problem solving and, 328
  processing speed, 319–20
  reasoning and, 327
  social cognition and, 3–6, 158–59
  statistical differentiation with social
    cognition, 3–4
  verbal learning, 324–25
  vigilance and, 319–20
  visual learning, 324–25
  working memory in, 329–30
Neurocognitive Enhancement Therapy
    (NET), 294
neurocognitive remediation, 286
neuroleptics, 177
  atypical, 358–59
  use of, 358

neuroscience. *See also* social cognitive
    neuroscience
  cultural, 70
  social, 54
neurosteroids, 188
new goal events, 20
new path events, 20
Nienow, T. M., 162
nigrostriatal dopaminergic blockade,
    177
NIMH. *See* National Institute of Mental
    Health
Njomboro, P., 8
N-methyl-D-aspartate (NMDA) agonists,
    188
nonconscious mimicry, 60
nonliteral meaning, 24
nonverbal behavior
  mimicry and, 51
  in social perception, 51
nonverbal ToM tasks, 27

object labeling, 30
obsessive-compulsive disorder (OCD),
    185
occipitotemporal cortex, 102
OCD. *See* obsessive-compulsive disorder
Onishi, K. H., 28
orbitofrontal cortex lesions, 124
Orientation Remediation Module, 343
Ostrom, T. M., 2
others
  cross-cultural variation in processing of,
    71–77
  mentalizing and, 97
  social cognitive brain and, 97–101
  ToM and, 97
overmentalizing, 205–6
  undermentalizing and, 207
ownership, 94–95

paid work programs, 188
pain, 77
PANAS. *See* Positive and Negative Affect
    Scale
PANSS. *See* Positive and Negative
    Syndrome Scale

paranoia, 385
  anomalous perceptions in, 228–29
  attributions and, 229–31
  cross-cultural variation in, 216
  defensiveness and, 229–31
  defined, 216
  definitional issues, 215–17
  emotional factors in, 225–33
  JTC and, 224–25
  longitudinal data on, 217
  moderate, 220
  poor-me, 218–19
  psychotic, 218–19
  in SCIT, 390–91
  self-esteem and, 225, 231–33
  severe, 220
  as social adaptation, 219–23
  social adversity and, 220
  social cognition and, 223–25
  subclinical, 218–19
  ToM and, 223–24
Paranoid Personality Disorder, 216
paranoid schizophrenia, 2, 206–7
paranoid spectrum, 217–19
Park, B., 52
Parmenides, 120
passivity experiences, 197
passivity phenomena, 204, 208
Pavlov, I. P., 121
peer relations, 33
Pelham, B. W., 404
Penn, D., 292, 409–10
perception, 159. *See also* social perception
  affect, 289–90
  anomalous, 228–29
  context in, 70
  emotion, 156, 321–24, 384
  experience and, 22–23
  face, 3, 102–4, 134
  information based on, 198, 204
  knowledge and, 22
  mind, 53
  person, 41, 57, 122
  threat, 222
  visual, 70
Perner, J., 23
persecutory delusion, 216

personality, 96
personalizing bias, 269
person perception, 41, 57, 122
perspective taking, 55, 348
  cross-cultural variation and, 71–72
persuasion, 57, 98
pet therapy, 188
philosophy of mind, 120–21
physical abuse, 221
Piaget, J., 121
Pilowsky, T., 201
Pinkham, A. E., 402
PIT. *See* Pragmatic Inference Task
planning, 133
plasticity, 70, 84–85, 337
Plato, 120
pleasure
  anticipatory, 182–83
  consummatory, 182–83
  remembered, 182–83
PMC. *See* premotor cortex
PM paranoia. *See* poor-me paranoia
political party affiliation, 51
Pomarol-Clotet, E., 3
PONS. *See* Profile of Nonverbal Sensitivity
    Test
poor-me (PM) paranoia, 218–19
Positive and Negative Affect Scale
    (PANAS), 176
Positive and Negative Syndrome Scale
    (PANSS), 175, 182, 200, 216
posterior cingulate cortex, 74, 83, 96
posterior ventrolateral PFC, 100
posttraumatic stress disorder (PTSD), 185,
    216
PowerPoint, 389
PPI. *See* psychophysiological interaction
practice partners, SCIT, 397–98
Pragmatic Inference Task (PIT), 249
preattributional process, 53
precentral gyrus, 270
precuneus, 96
preference-conditioning tasks, 184
prefrontal activity, 85
prefrontal cortex, 5, 25, 108. *See also*
    specific regions
  in social cognition, 132–34

prejudice, 43
premotor cortex (PMC), 95
    right, 72
    ventral, 271
pretend play, 98
primary auditory cortex, 84
primates, 131
priming, 78
    in social perception, 52
problem solving, 133
    CET training, 343
    in INT Module C, 328
Problem Solving Skill Training (PST), 291
processing skills, 285–86
    speed, 319–20
process orientation, 43–44
prodromal phase, 245
Profile of Nonverbal Sensitivity Test
    (PONS), 255
proof-of-concept studies, 286–88
    affect recognition improvement, 287
    emotion training studies, 287–88
    facial identification training, 287
    Micro-Expressions Training Tool, 288
    social cue recognition, 287
    ToM impairment modifiability, 288
prosocial behavior, 55, 76
prosody, 174, 179
    tasks, 180
prosopagnosia, 6, 136
PST. See Problem Solving Skill Training
psychology. See also Integrated
    Psychological Therapy; social
    psychology
    clinical, 44
    comparative, 23, 44
    evolutionary, 121
    in social cognitive neuroscience, 120–26
    unobservable, 21
The Psychology of Interpersonal Relations
    (Heider), 46
psychometric properties, 9–10
psychopharmacology, 358–59
psychophysiological interaction (PPI), 95
psychosis, 176, 220
    clinical high risk of, 246, 251–54, 257
    family high risk of, 254–56

first-episode, 246–50
    longitudinal studies on, 359
    reversibility of, 359
Psychosis Screening Questionnaire, 217
psychotherapy, 358
psychotic paranoia, 218–19
PTSD. See posttraumatic stress disorder
Pugh, K., 229
puppets, 22

Quality of Life scale (QOL), 154

rACC. See rostral anterior cingulate cortex
racism, 43
Rameson, L. T., 111
Ramon y Cajal, Santiago, 139
rapid facial mimicry, 177
Rassovsky, Y., 164, 165
reaction time, 72
    in self-face recognition, 78
Reading the Mind in Eyes (RME) test,
    73–74, 198, 201, 204
reappraisal, 106–7
reasoning, 327
recall, 57
receiving skills, 285–86
recursive thinking, 98
region of interest (ROI) approach, 109
reliability tracking, 31
remembered pleasure, 182–83
Repacholi, B. M., 21
representational aspect of mentalizing, 198
representational understanding, 26
reward processing, 184
right angular gyrus, 270
right anterior insula, 79
right frontal cortex, 79
right fusiform gyrus, 79
right inferior frontal gyrus, 96
right inferior parietal lobe, 72, 79
right lingual gyrus, 270
right middle frontal cortex, 80
right middle frontal gyrus, 73
right middle temporal gyrus, 270
right premotor cortex, 72
RME test. See Reading the Mind in Eyes
    test and Eyes test

Roberts, D. L., 292
Rogers, T. B., 81
ROI approach. *See* region of interest
    approach
Rosenberg Self-Esteem Scale, 83
Rosenthal, R., 51–52
Ross, C. E., 220
rostral anterior cingulate cortex (rACC),
    109
Rusch, N., 163
Russell, J. A., 207, 287–88

S. M., 123
    findings from, 138
sadness, 50
Saeedi, H., 163
SANSS. *See* Scale for the Assessment of
    Negative Symptoms
sarcasm, 98
Sarfati, Y., 288
SAT. *See* social attribution task
Satisfaction with Life Scale (SWL), 154
Savitsky, K., 54
Scale for the Assessment of Negative
    Symptoms (SANSS), 175
Scale of Prodromal Symptoms (SOPS), 245
scapegoating, 363
SCET. *See* Social Cognition Enhancement
    Training
Schaub, D., 201
schemas, 42
    chronically accessible, 52
    social, 328–29
schizophrenia, 41–42, 93
    amygdala in, 265–66
    attribution biases in, 46–48
    chronic, 1–2, 247
    cognitive biases in, 363–75
    comorbid intellectual disabilities, 340
    conscious will in, 58–59
    controlled processing in, 44
    criteria for, 151
    dual-processing models, 56–57,
        271–72
    early course, 245–46, 296
    emotion expression in, 174–78
    emotion processing in, 48–50

emotion recognition in, 179–81
executive functioning in, 44
facial affective flattening in, 174–76
functional impairment in, 151–52
functional outcome in, 153–56
lateral fusiform gyrus in, 263
metacognitive experiences and, 57–58
metamemory problems in, 372–73
misattributions and, 49
mood in, 374–75
paranoid, 2, 206–7
prodromal phase, 245
recovery-oriented treatment
    development, 152
research implications, 405–12
research topic breadth, 56–59
research topic depth, 45–56
self-esteem in, 374–75
self-serving bias in, 270–71
social perception in, 50–52
STS volumes in, 264
ToM in, 53–55, 196–99
schizotypy, 257
Schnall, S., 49
Schwartz, B. L., 178
scientific theory, 28
SCIT. *See* Social Cognition and Interaction
    Training
SCRT. *See* Social Cue Recognition Test
SCST. *See* Social Cognitive Skill Training
SDFF. *See* similarities and differences with
    family and friends
second-order ToM, 33
self
    construction of, 96
    in Eastern cultural context, 72
    in social cognitive brain, 94–96
    in Western cultural context, 71–72
self-attribution, 95
self-awareness, 131, 132
self-competence, 83
self-concept
    cross-cultural variation in, 77–84
    in Eastern culture, 77
    in Western culture, 77
self-construals, 70
    scale, 83

self-esteem
   low, 375
   MCT and, 361, 374–75
   paranoia and, 225, 231–33
   in schizophrenia, 374–75
self-face recognition
   cross-cultural variation in, 78–80
   in Eastern culture, 78
   ERPs in, 80
   fMRI of, 79
   left-hand advantage in, 96
   reaction time in, 78
   social contexts in, 78–79
   in Western culture, 78
self-identification, 96, 97
self-judgments
   in Eastern culture, 82–83
   VMPFC in, 81
   in Western culture, 82–83
self-knowledge
   conceptual, 97
   mPFC in, 99
self-labeling tasks, 96
self-liking, 83
self-other distinction, 94
self-reference task, 81
self-reflection, 54
self-regulation, 131, 132
self-related memory, cross-cultural variation in, 81–84
self-relevant processing, 131
self-representations, attributions and,
   226–27
self-serving bias, 270–71
self-thought monitoring, 96
sending skills, 285–86
Sendiony, M. F., 217
sentential complementary syntax, 27
Sergi, M. J., 4, 164
severe paranoia, 220
sexual orientation, 51
Shamay-Tsoory, S. G., 201, 206, 402
shame, 50
Silverstein, S., 164
similarities and differences with family and
   friends (SDFF), 83
Simmel, M., 404

simulation theory, 28, 54, 100
Singelis, T. M., 83
SIPS. See Structured Interview for
   Prodromal Syndromes
situational causal attributions, 56
situation factors, 48
Skinner, B. F., 121
sleep loss, 228
SLOF. See Specific Level of Functioning
   Scale
SMA. See supplementary motor area
SNF. See Swiss National Foundation
social adaptation
   CET training, 343
   paranoia as, 219–23
social adversity, paranoia and, 220
social anxiety disorder, 185
social attribution task (SAT), 404, 406
social cognition, 33, 41
   added value of, 158–60
   affective capacity, 71
   amygdala in, 137–40
   attribution and, 330–32
   brain regions involved in, 84, 131–40
   clinical high risk of psychosis, 251–54
   cognitive capacity, 71
   connectivity and, 139–40
   cross-cultural variation in, 70
   dealing with, in MCT, 370–72
   definitions of, 2–3, 42–45, 402–5
   in developing brain, 127–31
   domains of, 6–7, 313
   DP models for, 409–10
   ecological validity, 9–10
   emotion processing in, 48–49
   emotion regulation and, 330–32
   in family high risk of psychosis, 254–56
   in first-episode psychosis, 246–50
   functional outcome and, 4–5, 156–58,
      160
   interdisciplinary cross-fertilization in,
      44
   in INT Module A, 321–24
   in INT Module B, 325–27
   in INT Module C, 328–29
   in INT Module D, 330–32
   INT targeting of, 313

social cognition (*Cont.*)
IPT targeting of, 312
MCT and, 369–72
measurement of, 7–10
as mediator, 160–67
modeling studies, 160–67
neural substrates, 5–6
neurocognition and, 3–6, 158–59
paranoia and, 223–25
prefrontal cortex in, 132–34
processes involved in, 127
process orientation in, 43–44
psychometric properties, 9–10
real-world applications, 44–45
social brain in, 131–32
in social psychology, 42, 403–4
in sociocultural contexts, 69–71
special nature of, 136
statistical differentiation with
neurocognition, 3–4
structure of, 8–9
structures involved in, 127
temporal lobe in, 134–36
theory, 369–70
unabashed mentalism and, 42–43
Social Cognition and Interaction Training
(SCIT), 178, 289, 370, 410
check-in, 387
checking it out phase, 386, 395–96
description of, 387–96
development of, 298–99
effect durability, 299
efficacy of, 301–2
emotion defining in, 389
Emotion Morph Slides, 390
emotion reading in, 389
emotions in, 386
emotion training, 387
evidence gathering, 394–95
experimental trials of, 299–300
fact and guessing separation in, 393–94
family-assisted, 300–301
figuring out situations phase, 386, 391–96
homework, 397
integration, 395–96
introduction, 386
JTC in, 391

overview of, 385–87
paranoia in, 390–91
participant selection, 398–99
phases, 385
practical issues, 398–99
practice partners, 397–98
randomized controlled trials of,
300–302
research on, 298–302
suspicious feelings section in, 390–91
symptom heterogeneity, 396–97
theoretical orientation, 384–85
thinking up other guesses section,
392–93
triangle, 388
troubleshooting, 396–98
Social Cognition Enhancement Training
(SCET), 290
social cognitive bias, 404–5
social cognitive brain. *See also* human
brain
capacity in, 110–11
emotional expressions and, 104–5
emotion and, 101–10
face perception and, 102–4
incidental emotional regulation,
108–10
intentional emotion regulation, 105–8
others and, 97–101
self in, 94–96
in social cognition, 131–32
in sociocultural contexts, 69–71
tendency in, 110–11
social cognitive impairment models,
271–73
social cognitive neuroscience
approaches, 123–27
attributional style and, 269–71
emotion processing in, 263–66
historical context, 120
psychological approaches, 120–26
ToM and, 267–69
Social Cognitive Skill Training (SCST)
development of, 292
evaluation of, 293
feasibility of, 292–93
tolerability of, 292–93

social cognitive training, 345–51. *See also specific treatments*
  group content, 345–46
  group structure, 346–49
  overview, 345
  recovery plans, 349–51
social cognitive treatment. *See also specific treatments*
  broad-based, 293–94
  comprehensive, 292–93
  dual-processing model and, 410–12
  neurocognitive remediation, 286
  outcome measures, 306
  proof-of-concept studies, 286–88
  research on, 294–304
  roots of, 285–86
  social skills training, 285–86
  targeted, 289–92
social context, 78–79
social cue recognition, 287
Social Cue Recognition Test (SCRT), 251
social functioning perspective, 50
Social Functioning Scale, 154
social groups, 77
social hierarchy, 69
social information processing, 100
social intelligence, 93
social interactions, 70
social judgments, 41, 252
  emotion processing and, 49
  thin slicing in, 51–52
social knowledge
  in clinical high risk of psychosis, 251–52
  in family high risk of psychosis, 255
  in first-episode psychosis, 248
social networks, 32–33
social neuroscience, 54
social perception, 152
  in clinical high risk of psychosis, 251–52
  in family high risk of psychosis, 255
  in first-episode psychosis, 248
  in INT Module B, 325–27
  nonverbal behavior in, 51
  priming in, 52
  in schizophrenia, 50–52
  targeted treatment, 290
social psychology, 41, 121–22

  attribution biases in, 47–48
  clinical psychology and, 44
  social cognition in, 42, 403–4
social reasoning, 28
social referencing, 29
social schema, 328–29
social skills training, 285–86
social stimulation, 301
social understanding
  aggression and, 33
  of infants, 29
social wisdom, 338–39
sociocultural contexts
  social brain in, 69–71
  social cognition in, 69–71
sociocultural factors in ToM, 28
somatic marker hypothesis, 124
SOPS. *See* Scale of Prodromal Symptoms
Southgate, L., 229
Specific Level of Functioning Scale (SLOF), 154, 156
speech channel, 179–80
speed of processing, 319–20
Spence, S. A., 94
split-brain patients, 140
Spunt, R. P., 101
stable differences, 30
stereotypes, 122
STG. *See* superior temporal gyrus
stress-inoculation training, 331
Stroop tasks, 222
Structured Interview for Prodromal Syndromes (SIPS), 245
STS. *See* superior temporal sulcus
subclinical paranoia, 218–19
subjectivity, 23, 58
subordination, 75
Sui, J., 80
suicide, 184–85
superior frontal gyrus, 72
superior temporal gyrus (STG), 134
superior temporal sulcus (STS), 5, 73–74, 95, 134, 135, 263
  hyperactivation of, 265
  left, 72, 73
  in schizophrenia, 264
  in ToM tasks, 267, 269

supplementary motor area (SMA), 95
suppression, 106
Supreme Court, 44–45
surprise, 50
suspicious feelings section, 390–91
Swendsen, J., 228
Swiss National Foundation (SNF), 312
SWL. *See* Satisfaction with Life Scale
symptom heterogeneity, 396–97
syntax
    sentential complementary, 27
    ToM development and, 27
systematically distorted output, 402

TABS. *See* Test of Adaptive Behavior in
    Schizophrenia
TAR. *See* Training in Affect Recognition
targeted treatments, 289–92
    affect perception, 289–90
    social perception, 290
    ToM, 291
task management, 133
TAU. *See* treatment as usual
Taylor, M. A., 2, 42
tempoparietal junction (TPJ), 73–74, 99,
    132
    hyperactivation, 269
    hypoactivation, 269
    in ToM tasks, 267, 269
Temporal Experience of Pleasure Scale
    (TEPS), 186
temporal lobe, 134–36
tendency
    capacity and, 110–11
    social cognitive brain and, 110–11
TEPS. *See* Temporal Experience of
    Pleasure Scale
Test of Adaptive Behavior in Schizophrenia
    (TABS), 154, 156
theory of mind (ToM), 3–4, 6, 19, 131, 132,
    152, 233, 384. *See also* mentalizing
    in action, 29–33
    aggression and, 33
    application of mental states, 205–7
    attribution of mental states in, 202–4
    cartoon-based tasks, 73
    in clinical high risk of psychosis, 252

components of, 8–9
conversation and, 26–27
cross-cultural variation in, 73–74
deception and, 33
developmental course of, 19–25
domain-general accounts, 25
domain-specific accounts, 25
executive function skills in, 25–26
false-belief paradigm in, 53
in family high risk of psychosis,
    255–56
in first-episode psychosis, 248–49
first-order tasks, 200, 371
fMRI and, 98–99
impairment modifiability, 288
in INT Module B, 325–27
language development and, 26–27
lies and, 33
MCT and, 369–72
meta-analyses, 197
mPFC in, 267–68
nonverbal, 27
others and, 97
paranoia and, 223–24
presentation modality, 98
representational understanding and, 26
representation of mental states in,
    199–202
in schizophrenia, 53–55, 196–99
as scientific theory, 28
second-order, 24, 33, 371
simulation theory, 28, 54, 100
social cognitive neuroscience and,
    267–69
social networks and, 32–33
sociocultural factors in, 28
STS in, 267, 269
syntax and, 27
targeted treatment, 291
task design, 98
theories of development, 25–29
theory theory of, 28, 54
TPJ in, 267, 269
word-based tasks, 73
thinking up other guesses section, 392–93
thin slicing, 51–52
thought-confidence, 57

threat anticipation, 221–23
threat detection, 131, 132
    amygdala in, 137
threat perception, 222
three-dimensional-symptom model, 200
TMS. *See* transcranial magnetic
    stimulation
ToM. *See* theory of mind
Tomasello, M., 27
Tong, F., 78
Tower of Hanoi task, 129
TPJ. *See* temporoparietal junction
Training in Affect Recognition (TAR),
    289–90
trait-based impressions, 42
transcranial magnetic stimulation (TMS),
    74, 177
treatment as usual (TAU), 289, 299
treatment methods. *See* social cognitive
    treatment
Treatment Units for Research on
    Neurocognition in Schizophrenia
    (TURNS), 152
Trémeau, F., 175
Trower, P., 218
trust
    amygdala and, 137
    context and, 32
    selective, 31–32
Tudusciuc, O., 401
TURNS. *See* Treatment Units for
    Research on Neurocognition in
    Schizophrenia

UCSD Performance-Based Skills
    Assessment (UPSA), 154, 155
Udachina, A., 219, 402, 406
ultra-high risk (UHR), 246
unabashed mentalism, 42–43
undermentalizing, 206
    overmentalizing and, 207
unmotivated cognitive style, 339
unobservable psychology, 21
UPSA. *See* UCSD Performance-Based
    Skills Assessment
Urbach-Wiethe disease, 125
urban legends, 366

Vadher, A., 216
valence, 187
Validation of Everyday Real-World
    Outcomes, 156
Van der Gaag, M., 290
van Hooren, S., 4
Van Overwalle, F., 98–99
Vaskinn, A., 162
Vauth, R., 4, 163
ventral lateral prefrontal cortex (VLPFC),
    109, 110
ventral medial prefrontal cortex (VMPFC),
    96, 125, 272
    in Eastern cultural individuals, 82
    in self-judgments, 81
    in Western cultural individuals, 82
ventral premotor cortex, 271
ventral temporal cortex, 135
verbal learning, 324–25
vibrotactile stimuli, 84
victimization, 221
vigilance, 320–21
visual appreciation joke task, 207
visual learning, 324–25
visual perception, 70
vividness heuristics, 374
VLPFC. *See* ventral lateral prefrontal
    cortex
VMPFC. *See* ventral medial prefrontal
    cortex
vocational rehabilitation, 294
VOICE-ID, 180
von Ehrenfels, C., 121
von Langer, Johann Peter, 367
Vorontsoya, N., 229

Wallace, C. J., 285
Walter, H., 206, 268, 269
Wang, L., 76, 81
weak central coherence, 128
Wegner, Daniel, 58
Wellman, H. M., 32
Wessely, S., 224
Western culture, 70
    boss effect in, 79
    self-concept in, 77
    self-face recognition in, 78

Western culture (*Cont.*)
  self in, 71–72
  self-judgments in, 82–83
  VMPFC in, 82
white lie, 98
Whorfian hypothesis, 27
willed action, 202
Williams, L. M., 4, 204
Williams syndrome (WMS)
  autism and, 130
  in developing brain, 129–31
Wimmer, H., 23
Windschitl, P. D., 54

Wirtz, M., 163
Wisconsin Card Sorting Task, 129
Wittenbrink, B., 52
WMS. *See* Williams syndrome
Woodward, Todd S., 7
word-based ToM tasks, 73
word learning tasks, 31
working memory, 25, 159
  in INT Module D, 329–30
World Health Organization, 216

Zimbardo, P. G., 228
zygomaticus muscle, 176